MW01201256

Operative Techniques in Gynecologic Surgery

Gynecology

Operative Techniques in Gynecologic Surgery

Gynecology

Series Editor

Jonathan S. Berek, MD, MMS

Laurie Kraus Lacob Professor
Stanford University School of Medicine
Director, Stanford Women's Cancer Center
Senior Scientific Advisor, Stanford Comprehensive Cancer Institute
Director, Stanford Health Care Communication Program
Stanford, California

Tommaso Falcone, MD, FRCS(C), FACOG

Professor of Surgery
Cleveland Clinic Lerner College of Medicine
Case Western Reserve University
Chairman of Department of Obstetrics and Gynecology & Women's Health Institute
Cleveland Clinic
Cleveland, Ohio

M. Jean Uy-Kroh, MD, FACOG

Assistant Professor of Surgery
Cleveland Clinic Lerner College of Medicine
Case Western Reserve University
Department of Obstetrics and Gynecology & Women's Health Institute
Director, Chronic Pelvic Pain Program
Cleveland Clinic
Cleveland, Ohio

Linda D. Bradley, MD, FACOG

Professor of Surgery
Cleveland Clinic Lerner College of Medicine
Case Western Reserve University
Vice Chair of Department of Obstetrics and Gynecology & Women's Health Institute
Director, Center for Fibroid and Menstrual Disorders
Cleveland Clinic
Cleveland, Ohio

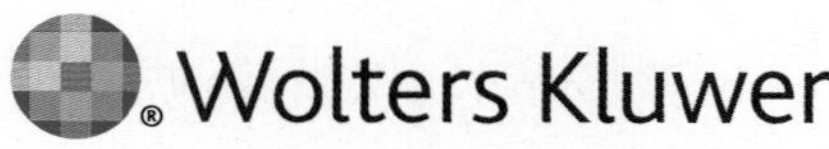

Philadelphia • Baltimore • New York • London
Buenos Aires • Hong Kong • Sydney • Tokyo

Executive Editor: Rebecca Gaertner
Acquisitions Editor: Chris Teja
Product Development Editor: Ashley Fischer
Editorial Assistant: Brian Convery
Marketing Manager: Rachel Mante Leung
Production Project Manager: David Orzechowski
Design Coordinator: Teresa Mallon
Artist/Illustrator: Jason M. McAlexander, MPS North America LLC
Manufacturing Coordinator: Beth Welsh
Prepress Vendor: Aptara, Inc.

9 8 7 6 5 4 3 2 1

Printed in China

978-1-4963-4288-1
1-4963-4288-7
Library of Congress Cataloging-in-Publication Data
available upon request

LWW.com

Contributing Authors

Mariam AlHilli, MD, FACOG
Department of Obstetrics and Gynecology
Section of Gynecologic Oncology
Cleveland Clinic
Cleveland, Ohio

Katrin S. Arnolds, MD
Section of Minimally Invasive Gynecologic Surgery
Women's Health Institute
Cleveland Clinic Florida
Weston, Florida

Cynthia Arvizo, MD
Department of Obstetrics and Gynecology
Cleveland Clinic
Cleveland, Ohio

Marjan Attaran, MD
Department of Obstetrics and Gynecology
Section of Reproductive Endocrinology and Infertility
Cleveland Clinic
Cleveland, Ohio

Rachel Barron, MD
Department of Regional Obstetrics and Gynecology
Cleveland Clinic
Cleveland, Ohio

Linda D. Bradley, MD, FACOG
Professor of Surgery
Cleveland Clinic Lerner College of Medicine
Case Western Reserve University
Vice Chair of Department of Obstetrics and Gynecology
Director, Center for Fibroid and Menstrual Disorders
Cleveland Clinic
Cleveland, Ohio

Robert DeBernardo, MD
Associate Professor of Surgery
Cleveland Clinic Lerner College of Medicine
Case Western University
Section of Gynecologic Oncology
Director, Minimally Invasive Surgery
Cleveland Clinic
Cleveland, Ohio

Jonathan D. Emery, MD
Assistant Professor of Surgery
Cleveland Clinic Lerner College of Medicine
Case Western University
Medical Director, Chagrin Falls Family Health Center
Cleveland Clinic
Cleveland, Ohio

Bianca Falcone, MD
Department of Obstetrics and Gynecology
Saint Barnabas Medical Center
Livingston, New Jersey

Tommaso Falcone, MD, FRCS(C), FACOG
Professor of Surgery
Cleveland Clinic Lerner College of Medicine
Case Western Reserve University
Chairman of Department of Obstetrics and Gynecology
Cleveland Clinic
Cleveland, Ohio

Rebecca Flyckt, MD, FACOG
Assistant Professor of Surgery
Cleveland Clinic Lerner College of Medicine
Case Western Reserve University
Section of Reproductive Endocrinology and Infertility
Director, Fertility Preservation Program
Cleveland Clinic
Cleveland, Ohio

Habibeh Ladan Gitiforooz, MD, MBA, FACOG
Assistant Professor of Surgery
Cleveland Clinic Lerner College of Medicine
Case Western Reserve University
Department of Obstetrics and Gynecology
Director, Global CME, Cleveland Clinic Abu Dhabi
Cleveland Clinic
Cleveland, Ohio

Oluwatosin Goje, MD, MSCR, FACOG
Assistant Professor of Surgery
Cleveland Clinic Lerner College of Medicine
Case Western Reserve University
Department of Obstetrics and Gynecology
Cleveland Clinic
Cleveland, Ohio

Jeffrey M. Goldberg, MD, FACOG
Professor of Surgery
Cleveland Clinic Lerner College of Medicine
Case Western Reserve University
Department of Obstetrics and Gynecology
Section Head, Reproductive Endocrinology and Infertility
Cleveland Clinic
Cleveland, Ohio

Rhoda Y. Goldschmidt, MD
Department of Obstetrics and Gynecology
Section of Benign Gynecology
Cleveland Clinic
Cleveland, Ohio

Lisa C. Hickman, MD
Department of Obstetrics and Gynecology
Cleveland Clinic
Cleveland, Ohio

Karl Jallad, MD
Department of Obstetrics and Gynecology
Section Female Pelvic Medicine and Reconstructive Surgery
Cleveland Clinic
Cleveland, Ohio

Swapna Kollikonda, MD
Department of Regional Obstetrics and Gynecology
Cleveland Clinic
Cleveland, Ohio

Alexander Kotlyar, MD
Department of Obstetrics and Gynecology
Cleveland Clinic
Cleveland, Ohio

Henry F. Kraft, CSFA
Department of Obstetrics and Gynecology
Cleveland Clinic
Cleveland, Ohio

Natalia C. Llarena, MD
Department of Obstetrics and Gynecology
Cleveland Clinic
Cleveland, Ohio

Megan Lutz, MD, MPH
Department of Obstetrics and Gynecology
Section of Benign Gynecologic Surgery
Cleveland Clinic
Cleveland, Ohio

Chad M. Michener, MD
Associate Professor of Surgery
Cleveland Clinic Lerner College of Medicine
Case Western Reserve University
Section of Gynecologic Oncology
Cleveland Clinic
Cleveland, Ohio

Stephanie Ricci, MD
Department of Obstetrics and Gynecology
Section of Gynecologic Oncology
Cleveland Clinic
Cleveland, Ohio

Michael L. Sprague, MD, FACOG
Clinical Assistant Professor of Surgery
Cleveland Clinic Lerner College of Medicine
Case Western University
Section of Minimally Invasive Gynecologic Surgery
Associate Director, Fellowship in Minimally Invasive Gynecologic Surgery
Cleveland Clinic Florida
Weston, Florida

Sharon Sutherland, MD, MPH
Assistant Professor of Surgery
Cleveland Clinic Lerner College of Medicine
Case Western University
Chief Quality Officer, Cleveland Clinic Akron General Health System
Cleveland Clinic
Cleveland, Ohio

Cecile A. Unger, MD, MPH
Assistant Professor of Surgery
Cleveland Clinic Lerner College of Medicine
Case Western Reserve University
Section of Female Pelvic Medicine and Reconstructive Surgery
Director, Transgender Medicine and Surgery
Cleveland Clinic
Cleveland, Ohio

M. Jean Uy-Kroh, MD, FACOG
Assistant Professor of Surgery
Cleveland Clinic Lerner College of Medicine
Case Western Reserve University
Section of Benign Gynecologic Surgery
Director, Chronic Pelvic Pain Program
Cleveland Clinic
Cleveland, Ohio

Roberto Vargas, MD
Department of Obstetrics and Gynecology
Section of Gynecologic Oncology
Cleveland Clinic
Cleveland, Ohio

Mark D. Walters, MD
Professor of Surgery
Cleveland Clinic Lerner College of Medicine
Case Western Reserve University
Vice Chair of Department of Obstetrics and Gynecology
Section of Female Pelvic Medicine and Reconstructive Surgery
Cleveland Clinic
Cleveland, Ohio

Stephen E. Zimberg, MD, MSHA, FACOG
Clinical Associate Professor of Surgery
Cleveland Clinic Lerner College of Medicine
Case Western University
Section Head, Minimally Invasive Gynecologic Surgery
Director, Fellowship in Minimally Invasive Gynecologic Surgery
Cleveland Clinic Florida
Weston, Florida

Foreword

Operative Techniques in Gynecologic Surgery is presented in four volumes—*Gynecology, Reproductive Endocrinology and Infertility, Urogynecology and Pelvic Reconstructive Surgery*, and *Gynecologic Oncology*. Their purpose is to provide clear and concise illustrations of essential operations representing the fundamental procedures for each of these subspecialties. This series is distinct from other textbooks in gynecology because of their focus as an illustrated practical guide to the surgical processes using easily accessible photographs and video clips.

In *Gynecology*, this first in the series, we depict the most common operations of our clinical specialty. The second does the same for *Reproductive Endocrinology and Infertility*, the third for *Urogynecology and Pelvic Reconstructive Surgery*, and the fourth for *Gynecologic Oncology*. We assembled a group of outstanding authors and contributors to produce these volumes, under the guidance of highly regarded expert senior book editors.

Gynecology—Tommaso Falcone, MD, is the Head of Gynecology at the Cleveland Clinic and is well known for his expertise in the operative management of benign gynecologic conditions. He and his co-authors, M. Jean Uy-Kroh, MD, and Linda D. Bradley, MD, have carefully assembled a very useful series of photographs and videos that highlight the fundamentals of the surgical operations in our field.

Reproductive Endocrinology and Infertility—Steven Nakajima, MD, is a Professor of Obstetrics and Gynecology at the Fertility and Reproductive Medicine Center, Stanford University School of Medicine, and his focus is on the procedural and operative aspects of. Along with the contributions from his colleagues, Travis W. McCoy, MD, and Miriam S. Krause, MD, this book will serve as a clear summary of the necessary procedures in this specialty.

Urogynecology and Reconstructive Pelvic Surgery—Christopher Tarney, MD, is an Associate Professor at the David Geffen School of Medicine at UCLA, where he is the Chief of Urogynecology and Reconstructive Pelvic Surgery. He and his colleague, Lisa Rugo-Gupta, MD, Clinical Assistant Professor, Stanford University School of Medicine, have contributed substantially to our understanding of the important discipline of Female Pelvic Medicine and Reconstructive Surgery.

Gynecologic Oncology—Kenneth Hatch, MD, is a well-known gynecologic oncologist who is a Professor at the University of Arizona School of Medicine. He is considered one of the primary experts in the surgical management of gynecologic malignancies. Dr. Hatch and his contributors will provide a precise visual explanation of the essential operative treatments in this subspecialty.

We intend this series to enhance the educational activities for our colleagues in the practice of Gynecology and dedicate this series to our patients in the hope that it will facilitate optimal care and improved outcomes for our patients.

Jonathan S. Berek, MD, MMS
Series Editor, *Operative Techniques in Gynecologic Surgery*
Laurie Kraus Lacob Professor
Stanford University School of Medicine
Director, Stanford Women's Cancer Center
Senior Scientific Advisor, Stanford Comprehensive Cancer Institute
Director, Stanford Health Care Communication Program
Stanford, California

Preface

We are confident this textbook will be widely read, intensely discussed, and most of all utilized as a dynamic compendium to improve the surgical care and outcomes of patients. This textbook includes a variety of visual formats with numerous high-quality images. It succinctly describes optimal technique and is beautifully illustrated. In addition, outstanding videos capture procedures step by step. You will feel that you are in the operating theatre with an experienced surgeon who meticulously instructs you through the case.

The authors were chosen for their surgical expertise and are thought leaders in gynecology. The body of this work epitomizes the surgical dictum, "Do as much as necessary and as little as possible." Our goal is to provide you the tools needed to teach modern gynecology, perform minimally invasive surgery, and to recognize and treat complications should they occur.

We are indebted to our families who understood the time commitment required to complete this project. We are indebted to our colleagues who submitted chapters and provided unabashed video critiques. And most importantly, we are indebted to our patients who continue to teach and inspire us. We appreciate the trust and confidence of the women we serve.

Tommaso Falcone, MD, FRCS(C), FACOG
M. Jean Uy-Kroh, MD, FACOG
Linda D. Bradley, MD, FACOG

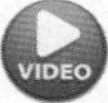

Please visit the eBook that accompanies this text to view the video(s) where this icon is indicated. Directions for accessing the eBook are located on the inside front cover.

Contents

SECTION I: BASIC SURGICAL SETUP

SECTION II: DIAGNOSTIC LAPAROSCOPY

SECTION III: UTERINE SURGERY

SECTION IV: CERVIX

SECTION V: ADNEXAL SURGERY

SECTION VI: SURGICAL MANAGEMENT OF ENDOMETRIOSIS

SECTION VII: VULVAR AND PERINEAL SURGERY

SECTION VIII: HYSTEROSCOPY, UTERINE STERILIZATION, AND ABLATION PROCEDURES

Section I

Basic Surgical Setup

1 Basic Setup and Equipment for Laparoscopic Surgery

Cynthia Arvizo, M. Jean Uy-Kroh

OPERATING ROOM SETUP

The operating room (OR) should be set up to allow mobility of members of the surgical team throughout the room, quick access to instruments, patient safety, and comfortable surgeon positioning. The OR table should be electric to allow for easy positioning of the patient during the case. Overhead lighting should be placed over the surgical field. The light source, monitor, and insufflator may be located on one mobile boom or suspended from the ceiling. A monitor should be placed directly in front of each surgeon to facilitate ergonomic operating. If only one monitor is available, the monitor should be placed between the patient's legs. Two separate sterile surgical fields are set for abdominal and vaginal instruments. Ideally, the scrub nurse is positioned between the patient's legs, or as close to the surgical field as feasible.

THE IMAGE

The imaging chain consists of seven devices: light source, light cable, laparoscope, camera head, camera control unit, digital cable, and the monitor. Malfunction of any of these components will lead to suboptimal image quality and disruption of the surgical case.

Troubleshooting during a surgical case is inevitable but sound knowledge of the imaging chain saves time.

Light Source and Light Cable

Good image quality is dependent on good lighting. The most widely available light sources use xenon, metal halide, or LED bulbs. LED bulbs are touted as more eco-friendly because they emit less heat and last longer than xenon bulbs. Light is transmitted from the light source through a light-guide cable. Two types of cables are available—fiber optic and liquid cables. Most ORs are equipped with fiber optic cables.

Laparoscope

Several laparoscope designs are available on the market. The two most common types of laparoscopes are a hollow rod with a series of lens connected to a video camera (rod–lens system) or digital systems with a charge-coupled device (CCD) at the end of the laparoscope. The digital laparoscope unites the video and light cable. A variety of scope diameters are available. Scope diameters as small as 1 mm exist, but most operative gynecologic surgery is performed with 5- or 10-mm zero-degree laparoscopes. Flexible and angled laparoscopes can significantly aid visualization, particularly when dealing with a bulky and enlarged uterus.

Camera, Camera Control Unit, and Monitor

The laparoscope attaches to the camera head, which is connected to the camera control unit (CCU) via the digital cable. Cameras are provided as one-chip or three-chip devices. Three-chip cameras are most commonly used today as they provide higher resolution than one-chip devices. An image passes through the lens on the camera head. A prism within the camera head splits light into three primary colors (red, blue, and green) each with a corresponding CCD. The CCD converts the image to an electric signal that is transmitted to the CCU. The CCU can then send the image as either analog or digital video outputs or signals for viewing and recording.

Insufflator

Surgery cannot be safely performed without adequate insufflation. An insufflator delivers carbon dioxide into the peritoneal cavity and maintains a set pressure and an inflow rate. Intracavitary pressure of 12 to 15 mm Hg produces sufficient pneumoperitoneum for most laparoscopic cases. Various insufflating systems offer additional features such as warmed, humidified carbon dioxide, concomitant smoke evacuation, and filtration. Leaky gaskets, cracked, poorly connected, or kinked tubing, and empty gas tanks are common causes of poor or absent insufflation.

INSTRUMENTS AND EQUIPMENT

Proper, well-functioning instruments allow for a smooth surgical case. In gynecologic laparoscopy, two sets of instruments are routinely utilized—vaginal and laparoscopic.

Vaginal Instruments

In general, the vaginal instruments aid in placing the uterine manipulator. The most basic set should include an open-sided speculum or Auvard weighted speculum, Sims vaginal retractor, single-toothed tenaculum, ring forceps, uterine sound, Hulka tenaculum, and cervical dilators.

There are several uterine manipulators available. The preferred manipulator is a cost-effective device that adequately manipulates and serves the needs for the particular surgery. The most basic manipulator is a reusable Hulka tenaculum. Other manipulators may provide additional functions such as a chromopertubation port, custom-sized colpotomy cup, built-in vaginal occluder, ante/retroflexion capabilities, and an angled curvature and sliding mechanisms to facilitate cervical insertion. Certain devices may be preferred for their durability with heavy specimens or they may work as accessories to surgical positioning units.

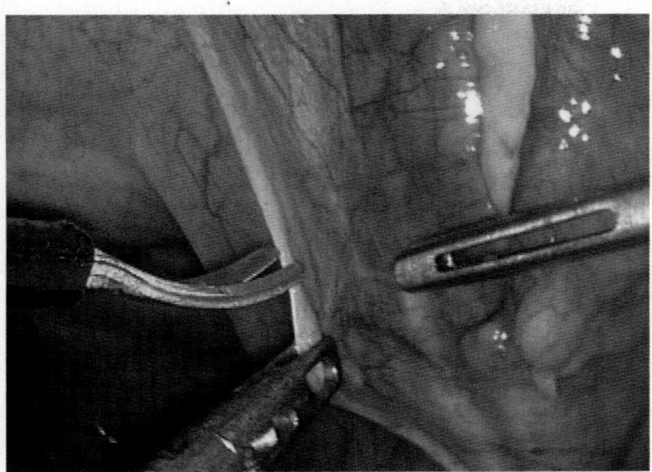

Figure 1.1. Scissors (top left). Atraumatic bowel grasper (top right). Allis forceps (bottom).

Laparoscopic Instrument

Trocars

Trocars range between 2 and 15 mm and are used to insert laparoscopes and instruments. They vary in material, reusability, tip type, valves, and specialized characteristics such as peritoneal balloons and insufflation mechanisms.

Graspers and Scissors

Most laparoscopic instruments are available in 3-, 5-, and 10-mm diameters. Additionally, bariatric instruments are available to accommodate the unique needs of high BMI patients. Each grasper serves a different, specialized purpose. For example, atraumatic graspers are used to gently manipulate tissue. The Maryland dissector is useful for fine tissue handling and coagulation. The Allis forceps firmly holds tissue and is ideal for creating tissue traction. A laparoscopic tenaculum manipulates the uterus and proves useful for traction during myomectomies. Atraumatic bowel grasper's smooth texture allows for safe retraction of the bowel. A variety of scissors with coagulative capabilities are employed for cutting tissue with and without the use of electrosurgery (Fig. 1.1).

Other Basic Instruments

Surgeon preference dictates the type of needle holders and knot pushers that are used for extracorporeal knot tying.

During gynecologic cases, safe specimen removal through small laparoscopic incisions is expedited with different instruments. Spoon forceps collect small specimens, such as clot or fragments of tissue. Specimen retrieval bags are either disposable or reusable plastic bags that minimize content contamination during the removal process. Smaller specimens may be delivered through trocars, but large specimens are brought up to the abdominal incision and the bag is opened to expose a part of the specimen.

Fascial closure systems introduce a needle with suture alongside the defect under direct visualization to close fascial defects greater than 10 mm. The needle is removed and reintroduced on the contralateral side. The suture is grasped, externalized, and tied.

Suction and Irrigation System

Suction and irrigation maintain a clear view and surgical field. The most rudimentary setup is a syringe attached to a hollow probe. When a surgery demands more rigorous assistance, a handheld, battery-powered system is connected to a standard OR suction. In addition, irrigation tubing connected to liter bags of Lactated Ringer's solution or saline is employed.

ENERGY SOURCES

The widespread use of operative energy sources necessitates a basic understanding of these energies and their devices. Radiofrequency (RF) electric, ultrasonic, laser, and plasma energy all generate heat, but they vary dramatically in their mechanics. The most commonly utilized energies, RF electrical energy and ultrasonic energy, are briefly described.

Radiofrequency Electrical Energy

RF electrical surgery delivers heat created by alternating current conducted through two electrodes. Monopolar instrumentation relies on a small "active" electrode and a larger "dispersive" or return electrode (Fig. 1.2). By definition, the patient is part of the electrical circuit. When a surgeon applies energy, electrons move through the tissue and generate heat. In addition to the type of current applied, surgical dwell time on tissue and the surface area of the active electrode collectively determine the thermal effect on both the target and surrounding tissues.

Three types of waveforms are routinely employed in the operating room are cut, coagulate, and blend. Cut current is a high-frequency, low-voltage continuous waveform that results in rapid tissue heating with little to no hemostasis. The electrode's proximity to the tissue leads to either vaporization (indirect contact tissue with resulting air gap) or dessication (direct contact with tissue). Coagulation current greatly interrupts the continuous waveform used in cutting mode and, as a result, produces a low-frequency, high-voltage waveform. Coagulation current's high voltage increases the potential for heat to deeply penetrate the tissue, thus causing "thermal spread." Blend current is an intermediate frequency, and is truly a "blended" form of cut current.

Unlike monopolar instruments, bipolar instruments rely on intervening tissue between the two electrodes to complete the electrical circuit. An example of this is the traditional bipolar Kleppinger forceps that is used to achieve hemostasis or tissue

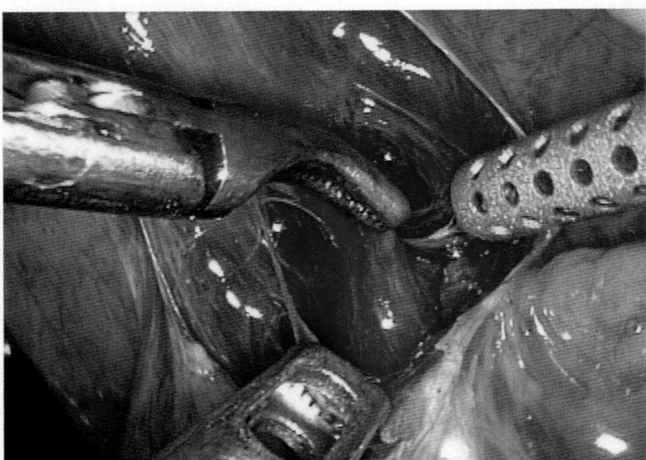

Figure 1.2. Maryland dissector (top left) with a fine grasping tip for tissue handling and monopolar radiofrequency energy application. Suction irrigator (top right). Allis forceps (bottom).

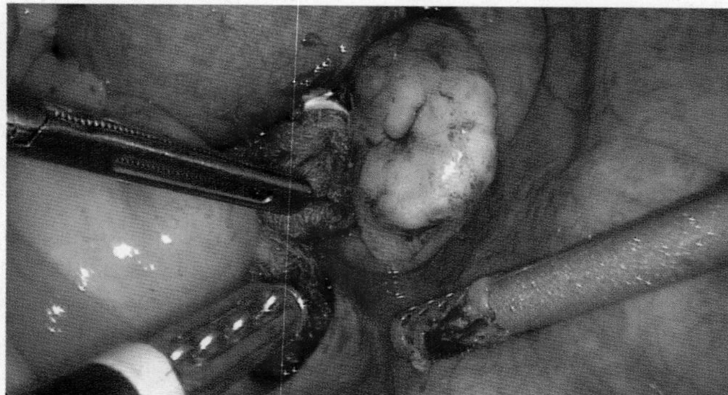

Figure 1.3. Kleppinger bipolar radiofrequency device (bottom left) with battery-powered suction irrigator (bottom right) and atraumatic grasper (top left).

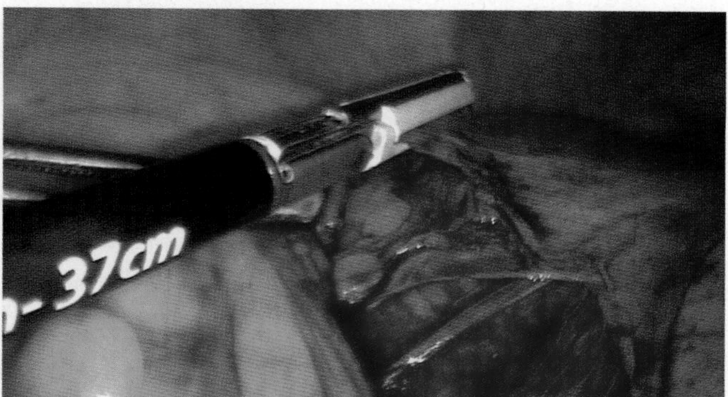

Figure 1.4. Ligasure (Valleylab) advanced bipolar device.

desiccation (Fig. 1.3). The thermal spread caused by the traditional bipolar instruments can be undesirable. Over time, "advanced bipolar" devices have emerged that combine various energy forms and rely on newer adaptive electrosurgical units (ESUs) that perceive and calculate tissue resistance encountered by the electrode tip. The ESU processes this information to modulate the power output to match the clinical scenario.

Other newer technologies fuse energies. Some examples include the LigaSure Advance (Valleylab) which integrates advanced bipolar and monopolar energies (Fig. 1.4). The Thunderbeat device (Olympus) combines ultrasonic and advanced bipolar technologies. In addition to devices, there has been an introduction in novel energy delivery systems. An example of this is the Valleylab waveform that modulates coagulation current instead of a continuous cut current. In theory the effect is reduced tissue drag, when compared to the standard coagulation current, and greater hemostasis than compared to the cut current.

Ultrasonic Energy

Ultrasonic energy exerts mechanical energy to create frictional heating. The active blade of the ultrasonic shears vibrates about 55,500 times per second causing low-temperature denaturation, while the nonactive blade holds tissue in place. Similar to RF energy, the cycling of the active blade determines the energy mode employed. Rapid cycling results in cutting with less hemostatic properties, whereas slow cycling is less precise but creates more energy dispersion.

KEY READINGS

Bittner JG, Awad MM, Varela JE. Laparoscopic hemostasis: energy sources. In: Soper NJ, Scott-Connor CEH, eds. *The SAGES Manual: Basic Laparoscopy and Endoscopy.* Vol. 1. 3rd ed. New York: Springer; 2012:105–120.

Law KS, Lyons SD. Comparative studies of energy sources in gynecologic laparoscopy. *J Minim Invasive Gynecol.* 2013;20(3):308–318.

Munro MG, Abbott JA, Vilos GA, Brill AI. Radiofrequency electrical energy guidelines for authors: what's in a name? *J Minim Invasive Gynecol.* 2015;22(1):1–2.

Schwaitzberg SD. Imaging systems in minimally invasive surgery. In: Swanstrom LL, Soper NJ, eds. *Mastery of Endoscopic and Laparoscopic Surgery.* Philadelphia, PA: Lippincott Williams & Wilkins; 2014: 47–61.

Basic Equipment and Setup for Robot-Assisted Laparoscopic Surgery Using the Intuitive Da Vinci Si Robot

2

Tommaso Falcone, Henry F. Kraft

GENERAL PRINCIPLES

There are several steps to efficient use of the robot:

1. Correct choice of equipment during surgery.
2. Correct placement of robotic ports for effective pelvic surgery.
3. Correct docking so as to maximize the full range of motion of the robotic arms.

This chapter will cover the use of a multi-port robot-assisted laparoscopic procedure.

INSTRUMENTS AND EQUIPMENT

Correct Choice of Equipment During Surgery

- It is critical to choose the correct instruments required for a procedure. Surgery must be cost-effective, so it is inappropriate to simply keep changing instruments during the procedure until you find the one that works. The surgical approach should be carefully planned and appropriate instruments chosen to reduce exchange of instruments and be cost-effective. Each surgical procedure has some basic instruments required—a grasper appropriate for the case, an energy form for hemostasis, and a cutting instrument such as scissors.
- Figure 2.1 shows some basic instruments.

Correct Port Placement

- After the patient has been properly positioned in dorsal lithotomy, prepped, and draped, and a proper time-out has been done, incision is made, and the ports are placed.
- There are different possibilities for placement of robotic ports based on pathology and type of procedure. The camera port can be placed at the umbilicus for most procedures. The assistant/accessory ports are placed in the left or right upper quadrant.
- However, if the uterus is large, a supra umbilical port is necessary.
- The camera port should be placed 2 to 4 cm higher than the umbilicus so as to maintain a 10 cm working distance between the tip of the endoscope and the fundus of the uterus.
- Likewise, the 8-mm robotic instrument ports should also be moved higher in tandem with the movement of the camera port.
- It is also noteworthy that all precautions should be taken to keep the tip of the endoscope from touching any of the surrounding tissue. It is hot and can cause thermal injury.

Scenario 1

- It is a standard four-arm configuration, where the camera port is placed at the umbilicus and the 8-mm robotic ports are placed each at least 8 to 10 cm lateral to the camera port.
- See Figure 2.2.

Scenario 2

- It is a three-arm configuration, where the camera port is placed at the umbilicus and only two robotic instrument arms are used. Each robotic instrument arm should be placed 8 to 10 cm lateral to the camera port.
- See Figure 2.3A.

Scenario 3

- Another approach is a four-arm configuration where robotic port no. 2 is placed higher (closer to the costal margin). This is particularly advantageous with smaller patients.
- See Figure 2.3B.

Scenario 4

- There are exceptions to introducing the assistant/accessory port in the upper abdomen. For tubal reanastomosis, a three-arm configuration is used as in Figure 2.3A. However, in this scenario, a 12-mm assistant/accessory port is placed in the lower quadrant so that small needles can be introduced and extracted under direct vision.

Docking the Robot

- After the ports are placed, and the patient is positioned in the proper amount of Trendelenburg, lower the operating room table to the lowest position possible.
- Place the patient's legs as close together as the yellowfin stirrups will allow—this will enable maximum access and visualization as the robotic patient cart approaches the OR table.
- Align the patient cart base pointing toward the patient, with a starting point 2 to 3 ft beyond the yellowfin stirrups, and oriented so as to be able to come straight toward the patient's umbilicus on a 45-degree angle to the patient's longitudinal axis.
- See Figure 2.4.
- If maneuvering the patient cart is difficult due to the confines of a small OR, it can be helpful to preemptively angle the OR table 15 degrees to one side or the other in order to facilitate advancing the patient cart on a 45-degree angle to the patient's umbilicus and longitudinal axis.

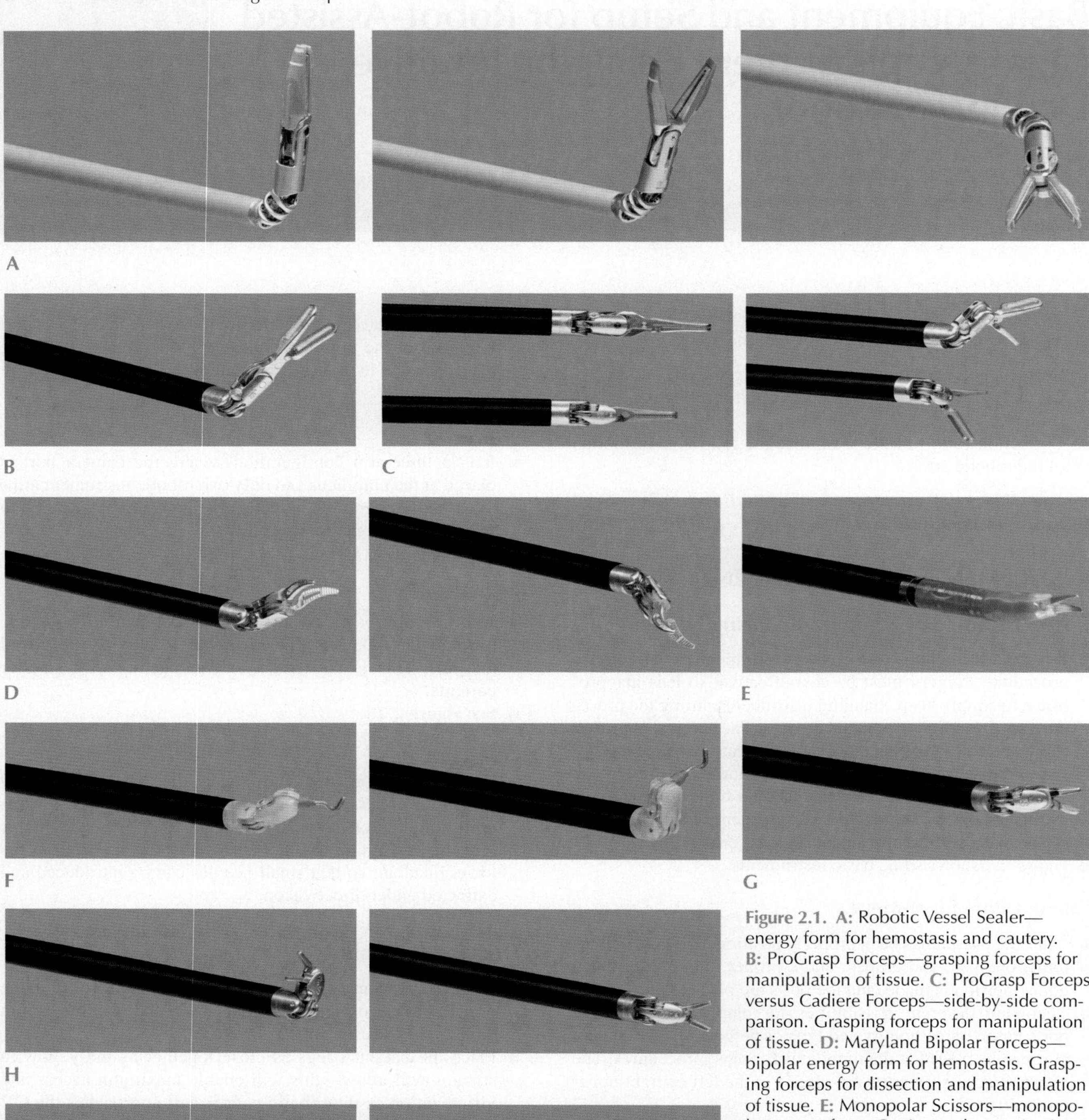

Figure 2.1. A: Robotic Vessel Sealer—energy form for hemostasis and cautery. B: ProGrasp Forceps—grasping forceps for manipulation of tissue. C: ProGrasp Forceps versus Cadiere Forceps—side-by-side comparison. Grasping forceps for manipulation of tissue. D: Maryland Bipolar Forceps—bipolar energy form for hemostasis. Grasping forceps for dissection and manipulation of tissue. E: Monopolar Scissors—monopolar energy form. Cutting and cauterization of tissue. F: Permanent Cautery Hook—monopolar energy form. Divides and cauterizes tissue. G: Mega Suturecut Needle Driver—dual function instrument. Both drives needle through tissue and cuts suture. H: Large Needle Driver—drives needle through tissue. Medium size jaws are more appropriate for smaller needles. I: Black Diamond Needle Driver—drives needle through tissue. Fine tip jaws needed for very small needles. (Reprinted with permission, Cleveland Clinic Center for Medical Art & Photography © 2015 all rights reserved.)

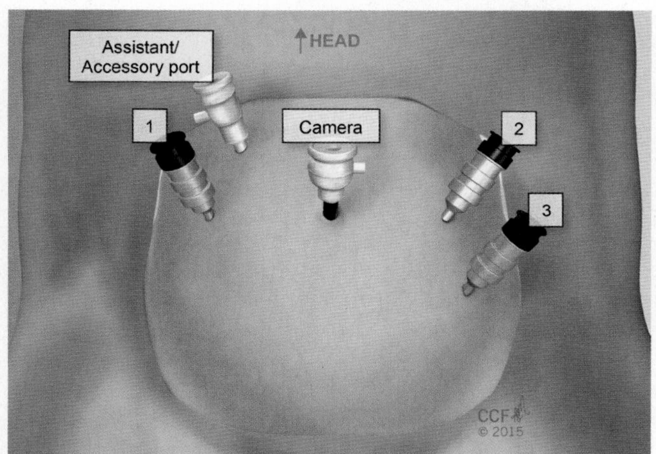

Figure 2.2. Port placement for standard four-arm side docking of the Intuitive Da Vinci Si robot. Numbers 1, 2, and 3 are 8-mm robotic instrument arm ports. (Reprinted with permission, Cleveland Clinic Center for Medical Art & Photography © 2015 all rights reserved.)

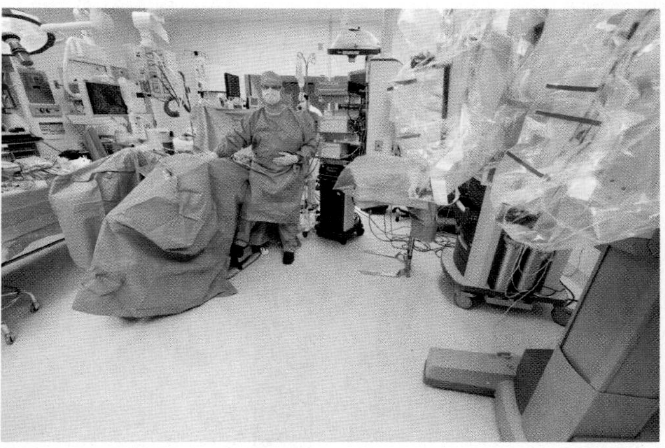

Figure 2.4. Demonstrates the 45-degree angle of approach for the patient cart toward the OR table. Surgeon directs the angle of approach. (Reprinted with permission, Cleveland Clinic Center for Medical Art & Photography © 2015 all rights reserved.)

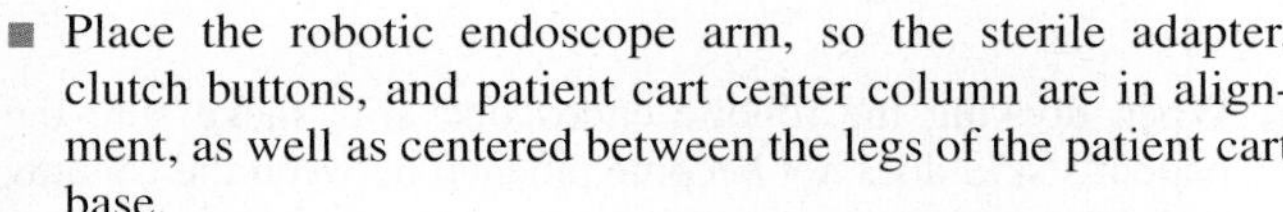

- Place the robotic endoscope arm, so the sterile adapter, clutch buttons, and patient cart center column are in alignment, as well as centered between the legs of the patient cart base.
- The camera arm setup joint (which is the articulating joint on the robotic endoscope arm closest to the patient cart center column) should be articulated to the same side as robotic instrument arm no. 1. There is no consideration necessary for the "sweet spot" (blue band) found on the camera arm setup joint when side docking.
- See Figure 2.5.
- Extend robotic instrument arms no. 1, no. 2, and no. 3, so they are evenly spaced at approximately a 45-degree angle on either side of the robotic endoscope arm.
- See Figure 2.6.
- Before advancing the patient cart toward the OR table, extend the robotic endoscope arm slightly forward of the robotic instrument arms, with a 45-degree forward tilt of the sterile adapter, as this will be a helpful indicator when approach to the OR table should be stopped and the brakes on the patient cart set.
- See Figure 2.7A.
- The OR table base (closest to the patient's foot) serves as a helpful landmark, approximately coinciding with the 45-degree angle of approach to the patient's umbilicus and longitudinal axis necessary for docking.
- See Figure 2.7B.
- Slight adjustments may be necessary if using the table base as a landmark due to variance in both the size and shape of the base of OR tables (company and model dependent).
- Patient body habitus plays a role in determining how close along the 45-degree angle the patient cart should be from the OR table.

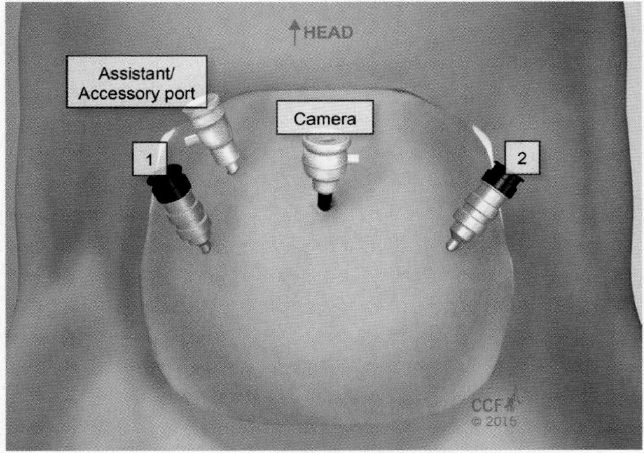

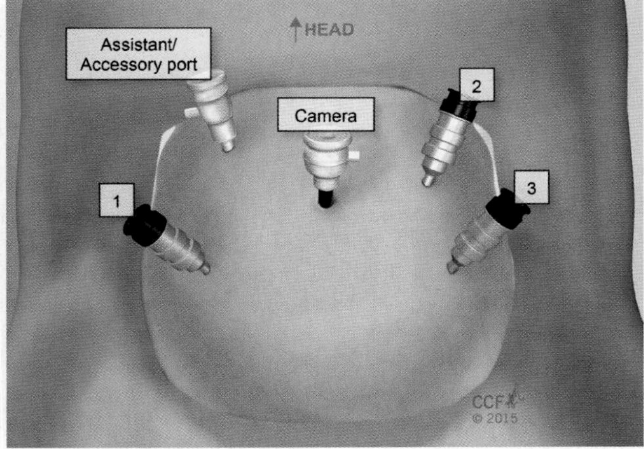

Figure 2.3. A and B: Alternate port placement. A: Three-arm port placement. Numbers 1 and 2 are 8-mm robotic instrument arm ports. B: Four-arm port placement for smaller patients. Numbers 1, 2, and 3 are 8-mm robotic instrument arm ports. (Reprinted with permission, Cleveland Clinic Center for Medical Art & Photography © 2015 all rights reserved.)

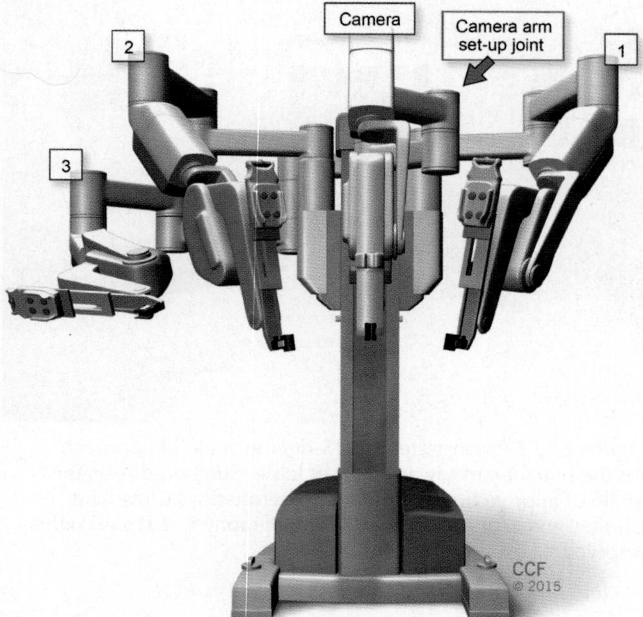

Figure 2.5. Starting position for robotic arms on patient cart. Note camera arm setup joint is angled opposite arm no. 3. (Reprinted with permission, Cleveland Clinic Center for Medical Art & Photography © 2015 all rights reserved.)

Attaching the Robot Arms to the Trocars

- The robotic endoscope arm should be docked first, in order to confirm that the 45-degree angle and the distance of the patient cart from the OR table are correct.
- Note the alignment of the camera port in the umbilicus, the anterior superior iliac spine (ASIS), the robotic endoscope arm, and the patient cart center column.
- See Figure 2.8.
- If any of those are not correct, this is the time to make the adjustments.

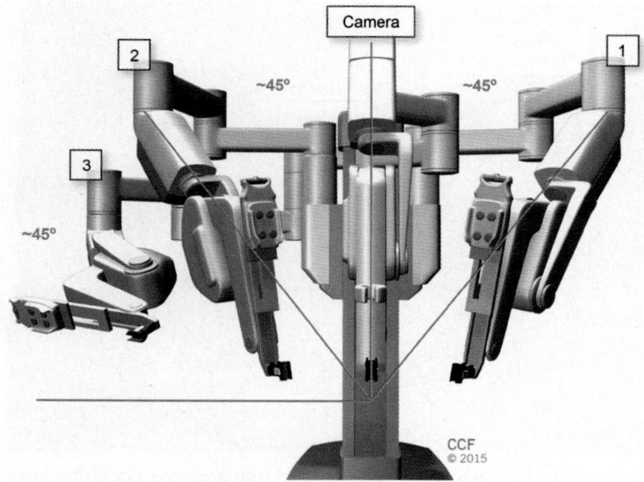

Figure 2.6. Forty-five–degree angle between each of the robotic arms. Note alignment of the endoscope arm sterile adapter and patient cart center column. (Reprinted with permission, Cleveland Clinic Center for Medical Art & Photography © 2015 all rights reserved.)

- When docking the robotic endoscope arm, make sure the patient's skin does not become pinched between the cannula and the quick click cannula mount.
- After the camera port (12-mm cannula) is docked to the robotic endoscope arm, ensure that the luer-lock on the side of the 12-mm cannula is rotated to the patient's left or right so as to avoid blunt force trauma to the abdomen.
- For patients that have a low BMI, a way to keep the robotic instrument arms from colliding with the robotic endoscope arm is to use an extra-long 12-mm endoscope cannula in the umbilicus.
- Insert it so that only the distal 2 cm of the cannula is visible in the abdominal cavity. This will raise the attachment point of the robotic endoscope arm to the 12-mm endoscope cannula, allowing for a greater range of motion for the robotic instrument arms intraoperatively.

A

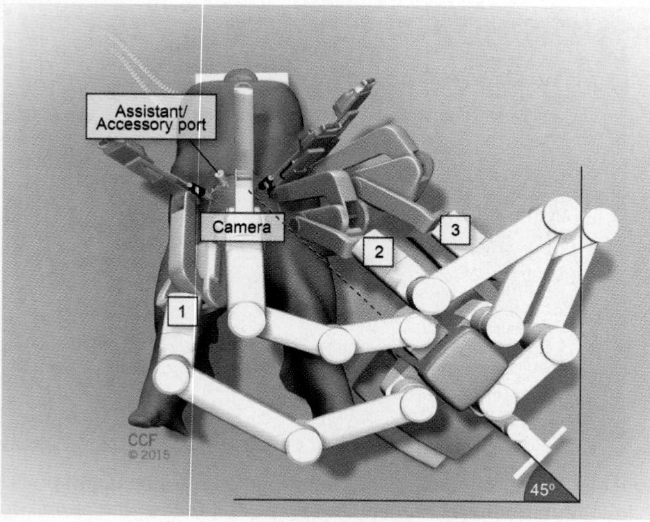

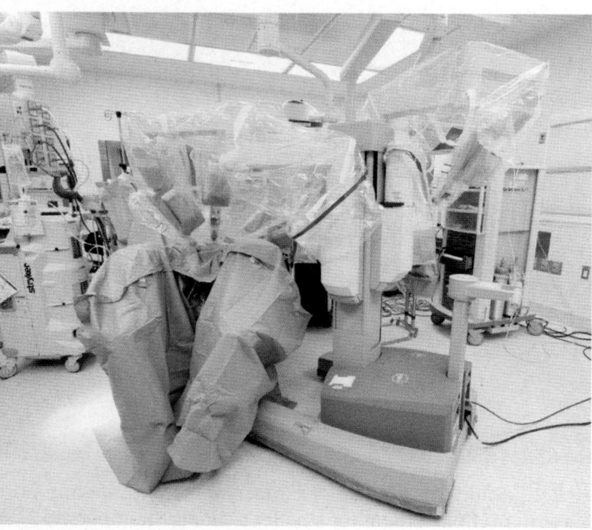

B

Figure 2.7. A: Patient cart base at a 45-degree angle to OR base. B: Robotic patient cart base at approximately 45-degree angle to the base of OR table. Yellowfin stirrups as close together as possible. Patient in desired amount of Trendelenburg. OR table in its lowest position toward the floor. (Reprinted with permission, Cleveland Clinic Center for Medical Art & Photography © 2015 all rights reserved.)

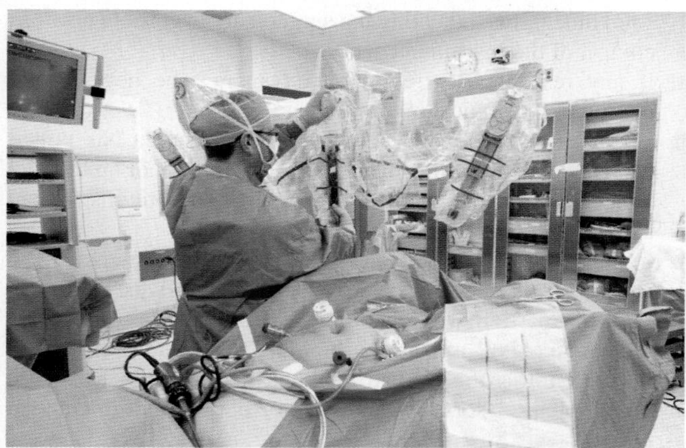

Figure 2.8. Note alignment of the camera port in the umbilicus, the ASIS (anterior superior iliac spine), the robotic endoscope arm, and the patient cart center column. (Reprinted with permission, Cleveland Clinic Center for Medical Art & Photography © 2015 all rights reserved.)

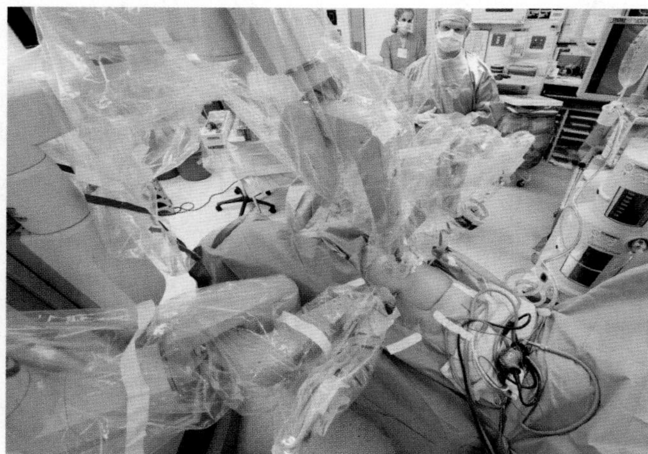

Figure 2.9. Robotic arms docked and robotic center established for the cannulas. (Reprinted with permission, Cleveland Clinic Center for Medical Art & Photography © 2015 all rights reserved.)

- Next, dock the robotic arms to their respective 8-mm robotic cannulas. This can be done at the same time if there are two people scrubbed at the time of docking.
- In our experience, during a tubal reanastomosis, using only robotic arms no. 1 and no. 3 allows more free space on the patient surface.
- Noteworthy, the difficulty in docking the 8-mm robotic ports can be greatly reduced by ensuring the drape is properly fitted on the quick click cannula mount and holding it there with your thumb.
- While holding the 8-mm robotic port perpendicular to the abdomen with one hand, press the port clutch button and bring the robotic arm in at the same perpendicular angle with the other hand. This will maximize visualization throughout the process.
- When the quick click cannula mount is properly interfaced with the 8-mm cannula, squeeze the front of the quick click cannula mount together with one hand, before squeezing the wings of the cannula mount together with your other hand.
- You will find docking the robotic arms to the robotic cannulas quick and easy using this technique.
- Lastly, "Burp" each of the robotic arms by pressing the robotic arm port clutch button. This is an important last step where the robotic center for each port is established.
- See Figure 2.9.

Introducing the Endoscope

- Connect the robotic camera to the robotic endoscope.
- Ensure the (sterile) draped camera cord does not fall as you bring the robotic camera and cord to the sterile field.
- Insert the distal end of the robotic endoscope carefully into the opening of the endoscope cannula, lifting the camera body toward the sterile adapter ring as you do.
- Be sure to orient the buttons on the endoscope camera housing so that they are facing the robotic endoscope sterile adapter.
- Place two fingers under the sterile adapter ring and gently lift as you insert the endoscope. This will aid in the ease of locking the endoscope into place.
- The last step in preparing the robotic arm endoscope for use is to secure the yellow rubber endoscope camera cord cable block in the robotic endoscope arm clip (found on the right side of the robotic endoscope arm, to the side of the sterile adapter).
- Press the robotic endoscope arm clutch button and advance the endoscope into the abdomen.
- While activating the endoscope clutch button, rotate the endoscope so as to visualize the distal end of the robotic instrument cannula before advancing either of the robotic instruments into the body.

Introducing the Robotic Instruments

- When inserting the robotic instruments into the robotic instrument arm cannulas, carefully place the working end of the instrument into the instrument cannula and then place the flat side of the instrument housing squarely against the sterile adapter.
- Gently slide the instrument forward until it clicks into place.
- Wait for the robot to cycle and recognize the instrument. This will be confirmed with a series of three beeps.
- Once the robot has recognized and confirmed the instrument, press the instrument arm clutch button and slowly advance the instrument, watching the laparoscopic monitor for the distal end of the robotic instrument to be visualized as it emerges through the distal end of the robotic instrument cannula.
- Continue to advance the instrument under endoscopic visualization until the instrument is at the target anatomy.
- In this example (robotic tubal reanastomosis), we performed this movement for both robotic arms no. 1 and no. 3, one at a time, slowly and cautiously.

Removal of Instruments and Guided Instrument Exchange

- To remove an instrument from the robotic instrument arm, ensure the distal end of the robotic instrument is in a straight and neutral position with the tips open.
- Then, squeeze the release levers found on the sides of the instrument housing, and pull the instrument back.
- See Figure 2.10.

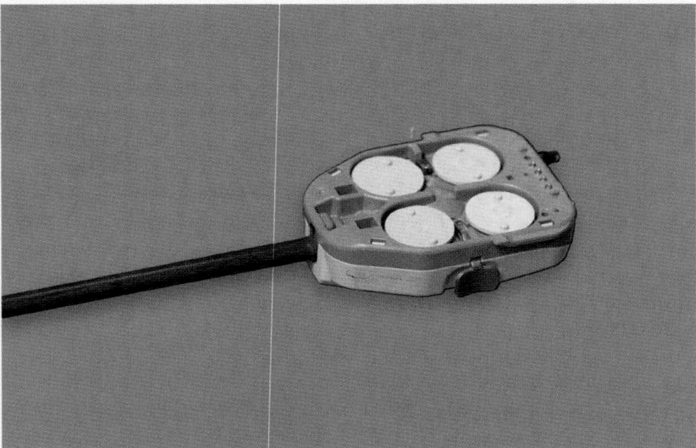

Figure 2.10. Flat side of the instrument housing unit—which interfaces with the robotic arm sterile adapter. Robotic instrument release lever (one of two) on the side of the instrument housing. (Reprinted with permission, Cleveland Clinic Center for Medical Art & Photography © 2015 all rights reserved.)

- After the initial pull, you will feel some assistance from the robot as the instrument retracts back into the instrument arm cannula.
- Squeeze the release levers and pull again to release the interface of the instrument with the robotic instrument arm sterile adapter.
- If you reinsert another robotic instrument for guided instrument exchange, you will notice once the robot has cycled and recognized the instrument (confirming with a series of three beeps), the lights at the proximal end of the robotic instrument arm sterile adapter will flash green and white in an alternating fashion. This indicates the robot remembers the position of the previous robotic instrument inserted into that instrument cannula.
- At this point, place two fingers directly on the flashing lights and slowly advance.
- If the instrument arm clutch button (located at the proximal end of the robotic instrument arm sterile adapter) is pushed, it will clear the memory of the previous position for that robotic arm instrument.
- In that situation, the distal end of the robotic instrument cannula must be visualized by the endoscope before advancing the instrument back to the target anatomy.
- Once the robotic instrument has reached its previous position in the body, the flashing green and white light will turn to a solid blue light (indicating the surgeon at the console now has control of the instrument arm).
- If any resistance is felt upon advancing the new robotic instrument, stop pushing immediately!
- Either the distal end of the instrument cannula has pulled back and is now no longer in a correct position, or an internal structure has come between the tip of the robotic instrument and the target anatomy.
- In either case, DO NOT advance the robotic instrument! The endoscope must be used to determine the source of the resistance.
- For this particular procedure (robotic laparoscopic tubal reanastomosis), a robotic bipolar Maryland Forceps is inserted into robotic instrument arm no. 3 and a robotic monopolar scissors is inserted into robotic instrument arm no. 1.
- For the reanastomosis of the fallopian tubes, robotic black diamond needle holders are inserted into both robotic instrument arms no. 1 and no. 3.

Undocking the Robot

- To undock the robot, it is critical that the robotic instruments be completely removed from the robotic cannulas before proceeding to undock the robotic instrument arms from the robotic cannulas!
- Once the robotic instruments have been removed, press the instrument arm clutch button and move the robotic instrument arm to a perpendicular position to the port site it is connected to.
- Spread the wings of the quick click cannula mount, which in turn will release the 8-mm robotic cannula from the quick click cannula mount.
- This can be done with the robotic instrument arm in any position, but is easiest when the robotic instrument arm is perpendicular to the port site.
- It may be necessary to place your thumb over the top of the 8-mm robotic cannula to aid in distracting the cannula from the robotic instrument arm.
- Once the robotic instrument arm has been released from the 8-mm robotic cannula, press the robotic instrument arm port clutch button and gently lift the robotic instrument arm away from the patient's body.
- To aid in both ease and safety in backing the robotic patient cart away from the operating table, gather the robotic instrument arms together close to the patient cart center column.

PEARLS AND PITFALLS

- If maneuvering the patient cart is difficult due to the confines of a small OR, it can be helpful to preemptively angle the OR table 15 degrees to one side or the other in order to facilitate advancing the patient cart on a 45-degree angle to the patient's umbilicus and longitudinal axis.
- Before advancing the patient cart toward the OR table, extend the robotic endoscope arm slightly forward of the robotic instrument arms, with a 45-degree forward tilt of the sterile adapter, as this will be a helpful indicator when approach to the OR table should be stopped and the brakes on the patient cart set.
- After the camera port (12-mm cannula) is docked to the robotic endoscope arm, ensure that the luer-lock on the side of the 12-mm cannula is rotated to the patient's left or right so as to avoid blunt force trauma to the abdomen.
- For patients that have a low BMI, a way to keep the robotic instrument arms from colliding with the robotic endoscope arm is to use an extra-long 12-mm endoscope cannula in the umbilicus.
  - Insert it so that only the distal 2 cm of the cannula is visible in the abdominal cavity. This will raise the attachment point of the robotic endoscope arm to the 12-mm endoscope cannula, allowing for greater range of motion for the robotic instrument arms intraoperatively.
- When the quick click cannula mount is properly interfaced with the 8-mm cannula, *squeeze the front of the quick click cannula mount together with one hand,* before squeezing the wings of the cannula mount together with your other hand.

3 Basic Equipment for Diagnostic Hysteroscopy

Linda D. Bradley

GENERAL PRINCIPLES

Definition

- Hysteroscopy is a minimally invasive transcervical procedure to provide panoramic visualization of the vagina, endocervix, endometrial cavity, and tubal ostia.

IMAGING, INSTRUMENTS, AND EQUIPMENT

- The basic hysteroscope may be flexible or rigid and is connected to a light source. It has an ancillary port to which distention fluid or CO_2 is used to distend the uterine cavity. A camera is frequently attached to the lens. When a video tower system is available, both the patient and nursing staff can be engaged in the procedure.
- In addition to an inflow tract, some hysteroscopes have an outflow tract.
- Hysteroscopes have variable lens ranging from 0, 12, 15, 30, to 70 degrees.
- There are variable diameters of diagnostic hysteroscopes available ranging from 2.9 to 10 mm (Fig. 3.1).
  - The most comfortable hysteroscopic diameters for office use are 4 mm or less. They usually require minimal or no cervical dilation.
- Rigid hysteroscopes have a rod lens and offer the clearest view.
- Flexible hysteroscopes incorporate a distal tip that is flexible and defects over a range of 120 to 160 degrees (Fig. 3.2). They utilize a fiber optic or digitally enhanced lens system.
  - The flexible hysteroscope has the smallest diameter compared to a rigid system. Its lens is 0 degrees.
  - Several benefits of the flexible hysteroscope include:
    - A longer working length which is ideal for obese women who may have a longer vaginal length.
    - Due to its flexibility compared to a rigid hysteroscope, the flexible hysteroscope can circumnavigate a tortuous endocervix and go around lesions within the uterine cavity.
- Hysteroscopy can be performed for diagnostic or therapeutic indications.
- Diagnostic hysteroscopy with small-caliber hysteroscopes ideally can be performed in the office. However, diagnostic hysteroscopy can also be performed in an ambulatory surgical center or operating theatre.
- Smaller-caliber, flexible, disposable, or rigid hysteroscopes decrease patient discomfort, need for dilation, and facilitate use in an office setting.
- Some diagnostic hysteroscopes have an ancillary port that will permit small surgical instruments to be inserted through an operating channel (Figs. 3.3 and 3.4). These instruments include:
  - Graspers—to grasp lost IUD strings that are in the endocervix or uterine cavity, foreign body (suture, dislodged tip of an IUD) (Fig. 3.5).
  - Biopsy forceps—to take targeted biopsies (Fig. 3.6).
  - Scissors—to cut thin adhesions (endocervix or endometrial), excise a polyp, cut a small septum (Fig. 3.7).

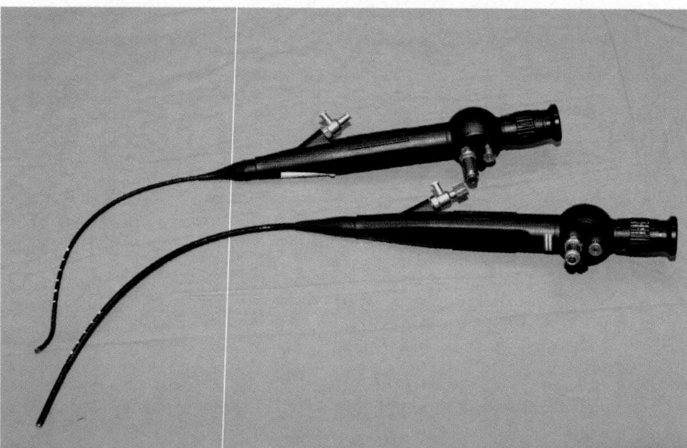

Figure 3.1. Comparison of two sizes of flexible hysteroscopes—(upper) 3.1 mm flexible; (lower) 5 mm flexible.

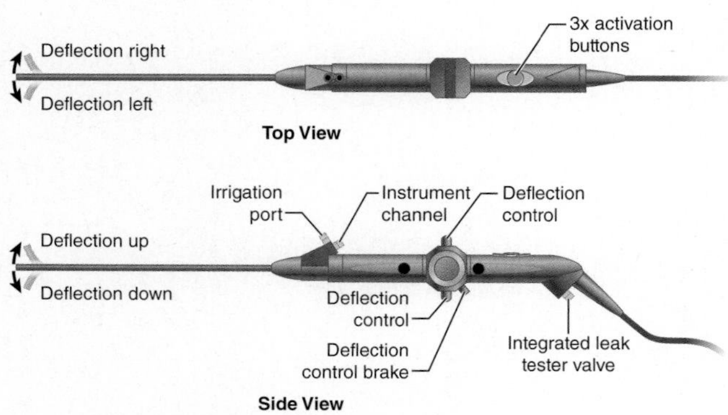

Figure 3.2. Demonstration of distal tip movement.

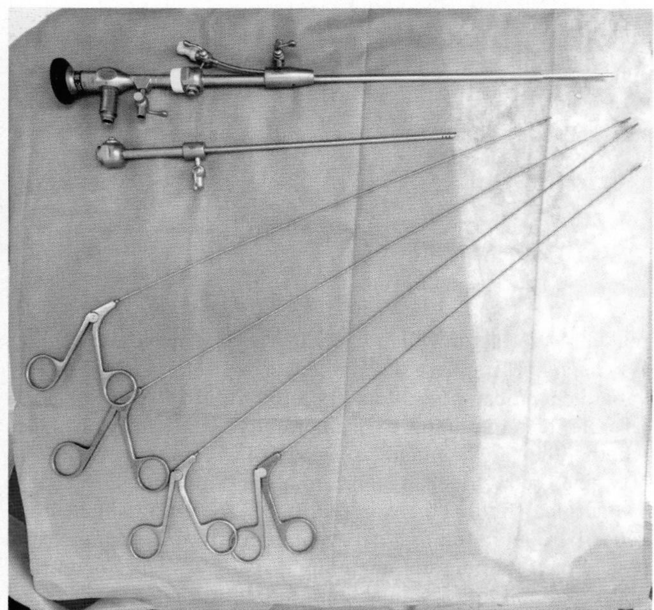

Figure 3.3. View of hysteroscope and ancillary equipment.

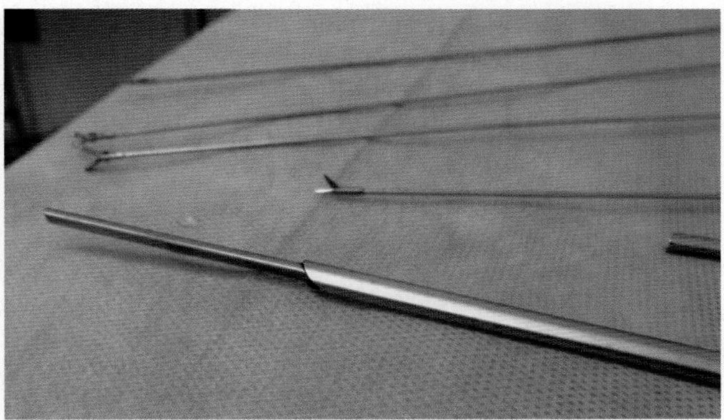

Figure 3.4. Close-up view of hysteroscope and ancillary equipment.

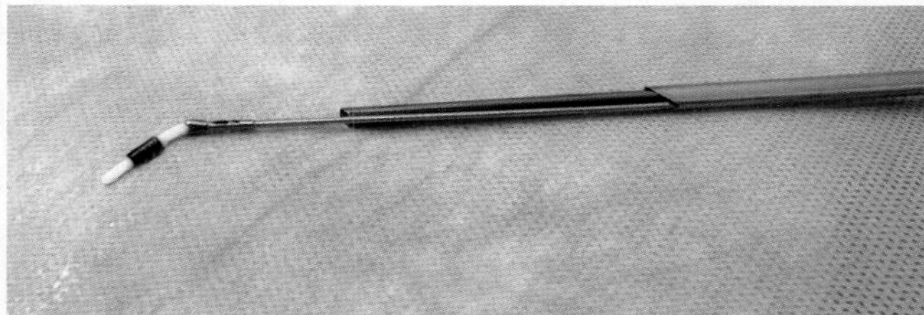

Figure 3.5. Hysteroscopic grasper holding fragmented IUD.

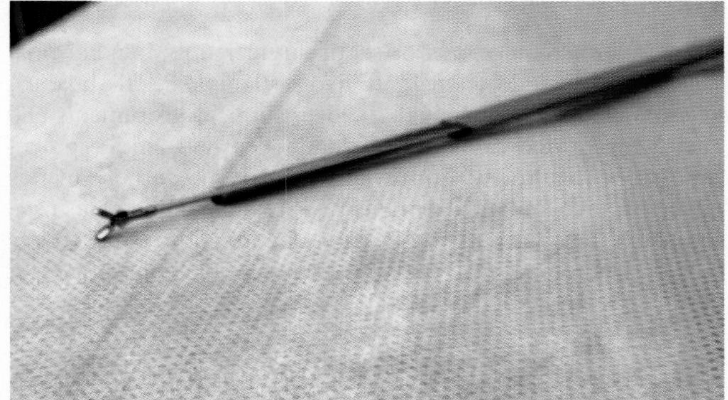

Figure 3.6. Hysteroscopic graspers.

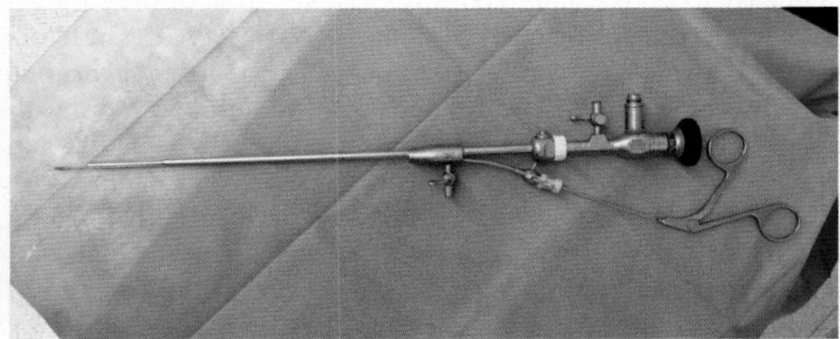

Figure 3.7. Scissors introduced through accessory port.

4 Basic Surgical Equipment for Abdominal Surgery

Bianca Falcone, M. Jean Uy-Kroh

GENERAL PRINCIPLES

A laparotomy requires a basic set of surgical tools. Fundamental instruments include scalpel, retractors, clamps, needle holders, scissors, and surgical sponges. Electrosurgical instruments and suctioning devices may also be employed and unique procedures may require additional instruments. The purpose of this chapter is to identify and demonstrate essential implements used in abdominopelvic surgery. It is not an attempt to exhaustively catalog laparotomy instruments, but rather an attempt to depict common instruments in use.

INSTRUMENTS AND EQUIPMENT

Retractors

The ideal abdominal retractor occupies minimal space, is quick and easy to set up, and maximizes visualization of the surgical site while protecting vital structures. A variety of retractors exist and surgeon's preference and surgical need determine which type is used. The framed, oval, or circular Bookwalter retractor is affixed to the surgical table by steel posts and hovers above the incision. Adjustable ratchet mechanisms are attached to the frame and secure a variety of self-retaining blades that expose the surgical site. It has the advantage of occupying minimal abdominal cavity space at the expense of a slightly cumbersome setup (Fig. 4.1 and Tech Fig. 8.1.12). In contrast, the Balfour retractor is a self-retaining, spreadable retractor. Its two blades are placed within the abdominal incision and the two blades are then pushed apart to expose the surgical site. Most commonly, a bladder blade is attached to the most inferior aspect of the retractor set. For increased exposure, additional handheld retractors can be utilized. Options include a right-angle retractor (Fig. 4.2), Dever retractor, and malleable retractor which exist in varying sizes and widths. As the name implies, the malleable retractor is particularly valuable as it can be bent and tailored to fulfill specific needs. Of note, it is important to use correctly sized retractor blades whether they are handheld, or as part of a retractor set; improperly sized retractors can cause injury and inadequately expose the surgical field. For example, oversized lateral blades can cause iatrogenic femoral neuropathy due to the extra pressure placed over the femoral nerve and psoas muscles. In contrast, obese patients may require appropriately longer, specialized bariatric retractor sets.

Clamps

A variety of clamps are required for grasping tissue. Generally, clamps can be subdivided into atraumatic versus traumatic. Hemostatic clamps are a separate subdivision; however, they may be considered atraumatic due to their use in fine dissection.

Atraumatic Clamps

- Babcock clamp
  - The smooth, cylindrical tip of the Babcock clamp makes it ideal for gently grasping fallopian tubes or bowel without causing damage.
- Kelly clamp
  - The Kelly clamp is the most basic hemostatic clamp that is used to secure bleeding vessels. This clamp is commonly used to isolate the infundibulopelvic ligament during abdominal hysterectomy.
- Tonsil clamp
  - A tonsil clamp is a hemostatic clamp. It is often utilized to secure a vessel or dissect around it. It can also be used for passing suture ties or vessel loops.

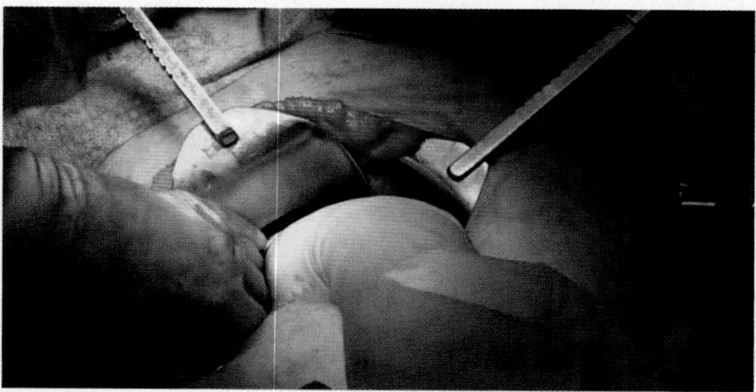

Figure 4.1. Bookwalter retractor setup with retracting blades.

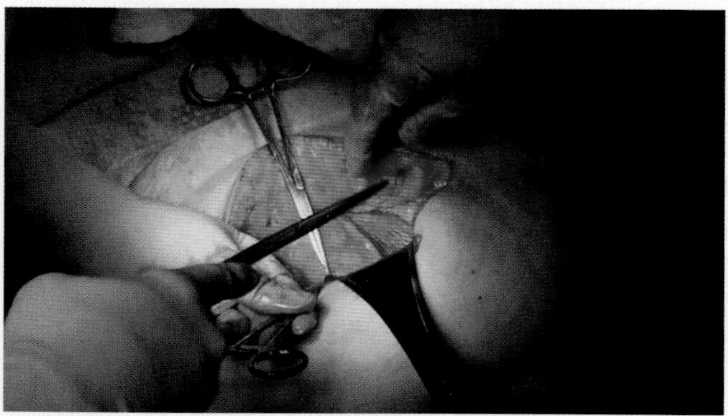

Figure 4.2. Handheld right-angle retractor, tonsil grasping peritoneum, Metzenbaum scissors in use.

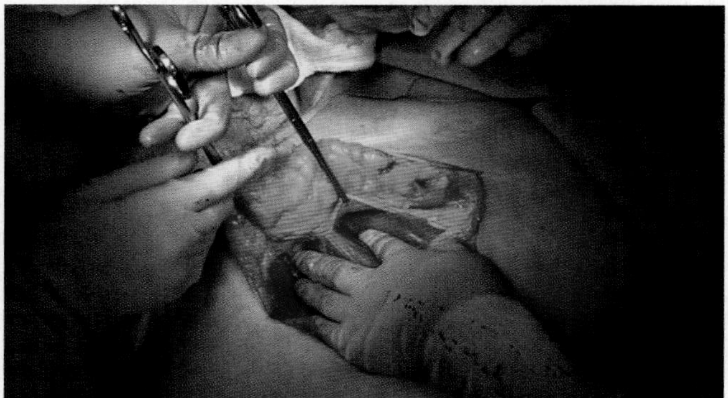

Figure 4.3. Kocher clamps grasping the most inferior aspect of fascial incision.

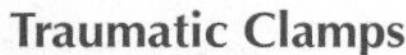

Traumatic Clamps

- Allis clamp
  - This minimally traumatic clamp is characterized by a single row of fine serrations on each tip.
- Kocher clamp
  - This moderately traumatic clamp has interlocking teeth at the tip and large horizontal serrations along the jaws. They are typically used to grasp fascia (Fig. 4.3).
- Heaney clamp
  - The Heaney clamp may be straight or curved. It possesses interlocking teeth and ridges or grooves that prevent tissue slippage. Because of these features, it is often used to clamp thick parametrial or paracervical tissue to create large pedicles during hysterectomy (see Tech Fig. 8.1.38).

Tissue Forceps

Smooth

- DeBakey forceps
  - The longer length of a DeBakey forceps allows secure handling of tissue that is deeper in the abdominal cavity. The tips are elongated with fine grooves ideal for precise atraumatic tissue manipulation (Fig. 4.4).

Toothed

- Adson forceps
  - Adson forceps are more commonly used when closing surgical incisions. The teeth are used to elevate and reapproximate the skin without causing trauma. The classic Adson forceps has two small teeth at the tips which allude to its alternate name of a "rat tooth" forceps.

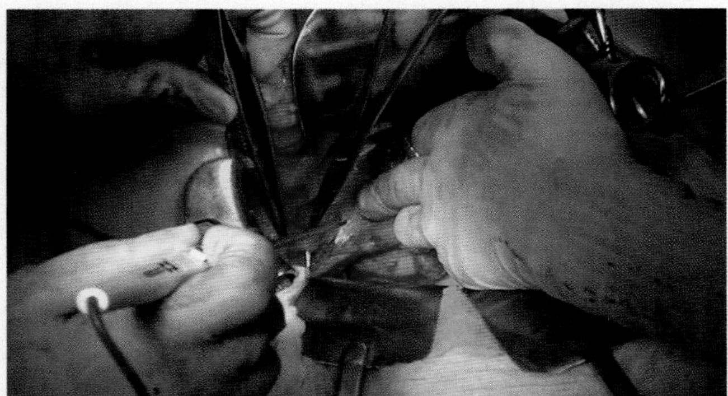

Figure 4.4. DeBakey forceps, monopolar instrument, tonsil clamp.

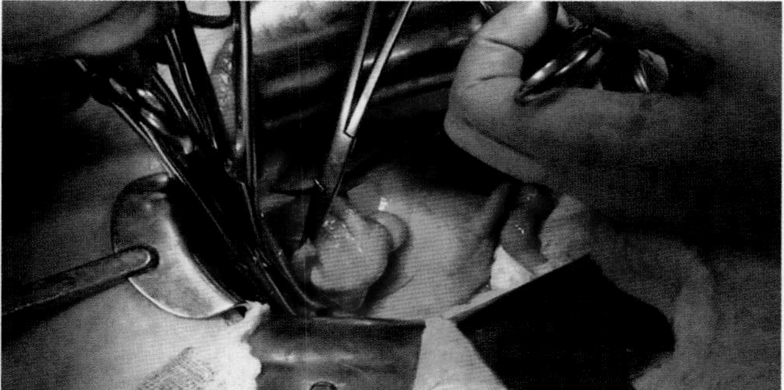

Figure 4.5. Two curved Heaney clamps secure a ligament, while curved Mayo scissors are placed between the clamps to incise the pedicle.

- Russian forceps
  - The wide, rounded tip with serrations is designed to increase the grasping force by increasing the grasping surface area.
- Bonney forceps
  - These forceps have the most aggressive toothed tips and textured grasping shaft that facilitate fascial closure.

Scissors

Generally, all scissors come in straight or curved variations. The scissors' curvature increases visibility and enables a smooth, horizontal incision in a deep wound. Suture scissors are recognizable by their blunted ends that prevent inadvertent puncture or laceration to distal organs and vessels. They are reserved for cutting suture alone and should not be used on tissue. There are three commonly used tissue scissors.

- Metzenbaum scissors are those of choice for delicate tissue dissection and excision.
- Mayo scissors are heavier scissors used for cutting ligaments, fascia, and large pedicles (see Fig. 4.5).
  - Jorgensen scissors are heavy scissors with a dramatically angled blade. They are typically used to cut the cardinal ligament during hysterectomy (see Tech Fig. 8.1.38).

Needle Holders

- Curved: Heaney needle holders have curved jaws and are useful specifically for vaginal suturing. The curve of the needle holder facilitates needle placement.
- Straight: The Bulldog needle holder is the favored needle holder in pelvic surgery. It is versatile as it can be used with a range of needles and in multiple anatomical locations. The Ryder needle holder is another straight needle holder that is used when fine, small needles are required.
- Both the straight and curved needle holders are available in long and short lengths. This allows the surgeon to choose her preference depending on needle size as well as suture location. For example, a longer needle holder would be ideal for deeper suturing.

ENERGY SOURCES

Radiofrequency Electrical Energy

- Electrical energy in the form of monopolar or bipolar energy can be used to vaporize, linear vaporize (cut), coagulate, desiccate, or fulgurate tissue.
- Monopolar energy requires an adhesive dispersive pad that is placed on the patient's body in order to create a closed circuit. There are various blade tips (i.e., extended tip) that fit into the universal hand piece.
- Bipolar energy allows less spread of thermal energy than monopolar.

KEY READINGS

Baggish MS, Karram MM. *Atlas of Pelvic Anatomy and Gynecologic Surgery.* 2nd ed. St Louis, MO: Elsevier Saunders; 2006.

Malt RA. *The Practice of Surgery.* Philadelphia, PA: WB Saunders; 1993.

Nemitz R. *Surgical Instrumentation: An Interactive Approach.* 2nd ed. St Louis, MO: Elsevier Saunders; 2014.

Nichols DH. Instruments and sutures. In: Nichols DH, ed. *Gynecologic and Obstetric Surgery.* St Louis, MO: Mosby-Yearbook; 1993, p.120.

Sutton PA, Awad S, Perkins AC, Lobo DN. Comparison of lateral thermal spread using monopolar and bipolar diathermy, the Harmonic Scalpel™ and the Ligasure™. *Br J Surg.* 2010;97:428–433.

Wells MP. *Surgical Instruments.* 3rd ed. St. Louis, MO: Elsevier Saunders; 2006.

Section II

Diagnostic Laparoscopy

5 Diagnostic Laparoscopy

Rachel Barron

GENERAL PRINCIPLES

Diagnostic laparoscopy is the surgical examination of the pelvis and abdomen with the intent to diagnose various pathologies.

Differential Diagnosis

- Ruptured ectopic pregnancy
- Adnexal masses—benign versus malignant
- Adnexal torsion
- Endometriosis

Anatomic Considerations

- Aorta
  - The aortic bifurcation is located cephalad to the umbilicus in 90% of nonobese, supine patients.
  - In a patient with body mass index (BMI) <25 kg/m^2, the abdominal wall is approximately 2 to 3 cm thick. At a 90-degree angle, the distance to the bifurcation is between 6 and 8 cm and directly correlates to the patient's BMI. Therefore, an entry angle of 45 degrees is recommended to avoid vascular injury.
  - In a patient with BMI >25 and >30 kg/m^2, the distance from the umbilicus to the aortic bifurcation averages 10 and 13 cm, respectively.
- Inferior epigastric vessels
  - See Figure 5.1.
  - The deep inferior epigastric vessels originate from external iliac vessels and travel along the anterior abdominal wall on the inferior side of the rectus abdominus.
    - Their path begins medial to the insertion of the round ligament into the deep inguinal ring.
    - At the level of pubic symphysis, the vessels are lateral to the rectus abdominis.
    - At the level of the anterior superior iliac spine (ASIS), the vessels are an average of 3.5 (2.6 to 5.5) cm from the midline.
  - During laparoscopy, the deep inferior epigastric vessels can be identified in the lateral peritoneal umbilical folds bilaterally.
- Iliohypogastric and ilioguinal nerves
  - The iliohyogastric nerve provides sensory innervation to the oblique abdominal muscles and the suprapubic skin.
  - The ilioguinal nerve provides sensory to the transversus abdominis, internal oblique, skin of medial thigh, and the vulva.
  - Classically, when a nerve has been injured or entrapped, patients report a burning sensation near the incision sites that radiates toward the groin.
  - Both nerves originate from L1 vertebra, after emerging from the lateral border of the psoas muscle. They wrap around the iliac crest to pierce through the transversus abdominis and internal oblique.
    - The ilioinguinal nerves emerge 3.1 cm medial and 3.7 cm inferior to the ASIS. The iliohypogastric emerges 2.1 cm medial and 1 cm inferior to the ASIS.
    - Both nerves emerge near classic locations for lateral trocar placement.

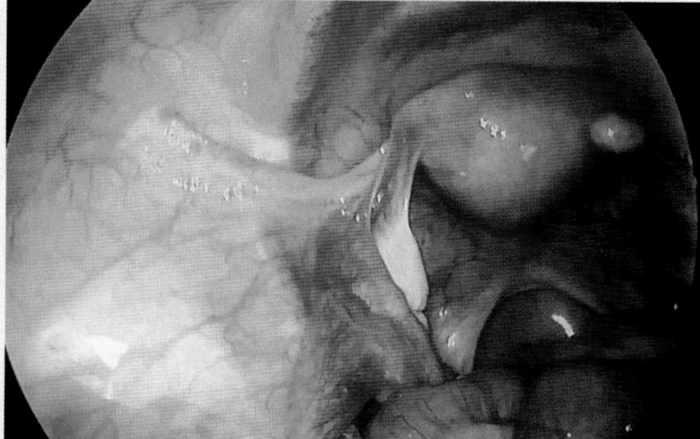

Figure 5.1. Laparoscopic view of the anterior abdominal wall: Inferior epigastrics traveling through lateral umbilical fold.

IMAGING AND OTHER DIAGNOSTICS

- Transvaginal pelvic ultrasound is the imaging modality of choice.
  - The primary entry site may be altered by a pelvic mass, an enlarged uterus, or suspected adhesions revealed by ultrasound.
  - A visceral slide test performed with ultrasound can be used to preoperatively identify dense subumbilical adhesions in a high-risk patient. During this test, an echogenic area of bowel or omentum is identified near the umbilicus on ultrasound. The patient then performs exaggerated inhalation and exhalation. Longitudinal movement of this location greater than 1 cm corresponds to a low risk of obliterating subumbilical adhesions.
- A urine pregnancy test is recommended for premenopausal patients who have a uterus and have not undergone a sterilization procedure.
  - A positive pregnancy test does not contraindicate surgery, but intrauterine procedures should not be performed.

PREOPERATIVE PLANNING

- Obtain a surgical history. History of a prior laparotomy or multiple surgeries is a significant risk factor for laparoscopic complications.
- Obtain a medical history, especially note cardiovascular and pulmonary diseases.
  - Trendelenburg position may be limited in a patient with poor cardiopulmonary function or extreme obesity. It is important to preoperatively counsel these patients about these inherent limitations and the possibility of conversion to laparotomy.

SURGICAL MANAGEMENT

Positioning

- Proper patient positioning is essential to ensure patient safety.
- Position the patient in low lithotomy position using adjustable stirrups. These stirrups allow for quick and easy position changes and should neutralize pressure points from the patient's own leg weight.
- See Figure 5.2.
- Ideal low lithotomy position:
  - The hips are flexed with minimal internal or external rotation. Hip flexion should not be less than 60 degrees and preferably set at 80 to 90 degrees in high lithotomy to avoid compression of the femoral nerve. The hips should also not be extended beyond 170 degrees in low lithotomy as this places strain on the lumbar spine.
  - Similarly, avoid excessive abduction of the legs. The angle between thighs should be limited to 90 degrees.

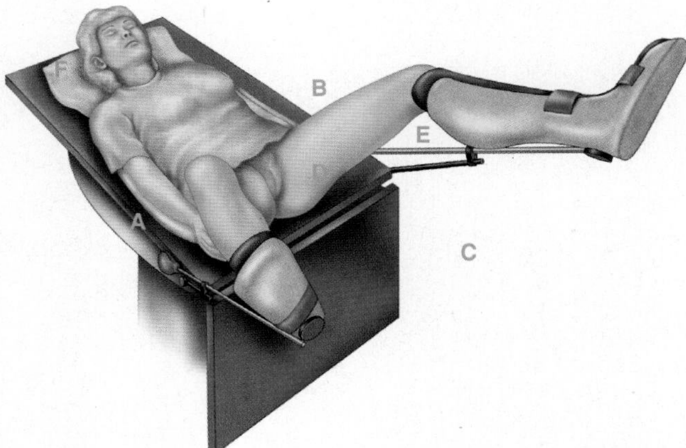

Figure 5.2. Proper positioning in dorsal lithotomy using padded stirrups. A. The patient's elbow is tucked at her side with her hand in neutral position. Additional foam padding is placed on the most lateral aspects of the elbows and hand prior to securing or "tucking" the arm. B. Hip flexion: This angle can vary widely for laparoscopic and vaginal surgeries. However, at its maximum limits should range from 60 to 170 degrees with flexion preferably at 80–90s degrees in high lithotomy. C. Hip abduction: The angle between the thighs should be less than 90 degrees. D. Hip rotation: Maintain minimal rotation. E. Knee flexion: Thigh-to-calf angle should range between 90 and 120 degrees. Additional foam padding is placed on the lateral aspect of each knee to protect the peroneal nerve. F. Note an egg crate or additional gel table padding is placed to reduce patient slippage.

  - Knees should be flexed and padded with foam to avoid lateral compression which can result in a peroneal nerve injury. Knee flexion should be 90 to 120 degrees. Increased knee flexion can put strain on the femoral nerve and promote venous stasis in the lower leg.
  - Use an egg crate or gel cover on the top of the surgical table and in direct contact to the patient's back to prevent the patient from slipping while in the Trendelenburg position. Avoid using shoulder supports to stabilize the patient as these supports can cause brachial plexus injury. A padded chest strap or large Velcro strap can be placed across the patient's chest and secured to the surgical bedframe to prevent slippage in the obese, but should also allow for maximum ventilation.
- Tuck the arms to the patient's side using disposable positioning systems, sheets, foam, or a combination of the above. Place the wrist in a neutral position with the thumb anterior. Place padding under the wrist and elbow to avoid ulnar nerve compression. Take great care not to compress peripheral intravenous access and to cushion the patient's fingers from the table joint. In obese patients, use low-profile surgical sleds or bed extensions to provide extra support and space to accommodate increased patient habitus.
  - This position allows the surgeon closer proximity to the patient and protects the patient's hands, wrists, and joints.
- Ensure the bed is level and the patient is lying flat.
  - Avoid Trendelenburg position initially as this position shifts the aortic bifurcation closer to the umbilicus and increases the risk of aortic injury.
- Confirm a nasogastric tube and Foley catheter are inserted as distention of these organs increases the risk of injury during surgical entry.
- Place a uterine manipulator to facilitate uterine mobility.
  - Complex manipulators have been designed to aid in more complicated operative procedures. In the case of a diagnostic procedure, consider a reusable low-cost option such as a cervical dilator secured to a tenaculum or a Hulka tenaculum.

Approach

- Entry into the peritoneal cavity and establishment of pneumoperitoneum is the essential first step to all laparoscopies. It also carries the highest risk.
- The primary entry site is typically at the umbilicus or Palmer's point.
  - Palmer's point is located 3 cm below the costal margin in the midclavicular line. This site has significantly less adipose tissue compared to the periumbilical area and typically has a smaller skin to peritoneum distance. It may be preferable in obese patients.
    - Palmer's point can be utilized when there is concern for adhesions from prior laparotomy (including cesarean section), large fibroid uterus, pelvic mass, or prior umbilical hernia repair with mesh.
    - The stomach and liver are the closest structures and are at increased risk of injury.
    - Relative contraindications to Palmer's point include splenomegaly, hepatomegaly, and a known left upper quadrant mass. Adhesions from prior upper abdominal surgery should also be considered.

- A supraumbilical site can also be used for the same preoperative risks. This site is located 3 to 5 cm above the umbilicus in the midline.
- Adhesions in the infraumbilical area can be as high as 50% after prior low transverse laparotomy and up to 90% after prior midline laparotomy.

- Entry techniques in laparoscopy are typically classified as closed or open entry. Open entry refers to a mini-laparotomy or Hasson approach. Closed entry is the blind insertion of an instrument into the peritoneal cavity. The most common methods of both types of techniques will be described below.
  - Multiple studies have affirmed that over 50% of major complications, specifically bowel and vascular injury, occur at initial entry.
  - No method has been proven to be superior at preventing injuries. We recommend perfecting one technique to acquire mastery and proficiency, then gradually adding other techniques to your surgical repertoire.
  - Consistency, experience, and good technique lead to safe entry, no matter the approach.

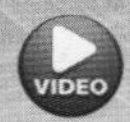

Procedures and Techniques (Video 5.1)

Veress needle

The Veress needle is a thin long needle with a spring-loaded blunt tip that is used for closed entry. Once this needle is passed into the peritoneal cavity, it is then used to insufflate the abdomen prior to trocar insertion.

- To insert the Veress needle, grasp and elevate the abdominal wall. A small skin incision may be made.
- With the valve open and the needle at a 45-degree angle, apply gentle inward pressure to pass the needle through the abdominal wall.
- A double-click sensation will be felt as the blunt tip passes through the rectus fascia and then the peritoneum.
- Confirm entry into the peritoneal cavity prior to initiating insufflation.
  - Aspiration test—Attach a 5-mL syringe with normal saline to the Veress needle. Aspirate to ensure no blood or fecal matter returns.
  - Hanging drop test—Remove the syringe leaving a drop of saline at the Veress hub. With the Veress needle valve open, the saline should freely flow into the needle confirming its placement in the low-pressure peritoneal cavity.
  - Initial opening pressures should measure ≤9 mm Hg (up to 10 mm Hg in obese patients).
  - A prospective study of 348 cases evaluated the first four mentioned methods and found a low sensitivity and low positive predictive value for all tests, but they noted initial pressures were the best at evaluating for extraperitoneal location. The aspiration test, while not sensitive, still has merit as any finding of fecal matter or blood allows for rapid recognition of an injury.
- Following Veress placement into the peritoneal cavity, the abdominal cavity is then insufflated to 15 to 20 mm Hg. Following insufflation, the initial trocar is placed.

Primary direct trocar placement

- Similar to the Veress needle for closed entry, a trocar can be directly inserted into the abdominal cavity without establishing pneumoperitoneum.
- Make a small incision at the entry site. Grasp and elevate the abdominal wall and insert the trocar at 45 degrees.
- If a noncutting trocar is used, advance the trocar by applying a twisting motion with simultaneous inward pressure. There will be two distinct losses of resistance that correlate to traversing the fascia and the peritoneal layers.
- Remove the obturator and insert the laparoscope to visually confirm peritoneal entry.
- Multiple studies have shown equivalent or lower rates of injury and complications for direct trocar compared to Veress needle entry making it a safe alternative.
- An **optical trocar** may also be used for direct entry.
  - The optical trocar tip is made of clear, hydrophobic plastic and allows for visualization of each abdominal layer as opposed to tactile confirmation.
  - The rates of blind versus optical entry injury are equivalent.
  - However, the optical method allows for faster recognition of penetrating injuries.

Angle of insertion for closed entry

- The instrument must be inserted at a trajectory that guides it into a safe anatomical location to avoid puncture injury but also is short enough that the instrument penetrates the peritoneum.
- A 45-degree angle of insertion at the umbilicus aims the trocar toward the hollow of the lumbar and sacral spine. This area carries minimal risk of major vessel injury. At this angle, failed peritoneal entry is also uncommon in nonobese patients.
- However, obesity increases the distance for peritoneal entry, therefore, making preperitoneal insufflation a more common complication. Hurd et al. preformed an anatomic analysis using CT and MRI scans of the abdomen. He measured from the umbilicus to anterior peritoneum and great vessels. Based on his findings, he proposed 90-degree angle of instrument insertion in obese patients. In their analysis, they found that due to a significant increase in the abdominal wall width, the retroperitoneal vessels were at a safe distance from the trocar insertion at 90 degrees, but this angle avoided preperitoneal placement of the entry instrument.
- This has been the traditional teaching for many years; however, it was recently challenged by Stanhiser et al. Preforming similar measurements using CT scans, they purposed that using standard trocars (10 cm) and standard Veress needle (12 cm), a 45-degree angle could be used up to a BMI of 65. This angle in the very obese would allow for increased safety from vascular puncture in a patient population where emergent laparotomy carries increased difficulty and risk.

Open entry (Hasson technique)

- Make a vertical or horizontal small incision at the umbilicus to accommodate the diameter of a trocar.
- Grasp the base of the umbilical fascia stalk with a Kocher clamp.
  - Bluntly dissect the subcutaneous fat from the fascia. Then regrasp the more caudal fascia with a second Kocher clamp.
  - Elevate the clamps, pulling the abdominal wall away from the intra-abdominal contents.
- Make a 10- to 12-mm horizontal fascial incision with a scalpel.
- Place two separate absorbable sutures though the cephalad and caudad aspects of the fascial incision, respectively.
- Using S-retractors, bluntly retract the preperitoneal adipose tissue to visualize the peritoneal tissue. Enter the peritoneum either bluntly or sharply with hemostats and Metzenbaum scissors.
- Once entry into the peritoneal cavity is confirmed visually, assess for signs of accidental injury and digitally palpate the surroundings for adhesions.
- Finally, place the Hasson trocar with a blunt obturator and secure it to the fascia using the two fascial sutures.

Placement of secondary trocars

- See Tech Figure 5.1.
- The number and placement of additional trocars are determined by the needs of the procedure. For diagnostic procedures, a single secondary trocar may be sufficient to manipulate the viscera and adequately visualize all structures.
- Use a scalpel to make a small stab skin incision large enough to accommodate the trocar diameter. Holding the trocar in the surgeon's dominant hand, engage the fascia at a 90-degree angle to allow for maximum mobility of the port site.
  - Advance the trocar into the peritoneal cavity with a gentle downward twisting motion, while keeping the tip always in view and in control to prevent accidental puncture. After the fascia is punctured, aim the trocar toward the pelvis while completing insertion.
  - The ASIS is an often used reference point. Placing accessory trocars approximately 3 cm superior and medial to this anatomical point on the insufflated abdomen decreases injury to ilioinguinal and iliohypogastric nerves and the inferior epigastric vessels.

- Two cadaver studies by Whiteside and Rahn mapped the course of these nerves before and after insufflation. Both studies recommend accessory trocar placement 6 cm above the pubic symphysis or above the ASIS.

- The superficial epigastric vessels can be transilluminated and avoided, although obesity may limit visualization of these structures.
- Visualize the inferior epigastric vessels laparoscopically by identifying the lateral umbilical folds. If the vessels are obscured by adipose tissue, identify the vessels medial to their insertion of the round ligament and trace their cephalad path.
- Ports should be placed so that all instruments have at least a 60-degree angle of intersection in the pelvis.
    - Port sites should be placed at least 5 cm apart. A fist width can be used to estimate the needed distance between trocars. Instruments can be placed on the abdominal wall at the proposed trocar sites and aimed at the pelvic target to aid in optimal site selection to prevent collision of instruments in the operative field.

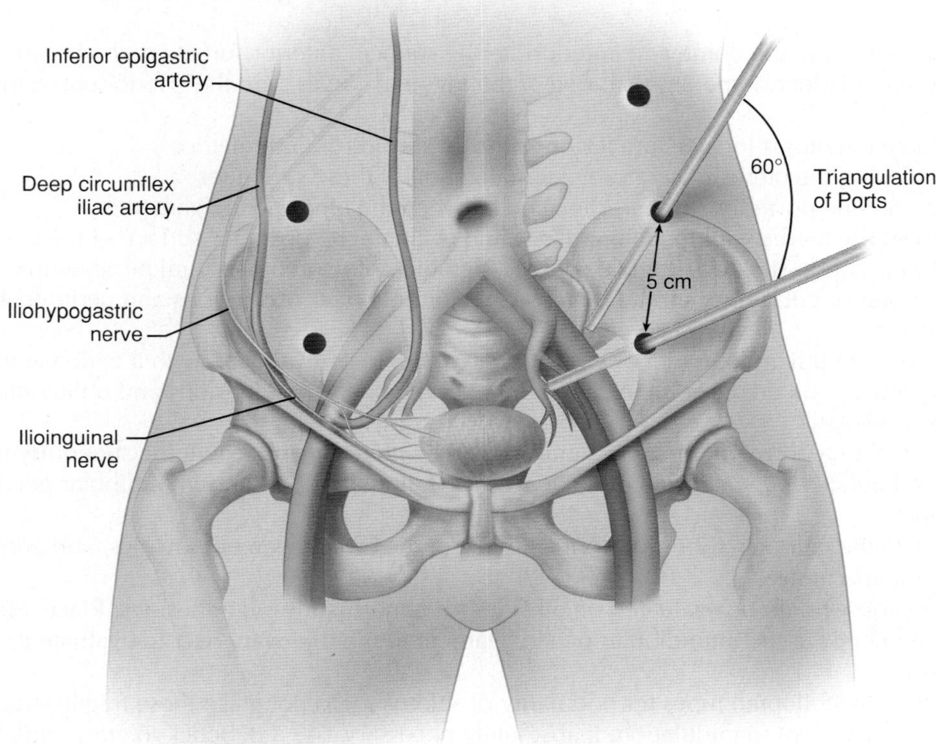

Tech Figure 5.1. Accessory port placement. **Left side:** Anatomy of the pelvic vessels, ilioinguinal nerve, and iliohypogastric nerve in relation to port placement. **Right side:** Ports must be place at least 5 cm apart on the abdominal wall to allow mobility of each instrument in the pelvis.

Pelvic survey

- Inspect the pelvis in a systematic manner. Begin with the area of primary entry and the area just posterior to the abdominal wall entry, regardless of the entry method. Assess for any evidence of injury.
- Evaluate the upper abdomen: the liver, gallbladder, diaphragm, stomach, and bowel. Take particular note of perihepatic adhesions, masses, or enlarged structures.
- Place the patient in Trendelenburg position to maximize exposure of the pelvis.
- Globally survey the pelvis to assess for abnormalities or adhesions.
  - If adhesions are present, address only those that require adhesiolysis in order to complete the pelvic survey.
- The systematic survey of all pelvic structures includes pelvic and abdominal walls. The pelvis is divided into zones based on anatomical boundaries to prevent exclusion of important structures.
  - See Tech Figures 5.2 and 5.3.
  - Using the same systematic approach, the findings for each area should be described in the operative report.
- Zone 1: anterior abdominal and pelvic structures with round ligaments limiting the lateral borders.
  - Evaluate the uterine dome and anterior uterine surface, anterior surface of the broad ligament, bladder dome, internal ring of the inguinal canals, and the inferior epigastric vessels.
  - Evaluate the uterus for size and lesions such as fibroids or endometriosis.
  - Retroflexing the uterus may improve visualization of these structures.
- Zone 2: midline posterior structures located between the uterosacral ligaments.
  - Antevert the uterus with the manipulator and evaluate the posterior surface of the uterus, posterior cul-de-sac, rectovaginal septum, sigmoid colon, and presacral peritoneum.
  - The posterior cul-de-sac should be inspected for endometriosis lesions and peritoneal windows.
  - The entire depth and breadth of the cul-de-sac should be evaluated with a wide view and also with a zoomed, close-up examination of the tissues, for adhesions and obliterating endometriosis.
- Zone 3: the area between the uterosacral ligaments inferiorly and extending superiorly to the lateral pelvic side walls including the ovaries, fallopian tubes, and infundibular pelvic ligaments.
  - Evaluate the fallopian tubes, posterior surface of the broad ligament, ovaries, and adnexal vessels, and ureters.
  - The ovaries should be evaluated on all sides for abnormalities or adhesions. Place a blunt probe inferior to the infundibular pelvic ligament to flip the ovary over to evaluate its inferior aspect.
  - Evaluate the fallopian tubes for nodularity or sclerosis. Do not grasp these fragile structures. Instead, use blunt manipulation. If absolutely necessary, use a Babcock to grasp only the mesosalpinx and limit traumatic manipulation.
- Zone 4: pelvic side walls superior to the adnexa.
  - The appendix should be identified and inspected, especially if the patient suffers from undiagnosed pelvic pain.
  - The survey should be completed before an operative procedure is initiated since manipulation of the tissues can cause bleeding and obscure initial findings.

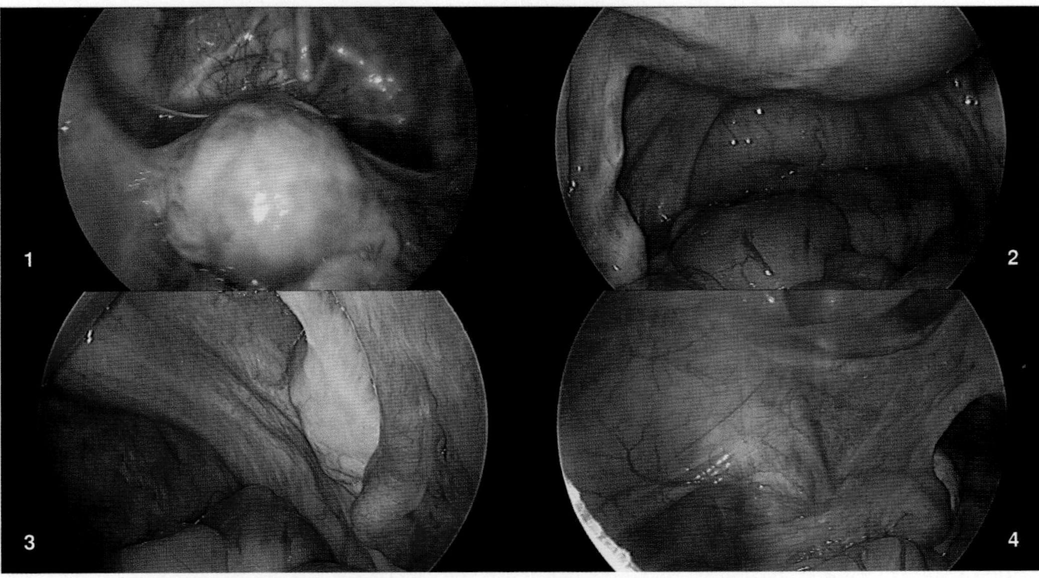

Tech Figure 5.2. Zones of the pelvis.

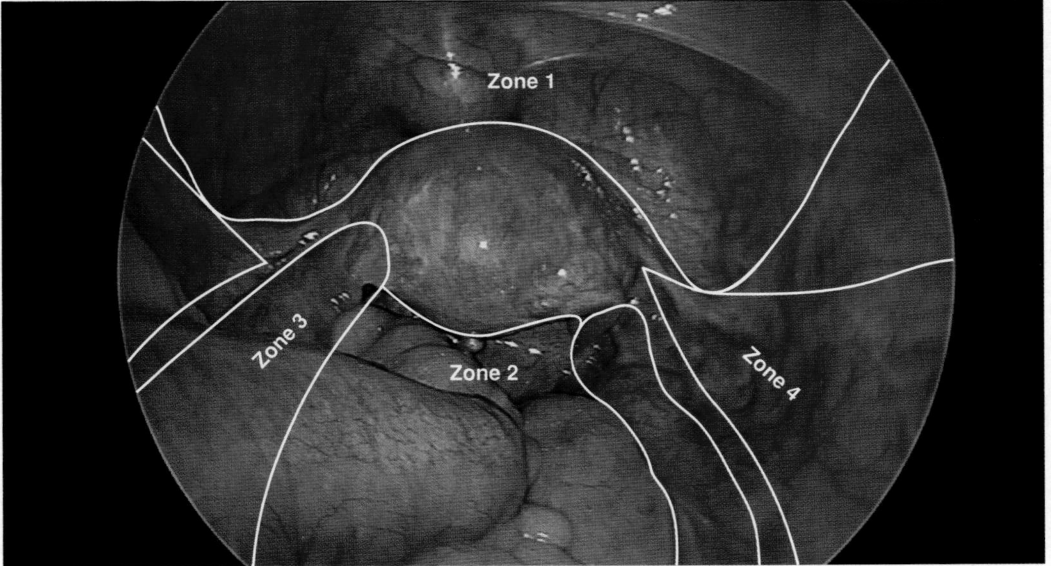

Tech Figure 5.3. Zones of the pelvis.

Port removal and closure

- Ports larger than 8 mm require fascial closure with either a suture closure device, such as a Carter Thomason device, or with direct closure using S retractors, Kocher clamps, and a delayed, absorbable suture. Always begin with the larger port sites and remember to switch the insufflation tubing to the smaller caliber ports to maintain pneumoperitoneum.
- Following completion of the laparoscopy, remove the ports under direct visualization to ensure no structures are inadvertently incorporated.
- To optimally evacuate the pneumoperitoneum, turn off the insufflation, and either suction the remaining intraperitoneal gas while the suction device is placed over a safe viscous or ask the anesthesiologist to have the patient take several deep breaths while the abdominal wall is compressed. Place the laparoscope in the final remaining port site and withdraw both the scope and port simultaneously, ensuring no bowel is entrapped within the abdominal wall.
- Reapproximate the skin with a small caliber, absorbable suture, or dermal glue.

PEARLS AND PITFALLS

- ○ Place an intrabladder Foley catheter to gravity drainage and a nasogastric tube to suction before every procedure. Decrease the potential for puncture injuries by ensuring viscous structures are decompressed prior to surgical entry.
- ✖ Proper patient positioning to avoid neuropathic and crush injuries and awareness of light cord contacts that can cause burn injuries and fire are integral aspects of laparoscopic surgery.
- ○ Palmer's point is an excellent alternative primary entry site. Consider this when there is a failed entry at umbilicus, in obese patients, or when there are suspected dense periumbilical adhesions.
- ✖ Do not initially position the patient in Trendelenburg position since it increases the risk of vascular injury upon initial entry.
- ○ Laparoscopic direct entry with optical trocar is the fastest method of entry and does not increase puncture risks.
- ○ Improves identification of abdominal wall layers particularly with thickened adipose layers.
- ○ Puncture injuries are typically recognized faster during this procedure; however, it does not improve incidence of missed injuries.
- ✖ When a difficult entry is encountered, immediately turn the insufflation valve to the "off" position or disconnect the gas from the needle or trocar. Accidental insufflation of a preperitoneal space will obscure normal anatomic planes and increase the morbidity of the procedure.
- ○ Factors that increase complications: number of attempts for surgical entry
- ○ Case complexity
- ○ Prior abdominal surgery: specifically, history of prior laparotomy
- ✖ Various entry techniques each have their own advantages but complete mastery of one technique is the safest and most important skill set to achieve instead of a diverse repertoire.

POSTOPERATIVE CARE

- Uncomplicated diagnostic surgery is safely performed as an outpatient procedure.
- Right upper quadrant pain from residual pneumoperitoneum is common for a few days and up to a week after surgery. Prescribe nonsteroidal anti-inflammatory and narcotic medications for incisional analgesia. Depending on the size of port sites, activity is not significantly limited following surgery and patients are instructed to resume their normal activities as tolerated.

If the patient is not improving on a daily basis, she should be evaluated in person.

COMPLICATIONS

- The majority of diagnostic laparoscopy complications occur during initial entry.
  - Entry complications comprise 50% of all laparoscopy complications but their incidence of 0.3% to 1% still makes these complications rare.
  - Injuries are mostly vascular and bowel punctures, but also include gas embolism, bladder injury, extraperitoneal insufflation, and failed entry.
- An open technique avoids the element of blind insertion and therefore was once thought to be the ideal method to prevent accidental puncture injuries. This has not been supported by literature. Many studies have shown a lower rate of vascular injuries, and gas embolism becomes nearly absent with open technique. Bowel injuries are equivalent or increased with an open technique. The increased incidence could be due to selection bias as surveys have shown surgeons favor an open technique for patients with a history of prior surgery when there are anticipated adhesions.
  - A Cochrane review concluded that there is no evidence that supports the superiority of any method as the safest form of entry.
  - Experience decreases the rate of complications; therefore, the current recommendation is to use the techniques that are most experienced and comfortable in performing.
- Vascular punctures to major vessels carry the highest mortality risk.
  - 75% of punctures are arterial and, of them, 25% were aortic and 20% were common right iliac artery injuries.
  - The instrument angle must be maintained in the midline during entry as a slight deviation can result in peritoneal entry many centimeters laterally and risks injury to the iliac vessels.
- Bowel injuries are more common than vascular injuries, and occur in approximately 0.4% of laparoscopic surgery.
  - Regardless of entry technique, studies estimate 30% to 50% of bowel injuries go unrecognized during the procedure. The resulting peritonitis and sepsis from delayed recognition has a mortality rate of 2.5% to 5%.
  - Optical trocars have not mitigated this risk and have a similar rate of missed bowel injury diagnosis.
- Obese patients are at an increased risk for failed entry.
  - An open technique can be more challenging due to an increased thickness of the abdominal wall, preperitoneal adipose tissue, and peritoneal layer.
  - A direct optical trocar entry can be helpful as well as a left upper quadrant entry.
  - Obese patient may also be limited in their Trendelenburg positioning due to ventilation challenges.

- Risk factors that are associated with an increased complication rate:
  - The number of attempts needed to successfully complete the primary entry is associated with an increase in accidental puncture.
  - Case complexity was a significant risk factor for major complications, minor complications, as well as conversion to laparotomy.
  - Prior abdominal surgery was the only other factor that increased the rate of major complications (defined as visceral punctures, serious bleeding, death).
  - Obesity does not always prove to be a risk factor in studies; however, increased rates of failed entry would suggest otherwise.

KEY READINGS

Ahmad G, O'Flynn H, Duffy JM, Phillips K, Watson A. Laparoscopic entry techniques. *Cochrane Database Syst Rev.* 2012;2:CD006583.

Bedaiwy MA, Pope R, Henry D, et al. Standardization of laparoscopic pelvic examination: a prosal of a novel system. *Minim Invasive Surg.* 2013;2013:153–235.

la Chapelle CF, Bemelman WA, Rademaker BM, van Barneveld TA, Jansen FW; on behalf of the Dutch Multidisciplinary Guideline Development Group Minimally Invasive Surgery. A multidisciplinary evidence-based guideline for minimally invasive surgery. Part 1: entry techniques and the pneumoperitoneum. *Gynecol Surg.* 2012;9:271–282.

Fuentes MN, Rodríguez-Oliver A, Naveiro Rilo JC, Paredes AG, Aguilar Romero MT, Parra JF. Complications of laparoscopic gynecologic surgery. *JSLS.* 2014;18(3):e2014.00058.

Hurd WH, Bude RO, DeLancey JO, Gauvin JM, Aisen AM. Abdominal wall characterization with magnetic resonance imaging and computed tomography. The effect of obesity on the laparoscopic approach. *J Reprod Med.* 1991;36(7):473–376.

Pickett SD, Rodewald KJ, Billow MR, Giannios NM, Hurd WW. Avoiding major vessel injury during laparoscopic instrument insertion. *Obstet Gynecol Clin N Am.* 2010;37:387–397.

Rahn DD, Phelan JN, Roshanravan SM, White AB, Corton MM. Anterior abdominal wall nerve and vessel anatomy: clinical implications for gynecologic surgery. *Am J Obstet Gynecol.* 2010;202:234.e1–e5.

Stanhiser J, Goodman L, Soto E, et al. Supraumbilical primary trocar insertion for laparoscopic access: the relationship between points of entry and retroperitoneal vital vasculature by imaging. *Am J Obstet Gynecol.* 2015;213:506.e1–e5.

Teoh B, Sen R, Abbott J. An evaluation of four tests used to ascertain veres needle placement at closed laparoscopy. *J Minim Invasive Gynecol.* 2005;12:153–158.

Tulikangas PK, Nicklas A, Falcone T, Price LL. Anatomy of the left upper quadrant for cannula insertion. *J Am Assoc Gynecol Laparosc.* 2000;7(2): 211–214.

Vilos GA, Ternamian A, Dempster J, Laberge PY. The Society of Obstetricians and Gynaecologists of Canada. Laparoscopic entry: a review of technique, technologies, and complications. *J Obstet Gynaecol Can.* 2007;29:433–465.

Whiteside JL, Barber MD, Walters MD, Falcone T. Anatomy of ilioinguinal and iliohypogastric nerves in relations to trocar placement and low transverse incision. *Am J Obstet Gynecol.* 2003;189:1574–1578; discussion 1578.

Section III

Uterine Surgery

Dilatation and Curettage of the Nonpregnant Uterus

6

Rhoda Y. Goldschmidt

GENERAL PRINCIPLES

Definition

- Dilatation and curettage, commonly called D&C, is the sampling of the uterine endometrial lining and contents of the uterine cavity. Dilatation, or dilation, refers to the opening of the cervical canal which is the portal into the uterine cavity. Curettage is the scraping of the endometrial lining of the uterine cavity.

Differential Diagnosis

- Abnormal uterine bleeding, perimenopausal bleeding, postmenopausal bleeding, fibroids, endocervical or endometrial polyps, cervical cancer, endometrial hyperplasia, uterine cancer, pyometra, hematometra, retained products of conception.

Anatomic Considerations

- In cases of Mullerian defects, such as uterus didelphys, bicornuate uterus, or septate uterus, D&C should be performed under ultrasound guidance.

Nonoperative Management

- IPAS is a double-valve manual vacuum aspiration syringe that can be used in the office, obviating the operating room.[1] The World Health Organization has approved its use for endometrial sampling in the setting of abnormal uterine bleeding.

IMAGING AND OTHER DIAGNOSTICS

- Pelvic ultrasound and/or saline-infused sonogram characterize the uterine contour, endometrium, intracavitary polyps and fibroid, as well as intramural, subserosal, and submucosal fibroids. Furthermore, the classic heterogeneous pattern of adenomyosis may be recognized.
- In rare cases, MRI may be used to detect the presence of Müllerian defects such as unicornuate uterus, uterus didelphys, bicornuate uterus, or septate uterus.

PREOPERATIVE PLANNING

- A complete history and physical examination is necessary to rule out pregnancy, to determine the ease or difficulty of uterine access, to illicit any medical comorbidities that will affect anesthesia, and to determine coagulation risks.
- Cervical stenosis prevents the passage of a 2.5-mm Pratt dilator. Stenosis can be anticipated if there is a history of prior cervical or uterine procedures such as a LEEP or cone biopsy, routine biopsies, cryotherapy, laser surgery, or endometrial ablation. It can result from lack of vaginal deliveries, infection, or estrogen deficiency.
- Treat cervical stenosis with preoperative Misoprostol 400 mcg, oral or sublingual, 12 hours prior to D&C. Various regimens have been recommended and may facilitate cervical access.[2,3] Alternatively, laminaria are osmotic dilators that can soften and dilate the cervix in order to prevent uterine perforation during the dilatation process. They are placed in the office at least 12 to 24 hours before the D&C is performed and removed intraoperatively.

SURGICAL MANAGEMENT

Positioning

- The patient is placed in the lithotomy position with her legs in candy cane or Allen stirrups. Be careful not to hyperflex the hips or hyperextend the knees (Fig. 6.1).

Approach

Perform a pelvic examination, carefully sound the uterus, serially dilate the cervix, and then systematically scrape the

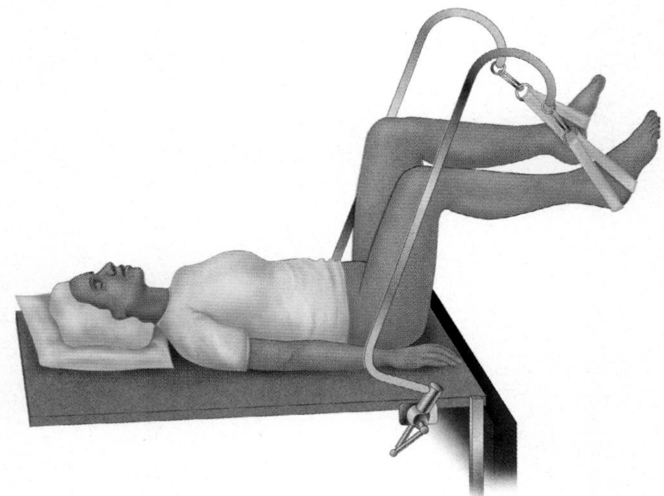

Figure 6.1. Lithotomy position. Hyperflexion of the hip and hyperextension of the knee are avoided to prevent injury of the femoral nerve and lumbosacral trunk.

uterine lining. If there is a high suspicion for the presence of uterine polyps, a polypectomy should be done before the curettage. If endometrial carcinoma is highly suspected, a fractional curettage is performed. Tissue is first obtained from the endocervical canal. Then, the endometrial canal is sampled. This is done in order to avoid contamination of the sites.

Perform pelvic examination prior to the procedure. It is imperative to determine whether the uterus is anteflexed or retroflexed to avoid uterine perforation. The degree of flexion is also important to note. Pratt or Hank dilators have the advantage of having tapered shank which accommodate the flexion of the uterus so that the instrument will not perforate a severely retroflexed or anteflexed uterus.

Procedures and Techniques

Visualize cervix

- After the patient has been prepped and draped in sterile fashion, place a weighted speculum posteriorly under the cervix and use a right-angle or single-bladed retractor to elevate the anterior vaginal wall (**Tech Fig. 6.1**).

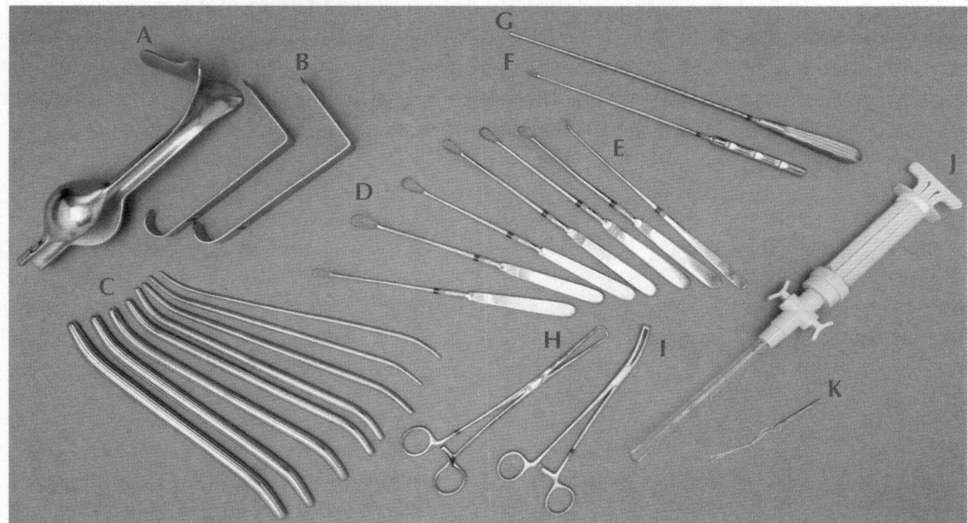

Tech Figure 6.1. Surgical instruments used in D&C: **A:** weighted speculum; **B:** side-wall retractors; **C:** Pratt dilators; **D:** Sharp curettes; **E:** Serrated curette; **F:** Duncan, rectangular curette; **G:** Uterine sound; **H:** Single-tooth tenaculum; **I:** Jacobs double-tooth tenaculum; **J:** IPAS; **K:** Laminaria.

Stabilize the cervix

- Grasp the anterior lip of the cervix with a single-tooth tenaculum.

Sound the uterus

- Gently sound the uterus with a Sims-graduated ball tip uterine sound.

Dilate the cervix

- Serially dilate the cervix using dilators.

Endometrial polypectomy

- In order not to miss an endometrial polyp, make a systematic sweep of the uterine lining with a ureteral stone forceps.

Uterine curettage

- Using a Heaney serrated curette, the uterine cavity is systematically scraped. In an anteflexed uterus, start at the 12-o'-clock position and scrape along the anterior uterine wall from the fundus toward the cervix. This motion is repeated in a clockwise fashion. It is better to start at the fundus and pull toward yourself rather than to scrape back and forth. As the tissue extrudes from the cervix, collect it in a spoon or directly onto a piece of Telfa that has been placed in the posterior fornix **(Tech Fig. 6.2)**.
- If cancer is suspected, perform an endocervical curettage using a Duncan rectangular curette before performing the uterine curettage. The entire length of the cervix, from the internal os to the external os, is scraped. Send the tissue specimens to pathology separately.

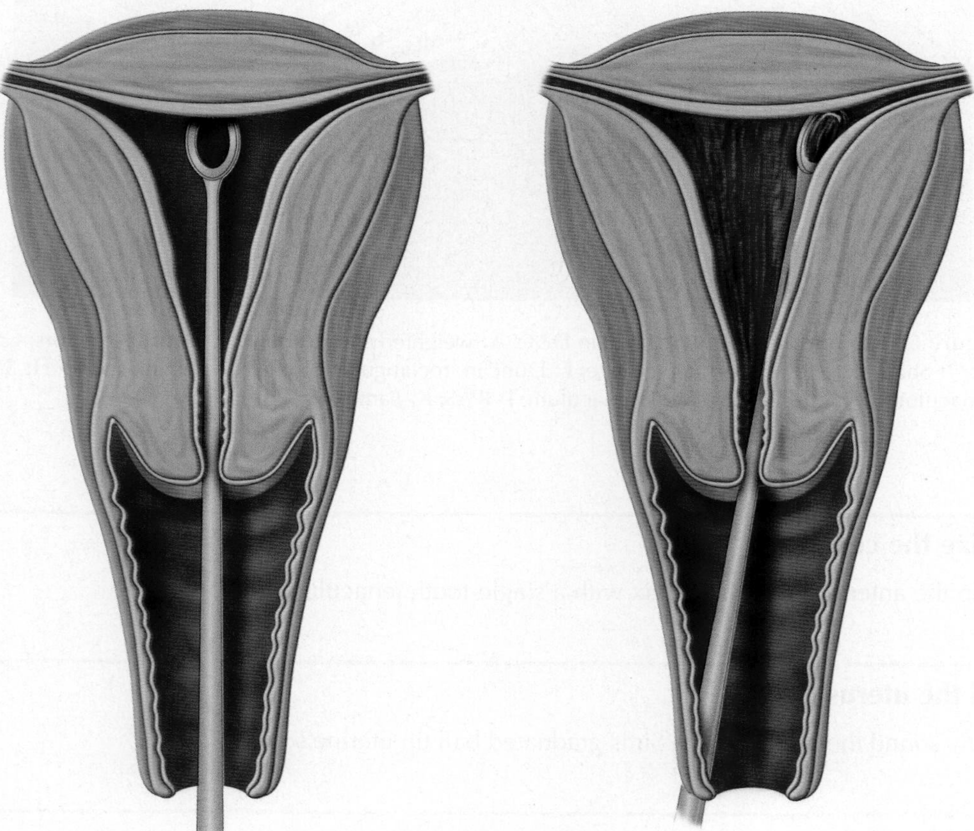

Tech Figure 6.2. Uterine curettage. The curette is gently advanced to the uterine fundus. Circumferentially, starting at 12 o'-clock, the sharp edge is brought forward toward the internal cervical os.

PEARLS AND PITFALLS

- ○ Cervical stenosis: In addition to preprocedure misoprostol treatment and laminaria, intraoperative dilute vasopressin solution may be injected into cervical stroma using 10 cc of solution.[4]
- ✖ Avoid overdilatation: Dilate just enough to accommodate the instruments needed. If hysteroscopy is to be performed, overdilatation will result in poor uterine distension as the hysteroscopic medium leaks out. If this occurs, the cervix may be tightened around the hysteroscope by clamping the cervix with a ring forceps or tenaculum or by placing a suture through the cervical tissue.
- ○ Cervical laceration: A single-tooth tenaculum can lacerate the cervical tissue causing bleeding and will not give you the necessary traction. Use a heavier tenaculum such as a Jacobs double-tooth tenaculum and take care to note the bladder margin at the anterior cervix.
- ✖ Avoid creating a false passage: Start with the largest curette that easily penetrates the cervix. Avoid very small dilators such as lacrimal duct dilators, as these instruments can be pushed through almost any tissue leading you to falsely believe that you have entered the uterine cavity.
- ○ Avoid uterine perforation: When dilating the cervix, do not apply excessive force. Hold dilators with your fingertips and not against the palm of your hand. When sounding the uterus, advance the sound slowly until resistance at the fundus is encountered.
- ✖ Asherman syndrome: Avoid aggressive curettage in a recently pregnant or infected uterus. A Foley balloon can be placed in the uterine cavity to prevent adhesion of the uterine walls. Remove 10 days after the procedure. Doxycycline 100 mg twice daily for 10 days is given concomitantly to prevent infection.

POSTOPERATIVE CARE

- Monitor the patient for bleeding, pain, and anesthesia complication in the PACU. Mild cramping and light spotting are to be expected for a few days. To avoid infection, nothing should be placed inside the vagina until menses resume or cleared by their physician. Patients are also instructed to avoid bathtub soaking, swimming, intercourse, and tampon usage for 14 days.

COMPLICATIONS

- The overall complication rate for D&C is less than 2%. Independent risk factors for D&C complication include retroverted uterus, postmenopausal status, and nulliparity.[5]
- Possible complications include uterine perforation; damage to internal organs such as bowel, bladder, ureters, major blood vessels; endometritis; hemorrhage; vaginal laceration; cervical laceration; pelvic pain; creation of a false passage; and Asherman syndrome. If uterine perforation is suspected, the surgeon must thoroughly evaluate the pelvic cavity to assess for additional injury. If the patient is hemodynamically stable and the surgeon is proficient in laparoscopy, a diagnostic laparoscopy is the preferred approach. The perforation should be examined to assess the entire extent of the injury/laceration, and the pneumoperitoneum should be decreased to 5 mm Hg and observed for several minutes. A hemodynamically stable uterine perforation requires no further surgical intervention. The patient should be informed of the complication and counseled on concerning signs and symptoms that should prompt medical care. If the perforation site is bleeding, the surgeon may utilize combination of suture, coagulation, or fulguration to achieve hemostasis. A thorough pelvic and vasculature survey must include a complete bowel evaluation. If the patient is hemodynamically unstable, surgical discretion is advised. A frank and clear discussion between the surgeon and anesthesiology team should include risks and benefits of exploratory laparotomy versus medical stabilization prior to laparotomy.

KEY REFERENCES

1. Lukman HY, DikranP. Trends in the evaluation of abnormal uterine bleedings with the introduction of manual vacuum aspiration. *East Afr Med J.* 1995;72(9):599–604.
2. Ghosh A, Chaudhuri P. Misoprostol for cervical ripening prior to gynecological transcervical procedures. *Arch Gynecol Obstet.* 2013;287(5): 967–673.
3. Temel M, Goynumer FG, Wetherilt L, Durukan B. Which route of misoprostol application is more advantageous prior to fractional curettage in postmenopausal patients? *Arch Gynecol Obstet.* 2009;279(5):637–642.
4. Christianson MS, Barker MA, Lindheim SR. Overcoming the challenging cervix: techniques to access the uterine cavity. *American Society for Colposcopy and Cervical Pathology*. 2008;12(1):24–31.
5. Hefler L, Lemach A, Seebacher V, Polterauer S, Tempfer C, Reinthaller A. The intraoperative complication rate of nonobstetric dilation and curettage. *Obstet Gynecol.* 2009;113(6):1268–1271.

7 Myomectomy

Chapter 7.1 Abdominal Myomectomy

Linda D. Bradley

GENERAL PRINCIPLES

Definition

- Abdominal myomectomy is performed via a laparotomy incision and is also referred to open myomectomy. It is the surgical removal of uterine leiomyomas which leaves the uterus intact. Reproductive-aged patients continue to have menstrual cycles and are able to theoretically able to conceive following abdominal myomectomy.
- Uterine leiomyomas are also called uterine fibroids, myomas, or fibromyomas. They are benign proliferative, unicellular, well-circumscribed, pseudoencapsulated, benign growths composed of smooth muscle and fibrous connective tissue. They are the most common benign growth of the uterus.
- The pathogenesis of leiomyomas remains unknown. However, several pathogenic theories may be associated with uterine fibroids including genetic predisposition, epigenetic factors, estrogens, progesterone, growth hormone factors, cytokines, chemokines, and extracellular matrix components.

Differential Diagnosis

- Adenomyosis
- Adenomyoma
- Leiomyosarcoma
- Diffuse leiomyomatosis
- Extrauterine pelvic tumors
- Ovarian mass
- Pregnancy

Anatomic Considerations

- Leiomyomas are unique and symptoms vary among women. The prevalence of uterine fibroids may approach 60% to 80%; however, the majority of women are asymptomatic.
- Asymptomatic women should be reassured and followed clinically.
- Thirty percent of women with fibroids may have significant symptoms.
- The size of leiomyoma may range from a few millimeters to more than 20 cm.
- The number of leiomyoma also varies. Most patients have fewer than 10 leiomyomas; however, several case reports of patients with more than 100 leiomyomas removed by abdominal myomectomy have been reported.
- The weight of each leiomyoma varies. The largest removed by case report was 65 kg.
- Uterine fibroids may impact fertility via the following mechanisms:
  - Mechanical blockage of the fallopian tube
  - Abnormal vascularization of the uterus
  - Abnormal endometrial development
  - Chronic intracavitary inflammation
  - Increased uterine contractions
  - Distortion of the endometrial cavity
- The FIGO classification system characterizes the variable anatomic locations of fibroids.
  - These benign growths may be located within various regions within the uterus and cervix including endocervical, intracavitary, submucosal, intramural, transmural, subserosal exophytic, pedunculated serosal, parasitic, and may prolapse through the cervix into the vagina.
  - Intramural fibroids are the most common location of fibroids. They reside in the myometrium. They may be of varying size and number. Proliferation of fibroids is associated with potential distortion of the endometrial cavity or the external serosal surface.
  - Submucous leiomyomas are commonly referred to as intracavitary fibroids. They are variably located within the endometrial cavity.
    - If they grow, they may efface the cervix and be seen in the internal cervical os.
    - Complete protrusion and prolapse through the cervix may occur such that the leiomyoma is seen dilating the ectocervix and be present within the vagina. Vaginal myomectomy is ideal for prolapsing leiomyomas.
  - Intracavitary fibroids may be associated with intense pelvic cramping, leukorrhea, foul-smelling vaginal discharge, or aberrant menstrual bleeding.
    - Intracavitary fibroids can be treated with hysteroscopic resection or hysteroscopic morcellation.
  - Subserous leiomyomas grow on the outer uterine surface leading to an irregular surface contour of the uterus.
    - They may develop a pedicle of varying width.
    - Fibroids attached to a stalk are mobile and may cause torsion with acute abdominal or intermittent abdominal

    - pain. Fever may occur if complete torsion and necrosis of the fibroid occur.
    - Most are asymptomatic and do not cause adverse pregnancy outcomes.
  - Exophytic fibroids may also attach to other peritoneal organs and develop a collateral blood flow. They are called parasitic fibroids.
    - The more common attachments of parasitic fibroids include bowel, omentum, and mesentery. Because these lesions are mobile, they may also be confused with an adnexal mass or abdominal mass of unknown etiology.
    - If they involve the broad ligament they are called intraligamentary leiomyomas. This anatomic variant is associated with deviation of the ureter. Much care must be taken when performing abdominal myomectomy with intraligamentary leiomyomas to prevent transection of the ureter.
- The size, number, and location of fibroids are unique to each patient and may be associated with a variety of clinical presentations including menstrual dysfunction, bulk symptoms, pelvic pain, increased abdominal girth, infertility, or pregnancy-related complications.
- Menstrual complaints may include heavy menstrual cycles, anemia and pica as a result of heavy menses, irregular bleeding, postcoital bleeding, dysmenorrhea, leukorrhea, and passage of large clots, chronic or acute anemia.
- Bulk symptoms may include increased abdominal girth, back pain, early satiety and cosmetic complaints from abdominal distention, constipation, urinary frequency, urinary urgency, urinary retention, unilateral or bilateral ureteral obstruction, and varying degrees of hydronephrosis.
- Pain including dysmenorrhea and dyspareunia.
- Enlarging uterus may also lead to an inability to visualize the cervix, making pap test, saline infusion sonography, and endometrial biopsy difficult.
- Reproductive-associated symptoms include infertility, recurrent miscarriage, premature delivery, preterm delivery, and abdominal pain during pregnancy due to leiomyoma degeneration.
- Degenerative changes may be seen within the fibroid including:
  - Hyaline degeneration—this represents the most common type of degeneration and is caused by excessive overgrowth of fibrous elements.
  - Cystic degeneration occurs after hyaline degeneration and results in myxomatous changes with the development of multiple cystic cavities within the fibroid.
  - Necrosis occurs with impaired blood flow to the fibroid. This is most often seen in pregnancy. The gross specimen when opened has a dull reddish color and is due to aseptic degeneration associated with local hemolysis.
  - Mucoid degeneration is associated with fibroid that are greater than 8 cm. This occurs more often with impaired arterial inflow to the fibroid.
  - Infectious degeneration is more often associated with pedunculated leiomyomas.
  - Calcific degeneration more commonly seen in postmenopausal women.
  - Sarcomatous degeneration is rare and occurs in up to 1/300 women undergoing surgery.
- Women desirous of pregnancy and who have indications for surgery should have the most minimally invasive uterine-sparing procedure performed by a skilled gynecologist.
- Size, number, and location of uterine leiomyoma determine which surgical procedure may be recommended and surgical skill set required.
  - These factors influence surgical approach, specifically whether a vaginal, hysteroscopic, abdominal, mini-laparotomy, laparoscopic, or robotic myomectomy is advisable.
  - Individual characteristics of uterine fibroids also influence length of surgery, surgical risks, intraoperative and postoperative blood loss, infectious morbidity, complications, and risk of recurrence.
- Surgical intervention may be indicated in patients with:
  - Failed medical therapy for the treatment of symptomatic disease
  - Intracavitary distortion leading to infertility or recurrent miscarriage
  - Unrelenting abdominal pain due to acute leiomyoma torsion, degeneration, or vaginal prolapse
  - Failure of medical therapy for intractable or heavy menstrual dysfunction
  - While uncommon, obstruction of ureters, renal insufficiency, marked hydronephrosis, or acute urinary retention may predispose to intervention
  - Concern for leiomyosarcoma

Nonoperative Management

Hysterectomy has been the traditional therapy offered to women with uterine fibroids, increasingly women are interested in less invasive therapy. Women with minimal fibroid symptomatology are advised to consider "watchful waiting" or monitoring that can include periodic clinical examination, imaging, and journaling of their symptoms. The frequency of office visits and testing should be based on clinical symptoms. Nonoperative management and alternative to hysterectomy procedures such as uterine fibroid embolization (UFE) and endometrial ablation options are only for women who do not desire future fertility but request uterine sparing procedures. Medical therapy including hormonal therapy, levonorgestrel intrauterine device, tranexamic acid, NSAIDs, and GnRH agonist therapy are well suited for women who wish to retain their fertility.

However, quality-of-life (QOL) indicators must be considered in women with uterine fibroids and clinicians inquire about them as they may help to determine whether nonoperative management, watchful waiting, or surgical intervention is needed. The patient should be queried about QOL-related factors including:

- Fears about her health
- Impact on her relationships
- Emotions
- Sexual functioning
- Body image
- Loss of control
- Hopelessness

A recent survey of 968 reproductive-aged women noted:

- Patients waited 3.6 years before seeking treatment
- 41% saw >2 health providers for diagnosis
- 28% missed work due to leiomyoma symptoms
- 24% believed that symptoms prevented career potential
- 79% expressed desire for treatment that does not involve invasive surgery

- 51% desired uterine preservation
- 43% wanted fertility preservation if they are less than 40 years of age

Nonextirpative uterine surgery should be considered for all women who desire pregnancy. Women of the African diaspora have the highest prevalence and burden of fibroid-related disease.

- Additionally, they have the greatest progressive symptomatology, younger age of onset, greater size, and number of fibroids when compared to other ethnic groups.
- The etiology and genetic predisposition for this racial difference are unknown.
- In certain geographic regions in the United States, the incidence of leiomyomas among women of the African diaspora is three to four times that of Caucasian women.

Uterine fibroid embolization (UFE) is a minimally invasive outpatient procedure performed by an interventional radiologist for the treatment of symptomatic uterine fibroids in women who do not desire fertility yet desire uterine preservation. Treatment is performed under conscious sedation and does not require an abdominal incision. Embolization results in ischemic infarction of the leiomyomata and decreased vascularity. Normal myometrium is spared.

Within 4 to 6 months the uterine fibroid diminishes in size, the fibroids undergo hyaline degeneration, and the volume and size of the uterus decrease. Shrinkage may continue up to 1 year after UFE. Among women with >90% fibroid infarction, there is more symptom relief and fewer subsequent treatments than in women with a lower infarction rate.

Magnetic resonance-guided focused ultrasound (MRgFUS) is a noninvasive outpatient treatment option for symptomatic uterine fibroids. It was approved by the FDA in 2004 for the treatment of uterine fibroids. Its labeling includes use for women who desire pregnancy. MRgFUS is an outpatient procedure that takes 2 to 4 hours and is performed under conscious sedation without an abdominal incision.

The objective of MRgFUS is to deliver focused high-energy ultrasound waves into the fibroid causing thermal coagulation of targeted tissue. With the patient lying prone, the ultrasound waves are focused by lenses or reflectors and pass through the skin and nontarget tissue and delivers sonications (heat) to targeted fibroids. It has been compared to the principle of focusing the sun's rays with a magnifying glass to burn a hole in a piece of paper.

Preprocedural magnetic resonance imaging (MRI) is required to determine suitable candidates for MRgFUS. Fibroids most amenable to MRgFUS treatment are those that are homogeneous and hyperintense (dark) on T2-weighted images. They should also enhance because degenerated/infarcted fibroids have lost their blood supply and will not respond to treatment.

Contraindications to MRgFUS include:

- Patients with pacemakers
- Prior UFE
- Sensitivity to MR contrast agents
- Severe claustrophobia
- Patient's body habitus exceeds the limitations of the MRI scanner
- Pedunculated fibroids
- Adenomyosis
- Abdominal scarring with bowel in the pathway of the ultrasound beam
- Intrauterine device (it would have to be removed prior to the procedure)
- Obese patients may have too much subcutaneous fat such that the fibroid would be out of the range of the ultrasound beam.
  - The ultrasound focus depth is limited to 12 cm for the standard protocols or to 7 cm if enhanced sonications are performed.
  - If the fibroid is out of these ranges due to obesity, then MRgFUS will not be successful.
- When compared to UFE there were more women excluded from MRgFUS. In fact, in one enrollment study, only 14% of women qualified for participation into. Limitations of the procedure include patients with multiple abdominal scars. Numerous scars may make it difficult to determine a safe pathway for treatment in order to avoid bowel, bladder, or pelvic adhesions. Dominant fibroids greater than 8 to 10 cm may take too long to sonicate in one setting.

Risks are very low but reports of skin burns to the abdomen, damage to structures near the fibroid, nerve stimulation causing temporary back or leg pain, and DVT.

Reported outcomes of MRgFUS include:

- Pelvic pain and pressure resolve most quickly
- Decrease pressure on the bladder
- Improvements in menstrual bleeding may take 4 to 6 months
- QOL indicators improved (heavy menstrual bleeding, nonbleeding symptoms of fibroids and QOL impact)
- Patients with fibroids that have the lowest signal intensity have better symptom relief and demonstrated a higher technical success.

Tranexamic acid is an oral, nonhormonal, antifibrinolytic medical therapy used only during menstruation in women with symptomatic fibroids–related ovulatory heavy menstrual bleeding. Women with heavy menstrual periods reportedly have high fibrinolytic activity due to increased endometrial levels of plasmin and plasminogen activators. Tranexamic acid works by reversibly blocking lysine binding sites on plasminogen, thus preventing plasmin from interacting with lysine residues on the fibrin polymer, causing subsequent fibrin degradation.

Tranexamic acid has been available for more than 40 years in clinical practice and often is prescribed as an over-the-counter therapy in many countries. In the United States, it requires a prescription. The recommended dose is: tranexamic acid 650 mg, take two tablets by mouth every 8 hours, to commence with the onset of menstrual bleeding for a maximum of 5 days. Its onset of action is rapid but requires every 8 hours dosing due to short half-life. Eliminated through the kidneys, it has a half-life of 2 to 3 hours.

Tranexamic acid reduces menstrual blood loss (MBL) by 26% to 60%. Numerous studies demonstrate that it is an effective treatment of heavy ovulatory menstrual bleeding in women with uterine fibroids; has low side-effect profile, favorable safety profile, and is well tolerated by patients.

Thromboembolic events have not been reported with oral treatment regimens for the treatment of heavy menstrual bleeding. When compared to placebo, NSAIDs, or oral cyclical luteal phase progesterone, tranexamic acid significantly improved QOL. Levonorgestrel-releasing intrauterine system reduced mean blood loss more than tranexamic acid in clinical trials. Tranexamic acid should not be prescribed to women with prior history of embolic disease, active thromboembolism, intrinsic risk for thrombosis, or currently using hormonal therapy.

Gonadotropin-releasing (GnRH) analogs (Lupron [TAP Pharmaceutical Products, Inc. Lake Forest, IL] may be considered for short-term use in women with symptomatic uterine fibroids and as adjunct to surgical therapy. GnRH agonists decrease uterine size and myoma volume by decreasing levels of estrogen and progesterone to menopausal values. They induce myoma degeneration, cause hyaline degeneration, decrease in the size of leiomyoma cells, reduce extracellular matrix, and decrease blood flow to the uterus. When used for short duration (<6 months), most women become temporally amenorrheic, have improvement in hemoglobin, and notice a decrease in uterine size by 40% to 60%.

GnRH analogs are often beneficial to women 50 years old or older. GnRH therapy given for 6 months will stop menstruation with improvement in bulk symptoms and cessation of menstruation. After 6 months of therapy, GnRH is stopped and the patient monitored for transition into natural menopause. If symptoms recur and patient has not entered menopause, then another 6 months of GnRH therapy instituted. Quite often these patients will enter natural menopause and not require surgical intervention and avoid surgery if menopause occurs shortly after completion of therapy.

Ulipristal is not currently available in this country; however, clinical trials are underway. Promising research in Europe has demonstrated the benefits of Ulipristal. Ulipristal is a synthetic steroid derived from 19-norprogesterone. It is a selective progesterone receptor modulator that binds to progesterone receptors. It exerts antiproliferative, pro-apoptotic, and antifibrotic action on leiomyoma cells. The binding and antagonist potency with glucocorticoid receptors is reduced compared to mifepristone.

- Recent randomized controlled trials comparing Ulipristal to placebo and Lupron have shown a statistically significant improvement in leiomyoma size, QOL indicators, and decrease in fibroid and uterine volume.
  - After 13 weeks, Ulipristal controlled uterine bleeding in 91% of 96 women who received Ulipristal 5 mg/d and uterine volume decreased 21%.
  - Compared to 92% of 98 women who took 10 mg/d and uterine volume decreased 12%.
  - Compared to 19% of 48 women who took placebo and had improvement of uterine bleeding with a 3% increase in uterine volume.

Levonorgestrel Intrauterine System

Increasingly, women with uterine fibroids, that do not distort the endometrial cavity and with a uterine size of less than 12 to 14 gestation weeks, with heavy bleeding have been rigorously evaluated. Improvement in primary outcome of patient-reported scores has noted improvements in domains (practical difficulties, social life, family life, work and daily routine, psychological well-being, and physical health). Dysmenorrhea improved in women using levonorgestrel intrauterine system. Menstrual blood flow decreased and 20% to 40% of women experience amenorrhea. More women using levonorgestrel intrauterine systems continued with therapy compared to routine medical therapy. Low rates of surgical intervention were noted.

IMAGING AND OTHER DIAGNOSTICS

- Several imaging modalities exist to detect uterine fibroids including transvaginal ultrasound (TVUS), saline infusion sonography (SIS), and MRI with gadolinium contrast. Less commonly is CAT scan employed.
- Most patients have an initial TVUS which can differentiate a pelvic mass from a pregnancy, adnexal mass, or uterine fibroids. However, results may be inconclusive in some patients. Transvaginal ultrasound alone may miss one-sixth intracavitary lesions in reproductive-aged women. This author believes that saline infusion sonography should be performed when the patient has complaints of heavy menstrual bleeding, intermenstrual spotting, leukorrhea, or recurrent pregnancy loss, as it is more sensitive in detecting intracavitary pathology.
- Fortunately, the cost differential between TVUS and MRI is decreasing, thus making MRI more accessible to more patients and physicians who care for women with fibroids.
- MRI with gadolinium contrast is the preferred imaging modality for abdominal myomectomy. It is more definitive in determining the size, number, and location of uterine fibroids, as well as how far from the serosal edge the myoma is located. Additionally, the lateral and posterior aspects of the pelvis can be better differentiated with MRI than with TVUS.
  - When intracavitary fibroids are larger than 3 to 4 cm, it may be difficult to distend the uterine cavity with SIS. In these situations, MRI of the pelvis is advised.
  - MRI can differentiate an adnexal mass from exophytic fibroids and is possible with MRI of the pelvis.
  - Cervical fibroids can be better delineated with MRI.
  - MRI of the pelvis can differentiate cellular degenerative changes including calcification, necrosis, and possible sarcomatous changes.

PREOPERATIVE PLANNING

- The patient should have a CBC with platelets, type, and screen available, and a negative pregnancy test on the day of surgery.
- If the blood loss is expected to be greater than 500 mL, consider using cell saver intraoperatively, consider perioperative autologous blood donation, and correct anemia.
- Short-term use of preoperative GnRH therapy considered in women who have symptomatic anemia and fail hormonal therapy or is contraindicated.
  - Short-term use of GnRH therapy effectively stops menstrual cycles and improves anemia. Surgery can be scheduled once anemia has resolved.
  - Short-term use of GnRH therapy considered in patients with anemia and who refuse blood products. Surgery is scheduled once anemia resolves.
- Moderate anemia can be improved with oral, IV iron therapy, iron rich foods, and supplementation with Vitamin C.
  - A consult with blood management is helpful in patients who do not tolerate oral iron therapy.
  - Iron stores can be repleted promptly with IV iron.
- Preoperative informed consent is critical. When possible the patient's partner or family member should be available for the consultation, with patient permission. Several components of informed consent must be discussed and documented:
  - Risk of conversion to hysterectomy:
    - Risk of intraoperative conversion to hysterectomy when diffuse leiomyomatosis is encountered.
    - Massive intraoperative or postoperative blood loss.
    - Inability to reconstruct the myometrial cavity.
    - Risk of conversion to hysterectomy if a large cervical leiomyoma is encountered. Removal of broad lower

uterine segment fibroids may detach the cervix or amputate the cervix from the body of the uterus.
    - Intraoperative frozen section reveals leiomyosarcoma.
- Need for intraoperative or post-operative blood or blood product transfusion.
- Risk of postoperative infection and prolonged hospitalization.
- Risk of ureter injury when a leiomyoma involves the broad ligament or cervical leiomyoma with distortion of the anatomic pathway of the ureter.
- Informed consent should also document risk of recurrence, subsequent infertility, need for C/section, uterine dehiscence/uterine rupture in pregnancy, postoperative adhesion formation, bowel obstruction, and more difficult abdominal surgery in the future as a result of postoperative adhesions.
- Additional preoperative planning essentials:
  - If the fibroid distorts and abuts or enters the endometrial cavity, removal must be judicious. Care taken to avoid removal of endometrium immediately adjacent to the fibroid. Removal of the endometrium may lead to hypomenorrhea, secondary amenorrhea, and intrauterine synechiae and infertility.
    - Placement of an intrauterine Foley catheter filled with methylene blue dye or intrauterine manipulator helps to identify entrance into the endometrial cavity.
    - If the endometrium is entered, it must be closed separately from the myometrium.
    - Consider postoperative hysteroscopy to evaluate the endometrium and exclude intrauterine adhesions.
  - It is imperative to determine if there are intracavitary fibroids present prior to abdominal myomectomy, especially in women with large intramural or subserosal fibroids.
    - If the endometrium is ill-defined, nonvisualized, or incompletely seen with preoperative imaging, diagnostic office hysteroscopy preoperatively should be performed to exclude intracavitary leiomyoma.
    - If office hysteroscopy is not available, then intraoperative diagnostic hysteroscopy should be performed prior to performing the abdominal myomectomy (same day of surgery).
  - Detection of tubal patency with preoperative hysterosalpingogram (HSG) is of equivocal use. There have been cases of tubal obstruction noted perioperatively but resolved when HSG was performed after abdominal myomectomy.
    - It is the opinion of this author that preoperative HSG is not useful and would not change recommendation for abdominal myomectomy.
    - Assisted reproductive technology may be indicated for tubal occlusion.
- Endometrial biopsy should be performed prior to abdominal myomectomy:
  - To exclude leiomyosarcoma
  - There is an increased risk of endometrial hyperplasia in women with uterine fibroids.
    - Higher concentration of estrone and estradiol sulfatase activity has been observed in the endometrium overlying a leiomyoma.
    - Cystic, simple, and complex endometrial hyperplasia has been reported in women with uterine fibroids.
- While office endometrial biopsy is helpful, remember that the sensitivity of detecting endometrial pathology is less in women with increased endometrial circumference, uterine size, or uterine sounding length. This is especially true in women with a uterine sounding length of greater than 12 cm.

SURGICAL MANAGEMENT

- Abdominal myomectomy is indicated in women with symptomatic uterine fibroids. Generally intramural and subserosal fibroids that cannot be treated with the laparoscopic or robotic approach are selected for open myomectomy.
  - Some patients with submucosal and intramural fibroids that protrude into the endometrial cavity are treated with abdominal myomectomy.
  - Patients with an intracavitary leiomyoma that cannot be removed with a one-staged hysteroscopic procedure (usually size >5 cm) may be treated with an abdominal myomectomy approach.
- Surgical management of uterine fibroids is dictated by fibroid size, number, direction of growth, location, patient's desire for definitive treatment and invasiveness of treatment, and surgeon's clinical expertise.
- Recent concerns have been raised about the potential of leiomyosarcomatous changes within uterine fibroids.
  - There is no set of testing that has high sensitivity in detecting sarcoma preoperatively, except for preoperative endometrial biopsy that demonstrates malignancy. However, MRI of the pelvis with and without contrast, LDH isoenzymes, and gross pathology can increase the suspicion of malignant degeneration.
    - Leiomyoma sarcomatous changes are defined by mitotic index (>10 mitotic figures per 10 high-power fields, presence of nuclear hyperchromatism, nuclear pleomorphism, giant cells, and other bizarre cell form changes).
- There are no national consensus guidelines for recommending abdominal myomectomy. However, the following clinical scenarios provide a practical clinical guide to recommend abdominal myomectomy to women:
  - Symptomatic patients with bulk symptoms, abnormal bleeding, and cosmetic concerns from increased uterine size.
  - Patients who do not meet inclusion criteria for minimally invasive options including laparoscopic or robotic myomectomy approach.
  - Patients who do not have access to physicians who perform minimally invasive myomectomy.
  - More than five uterine fibroids with variable individual size
  - Potential difficulty in reconstruction of the uterus with a laparoscopic or robotic approach in patients desirous of pregnancy
  - Large fibroids in the broad ligament that distorts the ureter
  - MRI pelvic imaging that is highly suggestive of hyaline degeneration with extensive liquefaction or gelatinous material that would be difficult to extract with minimally invasive techniques.
  - Extensively calcified leiomyoma that coexist more frequently with pedunculated subserous leiomyoma. Extensive degeneration of intramural fibroids may create a "womb stone" more often predisposed to older women and women from the African diaspora.

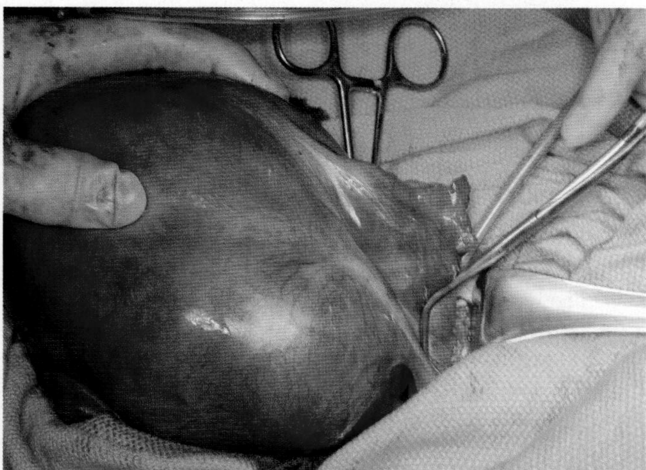

Figure 7.1.1. Satinsky clamp on ovarian vessels.

- Abdominal myomectomy is contraindicated:
  - with coexisting endometrial cancer, cervical cancer, or known leiomyosarcoma.
  - with fibroids that enlarge and become symptomatic in menopause.
- Controlling intraoperative blood loss is essential during abdominal myomectomy. The uterine anatomy and access to the uterine arteries may dictate choice of technique.
- Average blood loss for abdominal myomectomy varies between 200 and 800 mL. The risk of blood transfusion is 2% to 28%. Options to decrease intraoperative bleeding include:
  - Perioperative and intraoperative administration of intravenous tranexamic acid
  - Intramyometrial injection of a dilute solution of vasopressin
  - Temporary occlusion of the infundibular pelvic ligament blood vessels with Satinsky clamps (Figs. 7.1.1 and 7.1.2)
  - Tourniquets placed around the uterine arteries when feasible (Figs. 7.1.3 and 7.1.4)
  - Preoperative use of GnRH agonist for women with anemia. Some authors believe that routine use should be avoided as it may distort the cleavage planes and make enucleation of fibroids more difficult.
  - Perioperative uterine artery embolization

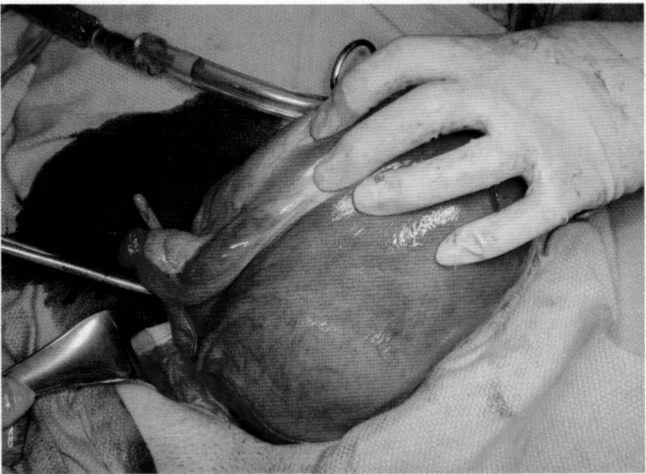

Figure 7.1.2. Satinsky clamps occlude infundibular ligaments.

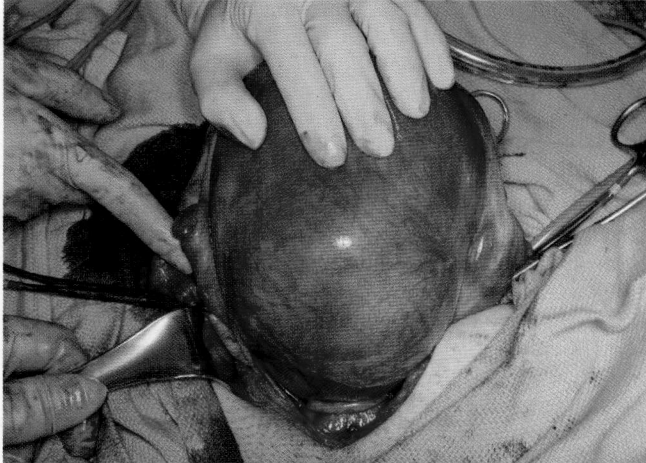

Figure 7.1.3. Red rubber catheter. Tourniquet around the lower segment.

Positioning

- The patient should be placed in the dorsal lithotomy position with the legs appropriately positioned and padded in Allen stirrups.
- Foam padding should be placed next to the patients' knees.
- PAS stocking should be placed prior to the induction of anesthesia.
- The arms should be placed horizontally on arm boards.

Approach

- There are no universal guidelines or high-quality data for the use of prophylactic antibiotics for abdominal myomectomy. Despite the lack of guidelines, this author utilizes preoperative and additional dosing if surgical case is greater than 4 hours of blood loss >1.5 L in order to avoid pelvic infection. This is important for women who desire pregnancy as pelvic infection may compromise future pregnancy.
- The team huddle is performed with the patient, nursing, entire surgical team, and anesthesia to discuss the proposed surgery.
  - This team huddle should outline anticipated length of surgery, anticipated blood loss, need for antibiotic prophylaxis, and answer patient-centered concerns.

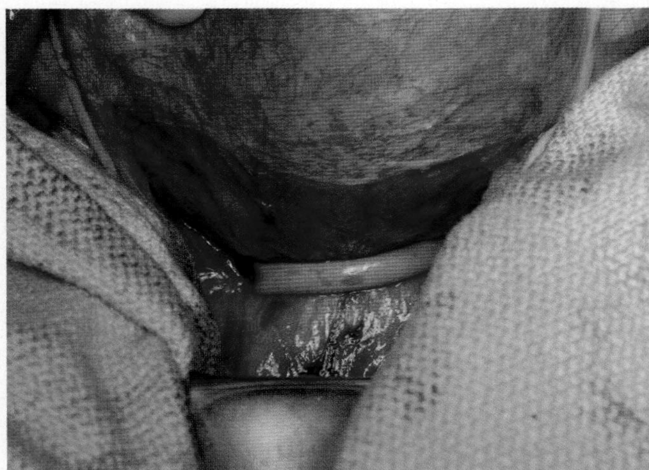

Figure 7.1.4. Red rubber catheter. Close-up of tourniquet.

    - Confirm that all needed instrumentation is available.
    - If cell saver will be used, then the blood bank team is also included in the discussion.
- After induction of anesthesia and legs appropriately placed, an abdominal bimanual and rectal examination performed.
- Uterine mobility should be accessed and will aid in the determination of the abdominal incision.
- This author advocate's placement of an intrauterine Foley catheter (10- to 30-cc balloon) filled with a dilute solution of methylene blue dye. If the endometrial cavity is entered, the blue color of the Foley can be seen and palpated confirming entrance into the endometrium.
    - Alternatively, a uterine manipulator be placed and methylene blue dye can be administered through the cannula to determine if the endometrial cavity has been entered.
    - Occasionally it is difficult to determine the boundaries of the endometrial cavity once extensive myomectomy has been performed.
        - The ability to palpate the intrauterine Foley catheter confirms that the endometrium has not been entered.
        - Or if the Foley catheter is seen, it can be deflated slightly to close the endometrial cavity, taking care not to incorporate the Foley catheter into the suture. As long as the Foley catheter fluid contact remains intact, the surgeon can be confident that the endometrium is not compromised.
    - It is important that the endometrial cavity not be incorporated into the myometrial closure; otherwise, menstrual aberrations including secondary amenorrhea, hematometria, or secondary infertility may occur.
    - Exploration of the upper and lower abdominal cavity performed to determine the mobility of the uterus exclude parasitic fibroids, presence of adhesions, endometriosis, adnexal masses, or unanticipated pathology.
    - When possible the uterus is exteriorized from the peritoneal cavity and an assessment of the number of fibroids and locations of the fibroids ascertained.
    - Self-retaining retractors are not routinely used as exteriorization of the uterus provides ample anatomic exposure.
    - The use of uterine artery tourniquets, placement of Satinsky clamps, or the use of myometrial vasopressin injection is individualized.
    - Minimal use of peritoneal packing decreases the risk of postoperative adhesions.
    - Traumatic instruments such as Kocher clamps and forceps with teeth on the serosa should be avoided. Rather, smooth pick-ups utilized on the serosa to minimize serosal trauma.
    - Meticulous hemostasis should be evident at the end of surgery.
    - Adhesion barriers should be considered at the conclusion of the surgery to decrease risk of postoperative adhesions.

Procedures and Techniques (Video 7.1)

Perform time out and place mechanical PAS stocking for thromboprophylaxis

Administer IV tranexamic acid for cases with anticipated blood loss of >500 mL

- Tranexamic acid 10 mg/kg/dose, in NaCl 0.9% in 100 mL (Cyklokapron)
  - Loading dose given intravenously 15 minutes prior to incision in the operating room. Maximum infusion rate of 100 mg/min.
  - Intraoperative maintenance dose, tranexamic acid 1,000 mg in NaCl 0.9% 100 mL (Cyklokapron), 1 mg/kg/hr, with maximum total dose 1 g. Use intraoperatively only and stop infusion at the end of surgery.
  - Tranexamic cannot be used in patients with prior embolic phenomena or who currently are receiving anticoagulation.
  - Misoprostol (400 mcg) intravaginally or rectally 1 hour prior to surgery.

Administer antibiotics at the induction of anesthesia

Place patient in Allen stirrups

Perform examination under anesthesia

Surgical prep

- The patient's mons pubis hair should be clipped in the operating room prior to the abdominal prep.
- A wide surgical prep including the abdomen, mons pubis, vulva, vagina, cervix, mid-thigh, and buttock. The extent of the prep will be dependent upon whether a low-transverse abdominal incision, vertical incision, or incision that extends above the umbilicus is utilized.

Sterile draping and additional considerations

- Sterile drapes placed to cover the abdomen and perineum.

Foley bladder catheter placement

- Insert a continuous indwelling bladder Foley catheter for continuous measurement of urine output.

Diagnostic hysteroscopy (if applicable)

- Ideally the endometrium should be evaluated prior to abdominal myomectomy. However, if preoperative evaluation demonstrated an ill-defined endometrium, poorly visualized endometrium, or inconclusive imaging of the endometrium, then diagnostic hysteroscopy should be performed in the OR if it was not performed in the office.
  - Diagnostic hysteroscopy excludes coexisting intracavitary fibroids or polyps and should be removed during surgery.
- Occasionally uterine enlargement and cervical distortion prevent office hysteroscopic evaluation of the endometrium.
- In the OR, a small rigid or flexible diagnostic hysteroscope can be used to evaluate the endometrium. Attach sterile IV tubing to the hysteroscope and manually infuse saline via 60-mL syringes for uterine distension.
  - If an intracavitary fibroid is identified, this author recommends its removal at the time of the abdominal myomectomy by opening the endometrial cavity, rather than performing hysteroscopic myomectomy with the abdominal myomectomy. The endometrium is reapproximated by repairing the myometrium at the interface of the uterine cavity and endometrial cavity with a running or interrupted suture of 3-0 polydioxanone (PDS™) avoiding placement of suture in the endometrial cavity.
  - If an endometrial polyp is detected, then the endometrial cavity can be opened and polyp removed concomitantly at the time of myomectomy, and cavity closed (as previously discussed).
- This step can be avoided if office or outpatient endometrial evaluation is negative for intracavitary pathology. Otherwise proceed to the placement of the intrauterine Foley catheter as described below.

Intrauterine Foley catheter placement

- Place a heavy-weighted speculum or open-sided speculum in the vagina to visualize the cervix.
- Grasp the cervix with a single-toothed tenaculum, dilate the cervix with Hegar dilators of size 4 to 6, enough to accommodate a 12- to 16-French intrauterine Foley catheter.
  - Use a Foley with a balloon that can expand to 10 to 30 mL. If the uterine cavity is greater than 12 cm, it is helpful to employ a Foley catheter guidewire to atraumatically guide and place the Foley in the uterine cavity until the fundus is reached.
  - Mix one ampule of methylene blue diluted with 50 cc of saline. After the intrauterine Foley catheter is placed, distend the balloon with the methylene blue solution until resistance is met.
  - With extensive myometrial dissection and multiple myometrial defects, sometimes it is difficult to discern if the endometrium is entered. Placement of a distended intrauterine Foley balloon helps identify endometrial landmarks. The author recommends this technique because it confirms entrance into the endometrial cavity if it occurs.
    - The distended balloon can be palpated during the myomectomy alerting the surgeon when in close proximity to the endometrium. If the surgeon is not sure of landmarks, the balloon can be further distended or deflated providing a tactile guide to determine the proximity of the endometrium.
    - If the pigmented blue tinged balloon is seen, it confirms that the endometrial cavity has been entered during the procedure.

- Additionally, if suture is inadvertently placed during myometrial closure in the endometrial cavity, the punctured balloon will rupture and dissipate the darkly pigmented methylene blue in the surgical site, providing visual feedback that the endometrial cavity has been breached and corrective measures taken to ensure that the endometrial cavity is not obliterated during myometrial closure.
- At the conclusion of the procedure, gently retract or pull the intrauterine Foley. If it is still intact, it will not slip out of the cervix and confirms that the endometrial cavity has not been entered or compromised.
- If the intrauterine Foley ruptures, consider diagnostic hysteroscopy after myometrial closure to exclude suture within the endometrium.

Surgical incision

- Depending upon the size of the uterine fibroid, the mobility of the uterus, or prior abdominal surgical incisions, a Pfannenstiel incision, Maylard incision, or vertical abdominal incision is made. This author prefers the Maylard incision when the uterine size is greater than 15-week gestational weeks and limited uterine mobility noted under anesthesia. This muscle splitting incision provides excellent lateral visualization.
- If the patient has had a prior vertical incision, then that incision may be used.
- Traditional entrance and safeguards are taken to enter the peritoneal cavity.

Exploration of the abdominal cavity

- Once the peritoneal cavity has been entered, the surgeon should determine, if the uterus is mobile, the presence of adhesive peritoneal disease, determine if there are adnexal masses, endometriosis, or unanticipated surgical findings.
- If the uterus is mobile, it should be elevated out of the peritoneal cavity.
- Advise the anesthesiologist that the uterus is being elevated out of the uterine cavity, especially if it is over 20 weeks gestational size, because changes in the hemodynamic state can occasionally occur when pressure is taken off of the great vessels.
- If uterine mobility limits extirpation of the uterus, then leave the uterus in the pelvis and extracts as many fibroids until uterine mobility permits exteriorization of the uterus and removal of remaining fibroids.

Evaluate and palpate location of all fibroids

- Choose an incision in which most fibroids can be removed with a single incision. Sometimes this is not practical as multiple incisions may be needed for safe removal.
- A transverse or vertical serosal incision can be utilized.
- Avoid incisions that will extend into the tubes, cornua, and uterine arteries.
- Palpate the myometrium throughout the procedure as additional smaller fibroids may be encountered after enucleation of larger myomas.
- Anterior incisions are associated with less risk of postoperative adhesions. However, if a fibroid is posterior it is recommended to make an incision posteriorly rather than tunnel through anteriorly.

Slowly inject a dilute solution of vasopressin

- Confirm with the anesthesiologist that vital signs are normal prior to proceeding with the slow injection of a dilute solution of vasopressin into the leiomyomas (**Tech Fig. 7.1.1**).
  - Vasopressin constricts smooth muscle in vascular capillaries, arterioles, and venules which helps decrease blood loss.
  - A dilute solution of vasopressin ([20 units = 1 ampule] mixed in 200 mL saline) is slowly injected into multiple uterine sites including the uterine serosa, intramyometrial or stalk of pedunculated leiomyomas until blanching occurs.
  - A 10-mL control-top syringe and 20- to 22-gauge needle is recommended for injection.
  - For every 10 mL injected with this ratio, one unit of vasopressin is administered.
  - Inform the anesthesiologist of the total amount used.
  - Vasopressin can be slowly injected into the planned serosal uterine incision and myometrium until blanching occurs. Multiple injection sites are made circumferentially in the myometrium. Always aspirate before injecting additional vasopressin. Wait 3 to 5 minutes for vasoconstriction before making the uterine incision.
    - This author injects one fibroid at a time.
    - Record the time of the injection. The half-life of vasopressin is 10 to 30 minutes and the duration of action is 2 to 8 hours. Vasopressin may be injected intermittently during surgery.
    - Avoid vasopressin in patients with coronary artery, vascular or renal disease as hypotension, bradycardia, arrhythmias, and death have been reported.

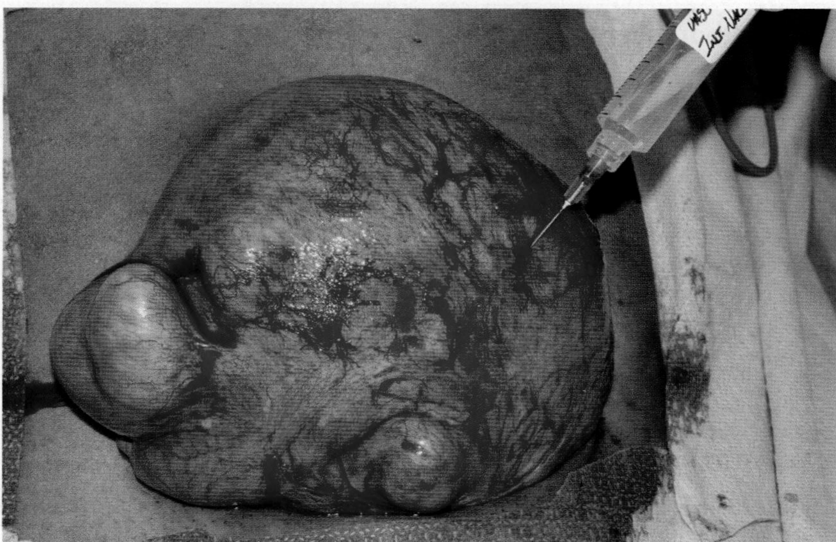

Tech Figure 7.1.1. Slowly inject dilute vasopressin solution.

Additional methods for hemostasis: tourniquets and clamps

- Factors that increase blood loss include size, number, and location of leiomyomas. Tourniquets may be used to decrease bleeding in patients who will have multiple leiomyomas removed.
  - Dissect the bladder peritoneum.
  - Identify a free space in the broad ligament by palpating the broad ligament above the internal os. Identify the ureter and uterine artery. Make a 1-cm incision with an electrosurgical instrument into this free space.
  - Pass a Penrose or red rubber catheter drain in this space and secure tightly posteriorly and secure with a Kelly clamp.
  - Tourniquets are removed at the completion of the myomectomy.
- The infundibular ligament with the ovarian artery and vein can be temporarily compressed with Satinsky clamps. They are removed after completion of the myomectomy.

Removal of myomas

- The easiest fibroids to treat are those that are pedunculated. The base of the pedunculated area should be injected with a dilute solution of vasopressin. The incision is made into the serosa over the leiomyoma until the pseudocapsule is reached. Using a towel clamp or single tooth tenaculum, the myoma can be bluntly dissected away from the stalk. Avoid transection of the fibroid from its stalk as brisk bleeding might occur and require many sutures for hemostasis.
- A monopolar instrument set on 30 to 40 W cutting current is used to make a vertical or horizontal serosal incision. The incision is extended until the pseudocapsule is reached (**Tech Figs. 7.1.2** and **7.1.3**). The length of the incision should incorporate the majority of the area involved with the fibroid.
  - Grasp the myoma with towel clamps and apply traction to fibroid. Separate the pseudocapsule from the myoma bluntly with an open 4 × 4 sponge or back of an empty knife handle (**Tech Figs. 7.1.4** to **7.1.6**). When the surgeon is in the appropriate plane the myoma literally peels away from the pseudocapsule and myometrium.

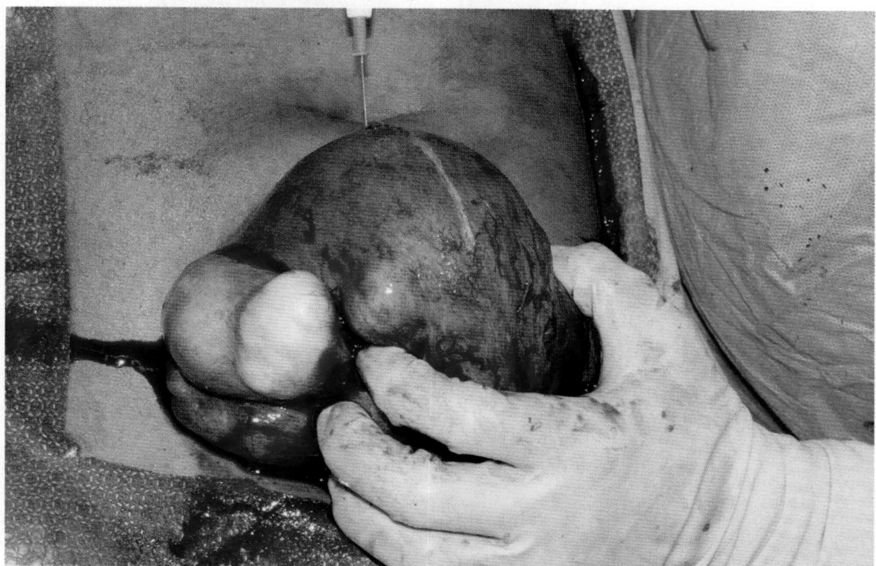

Tech Figure 7.1.2. Manual compression of fibroid facilitates incision with monopolar device.

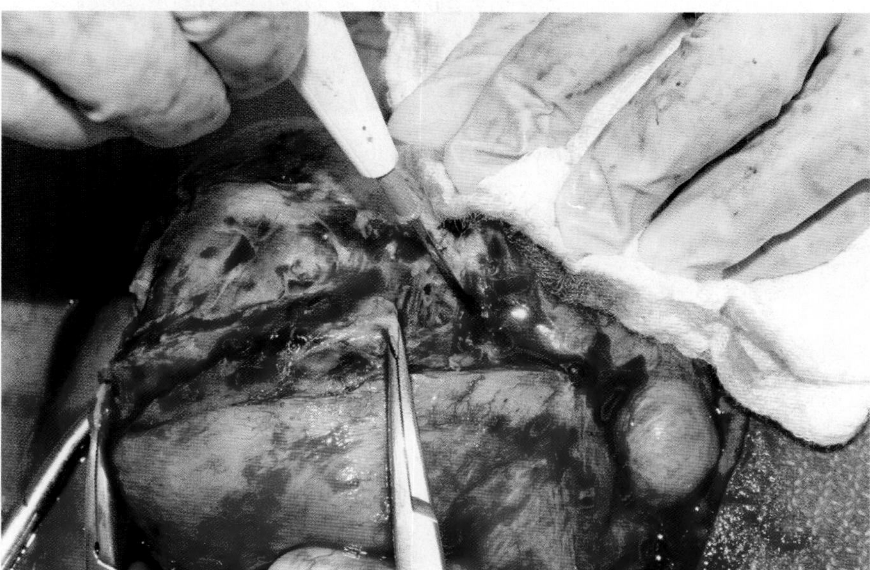

Tech Figure 7.1.3. Incision of pseudocapsule.

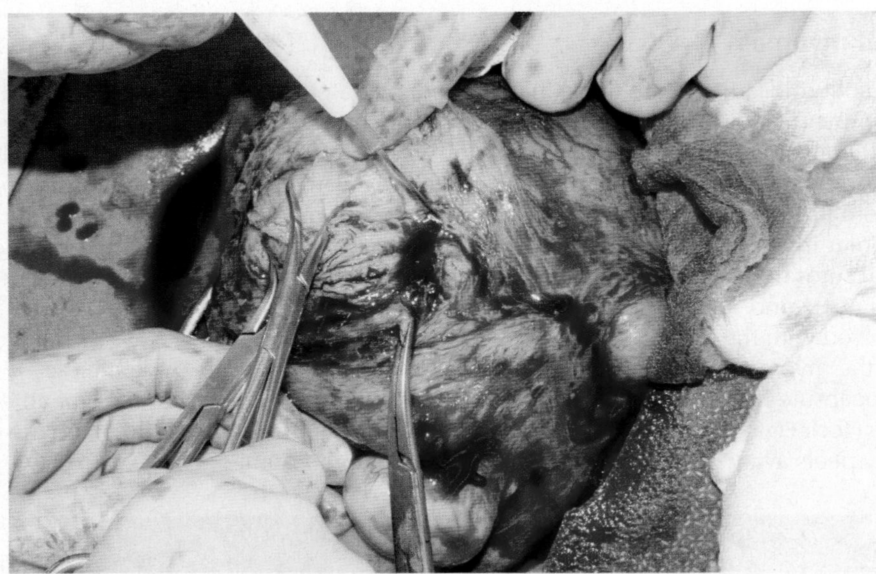

Tech Figure 7.1.4. Apply towel clamp to myoma to facilitate myoma enucleation. Grasp with towel clamp.

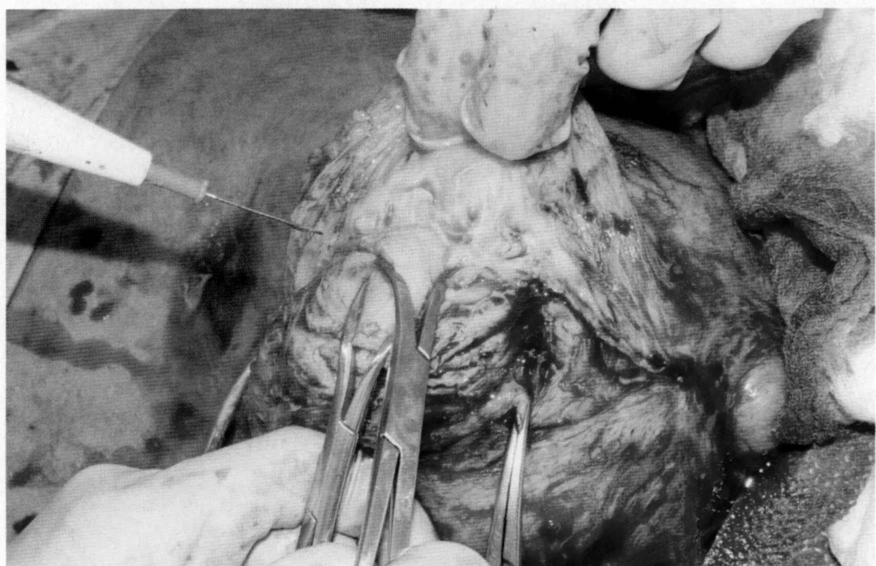

Tech Figure 7.1.5. Apply towel clamp to myoma to facilitate myoma enucleation. Dissection of myoma.

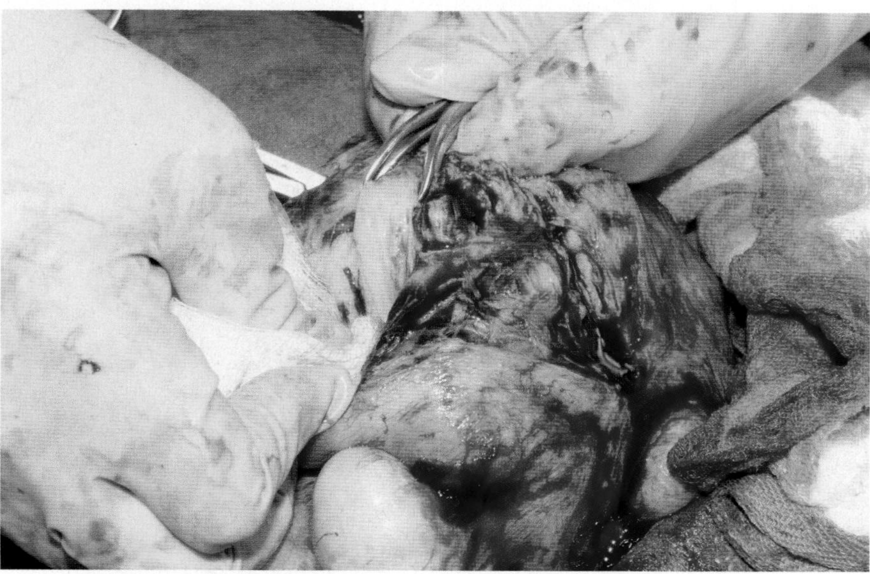

Tech Figure 7.1.6. Dissection with 4 × 4 sponge to develop surgical plane.

- Avoiding use of fingers to bluntly shell out the fibroids as more bleeding is encountered because the blood vessels are torn in the periphery and base of the leiomyoma.
- Push the surrounding tissue planes away from the fibroid. The towel clamps or Lahey clamps should be advanced as the fibroid begins to separate from the myometrium.
- The surgeon can squeeze the leiomyoma. This will help it bulge out further from the myometrial bed.
- With a large fibroid greater than 6 to 8 cm, a myoma cork screw may be used to apply traction to the myoma helping to enucleate the fibroid. Visible pseudocapsule that envelops the myoma may be cut in order to extricate the myoma.
- Small-surface blood vessels are coagulated with Bovie tip cautery. Hemostasis should be prioritized throughout the surgical procedure.
- If the leiomyoma protrudes into the endometrial cavity, identify the endometrium and separate it from the fibroid. The goal is to not have any endometrium removed with the leiomyoma.
- If the endometrial cavity is entered, it must be closed separately from the myometrium (Tech Fig. 7.1.7). Then the myometrium is reapproximated over the endometrium, avoiding closure of the endometrial cavity (Tech Figs. 7.1.8 and 7.1.9).

- Carefully palpate the myometrium after the dominant fibroid is removed in order to detect other lesions. The decision to close the defects immediately or after total enucleation of fibroids will depend upon the amount of bleeding that is encountered.

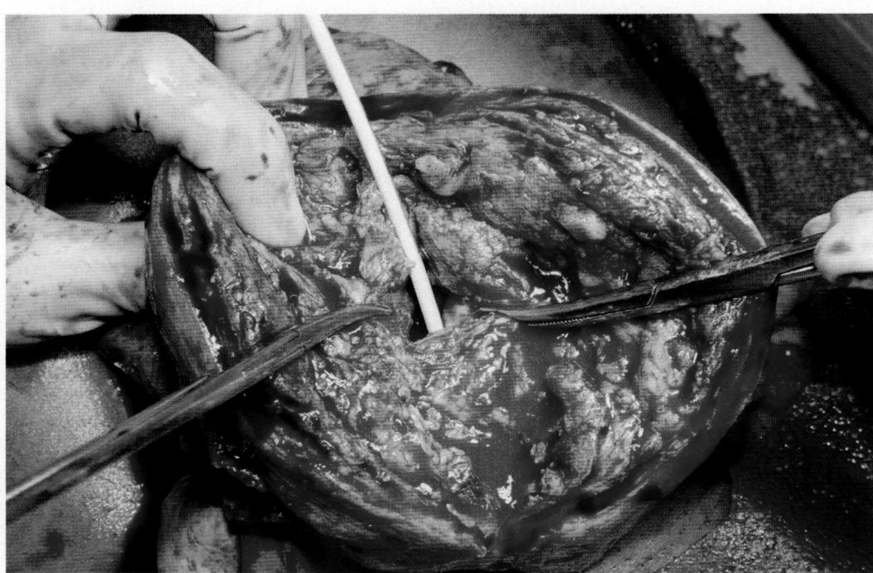

Tech Figure 7.1.7. Endometrium is opened and identified with a white probe.

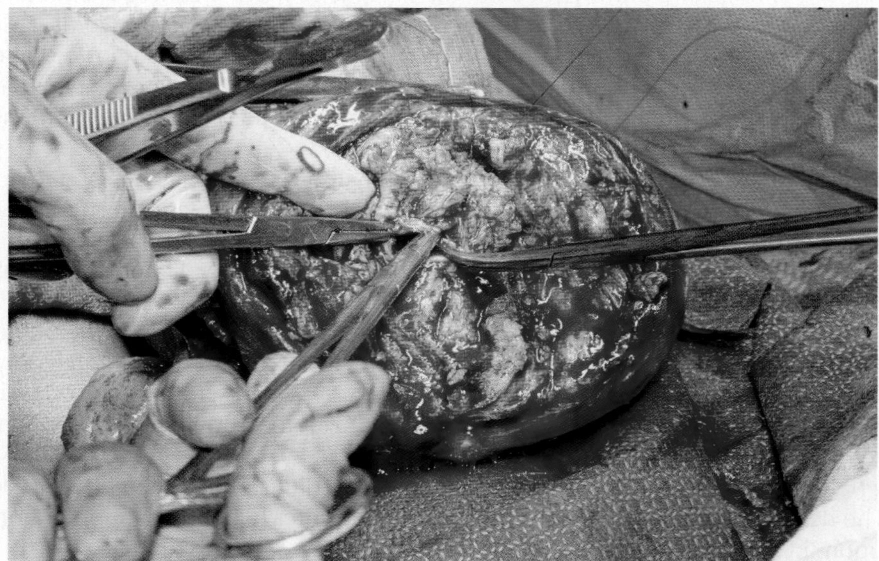

Tech Figure 7.1.8. Closure of the endometrial cavity taking care to avoid suture placement within the cavity. Reapproximate only endometrial edges.

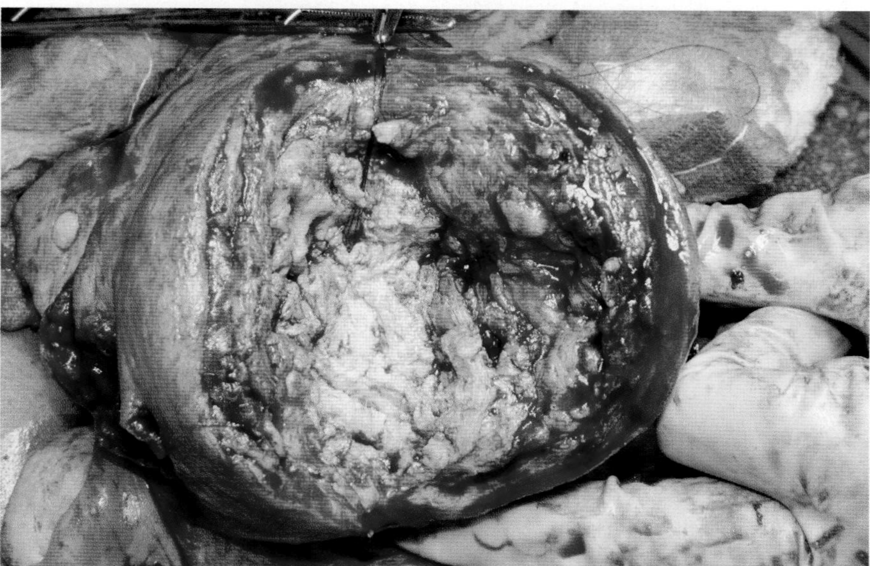

Tech Figure 7.1.9. Final closure of endometrial cavity.

Closure of the myometrial defects

If there are small residual areas of dead space, apply Arista™ (Bard), Floseal (Baxter International Inc., Hayward, CA), or Surgiflo (Ethicon, San Angelo, TX). They are thrombin-infused gelatin products and can be placed in the myometrial bed and dead spaces for additional hemostasis (**Tech Fig. 7.1.10**).

- Deeper intramural fibroids should be closed when possible with a three-layer closure, with zero-delayed reabsorbable suture beginning at the base and obliterating the space with a

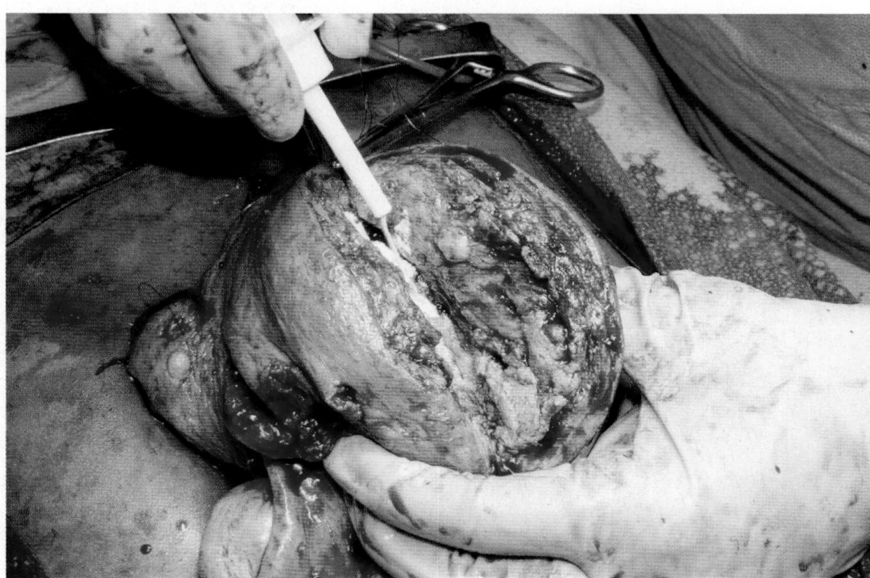

Tech Figure 7.1.10. Hemostatic agent is applied. In this case, Arista was used between the myometrial layers.

continuous-running suture or interrupted figure of eight sutures (**Tech Figs. 7.1.11** and **7.1.12**). During suturing, the assistant should squeeze the uterine walls together to help the surgeon close the myometrium effectively. Continue this deep-layer closure approximating the myometrium until the serosal edge is reached.

- The edges of the serosa are closed with an imbricating continuous, "baseball" stitch on the serosa. Synthetic absorbable 3-0 sutures are used including Vicryl, PDS, or Maxon suture, which are associated with delayed absorption and limited inflammatory response (**Tech Fig. 7.1.13**).
- Attempt to bury all surgical knots to a decrease adhesion formation.
- Place adhesion barriers such as Interceed™ (oxidized cellulose) over the suture lines, after irrigating the peritoneal cavity and ensuring hemostasis, if conditions ideal.

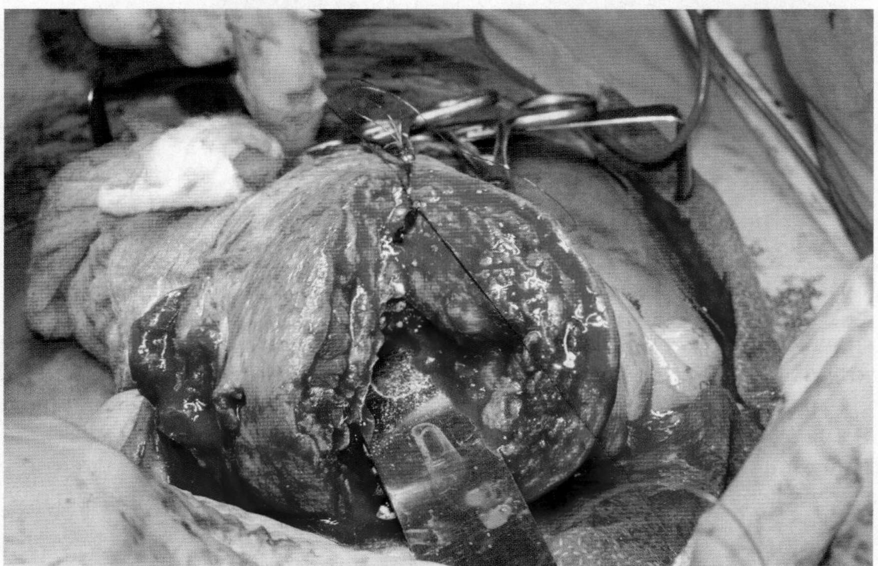

Tech Figure 7.1.11. First layer closure of the myometrium with delayed absorbable suture.

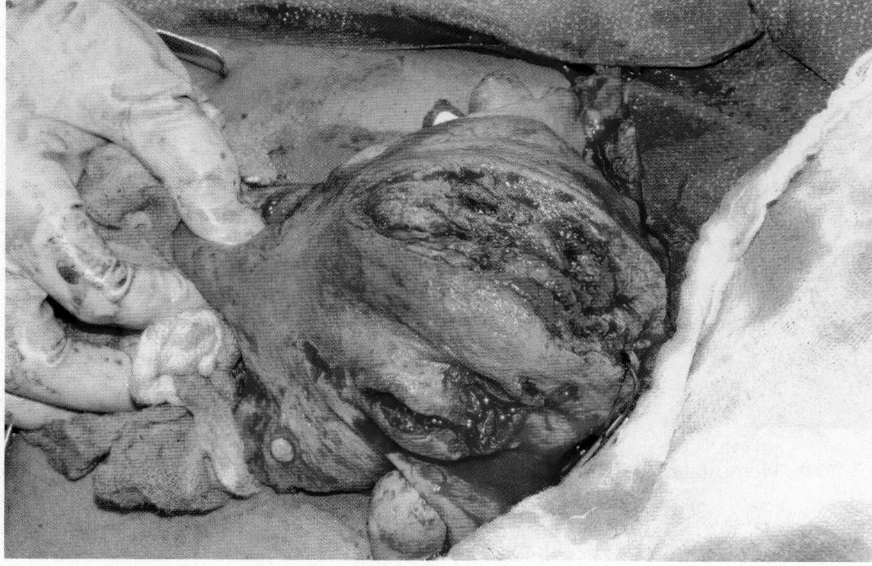

Tech Figure 7.1.12. Final multilayered closure of myometrium.

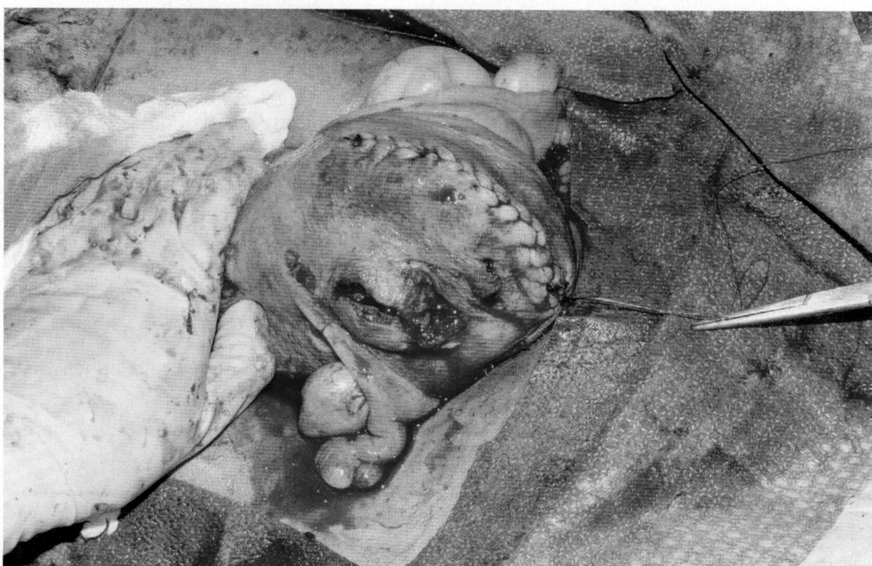

Tech Figure 7.1.13. Serosal closure.

- Send all leiomyomas for histological evaluation. Tabulate the number, size, and aggregate weight of all fibroids.
- The myometrium should be closed meticulously in a layered fashion. Surgeons must avoid placement of just a few two or three large through-and-through closures if the patient is interested in future pregnancy. A limited follow-up of patients who had abdominal myomectomy with meticulous closure and subsequent pregnancy observed that the majority of scars were symmetric and with uniform thickness compared with surrounding myometrium.
- Maintain awareness of the location of the fallopian tubes and avoid ligation of the fallopian tubes during myometrial closure.
- Copiously lavage the peritoneal cavity with saline or Ringer lactate solution after completion of the surgery.
- Once hemostasis is confirmed, application of an adhesion barrier is advised. Two current adhesion barriers are currently available for abdominal myomectomy. Seprafilm, a bioresorbable membrane (Genzyme Corporation, Cambridge, MA), and Interceed (oxidized regenerated cellulose) have been associated with decreased postoperative adhesion formation.

Abdominal closure

- Once completed, the nurses should perform the final instrument, needle, sponge, and ancillary equipment counts.
- The fascia and skin closure is performed per physician preference.

Perform vaginal sweep

- At the completion of surgery, remove the intrauterine Foley catheter.
- Perform a "vaginal sweep" to make sure that no foreign bodies are left in the vagina.

PEARLS AND PITFALLS

- ○ Confirm that abdominal myomectomy is indicated
- ✗ Recommending surgery for minimal clinical symptoms or for symptoms that will not be alleviated with surgery increases the risk of unnecessary operative complications
- ○ Exclude intracavitary fibroids even if the patient has multiple intramural and serosal fibroids
- ✗ Failure to remove intracavitary fibroids may cause menstrual dysfunction, infertility, or may leiomyoma prolapse after surgery
- ○ Identify ureter if fibroids distort the broad ligament and cervix
- ✗ Injury or transection of ureter
- ○ Meticulous myometrial and serosal closure
- ✗ Increased intraoperative and postoperative blood loss. Increased risk for postoperative adhesions
- ○ Place intrauterine Foley catheter in order to identify entrance into the endometrium
- ✗ Inadvertent closure of the endometrial cavity can be associated with secondary infertility, Asherman syndrome, and intracavitary distortion

POSTOPERATIVE CARE

- Postoperatively the patient is admitted to the hospital for 1 to 3 days until standard postoperative milestones are met.
  - Patient is ambulatory
  - Taking fluids
  - Pain is controlled
  - Afebrile and stable vital signs
- Serial CBC and platelet count until labs are stable. Additional postoperative labs followed if the patient has other comorbidities including renal, liver disease, or diabetes.
- Evaluate this patient for coagulopathy if large blood loss occurs.
- Early ambulation and early feeding are advisable. Both of these help to decrease atelectasis pneumonia, postsurgical embolism (DVT or pulmonary emboli), and decrease postoperative ileus.
- Utilize postoperative incentive spirometry.
- Approximately 12% to 67% of women have a nonlocalizing fever 48 hours after myomectomy. Generally, no focal findings are limited. However, standard fever works up and clinical examination is recommended.
- Consider withholding nonsteroidal pain medications if moderate or significant intraoperative bleeding.
- Follow serial CBC and coagulation panel if large intraoperative blood loss occurs. Evaluate the patient for disseminated intravascular coagulation if the patient continues to bleed postoperatively.
- Use of the patient-controlled analgesia (PCA) is often favored by patients and nursing staff for management of postoperative pain. Generally, after the first 24 hours, the PCA pump is discontinued and oral narcotic therapy and NSAIDs begin.
- When stable, the indwelling Foley catheter is removed the morning after surgery.
- The patient can be discharged home when afebrile, vital signs, and labs are stable, tolerates liquids, and able to ambulate.
- Homegoing discharge instructions should be reviewed with the surgeon. Additionally, homegoing written discharge instructions are given.
- Special emphasis must communicated with the patient prior to discharge:
  - Patient instructed to call if she has a persistent temperature of greater than 100 degrees.
  - Nausea, vomiting, leg pain, new onset anxiety, or shortness of breath.
- Reminder to keep the incision dry. Call if redness, discharge, wound separation, foul smell, change in color (dusky or black color), or increasing tenderness occurs.
- Avoid vaginal intercourse for four weeks.
- May shower immediately and cover the wound.
- No heavy lifting of more than 10 pounds.
- Resume hormonal contraception four weeks after surgery.
- Arrange for postoperative follow-up four weeks after surgery.
  - Review pathology.
  - Discuss route of delivery based on complexity of the abdominal myomectomy.
- Most patients return to work and full activities 4 to 6 weeks after surgery.
- Wait 3 to 6 months before attempting pregnancy.

OUTCOMES

- Morbidity and mortality are similar to an abdominal hysterectomy. However, complications such as vaginal vault prolapse and injury to the bladder and ureters are lower in patients undergoing abdominal myomectomy compared to abdominal hysterectomy.
- Bulk symptoms and heavy menstrual bleeding are greatly improved in 80% of women undergoing abdominal myomectomy when fibroids are completely removed.
- Approximately 36% of women develop postoperative adhesions.
- While generally improved, pelvic pain and dysmenorrhea may not be completely alleviated if coexisting adenomyosis or endometriosis exists.
- Prospective, randomized controlled studies are lacking regarding the impact of abdominal myomectomy on fertility. Fibroids can distort tubal anatomy and the uterine cavity. Male factors also impact fertility outcomes. Small series

document a 57% conception rate following abdominal myomectomy.

- The number of women who wish to conceive after abdominal myomectomy is unknown, thus making fertility outcomes difficult to calculate.
- Among women with recurrent pregnancy, loss or prior infertility successful pregnancies have been associated with abdominal myomectomy.
- The rate of recurrence of uterine fibroids is variable depending upon the length of time of follow-up after surgery.
    - Among patients followed for 7 to 10 years after surgery, 21% to 34% required subsequent surgery for fibroid-related symptoms.
    - Additional factor affecting recurrence of fibroids includes age of initial surgery, interval pregnancy after myomectomy, age of patient, race, and the number of fibroids removed.
- Despite these limitations, uterine sparing surgical options should be available to women who have this preference even if there are no plans for childbearing.

COMPLICATIONS

- Complications from abdominal myomectomy include:
    - Infectious morbidity
        - Respiratory
            - Atelectasis
            - Pneumonia
        - Urinary tract infection
        - Wound infection
        - Microscopic abscesses within the myometrium
        - Endometritis
    - Embolic
        - Deep venous vein thrombosis
        - Pulmonary embolism
    - Intraoperative and postoperative bleeding
        - Acute
        - Delayed
        - Coagulopathy
    - Infertility
        - Obstruction of the fallopian tube
        - Iatrogenic closure of the endometrium leading to secondary amenorrhea
        - Asherman syndrome due to complete or incomplete removal of the endometrium when performing myomectomy that involves myomas that abut the endometrium. Endometrium overlying the leiomyoma may be inadvertently removed.
    - Postoperative bowel adhesions
    - Uterine rupture during pregnancy or partial uterine dehiscence
        - If the patient becomes pregnant following the procedure, she should be informed to contact her obstetrician promptly if abdominal pain occurs during pregnancy.
        - Fetal loss
        - Postpartum hemorrhage
        - Hysterectomy
    - Death

KEY READINGS

American College of Obstetricians and Gynecologists. ACOG practice bulletin: alternative to hysterectomy in the management of leiomyomas. *Obstet Gynecol.* 2008;112:387–400.

Borah BJ, Nicholson WK, Bradley L, Stewart EA. The impact of uterine leiomyomas: a national survey of affected women. *Am J Obstet Gynecol.* 2013;209(4):319.e1–319.e20.

Gupta J, Kai J, Middleton L, Pattison H, Gray R, Daniels J; ECLIPSE Trial Collaborative Group. Levonorgestrel intrauterine system versus medical therapy for menorrhagia. *N Engl J Med.* 2013;368(2):128–137.

Kongnyuy EJ, Wiysonge CS. Interventions to reduce haemorrhage during myomectomy for fibroids. *Cochrane Database Syst Rev.* 2009;(3): CD005355.

Kroencke TJ, Scheurig C, Poellinger A, et al. Uterine artery embolization for leiomyomas: percentage of infarction predicts clinical outcome. *Radiology.* 2010;255:834–841.

Leminen H, Hurskainen R. Tranexamic acid for the treatment of heavy menstrual bleeding: efficacy and safety. *Int J Women's Health.* 2012;(4): 413–421.

Raga F, Sanz-Cortes M, Bonilla F, Casan EM, Bonilla-Musoles F. Reducing blood loss at myomectomy with use of a gelatin-thrombin matrix hemostatic sealant. *Fertil Steril.* 2009;92(1):356–360.

Roberts A. Magnetic resonance-guided focused ultrasound for uterine fibroids. *Semin Intervent Radiol.* 2008;25(4):394–405.

Spies, JB, Coyne K, Guaou Guaou N, Boyle D, Skyrnarz-Murphy K, Gonzalves SM. The UFS-QOL, a new disease-specific symptom and health-related quality of life questionnaire for leiomyomata. *Obstet Gynecol.* 2002;99:290–300.

Stewart EA. Clinical practice. Uterine fibroids. *N Engl J Med.* 2015;372(17): 1646–1655.

Van der Kooij SM, Ankum WM, Hehenkamp WJ. Review of nonsurgical/minimally invasive treatments for uterine fibroids. *Curr Opin Obstet Gynecol.* 2012;24:368–375.

Wellington K, Wagstaff AJ. Tranexamic acid: a review of its use in the management of menorrhagia. *Drugs.* 2003;63(13):1417–1433.

Widrich, T, Bradley LD, Mitchinson AR, Collins RL. Comparison of saline infusion sonography with office hysteroscopy for the evaluation of the endometrium. *Am J Obstet Gynecol.* 1996;174(4):1327–1334.

Chapter 7.2 Conventional Laparoscopy Myomectomy

Katrin S. Arnolds, Stephen E. Zimberg, Michael L. Sprague

GENERAL PRINCIPLES

Definition

- Uterine leiomyomas are the most common gynecologic tumor, with an incidence approximating 20% to 25% in women aged 18 to 65 years.[1] Uterine myomas are discreet, sharply circumscribed masses, and histologically appear as whorled bundles of smooth muscle. Most commonly, leiomyomas grow within the uterine corpus, but may also occur within the uterine ligaments, uterine cervix, or on other abdominal structures. Individual myomas are believed to be monoclonal and result from somatic mutations yielding dysregulation of genes involved in growth regulation. Growth of uterine leiomyomas lead to uterine enlargement, which may yield symptoms such as abnormal uterine bleeding, dysmenorrhea, dyspareunia, subfertility, pelvic pressure, urinary frequency, or defecatory dysfunction. Uterine myomectomy is the preferred surgical therapy for management of symptomatic uterine myomas in women who desire future pregnancy or uterine preservation. Laparoscopic myomectomy is a feasible, minimally invasive procedure and has been demonstrated to yield less pain, shorter hospital stays, improved cosmesis, less blood loss, and faster recovery compared to laparotomic procedures, and similar surgical outcomes with less overall cost compared to robot-assisted procedures.

Differential Diagnosis

- Adenomyosis
- Congenital uterine anomaly
- Endometrial polyp
- Hematometra
- Pregnancy
- Uterine leiomyosarcoma
- Uterine carcinosarcoma
- Endometrial carcinoma
- Metastatic disease
- Tubo-ovarian neoplasm

Nonoperative Management

- The goal of nonoperative management for uterine leiomyomas is to decrease symptomatology and improve the quality of life. To maximize patient satisfaction and compliance, therapies must be convenient for the patient and with minimal deleterious side effects. From a surgical perspective, medical therapies for uterine leiomyomas are frequently employed to raise preoperative hemoglobin levels or to reduce uterine volume to optimize a patient prior to surgical intervention.
- Observation, which entails no immediate intervention, is reasonable for patients who experience minimal symptoms or who elect not to receive treatment. Watchful waiting is a practical option to select women who are approaching menopause as uterine leiomyomas often regress as circulating levels of estradiol and progesterone naturally.
- Steroid hormones are commonly employed to manage bothersome symptoms attributable to uterine myomas. A common first-line therapy for management of abnormal uterine bleeding and dysmenorrhea is combination oral contraceptive pills (OCPs). Although the efficacy of combination OCPs for the treatment of symptomatic fibroids is uncertain and scientific evidence is scarce,[2] oral contraceptives may sufficiently reduce the bothersome symptoms attributable to leiomyoma uteri in certain women. The levonorgestrel intrauterine system (LNG-IUS) is another option for management of abnormal uterine bleeding and has been shown to decrease menstrual blood loss, reduce uterine volume, and lead to improvement in hemoglobin levels.[3] Of note, the presence of submucous myomas that significantly distort the uterine cavity is a relative contraindication for LNG-IUS.
- Administration of GnRH agonists results in downregulation of hypothalamic GnRH receptors, ultimately inducing a reversible hypogonadal state by 2 weeks. The GnRH agonist, leuprolide acetate, is approved by the Food and Drug Administration (FDA) to increase hemoglobin levels and decrease myoma size prior to myomectomy. Women who receive leuprolide acetate therapy typically develop amenorrhea within 3 months. The expected mean reduction in uterine volume is 36% by 3 months and 45% by 6 months following initiation therapy. Patients treated with GnRH agonists may experience menopausal symptoms such as hot flushes, vaginal dryness, mood changes, and a reversible decrease in bone density. Hormonal add-back therapy may be initiated to minimize side effects from GnRH agonists. Of note, preoperative treatment with leuprolide acetate may not improve blood loss during myomectomy.
- GnRH antagonists compete with endogenous GnRH for pituitary binding sites and have the advantage of a comparatively rapid onset of clinical effects without certain side effects observed with GnRH agonists. Evidence suggests that a 31.3% reduction in uterine leiomyoma size can be achieved by 14 days of treatment.[4] GnRH antagonists currently available in the United States require daily injections, which may be an obstacle for many patients.
- Mifepristone is a weak progesterone receptor agonist that has been demonstrated to reduce heavy menstrual bleeding and improve myoma-specific quality of life. Treatment with mifepristone yields a reduction of uterine volume by 26% to 74% in women with leiomyomas.[5] At present, mifepristone is not FDA-approved in the United States for the treatment of uterine leiomyomas.
- Ulipristal acetate (UPA) is an orally administered selective progesterone receptor modulator that inhibits proliferation of leiomyoma cells, but not in normal myometrial cells.[6] UPA has been shown to significantly reduce fibroid volume, decrease abdominal pressure, and decrease myoma-related pain. UPA has stimulatory effects on the endometrium and its progesterone antagonist action could result in an increased

risk for endometrial hyperplasia and endometrial carcinoma. However, studies have demonstrated that the incidence of endometrial hyperplasia and malignancy after treatment with UPA appears to be low. Pregnancies after UPA administration have been reported without maternal complications related to leiomyomas.

- Magnetic resonance–guided focused ultrasound surgery (MRgFUS) is an outpatient treatment option for uterine leiomyomas in premenopausal women. MRgFUS is a noninvasive, thermoablative technique in which waves of ultrasound energy converge on a small volume of tissue, which leads to the thermal destruction, coagulative necrosis, and reduction of leiomyoma of volume.[7] Pregnancies have been described after MRgFUS with no specific pattern of complications.
- Uterine fibroid embolization (UFE) reduces uterine arterial blood flow and results irreversible infarction of leiomyomas. The leiomyomas eventually decrease in size and bothersome myoma-related symptoms improve. Most commonly, the approach to percutaneous embolization is via the right or left femoral artery under local anesthesia. UFE may reduce menstrual loss by 85% and the mean dominant fibroid volume by 30% to 46%.[8] The safety of pregnancy after UFE has not been established to date; however, pregnancies after UFE have been reported.[9]

IMAGING AND OTHER DIAGNOSTICS

- Multiple imaging modalities are available for the evaluation of suspected uterine myomas, each with relative strengths and weaknesses. In addition to documenting the number and size of any myomas present, a primary objective of pelvic imaging prior to laparoscopic myomectomy is to rule out other pathologies such as adenomyosis and gynecologic malignancy.
- Pelvic ultrasound provides high-quality imaging of the uterus and adnexa and is oftentimes the primary imaging modality for the evaluation of patients with suspected uterine myomas (Fig. 7.2.1). Pelvic ultrasound is widely available, with advantages that include relatively low cost, high diagnostic accuracy, and lack of ionizing radiation. Ultrasound of the pelvis is performed using both transabdominal and transvaginal techniques to ensure the best-quality anatomic survey is obtained. It is important to note that, although effective at evaluating total endometrial thickness, transvaginal ultrasound has low sensitivity for detecting intracavitary masses and determining the type of submucous myomas. Saline-infused sonography (SIS) differs from nonenhanced transvaginal ultrasound in that saline is employed to distend the uterine cavity, which serves as a contrast medium and allows for detailed examination of the endometrium.
- Magnetic resonance imaging (MRI) of the uterus is the preferred imaging method for evaluating uterine myomas prior to laparoscopic myomectomy (Fig. 7.2.2). MRI allows for efficient, comprehensive evaluation of the uterus and clearly demonstrates the size and location of myomas present. Compared to SIS, MRI is superior at accurately estimating the degree of submucosal myoma ingrowth into the endometrial cavity, which is crucial for preoperative planning, as a surgeon may choose to excise certain submucous myomas in hysteroscopic fashion. MRI allows for assessment of the junctional zone, which is important for identifying adenomyosis. Compared to computed tomography and pelvic ultrasound, MRI is superior at differentiating benign uterine leiomyomas from uterine leiomyosarcomas.

PREOPERATIVE PLANNING

- Appropriate preoperative patient counseling is important to define a patient's goals from surgery and to establish reasonable expectations following laparoscopic myomectomy. In general, the intent of uterine myomectomy is to improve, not necessarily eliminate, bothersome symptoms attributed to uterine myomas. The risks of laparoscopic myomectomy should be emphasized, including perioperative blood loss possibly necessitating transfusion, postoperative adhesion formation which may yield pain or subfertility, and the rare

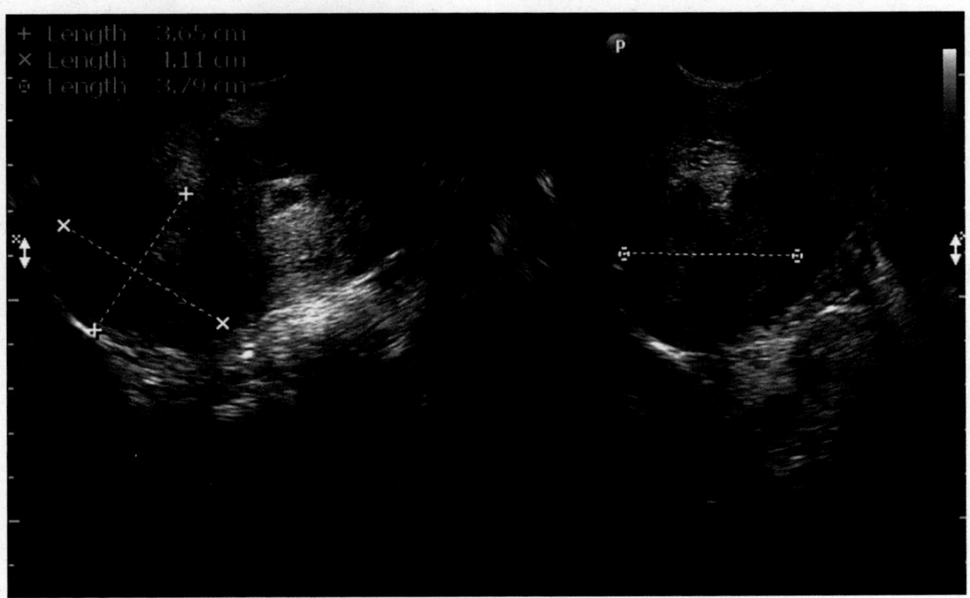

Figure 7.2.1. Pelvic ultrasound for evaluation fundal, subserosal myoma.

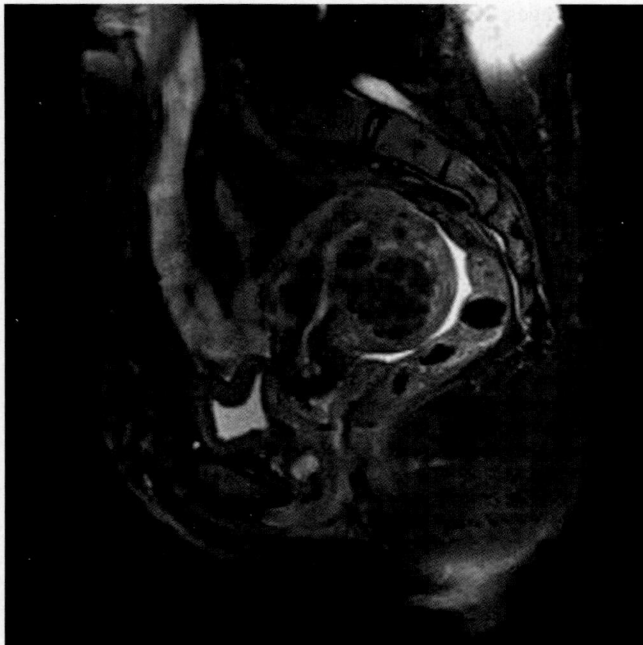

Figure 7.2.2. Pelvic MRI for evaluation of fundal, subserosal myoma.

need for hysterectomy if unexpected pathology or uncontrollable bleeding is encountered. Additionally, the patient should be informed of the possibilities of future myoma recurrence and of intrapartum uterine rupture. The patient should understand that any procedure that begins laparoscopically may require laparotomy to complete.

- Favorable surgical outcomes require that medical comorbidities are optimized prior to laparoscopic myomectomy. Commonly, patients with abnormal uterine bleeding have iron deficiency anemia, which should be corrected prior to surgery to minimize risk of perioperative transfusion and maximize wound healing potential. Options for iron repletion include oral iron therapy and intravenous iron infusions. Oftentimes, concomitant medical therapy is required to reduce abnormal uterine bleeding in order to achieve a net increase in hemoglobin. Pre-existing cardiopulmonary disease may lead to difficulty with ventilation or tolerance of Trendelenburg position and should be addressed prior to laparoscopic surgery. Poorly controlled diabetes mellitus may lead to poor wound healing and increased risk of perioperative infection.

SURGICAL MANAGEMENT

- Laparoscopic myomectomy should be avoided in patients with suspected gynecologic malignancy and contraindications to pneumoperitoneum or Trendelenburg positioning. Other limitations to laparoscopic myomectomy include the size and number of myomas to be excised and a surgeon's ability to efficiently perform laparoscopic suturing. In many instances, it is more difficult to remove numerous small myomas as opposed to fewer, larger myomas.

Positioning (Figs. 7.2.1 and 7.2.3)

- The patient is placed in dorsal lithotomy position with their legs in stirrups and their arms tucked in neutral positions at their sides. As Trendelenburg positioning will eventually be necessary for the completion of the surgery, it is prudent to take the opportunity to place the patient in Trendelenburg position prior to surgical preparation to ensure that patient does not shift on the operative table. Beanbag or foam egg crate mattress covers are effective measures to ensure the patient's position does not change during Trendelenburg positioning. Following surgical preparation of the abdomen and vagina, the patient is draped, a Foley catheter is introduced into the bladder, and a uterine manipulator is placed. We prefer to use a uterine manipulator through which fluid can be introduced into the uterine cavity and allow performance of chromopertubation.
- Placement of laparoscopic cannulas is dependent on the size and position of the myomas. In general, we place laparoscopic cannulas at the umbilicus, within the left and right epigastrum at the level of the umbilicus, and in the left lower quadrant to facilitate laparoscopic suturing in an ipsilateral approach from the patient's left side (Fig. 7.2.3). As total uterine length increases, port placement may need to shift cephalad, but the overall geometry of the port placement need not change. The diameter of each port depends on surgeon preference, myoma size, and quality of the laparoscopic instruments.

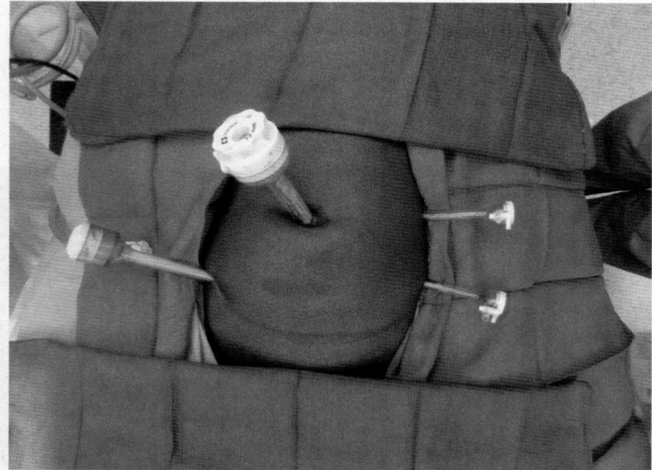

Figure 7.2.3. Typical port configuration for laparoscopic myomectomy.

Procedures and Techniques (Video 7.2)

Techniques to minimize perioperative blood loss

- Laparoscopic myomectomy can be associated with significant intraoperative blood loss, which may necessitate the perioperative transfusion of blood products. The knowledge of the various agents and techniques that reduce bleeding during laparoscopic myomectomy is essential to enhancing patient safety and surgical outcomes. Several pharmacologic agents have been found to reduce intraoperative blood loss during myomectomy. Preoperative administration of uterotonics such as methylergonovine, misoprostol, and prostaglandin E2 has been shown to decrease intraoperative blood loss by evoking myometrial contractions.[10] The intramyometrial injection of vasopressin leads to reduction of intraoperative blood loss by evoking local vasoconstriction. In our practice, 20 units of vasopressin are mixed with 100 mL of normal saline and injected to form a wheal over the underlying leiomyoma. The half-life of intramuscular vasopressin is 10 to 20 minutes and a surgeon should appreciate that the safe maximal dosage of vasopressin has not been established. Care should be taken to avoid intravascular injection, as there are rare cases in which injection of vasopressin evoked cardiovascular collapse. Intravenous administration of tranexamic acid (TXA) competitively inhibits the conversion of plasminogen to plasmin, thereby minimizing intraoperative blood loss during myomectomy by exerting an antifibrinolytic effect.[11] Of note, the use of intravenous oxytocin and locally injected bupivacaine with epinephrine have not been demonstrated to decrease blood loss during myomectomy.[12] Use of cell salvage devices decreases the need for perioperative allogeneic blood transfusion. Interventions that decrease blood flow to the uterus, such as uterine artery embolization, application of a pericervical tourniquet, and temporary clamping of the uterine artery, have been described with varying levels of efficacy.

Hysterotomy

- Hysterotomy planning is important. The planned incision must be of adequate length to allow for efficient enucleation of the myoma, but without undue trauma to healthy uterine tissue. The surgeon must ensure that vital structures such as the fallopian tubes and ascending uterine vessels are not at risk for injury (**Tech Fig. 7.2.1**). Transverse uterine incision facilitates ipsilateral

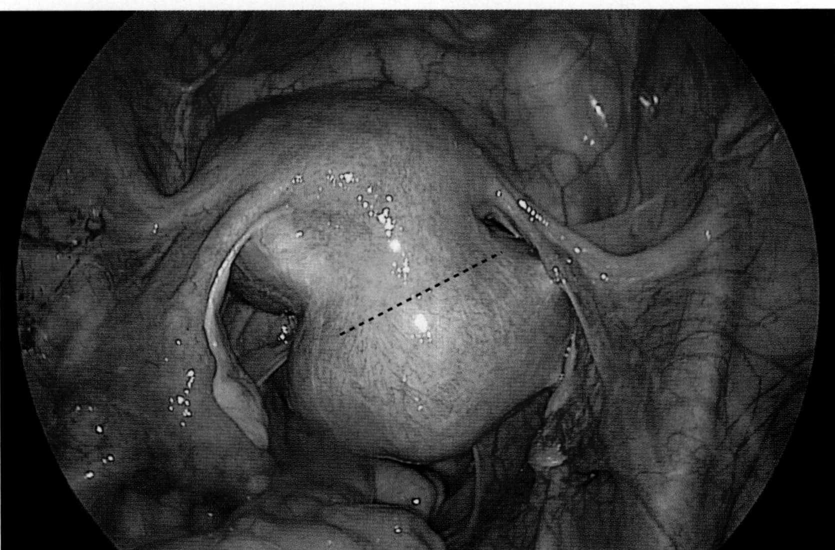

Tech Figure 7.2.1. Hysterotomy planning.

laparoscopic suturing. However, some myomas in the inferior aspects of the uterus may require a vertical or oblique incision to facilitate enucleation and hysterorrhaphy. Multiple myomas can be enucleated through a single hysterotomy when possible.

- Vasopressin (20 units mixed with 100 cc normal saline) is injected into the myometrium surrounding the myoma (Tech Fig. 7.2.2). Depending on the depth of the myoma, tissue blanching and wheal formation may be observed. Hysterotomy is performed using either a monopolar radiofrequency (RF) instrument or an ultrasonic scalpel. For both classes of instruments, the surgical goal is to rapidly incise tissue with the aim of minimizing unintended thermal injury. When using a monopolar instrument, the electrosurgical unit is set to output a low-voltage, continuous ("cut") waveform. The uterine tissue is incised by linear vaporization, a nontouch technique in which RF energy arcs from the tip of the active electrode to the target tissue, leading to rapid tissue division with minimal thermal spread. When using an ultrasonic scalpel, the device's maximum blade excursion setting should be used and care taken to minimize dwell time at the surgical site (Tech Fig. 7.2.3). Incidental bleeding from the serosa and myometrium can be controlled by judicious use of RF or ultrasonic energy. In

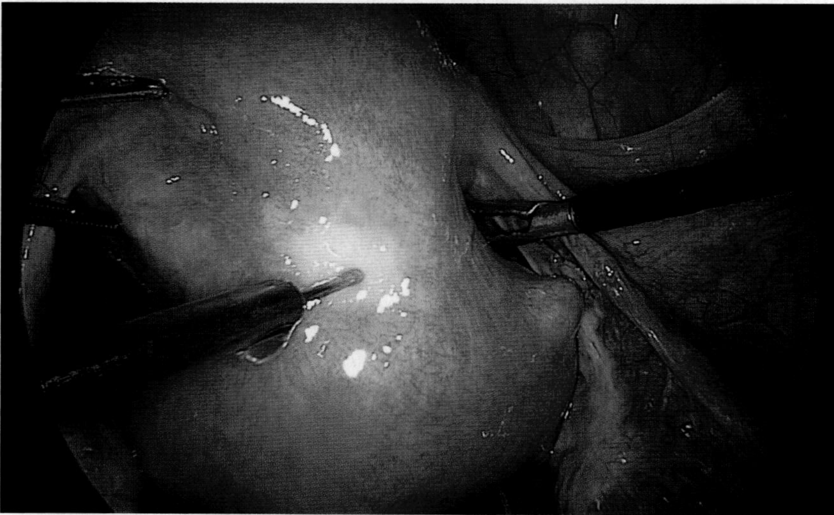

Tech Figure 7.2.2. Injection of dilute vasopressin solution into myometrium surrounding the myoma.

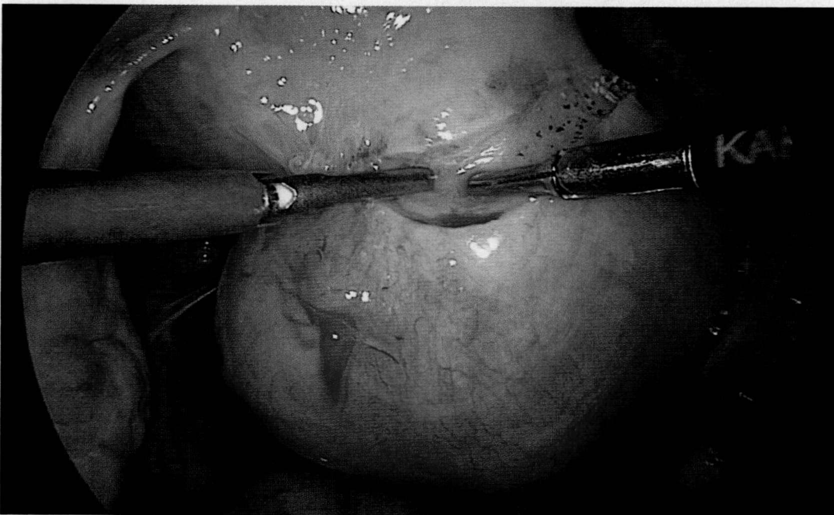

Tech Figure 7.2.3. Hysterotomy performed with ultrasonic scalpel.

general, excessive use of energy devices to control myometrial bleeding is ill advised due to the possibility of tissue necrosis and poor wound healing. If significant bleeding is encountered, hemostasis may be achieved by suture ligation or pressure application. Hysterotomy proceeds until the capsule of the myoma is observed (Tech Fig. 7.2.4).

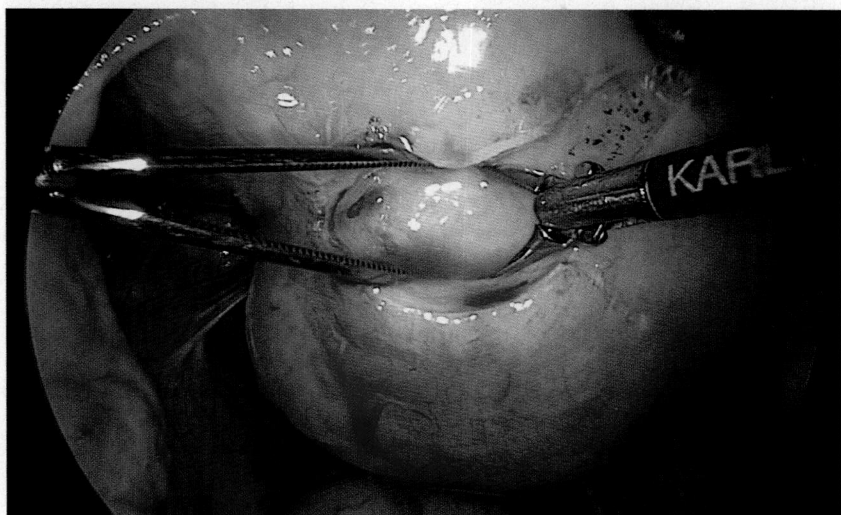

Tech Figure 7.2.4. Exposure of the myoma capsule following hysterotomy.

Enucleation of myoma

- The capsule of the myoma is incised (Tech Fig. 7.2.5) and dissection proceeds between the inner capsule and myoma edge (Tech Fig. 7.2.6). If developing the appropriate plane proves difficult, one can make a shallow incision in the myoma itself, which may help distinguish myoma from capsule. Application of traction on the myoma and countertraction on the capsule provides surgical exposure and aids in the enucleation of the myoma. Once excised, the

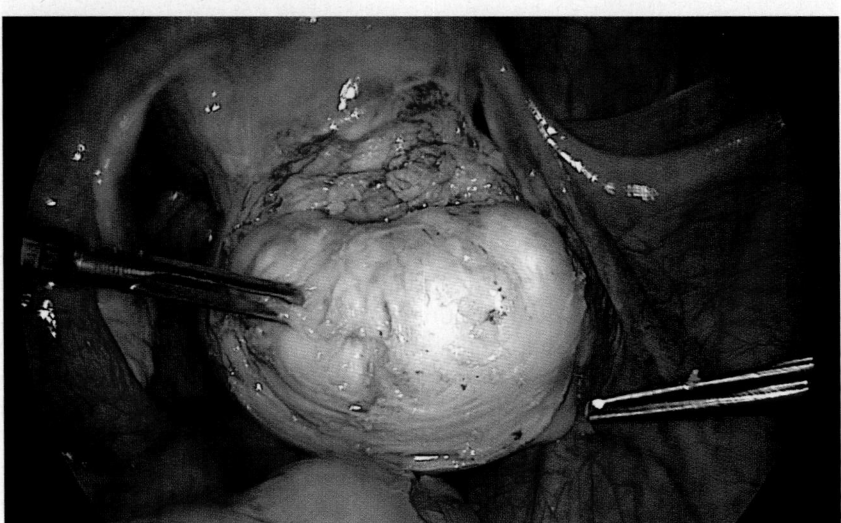

Tech Figure 7.2.5. Exposure of myoma following incision of myoma capsule.

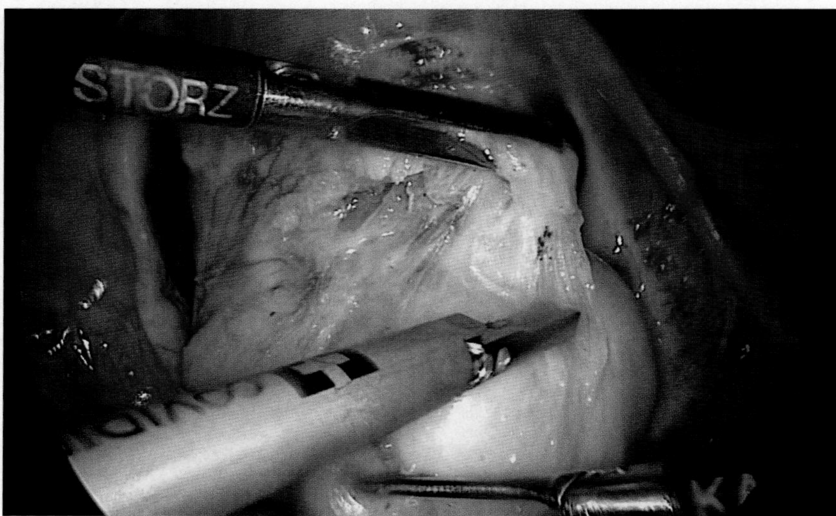

Tech Figure 7.2.6. Enucleation of myoma by dividing tissue investments between myoma and myoma capsule.

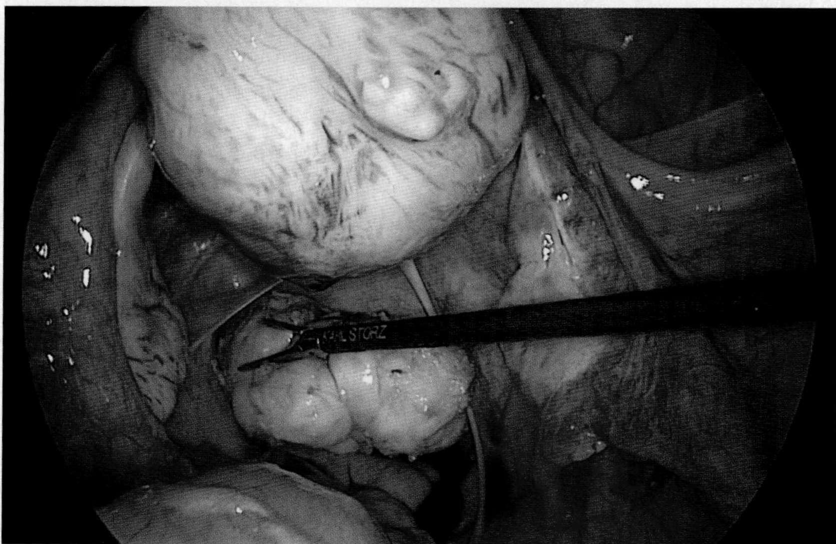

Tech Figure 7.2.7. Stowage of myoma in posterior cul-de-sac for later retrieval.

myoma is placed in the posterior cul-de-sac for later retrieval (**Tech Fig. 7.2.7**). It is important for the surgical team to keep an accurate count of the number of myomas excised to ensure all specimens are extracted from the abdomen at the end of the procedure. The myoma capsule need not be excised. Additionally, incising the endometrium should be avoided if possible. However, entering the cavity is unavoidable in the case of certain submucous myomas. If breach of the endometrial cavity is in question, a solution of methylene blue may be introduced into the endometrium through the uterine manipulator and any defects identified.

Hysterorrhaphy

- Using laparoscopic suturing techniques, the myometrium is approximated in multiple layers using 0 or 2-0 gauge, delayed absorbable suture in running or figure-of-eight fashion. Studies have established that the use of barbed suture is safe and effective for hysterotomy closure, with overall less time required for hysterorrhaphy (Tech Fig. 7.2.8).[13] Care must be taken to effectively approximate tissue and achieve hemostasis, without undue tension being placed on the myometrium which may lead to tissue strangulation. The serosa is approximated using either 2-0 delayed absorbable conventional or barbed suture in simple running or baseball stitch fashion. If the uterine cavity is entered during enucleation of a submucous myoma, the endometrium should be approximated with 3-0 delayed-absorbable, monofilament suture in simple running fashion. Chromopertubation, if indicated, may be performed after hysterorrhaphy completion (Tech Fig. 7.2.9).

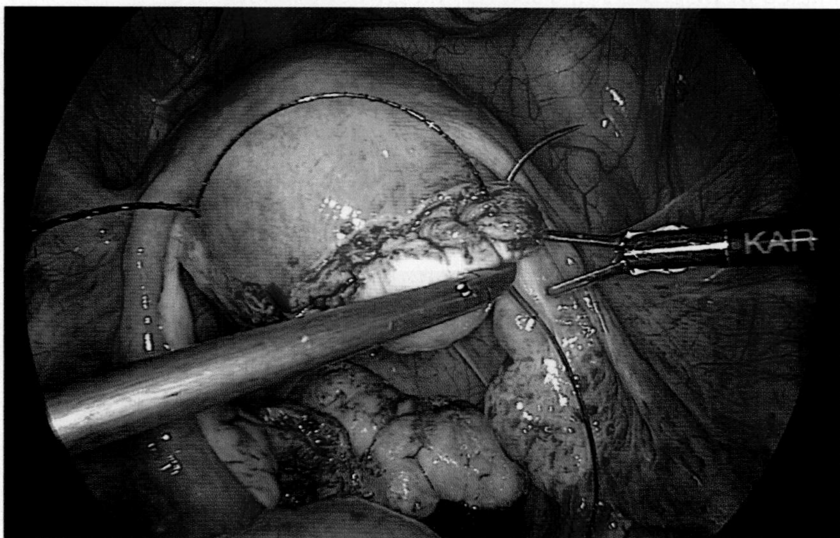

Tech Figure 7.2.8. Hysterorrhaphy using delayed-absorbable barbed suture.

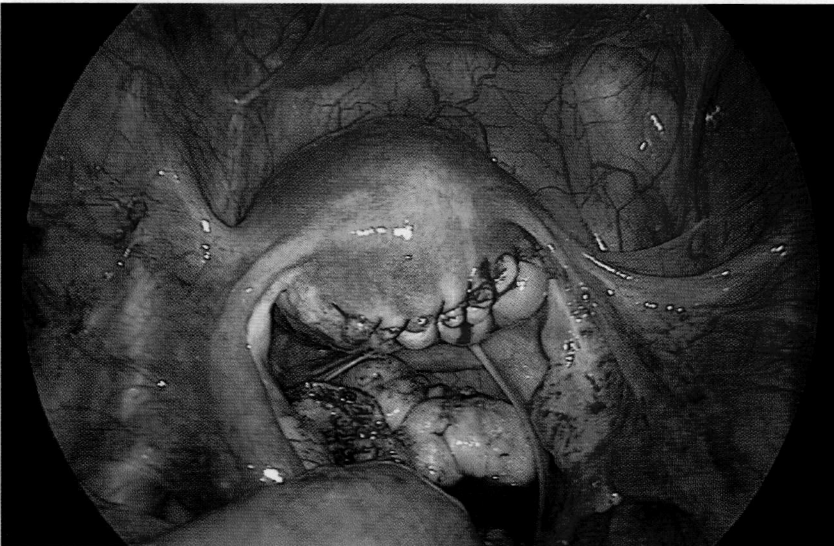

Tech Figure 7.2.9. Completion of hysterorrhaphy.

Myoma extraction

- The FDA has discouraged tissue extraction by laparoscopic power morcellation due to the risk of spreading unsuspected cancer during the process. Multiple groups are evaluating the potential utility of contained electromechanical morcellation, but data are sparse at present. However, other methods are available for extracting myomas following laparoscopic myomectomy.
- Minilaparotomy is efficient and effective for tissue extraction in most cases. Following hysterorrhaphy, the myomas are placed securely in a laparoscopic specimen bag (Tech Fig. 7.2.10). Depending on the patient's anatomy, myoma size, and prior surgical incisions, minilaparotomy is performed either through a transverse Pfannenstiel incision or an extended umbilical incision. The laparoscopic bag is brought through the incision and the myomas are removed (Tech Fig. 7.2.11). Again, it is important to confirm the number of myomas removed matches the number of myomas enucleated. For larger myomas, contained morcellation with a scalpel is feasible and can be facilitated by placement of a self-retaining wound retractor.
- Posterior colpotomy is a reasonable approach for extracting moderate-sized myomas in appropriately selected patients. Again, myomas are carefully placed within a laparoscopic retrieval bag. A posterior colpotomy is made from the medial aspect of one uterosacral ligament to the medial aspect of the contralateral uterosacral ligament using either a monopolar RF or an ultrasonic device. Posterior colpotomy is facilitated by elevating the posterior vaginal fornix cephalad, either by employing a uterine manipulator with a pericervical cup or an assistant

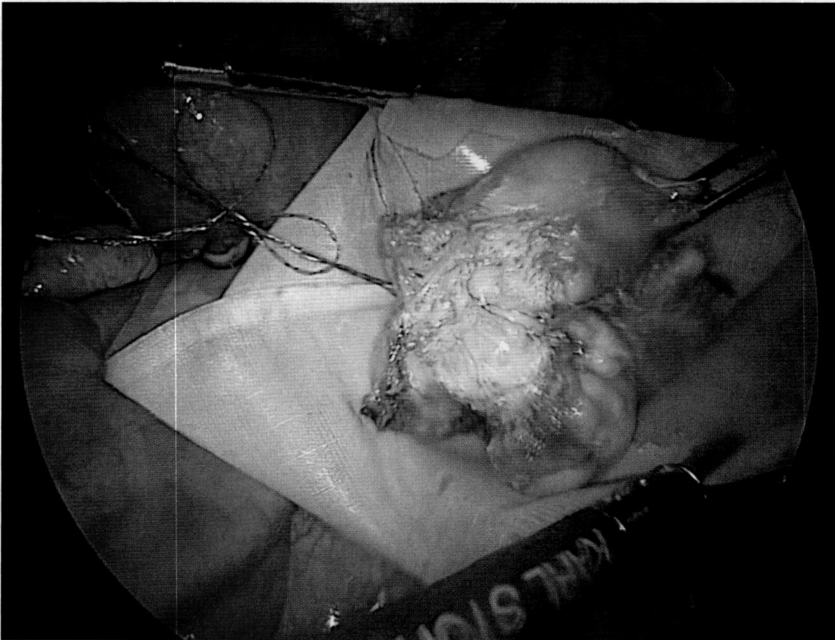

Tech Figure 7.2.10. Collection of myoma in laparoscopic retrieval bag in anticipation of contained transabdominal tissue extraction.

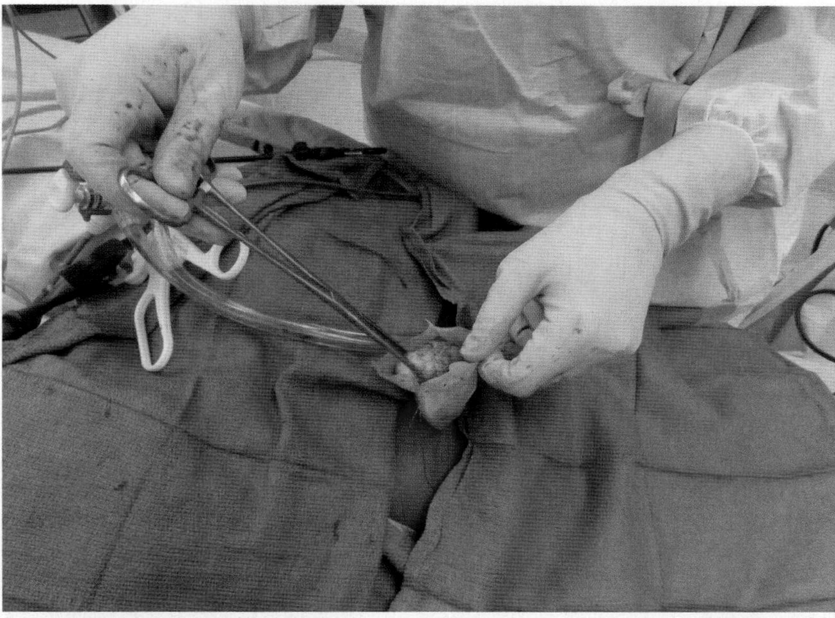

Tech Figure 7.2.11. Extraction of myoma through transverse mini-Pfannenstiel incision.

with a Breisky retractor placed within the posterior fornix (**Tech Fig. 7.2.12**). Ring forceps are introduced through the colpotomy and the string of the laparoscopic retrieval bag grasped (**Tech Fig. 7.2.13**). The myomas counted to confirm all specimens are extracted. The posterior colpotomy is repaired using 2-0 delayed-absorbable suture is running or figure-of-eight fashion using either laparoscopic or transvaginal suturing technique.

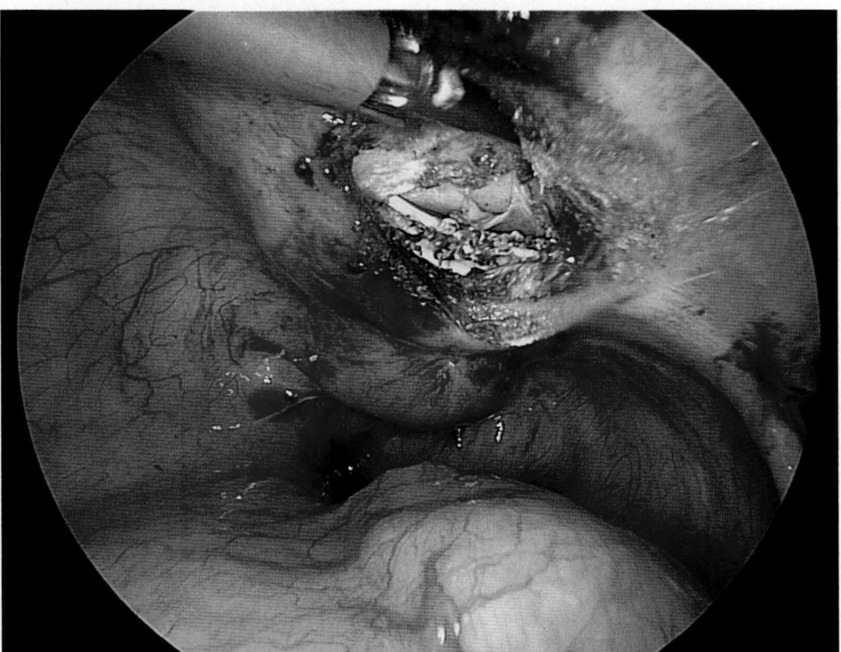

Tech Figure 7.2.12. Posterior colpotomy along pericervical cup.

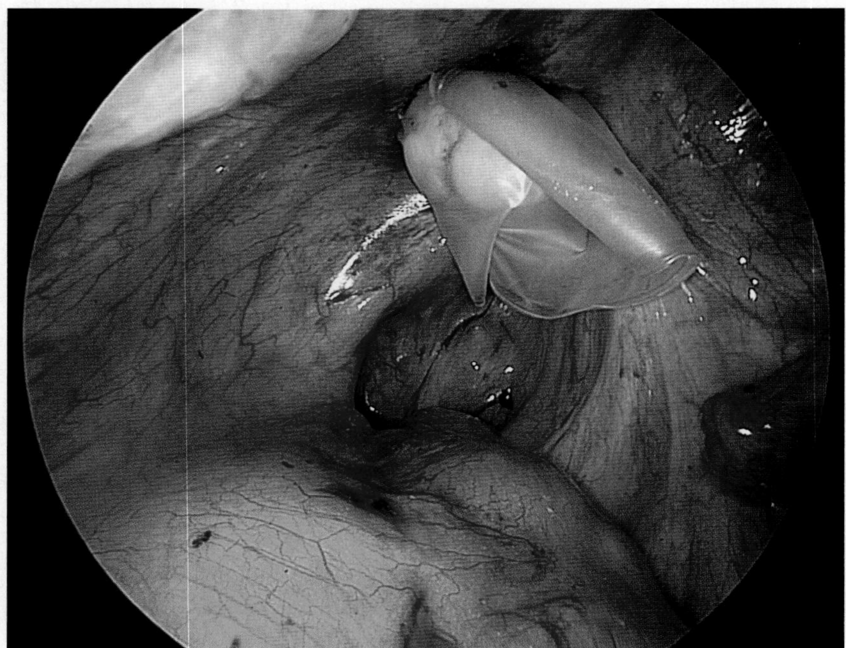

Tech Figure 7.2.13. Extraction of myoma tissue through posterior colpotomy.

Adhesion prevention

- Following tissue extraction, the pelvis is inspected laparoscopically. Meticulous hemostasis is achieved by holding pressure, use of RF energy, suture ligation, or hemostatic agent. An adhesion barrier such as oxidized regenerated cellulose is placed over each hysterotomy to decrease incidence of postoperative pelvic adhesion formation (Tech Fig. 7.2.14).

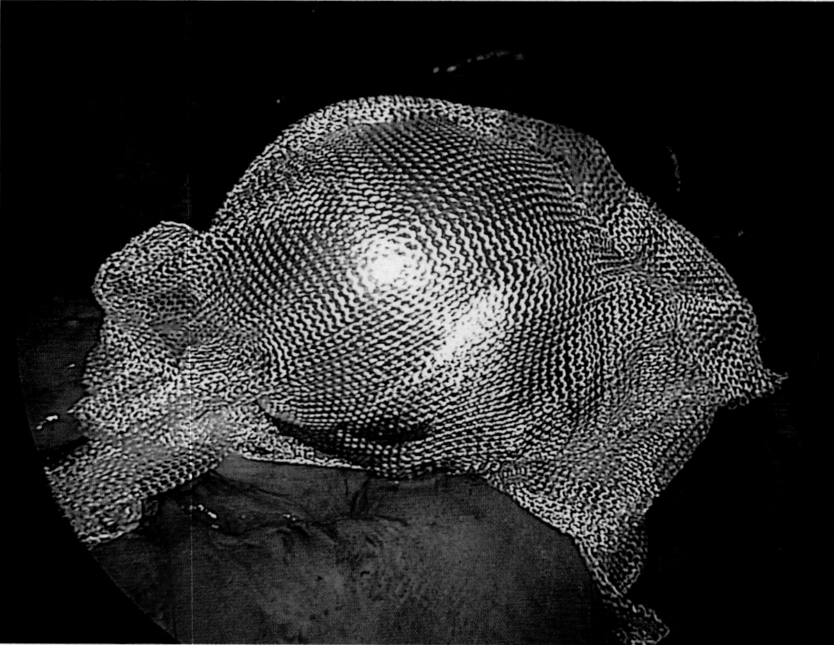

Tech Figure 7.2.14. Oxidized regenerated cellulose placed over hysterorrhaphy site for adhesion prevention.

PEARLS AND PITFALLS

CASE SELECTION

- Laparoscopic myomectomy is associated with a learning curve and perioperative outcomes are dependent on multiple factors. A surgeon should individualize their surgical approach for myomectomy based on factors including myoma size, number of myomas present, and their personal experience and skill level.

BARBED SUTURE

- The use of barbed suture facilitates efficient hysterotomy closure and can reduce the length of surgery in some cases.

UNDETECTED UTERINE PATHOLOGY

- MRI for preoperative evaluation of uterine fibroids is most likely to detect the presence of pathologies such as adenomyosis and sarcoma compared to other imaging modalities and is the preferred method for evaluating a patient considering surgical myomectomy.

POSTOPERATIVE CARE

- Patients who undergo laparoscopic myomectomy can typically be discharged home the same day. Common clinical scenarios that necessitate inpatient management include pain not controlled by oral pain medications, persistent nausea or vomiting, or for perioperative management of comorbidities. Patients are prescribed a narcotic pain medication, stool softener, antiemetic, and nonsteroidal anti-inflammatory medication. Patients are instructed to ambulate as tolerated, but refrain from strenuous activity for 2 weeks. Patients with tissue extraction via posterior colpotomy are instructed to refrain from vaginal intercourse for 6 weeks. Patients are counseled to expect mild uterine cramping and light bleeding per vagina. They are instructed to seek medical attention should they experience intractable pain, unrelenting nausea, fever greater than 38.3°C, excessive vaginal bleeding, lightheadedness, shortness of breath, or syncope. Patients are typically examined at 6 weeks following surgery. We advise patients to not conceive for 3 to 6 months following laparoscopic myomectomy.

OUTCOMES

- Studies report a steady increase in the cumulative recurrence rate of uterine myomas following laparoscopic myomectomy, specifically 11%, 36%, 53%, and 84% at 1, 3, 5, and 8 years, respectively.[14] However, recurrence does not always require further treatment. A study of 114 patients noted that at a 27-month interval after laparoscopic myomectomy, 33% of patients had recurrent leiomyomas; however, only 37% of the patients required additional surgical management.[15]

COMPLICATIONS

- Laparoscopic myomectomy has clear advantages over abdominal myomectomy by avoiding risks associated with laparotomy. A meta-analysis found that mean operative times were 13 minutes longer in the laparoscopic myomectomy group,[16] but the lengths of hospital stay and time required for recovery are significantly lower in laparoscopic myomectomies compared to laparotomic myomectomies. A multicenter study including 2,050 patients reported the total complication rate of laparoscopic myomectomy to be 11.1% with minor complications accounting for 9.1% and major complications for 2.02%.[17] The most serious reported complications were perioperative hemorrhage in 0.68% and postoperative hematomas in 0.48%.[17] A known complication of myomectomy is intra- and postoperative bleeding, and blood loss has been shown to be significantly less in laparoscopic myomectomy compared to abdominal myomectomy.[18]
- The formation of adhesions is a frequently encountered complication following myomectomy. Studies, in which a second-look laparoscopy was performed following laparoscopic myomectomy, have reported intra-abdominal adhesions to be present in up to 66% of women.[19] Adhesion prevention at time of myomectomy should be considered a priority and multiple agents have been found to reduce the rate of adhesion formation, such as oxidized regenerated cellulose, which was noted to significantly decrease the rate of adhesion formation to 12% at the time of second-look laparoscopy, compared to 60% without use of adhesion barrier.[20]
- Intrapartum uterine rupture is a rare and potentially life-threatening pregnancy complication after myomectomy and manifests with symptoms of vaginal bleeding, fetal distress on cardiotocographs, increased uterine contractions, pain, and loss of fetal station. Breach of the endometrium during myomectomy may increase this risk and, as such, women may be offered elective cesarean delivery of a subsequent pregnancy to minimize this risk. Expert opinion suggests that a multilayered uterine closure and avoidance of excessive use of RF energy on the myometrium are appropriate measures to reduce the risk of subsequent uterine rupture after myomectomy.[21] A study evaluated 359 women after laparoscopic myomectomy and 72 women became pregnant resulting in 76 pregnancies in which no case of uterine rupture or dehiscence occurred.[22] The authors supposed that their favorable results may be explained by the meticulous hemostasis that was obtained and by a layered closure of hysterotomies, as well the avoidance of excessive cautery. The true incidence of uterine rupture after myomectomy, whether laparoscopic

or abdominal, is unknown. No data suggest that one suturing technique or material is superior in minimizing this risk of uterine rupture.[23]

- A significant complication associated with minimally invasive myomectomy is dissemination of uterine tissue during enucleation and tissue extraction. Iatrogenic, parasitic myoma formation is a rare complication following myomectomy and has been observed in patients who underwent manual or electromechanical morcellation techniques. The enucleation and extraction of an unsuspected uterine sarcoma may lead to intra-abdominal spread of cancerous tissue and worsen a patient's long-term survival. Presently, the FDA warns that an estimated 1 in 350 women undergoing hysterectomy or myomectomy for treatment of uterine myomas are found to have an unsuspected uterine sarcoma. Patients should be informed of these risks and consent to tissue extraction by morcellation.

KEY REFERENCES

1. Buttram VC Jr, Reiter RC. Uterine leiomyomata: etiology, symptomatology, and management. *Fertil Steril.* 1981;36(4):433–445.
2. Moroni RM, Martins WP, Dias SV, et al. Combined oral contraceptive for treatment of women with uterine fibroids and abnormal uterine bleeding: a systematic review. *Gynecol Obstet Invest.* 2015;79(3):145–152.
3. Kriplani A, Awasthi D, Kulshrestha V, Agarwal N. Efficacy of the levonorgestrel-releasing intrauterine system in uterine leiomyoma. *Int J Gynaecol Obstet.* 2012;116(1):35–38.
4. Felberbaum RE, Germer U, Ludwig M, et al. Treatment of uterine fibroids with a slow-release formulation of the gonadotropin releasing hormone antagonist Cetrorelix. *Hum Reprod.* 1998;13(6):1660–1668.
5. Steinauer J, Pritts E, Jackson R, Jacoby AF. Systematic review of mifepristone for the treatment of uterine leiomyomata. *Obstet Gynecol.* 2004;103(6):1331–1336.
6. Trefoux Bourdet A, Luton D, Koskas M. Clinical utility of ulipristal acetate for the treatment if uterine fibroids: current evidence. *Int J Womens Health.* 2015;26(7):321–330.
7. Smart OC, Hindley JT, Regan L, Gedroyc WG. Gonadotropin-releasing hormone and magnetic-resonance-guided ultrasound surgery for uterine leiomyomata. *Obstet Gynecol.* 2006;108(1):49–54.
8. Gupta JK, Sinha AS, Lumsden MA, Hickey M. Uterine artery embolization for symptomatic uterine fibroids. *Cochrane Database Syst Rev* 2006;25(1):CD005073.
9. Pron G, Mocarski E, Bennett J, Vilos G, Common A, Vanderburgh L; Ontario UFE Collaborative Group. Pregnancy after uterine artery embolization for leiomyomata: the Ontario multicenter trial. *Obstet Gynecol.* 2005;105(1):67–76.
10. Baldoni A, Moscioni P, Colonnelli M, Affronti G, Gilardi G. The possibility of using sulprostone during laparoscopic myomectomy in uterine fibromyomatosis. Preliminary studies. *Minerva Gynecol.* 1995;47(7):341–346.
11. Peitsidis P, Koukoulomati A. Tranexamic acid for the management of uterine fibroid tumors: A systematic review of the current evidence. *World J Clin Cases.* 2014;2(12):893–898.
12. Bhave Chittawar P, Franik S, Pouwer AW, Farquhar C. Minimally invasive surgical techniques versus open myomectomy for uterine fibroids. *Cochrane Database Syst Rev.* 2014;(10):CD004638.
13. Tulandi T, Einarsson JI. The use of barbed suture for laparoscopic hysterectomy and myomectomy: a systematic review and meta-analysis. *J Minim Invasive Gynecol.* 2014;21(2):210–216.
14. Yoo EH, Lee PI, Huh CY, Kim DH, Lee BS, Lee JK, et al. Predictors of leiomyoma recurrence after laparoscopic myomectomy. *J Minim Invasive Gynecol.* 2007;14(6):690–697.
15. Nezhat FR, Roemisch M, Nezhat CH, Seidman DS, Nezhat CR. Recurrence rate after laparoscopic myomectomy. *J Am Assoc Gynecol Laparosc.* 1998;5(3):237–240.
16. Jin C, Hu Y, Chen XC, Zheng FY, Lin F, Zhou K, et al. Laparoscopic versus open myomectomy—a meta-analysis of randomized controlled trials. *Eur J Obstet Gynecol Reprod Biol.* 2009;145(1):14–21.
17. Sizzi O, Rossetti A, Malzoni M, et al. Italian multicenter study on complications of laparoscopic myomectomy. *J Minim Invasive Gynecol.* 2007;14(4):453–462.
18. Palomba S, Zupi E, Russo T, et al. A multicenter randomized, controlled study comparing laparoscopic versus minilaparotomic myomectomy: short term outcomes. *Fertil Steril.* 2007;88(4):942–951.
19. Hasson HM, Rotman C, Rana N, Sistos F, Dmowski WP. Laparoscopic myomectomy. *Obstet Gynecol.* 1992;80(5):884–888.
20. Mais V, Ajossa S, Piras B, Guerriero S, Marongiu D, Melis GB. Prevention of de-novo adhesion formation after laparoscopic myomectomy: a randomized trial to evaluate the effectiveness of an oxidized regenerated cellulose absorbable barrier. *Hum Reprod.* 1995;10(12):3133–3135.
21. Hurst BS, Matthews ML, Marshburn PB. Laparoscopic myomectomy for symptomatic uterine myomas. *Fertil Steril.* 2005;83(1):1–23.
22. Landi S, Fiaccavento A, Zaccoletti R, Barbieri F, Syed R, Minelli L. Pregnancy outcomes and deliveries after laparoscopic myomectomy. *J Am Assoc Gynecol Laparosc.* 2003;10(2):177–181.
23. Frishman GN, Jurema MW. Myomas and myomectomy. *J Minim Invasive Gynecol.* 2005;12(5):443–456.

Chapter 7.3 Robotic Myomectomy

Alexander Kotlyar, Rebecca Flyckt

GENERAL PRINCIPLES

Definition

Uterine leiomyomas are one of the most common problems encountered by the obstetrician/gynecologist with approximately 70% to 80% of reproductive-aged women eventually developing these benign myometrial tumors.[1,2] The majority of leiomyomas do not cause any symptoms and are often only noted incidentally on imaging or surgical pathology. However, as they enlarge, uterine myomas can lead to bulk symptoms, abnormal uterine bleeding, and dysmenorrhea. In a smaller percentage of cases, especially when submucosal fibroids are identified, pregnancy loss and infertility can occur.[3]

Differential Diagnosis

- Uterine adenomyoma or adenomyosis
- Pregnancy
- Hematometra
- Malignancy: uterine leiomyosarcoma or carcinosarcoma
- Endometrial carcinoma or metastases from primary malignancy
- Endometrioma

Anatomic Considerations

When planning a myomectomy, myoma location, number, and size are the key anatomic factors used to determine the most appropriate surgical approach. Uterine myomas are classified as being present just underneath the serosal surface (subserosal), within the myometrium (intramural), or beneath the endometrial lining (submucosal). Fibroids that are completely within the uterine cavity with little intramural involvement are called intracavitary. Submucous myomas can be further subclassified as type 0 (completely intracavitary), type I (>50% of the myoma is intracavitary), and type II (>50% of the myoma is intramural). For myomas that are type 0 or type 1, a hysteroscopic approach is preferred. However, for type II myomas, a nonhysteroscopic procedure is most appropriate.

Nonoperative Management

To treat uterine leiomyomas, multiple nonsurgical strategies are available and these can at times be very successful. These nonsurgical options include expectant management, medical management, uterine artery embolization, and high-frequency magnetic resonance (MR)-guided ultrasonography. The choice of the method is dependent upon judicious consideration of the patient's medical history, desire for future childbearing, risk of malignancy, and the chance for successful outcome based on myoma characteristics.

Medical management typically relies on hormonal methods to reduce abnormal uterine bleeding. Although many women obtain relief, especially when heavy menstrual bleeding is the predominant symptom, the chance for long-term treatment failure is relatively high. The first line in hormonal agents is combined estrogen–progestin oral contraceptives. Although these compounds will not restrict myoma growth or reduce uterine volume, in some patients they can effectively reduce monthly blood loss. Despite the presence of conflicting evidence, some studies have indicated that early exposure to combined oral contraceptives may actually increase the risk of fibroids later in life.[4] Progestational compounds such as depo-medroxyprogesterone and the levonorgestrel-containing IUD are also often used to manage symptomatic uterine fibroids. Although the levonorgestrel IUD is FDA-approved for the treatment of heavy menstrual bleeding, it is not indicated for the treatment of uterine myomas, and in fact, having a myoma with any significant intracavitary component is a relative contraindication to the placement of an IUD. These agents are effective for mild symptoms and help reduce heavy menstrual bleeding via endometrial and uterine atrophy. Lastly, a newer oral nonhormonal formulation (tranexamic acid, an antifibrinolytic) has been used successfully in women with myomas and can reduce the volume of monthly blood loss by up to 30%.

Gonadotropin-releasing hormone (GnRH) agonists are a highly effective treatment for both abnormal uterine bleeding related to myomas as well as bulk symptoms. These agents lead to a hypogonadotropic state which results in a substantial reduction in monthly blood loss within 3 months of administration. It must be noted that following the administration of a GnRH agonist, there is typically an initial increase ("flare") in the release of pituitary FSH and LH stores due to binding of the GnRH agonist to its pituitary receptors. These pituitary receptors subsequently become desensitized, with a resultant decline in FSH and LH secretion and clinical symptoms resembling menopause within a few weeks. Local effects on leiomyomas including direct inhibition of local aromatase p450 expression leading to decreased conversion of androgens to estrogens, which are thought to stimulate myoma growth. In addition, GnRH agonists can suppress myoma cell proliferation and induce apoptosis, which likely underlies their capacity to reduce myoma volume. A reduction in preoperative myoma size can make a laparoscopic approach more feasible and avert the need for laparotomy. GnRH agonists can also be useful for the short-term correction of anemia prior to surgery, as indicated by a Cochrane database review.[5] However, long-term use is not recommended due to the significant side effects of the hypoestrogenic state, such as bothersome hot flushes, and possible osteopenia and osteoporosis. It is not recommended to use these agents for longer than 6 months.[6]

The remaining nonsurgical options, as with medical options, can offer some relief but do also have associated limitations. Uterine artery embolization (UAE) or uterine fibroid embolization (UFE) is the first of these approaches. These methods involve instillation of occlusive material bilaterally into the arteries feeding the myoma beds.[7] This technique is not recommended for women who desire future childbearing as the effects on fertility and ovarian reserve are unclear. A newer method is the use of magnetic resonance imaging-guided focused ultrasound (MRGUS). Using MRI guidance, multiple ultrasound waves are focused to induce local tissue destruction. The latter method is best suited when the leiomyoma cannot be resected via other surgical methods.[6] MRGUS has been associated with complications such as skin burns, fibroid expulsion, and persistent neuropathy; it is not currently widely used.[8]

IMAGING AND OTHER DIAGNOSTICS

As with the evaluation of many forms of pelvic pathology, transvaginal ultrasound is often the initial basic imaging study obtained. Pelvic ultrasound allows for the basic identification and localization of leiomyomas (Fig. 7.3.1). Myomas typically appear as enlarged hypoechoic and/or heterogeneous masses with lobular contours. The amount of fibrous tissue versus smooth muscle tissue determines the degree of hypoechogenicity. Due to mass effects, myomas tend to compress the surrounding myometrial tissue, creating a pseudocapsule and a defined myoma border (Fig. 7.3.2). Due to myoma degeneration and necrosis, internal calcifications can cause shadowing and a

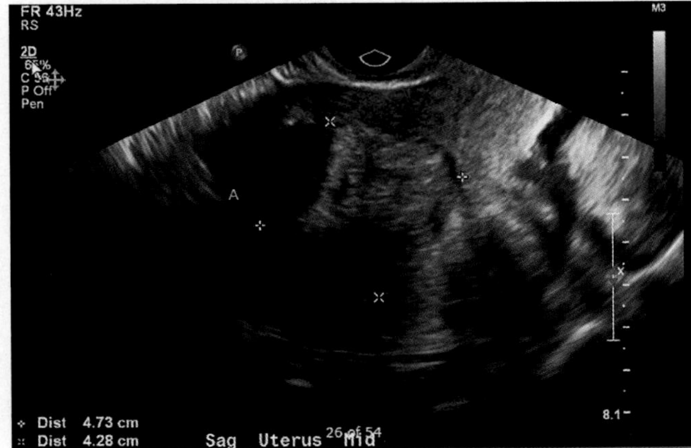

Figure 7.3.1. Transvaginal pelvic ultrasound demonstrating 4 to 5 cm posterior myoma displacing the endometrium anteriorly.

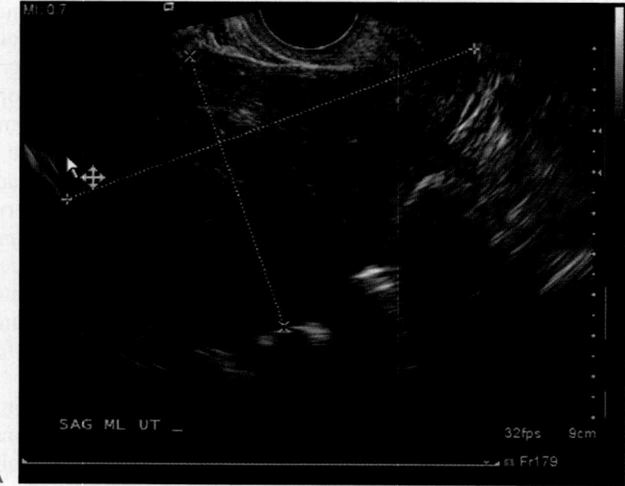

A

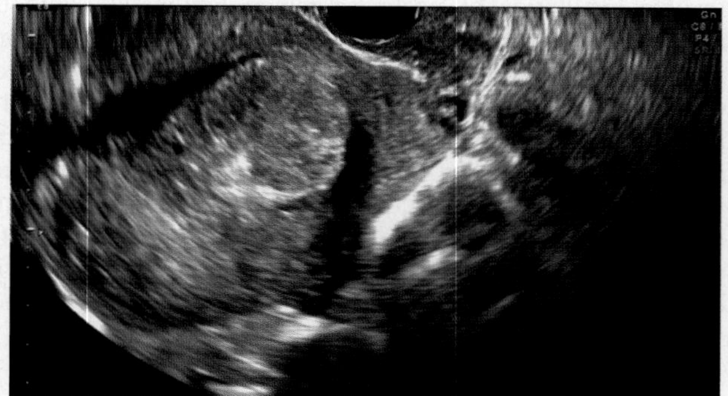

B

Figure 7.3.2. Transvaginal pelvic ultrasound with visualization of posterior myoma but indistinct margins and unclear cavity involvement.

"venetian blind" effect with ultrasound waves. Characterization of submucosal and intramural myomas can be further enhanced with the use of three-dimensional (3D) ultrasound; however, the utility of this feature is dependent on sonographer experience.

To evaluate the uterine cavity, saline infusion sonohysterography (SIS) can be used to determine the degree to which the uterine cavity is occupied or impinged upon by a submucosal myoma. Knowing the degree of penetrance of a myoma can influence the choice of operative approach. SIS has a greater sensitivity and specificity than transvaginal ultrasound (85.4% and 98.2% for SIS, respectively).[9]

Magnetic resonance imaging (MRI) is an additional imaging modality to complement the aforementioned ultrasonographic techniques and is routinely used at our institution to assist in preoperative planning for myomectomy. MRI relies on the use of a magnetic field to change the spin of hydrogen atoms present in tissue and measures the radiofrequency waves emitted by those atoms. The strength of the signal is affected by the number of hydrogen atoms (i.e., the water content of a particular tissue). Water content will affect the tissue's appearance on T1- and T2-weighted images, with tissues with high water content appearing brighter on T2-weighted imaging. T1-weighted images better depict fat and areas of hemorrhage. Myomas classically appear as dark, well-circumscribed areas on T2-weighted images. Cystic degeneration, however, leads to increased brightness in this image sequence.

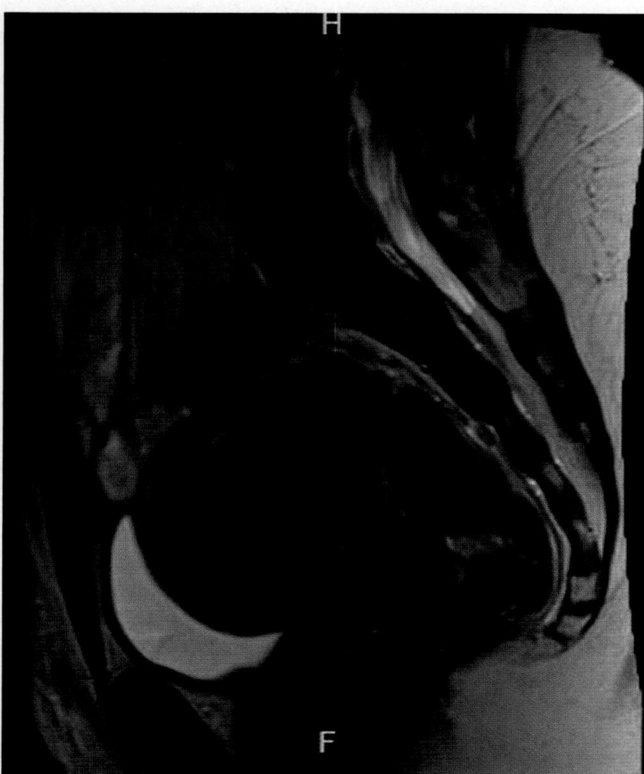

Figure 7.3.3. T2-weighted MRI images provide excellent fibroid "mapping" in preparation for a robotic approach. The endometrial cavity is well visualized using this technique and can be more easily avoided in the interest of future fertility.

MRI is useful for surgical planning, especially if a laparoscopic or robotic myomectomy is desired (Fig. 7.3.3). The advantages of MRI over TVUS is greater sensitivity (80% vs. 40%, respectively), especially when four or more myomas are present. Disadvantages include possible nonidentification of very small myomas (typically less than 0.5 cm^3) and significantly increased cost compared to ultrasound. Computed tomography is typically not used to image myomas given the inferior soft tissue contrast relative to MRI and TVUS. However, it may be useful in identifying ureteric compression if this is a concern.[10]

PREOPERATIVE PLANNING

Prior to performing any type of myomectomy, the surgeon must first address several issues:

- The most common preoperative issue is anemia resulting from heavy menstrual or abnormal uterine bleeding. Given the known bleeding dysfunction associated with uterine leiomyomas, the most common form identified is iron deficiency anemia. Milder forms of anemia can be treated with supplemental iron either in oral or IV form.
- As a second step in preoperative planning, treatment with a GnRH agonist such as leuprolide acetate can be considered for 3 months prior the procedure. This is used either to decrease uterine or myoma volume, or to reduce ongoing abnormal uterine bleeding and anemia.
- Ruling out malignancy is essential prior to performing any myomectomy. Women with risk factors (e.g., greater than

6 months of irregular menstrual cycles or known anovulation, polycystic ovarian syndrome, obesity or insulin resistance, or thickened endometrium) should be sampled to rule out endometrial cancer. This is typically done using office endometrial biopsy to detect any underlying endometrial hyperplasia or cancer.

- It is also essential to obtain appropriate imaging procedures to delineate the dimensions of the uterus and the number, size, and location of myomas, and other pelvic pathology. As outlined above, SIS or MRI is preferred versus traditional transvaginal ultrasonography.

SURGICAL MANAGEMENT

The decision to proceed with surgical treatment for uterine leiomyomas is based upon several factors. These include:

1. Any associated abnormal uterine bleeding or heavy menstrual bleeding that is not responsive to conservative measures
2. Ongoing growth following menopause or any suspicion of malignancy
3. Infertility secondary to distortion of the endometrial cavity or fallopian tubes
4. Recurrent pregnancy loss (especially with known distortion of the endometrial cavity)
5. Diminished quality of life due to pain or pressure symptoms
6. Chronic blood loss leading to ongoing iron deficiency anemia

In choosing robotic myomectomy versus other techniques, multiple factors must be considered as outlined in **Table 7.3.1**.

It is imperative to map the location, size, and relative proximity to the cavity for all uterine myomas. Robotic myomectomy is best suited for patients with subserosal, intramural, fundal, or pedunculated fibroids. It is also most appropriate when the patient has any single myoma less than 15 cm, and if there are five or fewer myomas present in the uterus. The main advantage of robotic myomectomy is the availability of a 3D view of the operative field and ease of instrument maneuvering and suturing. This is especially important for less-experienced surgeons who may find a total laparoscopic approach prohibitive, but who would still prefer to perform the surgery in a minimally invasive fashion. Robotic myomectomy, like other forms of minimally invasive approaches, provides the opportunity for decreased postoperative pain, faster return of bowel function, decreased length of hospital stay, and enhanced cosmesis versus an abdominal approach.[11]

Once the decision has been made to perform the myomectomy in a robotically assisted fashion, the patient is considered for pretreatment with a GnRH agonist. This pretreatment, as for laparoscopic, abdominal, and hysteroscopic approaches, is indicated when it is necessary to correct anemia and/or reduce uterine or myoma volume, but can also be associated with more difficult dissections and poor tissue definition, which can sometimes make a minimally invasive approach more challenging. We do not routinely use GnRH agonists in the absence of anemia when minimally invasive surgery is planned for the above reasons. Surgeons should always consent patients for a possible laparotomy due to bleeding or other intraoperative complications should the need arise.

Table 7.3.1 Comparison of Myomectomy Techniques

Procedure	Indication	Advantages	Disadvantages
Abdominal myomectomy	Large myomas that cannot be removed laparoscopically without significant morcellation or whose size prevents effective visualization and manipulation laparoscopically	Greater exposure and access facilitating hemostasis	Increased recovery time ~6–8 wks, postoperative pain, and increased risk of adhesion formation
Laparoscopic myomectomy	Subserosal, pedunculated or intramural fibroids	Decreased postoperative pain, reduced recovery time (~1–2 min), decreased blood loss given small area of entry	More technically complex, necessitating significant skill in laparoscopic surgery, especially if fibroids are greater than 15 mm
Laparoscopic-assisted myomectomy	Subserosal, pedunculated or intramural fibroids that typically cannot be removed with conventional laparoscopic myomectomy	Reduced recovery time (~1–2 wks), combines ability to use minimally invasive techniques while avoiding morcellation of larger fibroids	Minilaparotomy leads to increased pain postoperatively
Hysteroscopic myomectomy	Submucosal fibroids, especially if >50% is intracavitary	Fastest recovery, lowest cost	Limited spectrum of fibroids that can be resected; risk of fluid overload and electrolyte abnormalities with distension media
Robotic myomectomy	Subserosal, pedunculated, and intramural fibroids. Worthwhile when surgeon has limited comfort with conventional laparoscopic approach	3D view, increased dexterity with robotic instruments. Reduced recovery time (~1–2 wks)	Most expensive method, extended operating times, greater exposure to anesthesia

Positioning

In preparation for a robotic myomectomy, standard laparoscopic equipment is required along with the addition of the patient-side robot, the vision cart, and the robot–operator console.

The patient is positioned as for a conventional laparoscopic case, i.e., in dorsal lithotomy with Allen or yellowfin stirrups with arms tucked at the sides in a neutral position and all bony prominences appropriately padded. A gel pad or other cushioning device is placed underneath the patient to prevent the patient from sliding cephalad along the table while in Trendelenburg. Chest straps can also help in preventing patient drift during the case. Although some texts recommend routine use of maximum Trendelenburg position (as the table cannot be readjusted once the robot is docked if visualization is suboptimal), our experience is to use only as much Trendelenburg positioning as needed to perform the procedure.

Approach

Multiple robotic approaches have been described, including the use of parallel, between the legs, and side docking for gynecologic procedures (which is thought to provide improved access to the uterine manipulator). Our preference is to side dock the robot. In addition, there are various strategies for port placement, with the camera positioned intra-, infra-, or supra-umbilical depending on uterine size and surgeon preference. Our preference is to place the robotic camera intra- or slightly infraumbilically. The use of accessory ports is similarly a matter of surgeon preference and ease of the procedure. Our approach is described below. The most important factor is to determine prior to the procedure what the preferred approach will be, as there is some difficulty in placing additional ports or changing configuration once the robot is docked. Again, imaging and examination is key in preparing these steps.

Procedures and Techniques (Video 7.3)

Since the application of the daVinci robotic surgery system for use in myomectomy, multiple variations in technique have developed. In this section, we will discuss the methods typically used at our institution.

Uterine manipulator insertion

Once the patient has been prepped and draped as for a conventional laparoscopic myomectomy, the uterine manipulator is inserted. This is done to optimize exposure for myoma enucleation as well as to provide a conduit for instilling dye into the uterus to define and avoid the endometrial cavity during close dissection.

We typically place a uterine manipulator such as a RUMI (Cooper Surgical) manipulator. Once the Foley catheter is placed and the cervix is visualized with either a bivalve speculum or Spaniard–Auvard weighted speculum, a single-tooth tenaculum is placed on the upper lip of the cervix for traction and the uterine manipulator is inserted.

To insert the RUMI uterine manipulator, one first sounds the uterus. Then the balloon tip of the RUMI uterine manipulator is inserted through the cervix into the cavity. Once the full length of the balloon tip is inside the endometrial cavity, the balloon is inflated with approximately 7 mL of normal saline. Once the balloon is in place, the uterine manipulator is checked to confirm that it is secure (Tech Fig. 7.3.1).

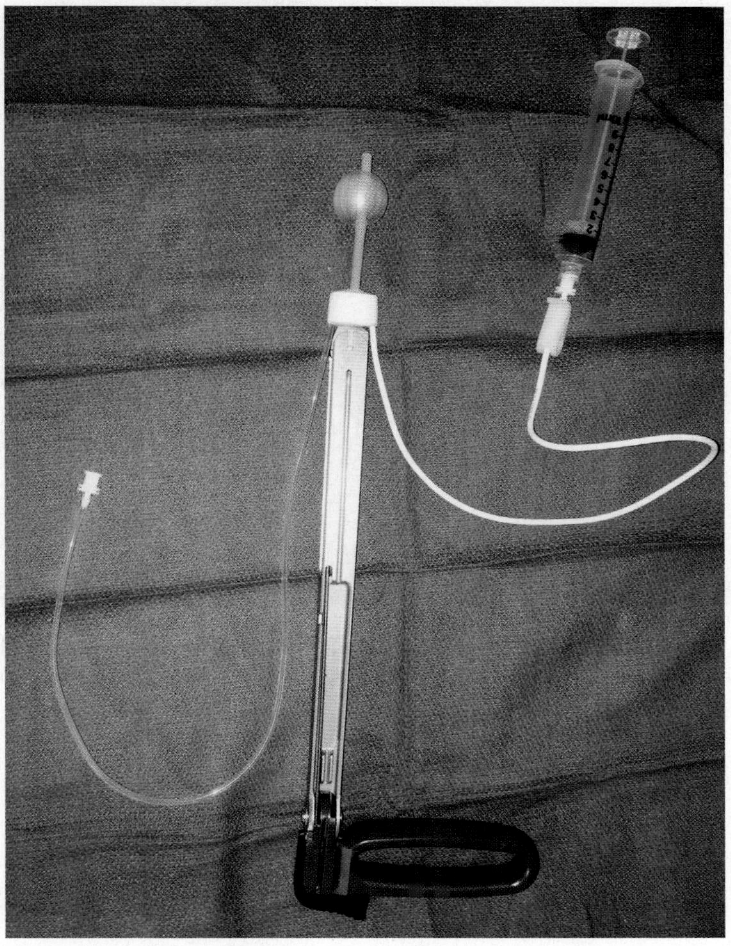

Tech Figure 7.3.1. RUMI and RUMI insertion.

Trocar placement and docking of the daVinci Robot

Trocar sites are placed as depicted in Tech Figure 7.3.2. Prior to insertion of each trocar, 0.25% bupivacaine is injected subcutaneously and an infraumbilical skin incision is made with a size-11 scalpel to allow placement of the umbilical trocar, which will ultimately accommodate the robotic camera. We typically start with a 5-mm trocar to survey laparoscopically and ensure the procedure is appropriate for the surgical robot. Once the initial infraumbilical incision has been made, an optical trocar such as the Xcel trocar (Ethicon) is used to enter the abdomen. If the survey confirms the pelvis is suitable for a robotic approach, we then exchange the 5-mm for a 12-mm trocar which can accommodate the robotic camera.

In addition, two to three 8-mm robotic trocars are placed at an angle approximately 15 degrees inferiorly and 8 to 12 cm lateral to the umbilical port site. An assistant port was then typically placed in the right lower quadrant and it is through this port that needles can be introduced and extracted with direct visualization (Tech Fig. 7.3.2). This arrangement was more prevalent when power morcellation was used for removal of the fibroid. However, given the recent controversy regarding morcellator use, we now place a GelPOINT suprapubically and forego the right lower quadrant accessory port so that the GelPOINT can be used to both pass needles and for tissue extraction at the conclusion of the case. If a suprapubic incision is not desirable, the right lower quadrant accessory port can be used to pass needles and the GelPOINT can be placed into the larger umbilical incision for tissue extraction at the conclusion of the case (Tech Fig. 7.3.3).

Following trocar placement, the daVinci robot is docked. As described earlier, the patient should be placed in deep to maximum tolerated Trendelenburg position. The robot may be placed either in between the patient legs, between each of the stirrups, or on the patient's side. As the robot is advanced toward the patient, each arm is extended at the most proximal joint away from

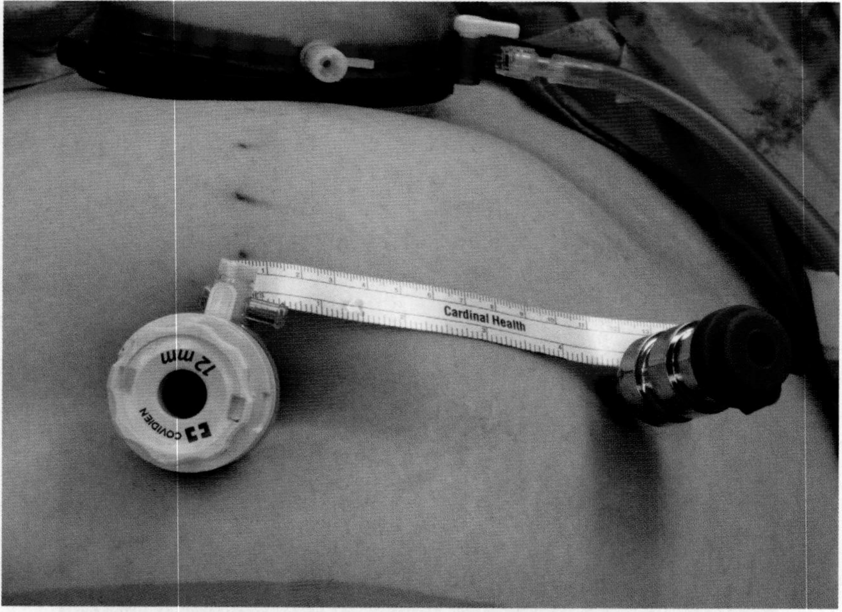

Tech Figure 7.3.2. Trocar placement: From the central 12 mm camera port, accessory robotic ports are placed 8 to 12 cm away to minimize the risk of interference between the camera and the robotic arms.

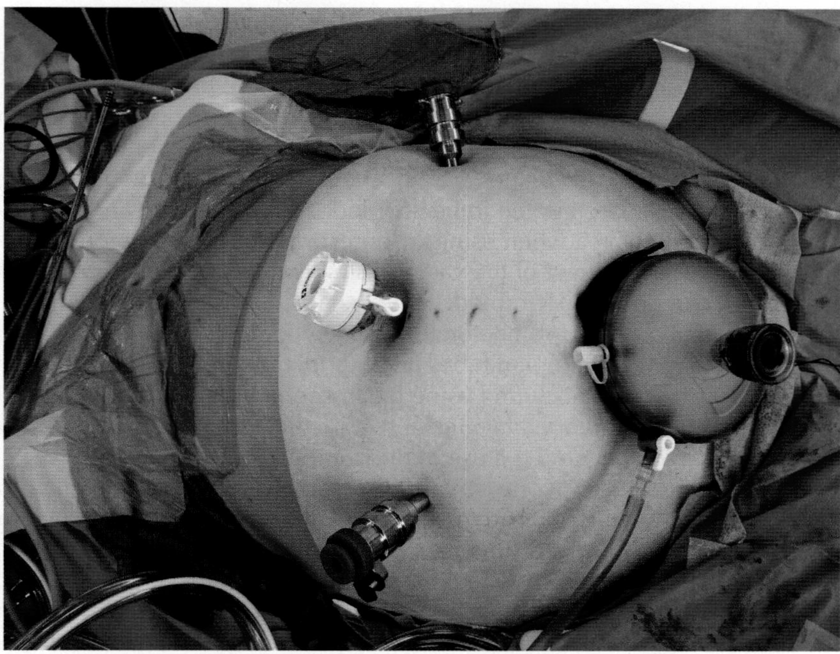

Tech Figure 7.3.3. GelPOINT placement: Note the placement of the GelPOINT in the midline suprapubic position.

the center of the robot. This provides adequate room in between each arm to allow for independent and unhindered movement for each instrument. Once all of the robotic arms are docked, the robotic camera and instruments are inserted into their respective trocars. Our preferred set of instruments include the tenaculum forceps, Maryland bipolar forceps connected to cautery, harmonic shears, and two needle drivers. In our experience, the third arm is rarely needed, especially if a skilled assistant is available to assist using the accessory port (Tech Fig. 7.3.4).

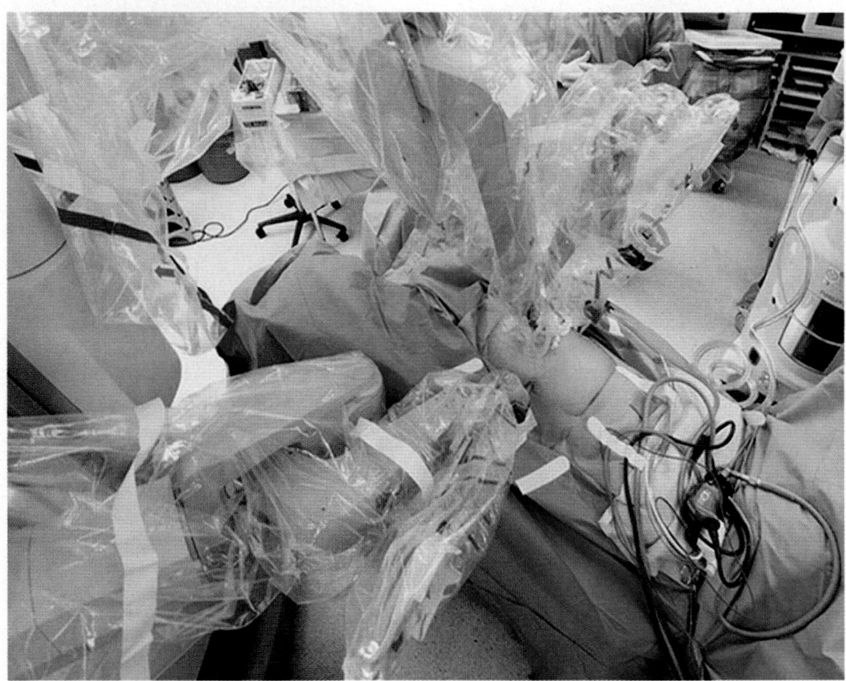

Tech Figure 7.3.4. Picture of robotic ports and placement of robotic arm over trocar.

Hysterotomy

Before making the hysterotomy, a solution of dilute vasopressin (20 units in 200 mL of normal saline) is injected into the serosa and myometrium surrounding the myoma. This is done by using a laparoscopic needle tip device attached to a syringe containing the vasopressin (**Tech Fig. 7.3.5**). Blanching will be noted if the correct planes are achieved. It should be noted that severe cardiopulmonary complications have been noted in healthy individuals such as cardiopulmonary arrest, hypotension, and pulmonary edema when using vasopressin, especially in more concentrated solutions. To further enhance the effect of the vasopressin, ligation of the vascular pedicle during the myoma enucleation can also be performed.[12]

Just as in open and laparoscopic myomectomies, it is key for the surgeon to be aware of the relationship of the myomas to the fallopian tubes and uterine arteries. To further limit bleeding, the uterine arteries can be temporarily occluded using laparoscopic Satinsky clamps. Techniques that have been successfully used are preoperative misoprostol, injection of bupivacaine with epinephrine, preoperative tranexamic acid, and the use of uterine tourniquets.

After injection of dilute vasopressin, one can proceed with the hysterotomy. A harmonic device is first applied with the "cut" setting to make the hysterotomy through the serosa and myometrium until the capsule of the fibroid is opened. The hysterotomy should be made in a horizontal fashion if possible, although suturing can be performed in a vertical plane if needed owing to increased maneuverability of the robotic instruments versus traditional laparoscopy (**Tech Fig. 7.3.6**). It is key to ensure that the hysterotomy not extend to the uterine vessels or fallopian tubes. Maintaining hemostasis is also critical throughout this procedure and bipolar electrosurgery can be used to control any acute bleeding.

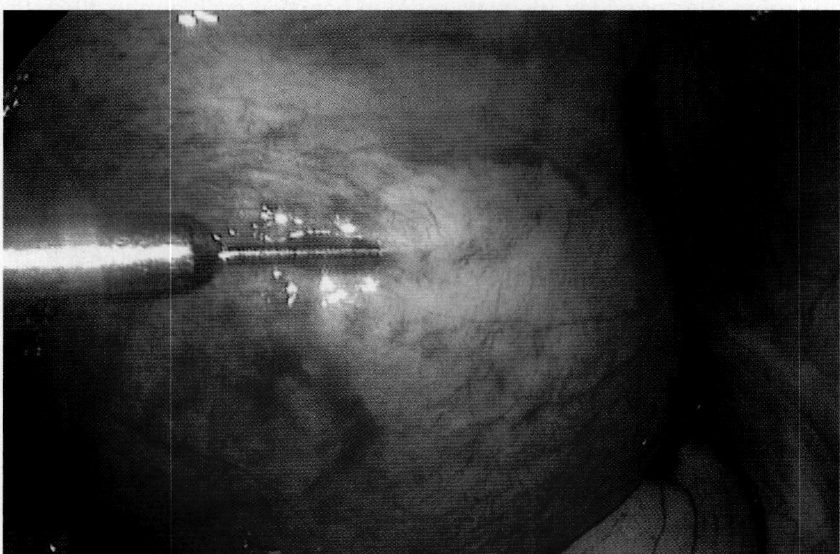

Tech Figure 7.3.5. Injection of vasopressin: A 1:10 dilution of vasopressin is injected in to the myoma bed, note the blanching which arises when injection is performed in the proper plane.

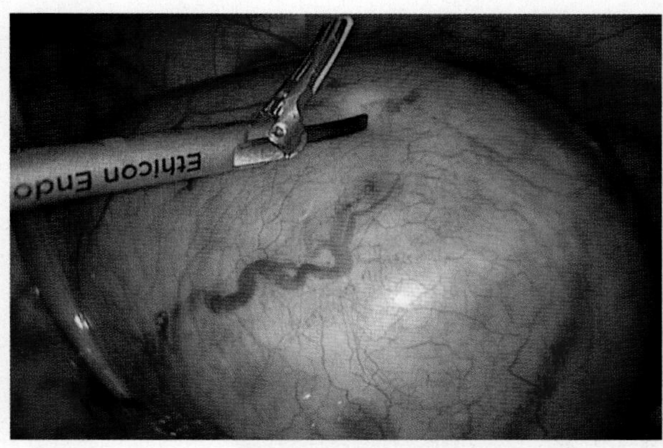

A

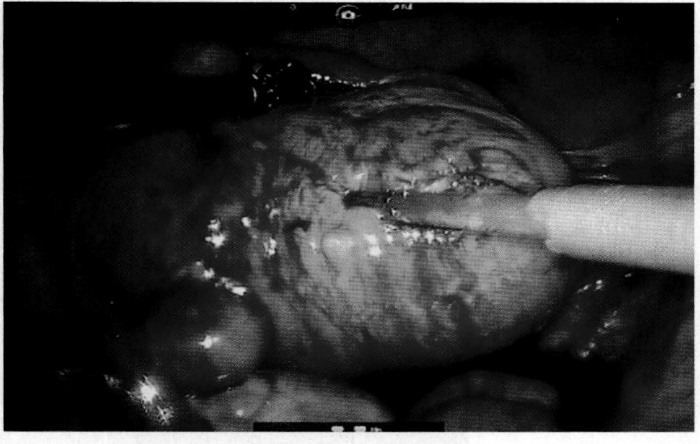

B

Tech Figure 7.3.6. A–B: In making the hysterotomy, a harmonic scalpel is used to cut the serosa and further dissect down to the myoma.

Myoma removal

Once the hysterotomy has been performed and the capsule is entered (exposing the smooth white myoma fibers), a robotic tenaculum is anchored into the myoma. Using blunt dissection, countertraction with the tenaculum, and judicious use of harmonic energy, the myoma is completely enucleated taking care at the base not to approach the endometrium. Once removed, the myomas can either be immediately removed or set aside in the posterior cul-de-sac or paracolic gutters if additional myomas need to be collected (Tech Figs. 7.3.7 to 7.3.9). It is essential that a written account of all the myomas removed be maintained by the surgical team to avoid any retained specimens in the abdomen at the conclusion of the case. It is not unusual that small myomas can roll cephalad and be lost behind the liver or under bowel loops. Discrete areas of myometrial or serosal bleeding can be coagulated using short bursts of bipolar current. Electrosurgery should be limited since excessive coagulation can compromise the integrity of the myometrium and hinder closure of the hysterotomy. It is also possible that excessive electrosurgery in myomectomy repair can relate to subsequent uterine rupture risk with pregnancy. Hemostatic methods that do not rely on cautery are products such as Floseal (Baxter, Deerfield, IL) or Surgiflo (Ethicon, Inc), which are frequently used by our group. These can be used as needed to maintain optimal hemostasis.

Pedunculated myomas are managed in a similar way. However, instead of subserosal injection of vasopressin, this injection is done into the stalk avoiding direct intravascular injection of vasopressin as much as possible. The myoma is removed by transecting the stalk using any number of methods of coagulation; our preference is to use the Ligasure device (Covidien) in such cases. Additionally, the remaining vascular pedicle can be oversewn at the conclusion to ensure hemostasis.

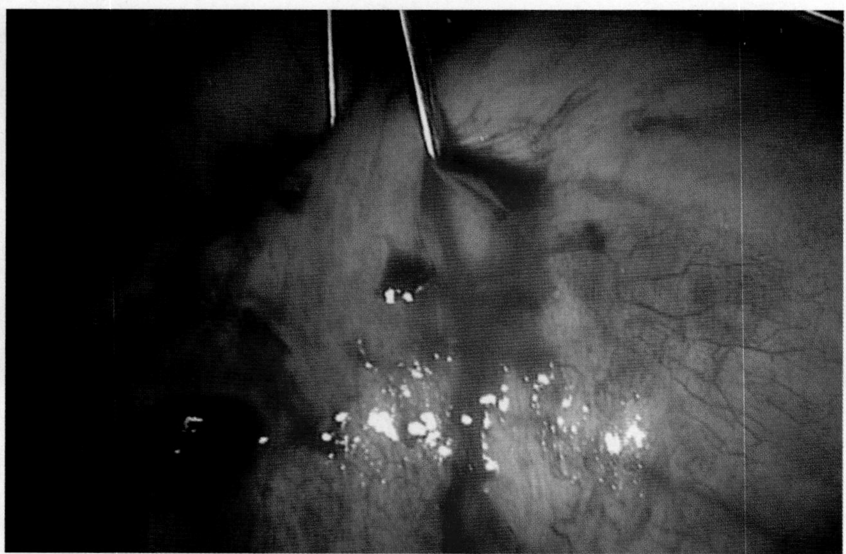

Tech Figure 7.3.7. During enucleation, traction is placed on the myoma using a laparoscopic tenaculum placed through the GelPOINT port.

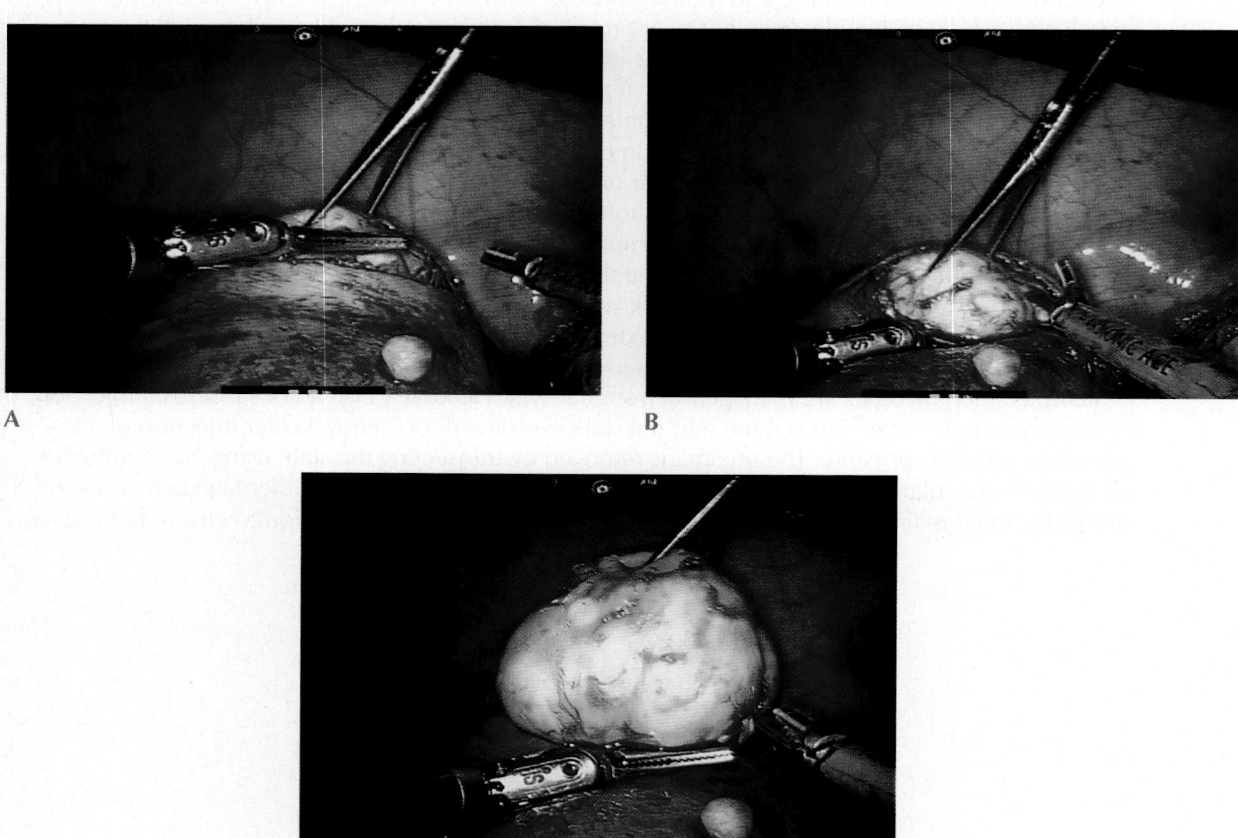

Tech Figure 7.3.8. A–C: Further enucleation using traction and countertractions. Hemostasis is maintained using the harmonic scalpel and bipolar electrosurgery.

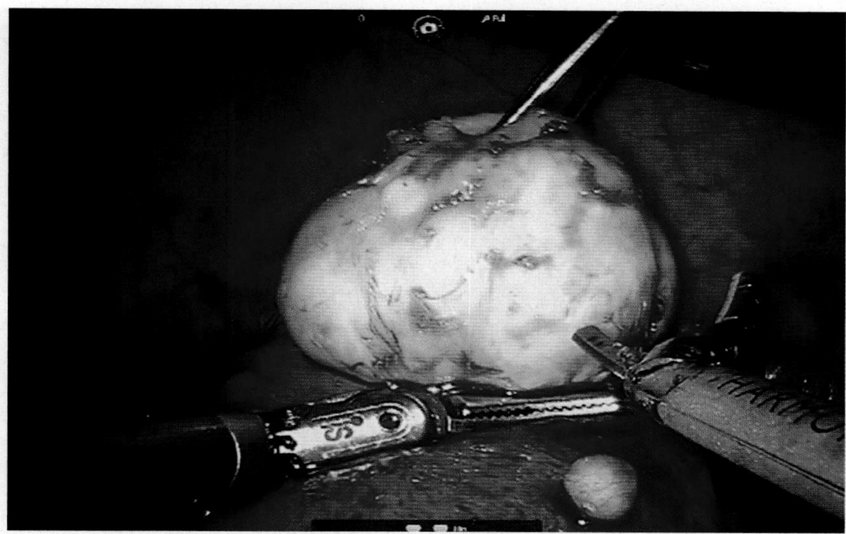

Tech Figure 7.3.9. Note the almost completely enucleated myoma with only a single pedicle of tissue remaining.

Deep intramural myomas and myomas of the broad ligament require the greatest amount of laparoscopic skill and especially skills at laparoscopic suturing. Furthermore, with myomas of the broad ligament, it is essential to maintain awareness of the position of the ureter and uterine vessels. Preoperative MRI can identify these myomas and these should be approached by surgeons skilled in advanced robotics, pelvic anatomy, and minimally invasive surgery.

Hysterotomy closure

Quick closure of the hysterotomy is essential for limiting blood loss during a myomectomy procedure. In this context, robotic surgery may offer advantages over the conventional laparoscopic approach given the increased ease and speed of suturing. This is especially important for surgeons with less experience in laparoscopic suturing and knot tying. Hysterotomy closure can be further facilitated via the use of barbed or quilled absorbable suture materials such as V-Loc™ (Covidien, Mansfield, MA) and Quill™ SRS (Angiotech Pharmaceuticals Inc., Vancouver, BC, Canada). These barbed sutures eliminate the need for the surgeon to tie knots and the barbs help distributed tension along the whole length of the suture (**Tech Figs. 7.3.10** to **7.3.12**).[13]

Regardless of the suture being used, hysterotomy closure is done in a manner similar to that of an open myomectomy. The closure is performed in several layers. If not using barbed suture, the deep layer is performed with either an interrupted or a running, locked technique using 0-polyglactin. Additional layers are placed as needed for approximation of tissue and strength. Once the uterus is well re-approximated, the uterine serosa is then closed using a running stitch of 2-0 or 3-0 polydioxanone. All sutures are initially introduced using the accessory port for suture passage. To help reduce the likelihood of adhesions, we typically place Interceed over the serosal defect if the incision line is completely hemostatic. Floseal or Surgiflo may also be used at this point in the case if there is ongoing diffuse oozing, but in those cases Interceed is not advised as it can increase adhesion formation in the setting of blood.

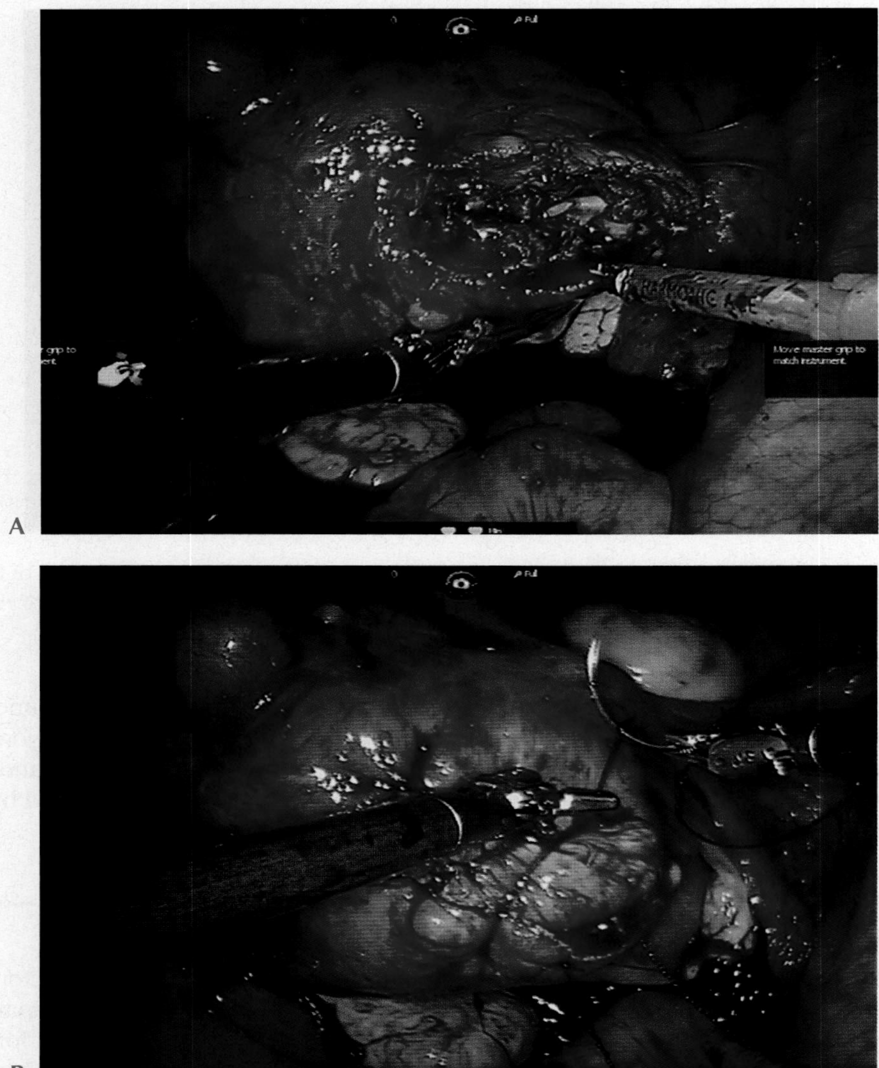

Tech Figure 7.3.10. **A:** Myoma bed following complete enucleation and prior to suturing. **B:** Start of hysterotomy closure with first layer using a single V-Loc suture. This initial layer is placed in a running, locked fashion.

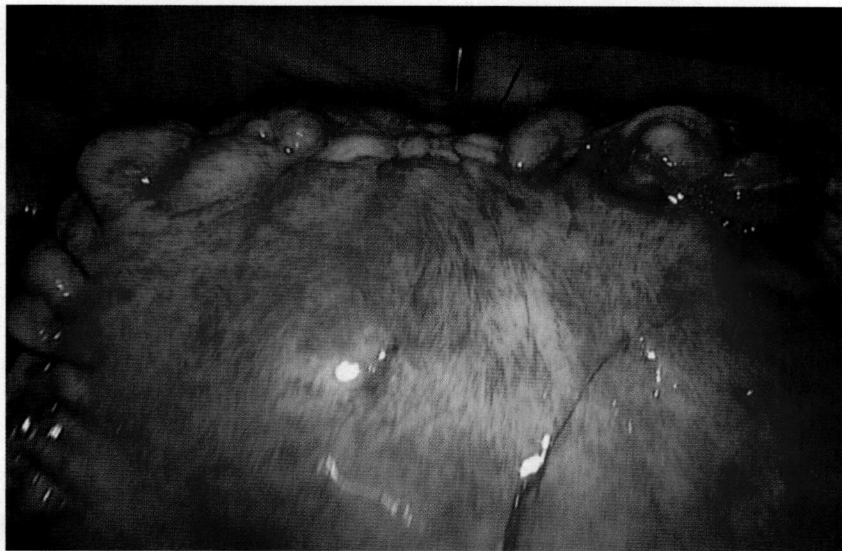

Tech Figure 7.3.11. Serosal closure is achieved using an additional V-Loc suture placed in a running, but unlocked fashion.

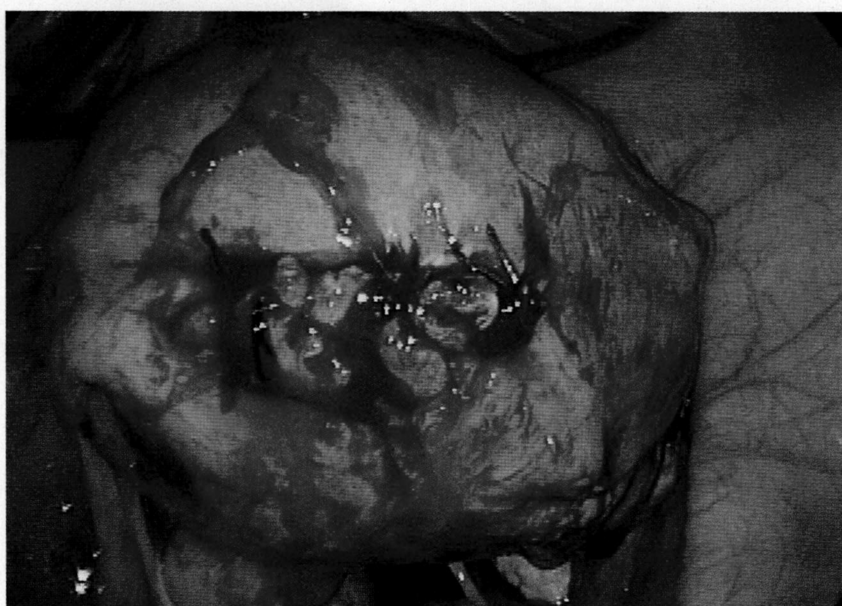

Tech Figure 7.3.12. Complete serosal stitch and completion of hysterotomy closure.

Myoma morcellation

Prior to a moratorium placed by the FDA on power morcellation in 2014, this technique was commonly used for tissue extraction at the conclusion of the case. The moratorium was placed based upon the risk of occult leiomyosarcoma in a morcellated specimen (which is approximately 1/300 to 1/500). Our current approach is to completely avoid power morcellation and use a suprapubically placed GelPOINT device for tissue extraction (Applied Medical, Rancho Santa Margarita, CA). Once all of the myomas have been removed from the uterus, the myomas are extracted either intact or via morcellation using a scalpel at the level of the skin incision where the GelPOINT device was placed. It should be noted that this incision is limited to 2 to 3 cm, so it is not a large additional incision and it is placed in a cosmetic location within the natural hairline (Tech Fig. 7.3.13). Some surgeons are performing this type of morcellation contained in a tissue extraction bag. There is no data as to whether these techniques alter the prognosis of a leiomyosarcoma once diagnosed.

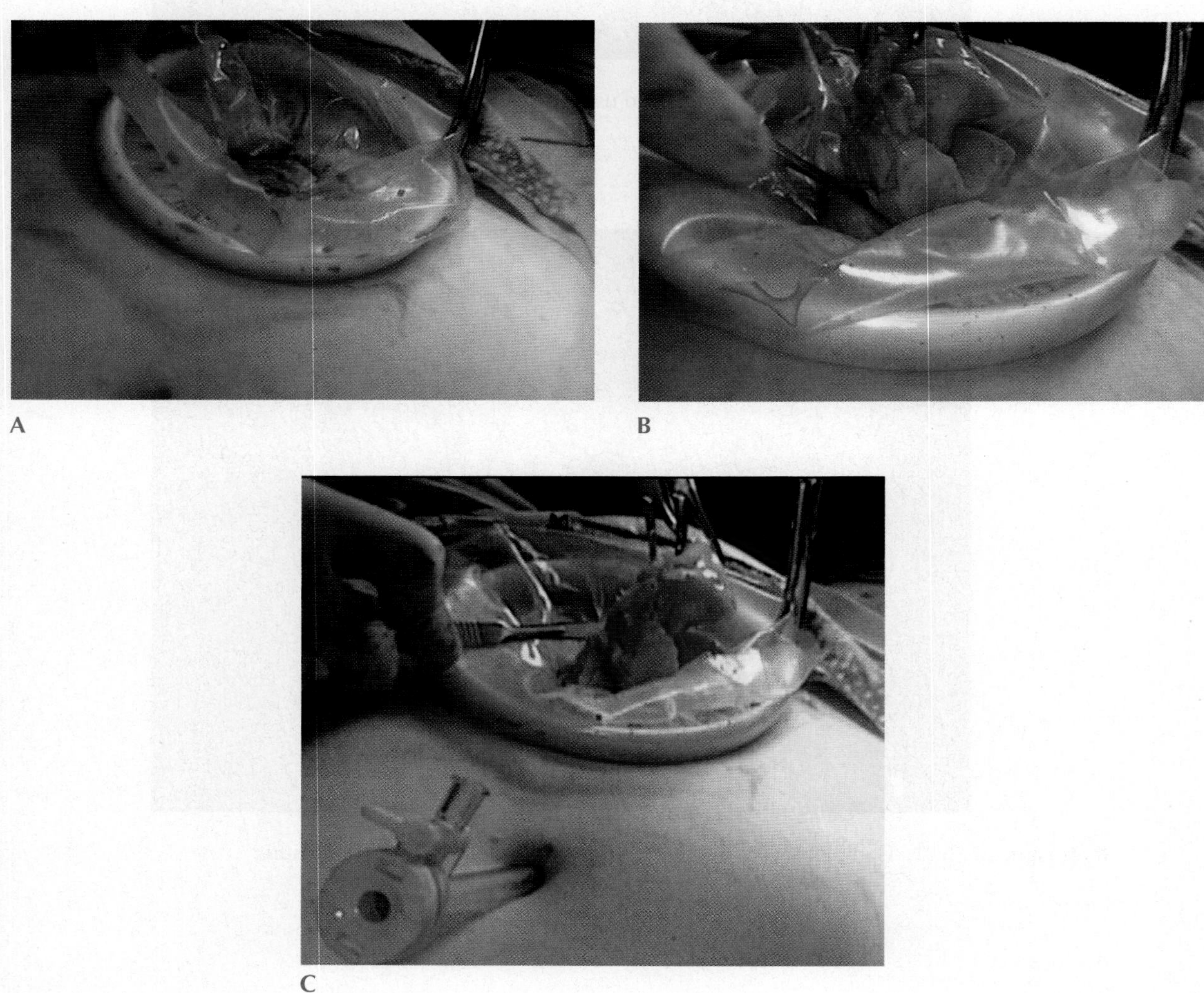

Tech Figure 7.3.13. **A–C:** Contained manual morcellation of the specimen within a bag at the level of the minilaparotomy site.

Robot undocking and closure

Once all the myomas have been removed and adequate hemostasis has been achieved, the rocked can be undocked. This is done by unlocking each of the robotic arms from each trocar by unclasping the distal arm knobs shown previously. Once each arm has been freed, the robot can be pulled away from the patient and each trocar can be removed under visual guidance. For any port larger than 10 mm, we typically close the fascia using a Carter–Thomason (Cooper Surgical) port closure device. Subcutaneous closure of the port sites is performed with interrupted stitches of 2-0 Polysorb. Skin closure can be performed with 4-0 or 5-0 absorbable suture, steri-strips, or surgical glue per the preference of the individual surgeon.

PEARLS AND PITFALLS

- O Address the patient's anemia prior to surgery. Anemia and uterine bulk can be minimized by administering a GnRH agonist 3 months prior to the myomectomy.
- ✖ If more than five fibroids are present or if there is a single myoma greater than 12 to 15 cm, consider an alternative to robotic myomectomy for all but the most skilled surgeons.
- O Most surgeons should only consider robotic myomectomy for a patient with a limited number of fibroids that are only subserosal, pedunculated, or intramural.
- ✖ Avoid power morcellation given the risk of malignancy and current FDA moratorium.
- O Limit operative blood loss using dilute vasopressin injection prior to hysterotomy.
- ✖ Consider cost and OR time when suggesting a robotic myomectomy and compare costs within your institution.
- O Use barbed suture such as a V-Loc to evenly distribute the tension on the suture and close the hysterotomy more quickly without the need to tie knots.
- O To remove the fibroids, perform a suprapubic minilaparotomy using a GelPOINT wound retractor which can double as an assistant port.
- ✖ Beware excessive use of cautery on the incision; instead select hemostatic agents such as FloSeal.

POSTOPERATIVE CARE

Postoperative treatment is identical for that of laparoscopic myomectomies. The main goal remains early mobilization and likely discharge later on the day of surgery or the following morning. During the follow-up appointment, it should be reviewed that due to her myomectomy, she may be at increased risk for uterine rupture. In counseling patients on their reproductive futures, a discussion should be initiated regarding potential recommendations for cesarean section depending on the extent of the dissection and disruption of myometrium. Recommendations should be made in the operative report for obstetricians to review.

OUTCOMES

Overall robotic myomectomy has favorable outcomes in comparison to laparoscopic myomectomy and especially to abdominal myomectomy. In our center's published experience, robotic myomectomy led to decreased blood loss compared with conventional laparoscopy and abdominal myomectomy, albeit with an increased surgical time.[14] Multiple studies have shown increased cost associated with the robotic approach; however, robotic surgery may afford opportunities for minimally invasive myomectomy to surgeons who otherwise would require an open procedure to complete the case. Long-term outcomes such as recurrence, fertility, and obstetric endpoints have yet to be determined.

COMPLICATIONS

In general, robotic myomectomy has a highly favorable complication profile. This is owing to the minimally invasive approach underlying this surgery. In our experience, operative blood loss is lower than for laparoscopic myomectomy and especially when compared with abdominal myomectomy.

KEY REFERENCES

1. Buttram VC Jr, Reiter RC. Uterine leiomyomata: etiology, symptomatology, and management. *Fertil Steril.* 1981;36:433–445.
2. Day Baird D, Dunson DB, Hill MC, Cousins D, Schectman JM. High cumulative incidence of uterine leiomyoma in black and white women: ultrasound evidence. *Am J Obstet Gynecol.* 2003;188:100–107.
3. Fernandez H, Sefrioui O, Virelizier C, Gervaise A, Gomel V, Frydman R. Hysteroscopic resection of submucosal myomas in patients with infertility. *Hum Reprod.* 2001;16:1489–1492.
4. Marshall LM, Spiegelman D, Goldman MB. A prospective study of reproductive factors and oral contraceptive use in relation to the risk of uterine leiomyomatas. *Fertil Steril.* 1998;70(3):432–439.
5. Lethaby A, Vollenhoven B, Sowter M. Pre-operative GnRH analogue therapy before hysterectomy or myomectomy for uterine fibroids. *Cochrane Database Syst Rev.* 2001;(2):CD000547.
6. Wallach EE, Vlahos NF. Uterine myomas: an overview of development, clinical features, and management. *Obstet Gynecol.* 2004;104(2):393–406.
7. Gupta JK, Sinha A, Lumsden MA, Hickey M. Uterine artery embolization for symptomatic uterine fibroids. *Cochrane Database Syst Rev.* 2012;(5):CD005073.
8. Quinn SD, Vedelago J, Gedroyc W, Regan L. Safety and five-year re-intervention following magnetic resonance-guided focused ultrasound (MRgFUS) for uterine fibroids. *Eur J Obstet Gynecol Reprod Biol.* 2014;182:247–251.
9. Grimbizis GF, Tsolakidis D, Mikos T, et al. A prospective comparison of transvaginal ultrasound, saline infusion sonohysterography, and diagnostic hysteroscopy in the evaluation of endometrial pathology. *Fertil Steril.* 2010;94:2720–2725.
10. Swayder J, Sakhel K. Imaging for uterine myomas and adenomyosis. *J Minim Invasive Gynecol.* 2014;21(3):362–376.
11. Flyckt R, Falcone T. Myomectomy: surgical approaches. *Female Patient.* 2011;36:24–32.
12. Soto E, Flyckt R, Falcone T. Endoscopic management of uterine fibroids: an update. *Minerva Gynecol.* 2012;64(6):507–520.
13. Quass A, Einarsson JI, Srouji S, Garguilo A. Robotic myomectomy: a review of indications and techniques. *Rev Obstet Gynecol.* 2010;3(4):185–191.
14. Barakat EE, Bedaiwy MA, Zimberg S, Nutter B, Mossier M, Falcone T. Robotic-assisted, laparoscopic abdominal myomectomy: a comparison of surgical outcomes. *Obstet Gynecol.* 2011;117(2):256–265.

Hysterectomy

8

Chapter 8.1 Abdominal Hysterectomy

Stephanie Ricci

GENERAL PRINCIPLES

Definition

Abdominal hysterectomy is defined as the surgical removal of the uterus via a laparotomy incision. A total hysterectomy removes both the uterus and cervix. A subtotal or supracervical hysterectomy removes the uterus only. The ovaries may remain *in situ* for both kinds of hysterectomy. The decision to retain or excise ovaries is a complex decision to be made by the patient and her physician after extensive counseling.

Differential Diagnosis

- Uterine leiomyomas
- Abnormal uterine bleeding
- Endometriosis
- Pelvic inflammatory disease
- Pelvic organ prolapse
- Malignant or premalignant disease

Nonoperative Management

Alternative therapies to surgical management are highly dependent on the underlying disease. For example, symptomatic uterine fibroids can be treated with uterine fibroid embolization techniques. Endometrial ablation or intrauterine progestin delivering devices are often used to reduce menorrhagia. Similarly, medical therapy including progesterone and gonadotropin-releasing hormone agonist regimens are used to treat pelvic pain caused by endometriosis. Progestins are also used in the treatment of endometrial hyperplasia in select cases. Furthermore, the need for surgical treatment of pelvic organ prolapse can sometimes be mitigated with the use of pelvic floor strengthening exercises.

IMAGING AND OTHER DIAGNOSTICS

- Depending upon the reason for hysterectomy, the use of preoperative imaging and diagnostics will differ. For surgical planning of an abdominal hysterectomy, the best tool to determine uterine size in addition to pelvic examination is pelvic ultrasound. This imaging provides an inexpensive and accurate assessment of uterine size, endometrial stripe thickness, and the adnexa. For peri- or postmenopausal women who are undergoing hysterectomy for abnormal uterine bleeding, preoperative endometrial sampling to rule out malignancy is imperative. Unless malignancy is suspected, the use of pelvic MRI prior to abdominal hysterectomy for benign disease is unlikely to provide additional information.

PREOPERATIVE PLANNING

- It is essential to have a comprehensive discussion with the patient regarding perioperative complication risk, choice of abdominal incision, and whether the ovaries, fallopian tubes, and cervix will be removed. These decisions should be well documented both in the patient's medical record as well as on the surgical consent form. The patient should be counseled that decisions made preoperatively are subject to change intraoperatively for patient safety.
- Preoperative optimization strategies for women undergoing gynecologic surgery include medical consultation for patients with medical comorbidities and regarding perioperative medication management, pregnancy testing in all women of reproductive age, up-to-date screening with pap testing, mammography and colonoscopy, and endometrial sampling in perimenopausal/postmenopausal women with abnormal uterine bleeding. Further testing with EKG and CXR are recommended for women >50 years. Laboratory testing including complete blood count, electrolytes, creatinine, and type and screen are not required, however, may be useful in the postoperative setting.
  - The *type of abdominal incision* is based on several factors that include uterine size and the anticipation of anatomic abnormality such as extensive adhesions. If a woman has a prior vertical abdominal scar, most surgeons prefer to use this incision (Figs. 8.1.1 and 8.1.2). However, if uterine size and the absence of adhesiophylic pathology permit, a transverse abdominal incision is a good option that improves cosmesis and decreases both postoperative pain and the incidence of incisional hernias. Although earlier studies demonstrated an increase in vertical incision dehiscence rates, compared to transverse abdominal incision, more recent studies have found no difference in dehiscence rates between these two incisions.[1]

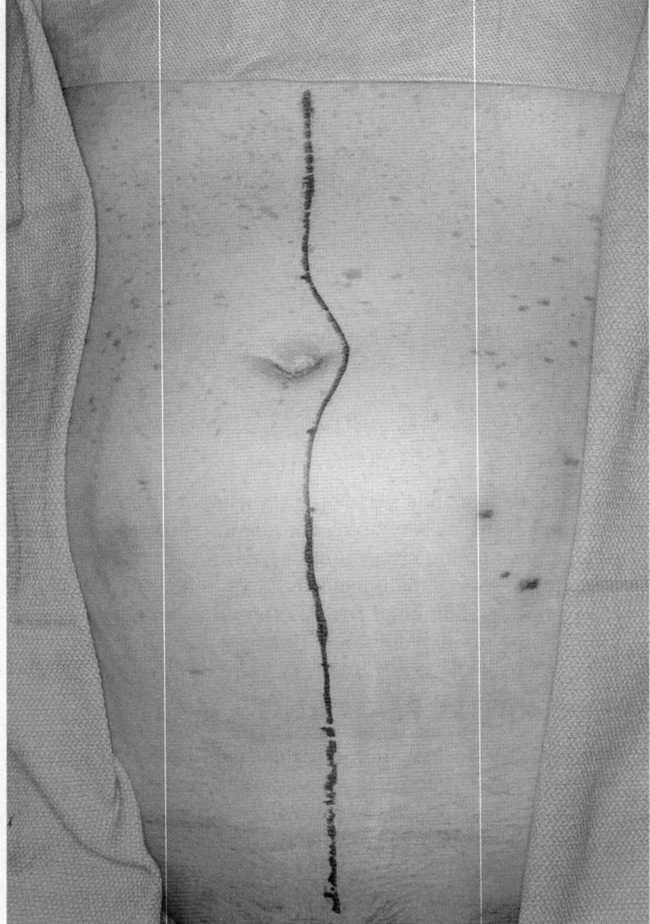

Figure 8.1.1. Vertical midline incision.

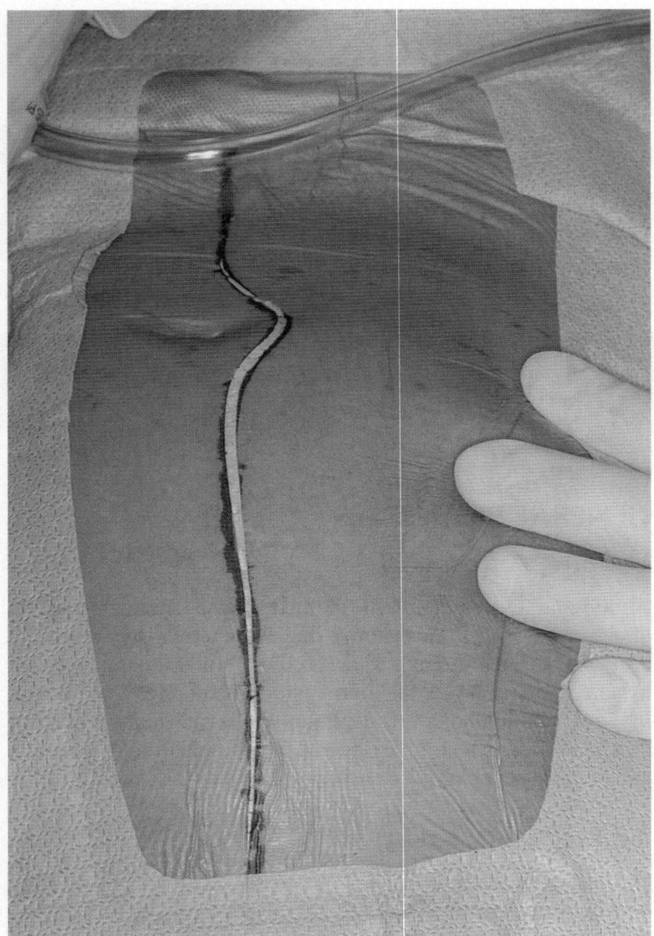

Figure 8.1.2. Vertical midline incision—skin incision.

- The *decision to remove both fallopian tubes and ovaries* at the time of hysterectomy is complicated and requires a frank discussion between the patient and her surgeon. Benign indications for oophorectomy at the time of hysterectomy include endometriosis, tubo-ovarian abscess, and pelvic pain. In 2005, a nationwide study reported that unilateral or bilateral salpingo-oophorectomy was performed in 68% of women undergoing abdominal hysterectomy in the United States.[2] Historically, the rationale for elective oophorectomy at the time of hysterectomy was ovarian cancer prevention in women nearing menopause. More recently, the thought has shifted to favor ovarian conservation, as new evidence suggests there are long-term health benefits associated with ovarian preservation and more risks than previously appreciated with elective oophorectomy.[3] Furthermore, the incidence of ovarian cancer in the general population remains low and does not warrant elective oophorectomy at the time of hysterectomy.
- In contrast, there are no proven medical or surgical benefits to performing a subtotal hysterectomy if the cervix can easily be removed with the uterus. *Retaining the cervix* commits the patient to continued cervical cancer screening and may result in posthysterectomy bleeding. The only absolute contraindication to supracervical hysterectomy is a malignant or premalignant condition of the uterus or cervix.

SURGICAL MANAGEMENT

- Women undergoing abdominal hysterectomy require *venous thromboembolism (VTE) prophylaxis.* Guidelines for perioperative thromboprophylaxis published by both the American College of Obstetricians and Gynecologists and the American College of Chest Physicians consistently define patients undergoing abdominal hysterectomy as at least moderate risk of VTE.[4,5] Therefore, mechanical VTE prophylaxis with sequential compression devices should be used in all women undergoing abdominal hysterectomy. Consideration for pharmacologic prophylaxis with heparin should be based upon risk factors further delineated in the aforementioned guidelines. Many institutions have developed routine, perisurgical thromboprophylaxis protocols, and administer both mechanical and pharmacologic therapies for women undergoing abdominal hysterectomy.[4]
- *Prophylactic antibiotics* to prevent surgical site infection are given as a single intravenous injection prior to induction of anesthesia. The greatest efficacy for antibiotic administration is within an hour prior to bacterial inoculation (i.e., abdominal incision).[6] For women greater than 50 kg, a dose of 2 g cefazolin is routinely used (1 g for women with BMI <30). If bowel penetration is anticipated, metronidazole 500 mg may be given in addition to cefazolin. Alternatively, cefoxitin 2 g can be administered to cover a broader spectrum of bacteria. Women

Table 8.1.1 Prophylactic Antibiotic Regimens for Abdominal Hysterectomy

Antibiotic	Dose (Intravenous)	Re-Dose Time (hrs)
Cefazolin/Cefoxitin	1 or 2[a] g	3
Clindamycin plus gentamicin	600 mg 1.5 mg/kg (240 mg max)	3 6
Clindamycin plus quinolone	600 mg 400 mg	3 6
Clindamycin plus aztreonam	600 mg 1 g	3 3
Metronidazole plus gentamicin	500 mg 1.5 mg/kg (240 mg max)	6 6
Metronidazole plus quinolone	500 mg 400 mg	6 6

[a]Use 2 g dose for obese patients—i.e., weight greater than 100 kg or BMI greater than 30.

who are penicillin-allergic require a combination of clindamycin (600 mg) and gentamicin (1.5 mg/kg; max 240 mg). For lengthy procedures, additional intraoperative doses of antibiotic are given at intervals of one or two times the half-life of the drug to maintain adequate levels throughout the operation **(Table 8.1.1)**. For cefazolin, a second dose is necessary at 3 hours. An increased blood loss greater than 1,500 mL also warrants a second dose of antibiotic.[3]

- Bowel preparation is not indicated in women undergoing abdominal hysterectomy unless there is a high probability of bowel injury secondary to adhesions. In these cases, it is reasonable to consider using a parenteral antibiotic regimen that is effective in preventing infection among patients undergoing elective bowel surgery. There is no evidence that mechanical bowel preparation further reduces infection risk.[3]

Positioning

- After the patient is brought to the operating room, preoperative prophylactic antibiotics and subcutaneous heparin are administered prior to the start of the procedure. Sequential compression devices are placed bilaterally on the patient's lower extremities. The patient may be positioned in either the dorsal supine or lithotomy position using Allen stirrups with careful attention to pressure points to avoid neurologic injury. A "time-out" is performed in which the surgeon, anesthesia, and operating room staff confirm and agree upon the patient's identity, indicated treatments and surgery including any procedure laterality (i.e., right salpingo-oophorectomy) followed by an examination under anesthesia. The vagina, perineum, and abdomen (from the anterior thighs to xiphoid) are then prepared with antiseptic solution and draped in a sterile fashion. In sterile fashion, a Foley catheter is placed in the bladder and drained to gravity. The surgeon then changes her gloves before moving to the abdomen.

Approach

- The skin incision may be transverse or midline vertical and is determined by a variety of factors, such as the presence of a prior surgical scar, need for upper abdomen exploration, uterine size, shape, and mobility, and desired cosmetic results. If a prior incision exists, most surgeons prefer to use this incision. If the *prior scar is cosmetically unacceptable,* it may be excised at the beginning or end of the procedure. This is accomplished by elevating the old scar with Allis clamps and creating an elliptical incision around the old scar.
- If a transverse abdominal incision is desired, consider a few options. The most commonly used transverse incision is a Pfannenstiel incision; however, this incision provides the least amount of exposure because the recti remain intact. Transverse Cherney and Maylard incisions improve exposure because the rectus muscles are transected. A Cherney incision transects the rectus muscles at their tendinous insertions into the symphysis pubis, while the Maylard incision is a true transverse transection through all layers, including the rectus muscles, and necessitates identification and suture ligation of the deep, inferior epigastric vessels.

Procedures and Techniques (Video 8.1)

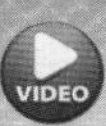

Incision and exploration

- Using a vertical abdominal approach, a midline vertical skin incision is made from the umbilicus down to the pubic symphysis (see Figs. 8.1.1 and 8.1.2). The underlying subcutaneous tissues are then divided down to the fascia (**Tech Figs. 8.1.1** and **8.1.2**). The fascia is incised in the midline over the rectus diastasis and along the length of the incision (**Tech Figs. 8.1.3** to **8.1.6**). The underlying posterior sheath is then elevated and entered sharply with

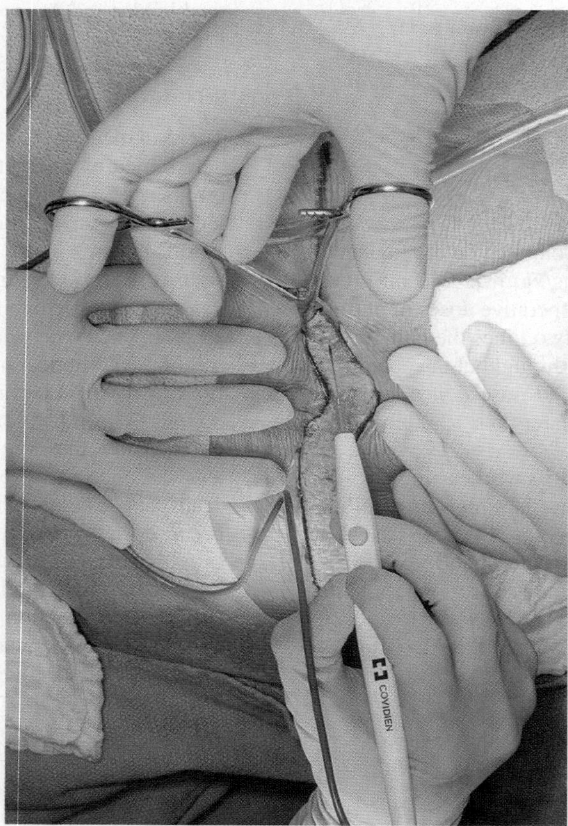

Tech Figure 8.1.1. Dissection through subcutaneous adipose.

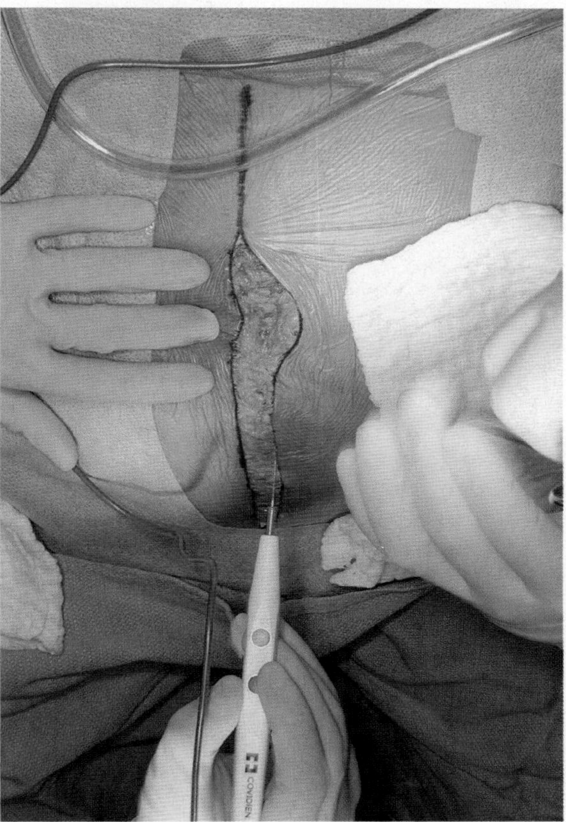

Tech Figure 8.1.2. Dissection through subcutaneous adipose.

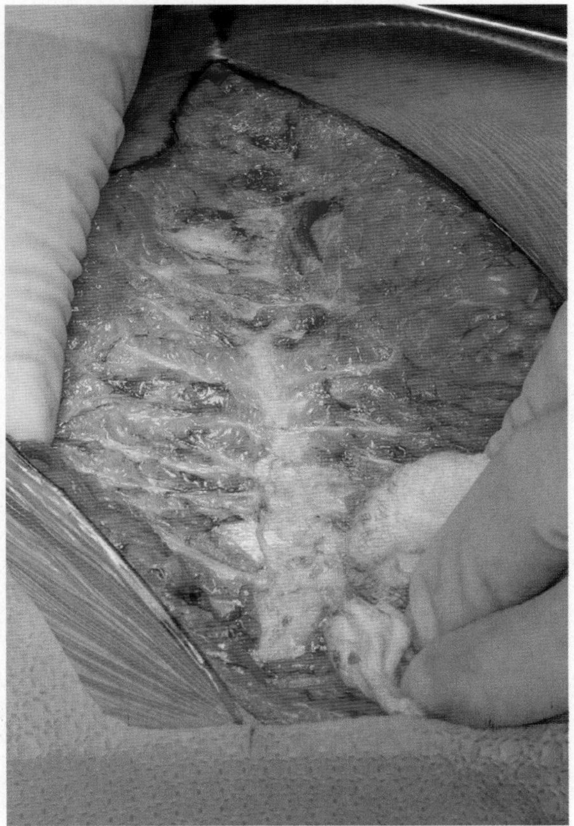

Tech Figure 8.1.3. The fascia is revealed.

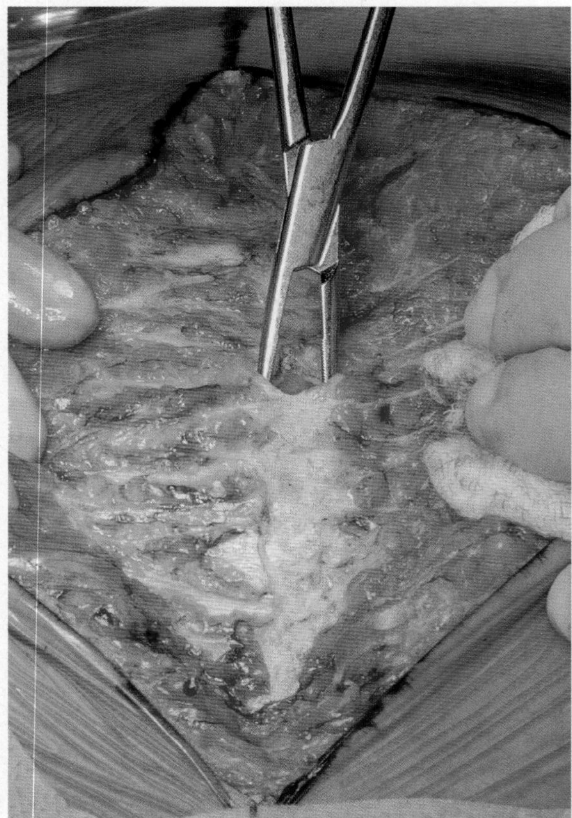

Tech Figure 8.1.4. Fascia is incised in the midline.

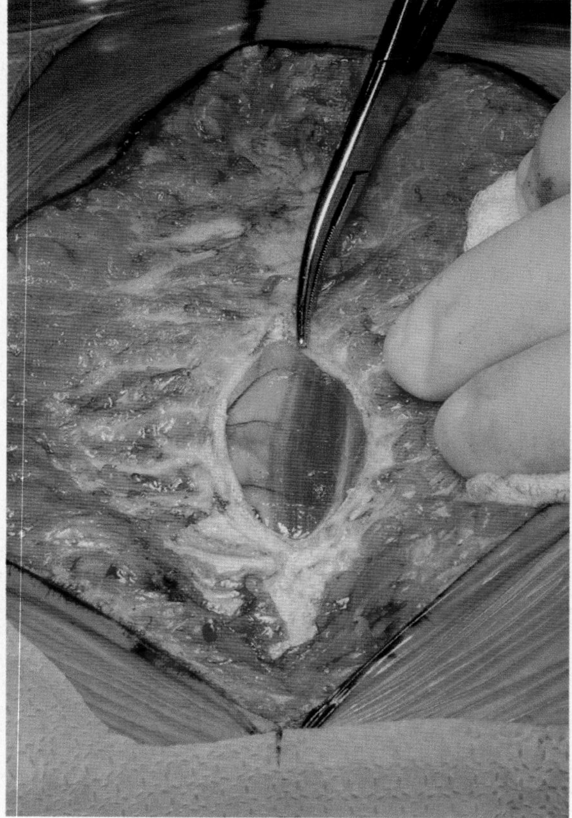

Tech Figure 8.1.5. Underlying rectus muscles are revealed.

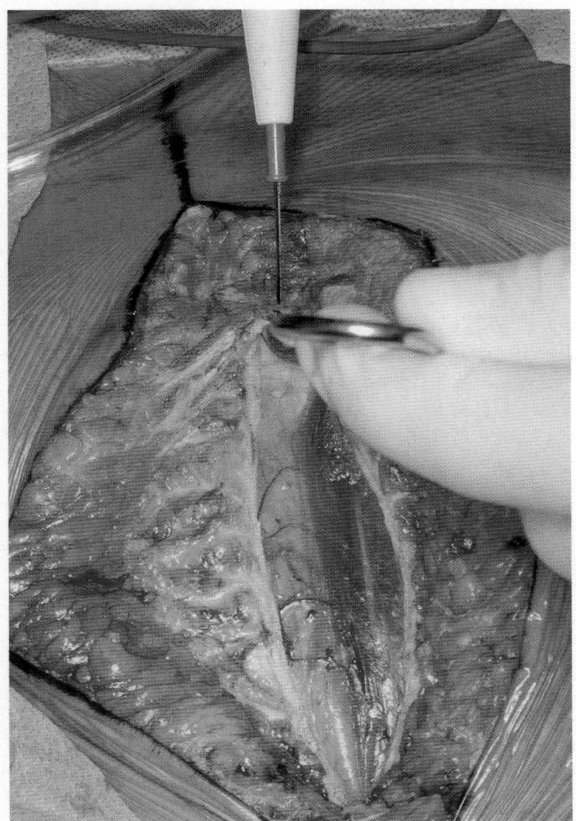

Tech Figure 8.1.6. The midline fascial incision is extended superiorly.

Metzenbaum scissors (Tech Figs. 8.1.7 and 8.1.8). The peritoneum is grasped with smooth pick-ups or Kelly clamps, elevated, and entered sharply with the knife to gain uncomplicated entry into the abdominal cavity (Tech Fig. 8.1.9). The incision is then extended along its entire length paying careful attention to the location of the bladder.

- A Pfannenstiel incision is a transverse incision made at a level suitable to the surgeon. It usually measured 10 to 15 cm transversely and extends through the skin, subcutaneous fat, and to the level of the rectus fascia. The rectus fascia is then incised transversely on either side of the midline with a scalpel and extended laterally with curved Mayo scissors. Kocher clamps are then placed on the inferior aspect of the fascial incision. While pulling vertically on the Kocher clamps with one hand, the surgeon uses her opposite hand to simultaneously and bluntly dissect the anterior rectus sheath from the underlying rectus muscle. The anterior aspect of the fascial incision is similarly dissected. The rectus muscles are then separated in the midline, and the peritoneum is opened vertically.
- As with a Pfannenstiel incision, the skin and fascia are divided transversely with the Cherney incision; however, the rectus muscles are divided at their tendinous insertion into the symphysis pubis with a monopolar instrument or scalpel. The recti are then retracted cephalad to improve exposure. Similarly, the Maylard incision requires a transverse incision through skin, subcutaneous tissue, and fascia. However, once the fascia is transversely incised, it is not detached from the underlying muscle. The surgeon must identify the lateral borders of the rectus muscles, then identify, clamp cut, and suture ligate the inferior epigastric vessels lying on the posterior lateral border of each muscle. After these vessels are secured, the rectus muscles are transected using a monopolar instrument.

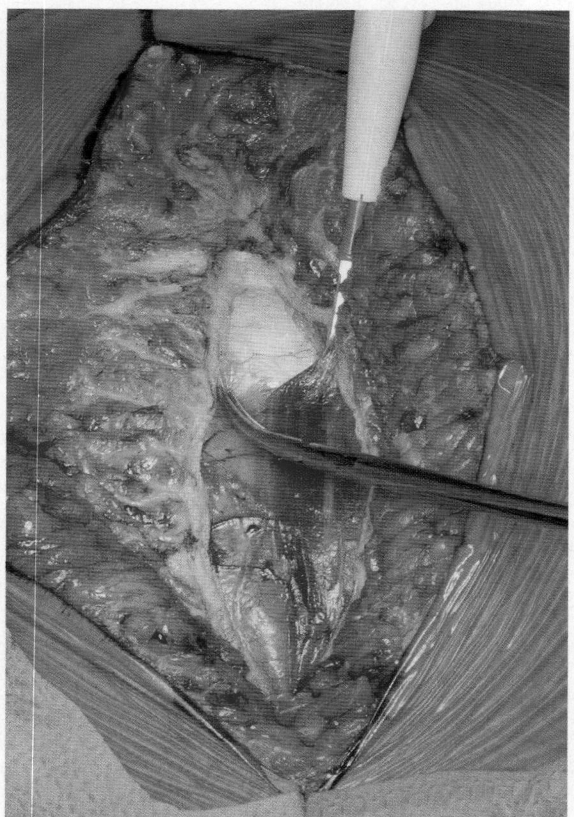

Tech Figure 8.1.7. The underlying peritoneum is exposed.

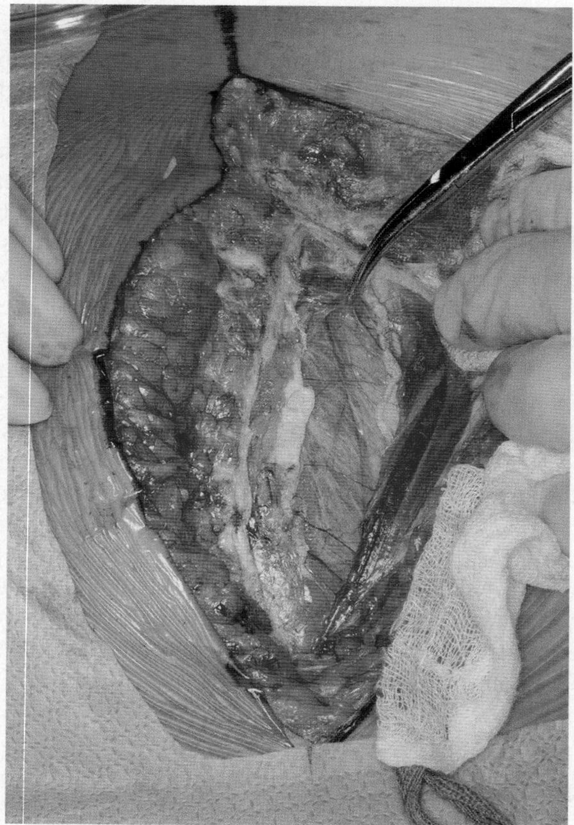

Tech Figure 8.1.8. The underlying peritoneum is exposed.

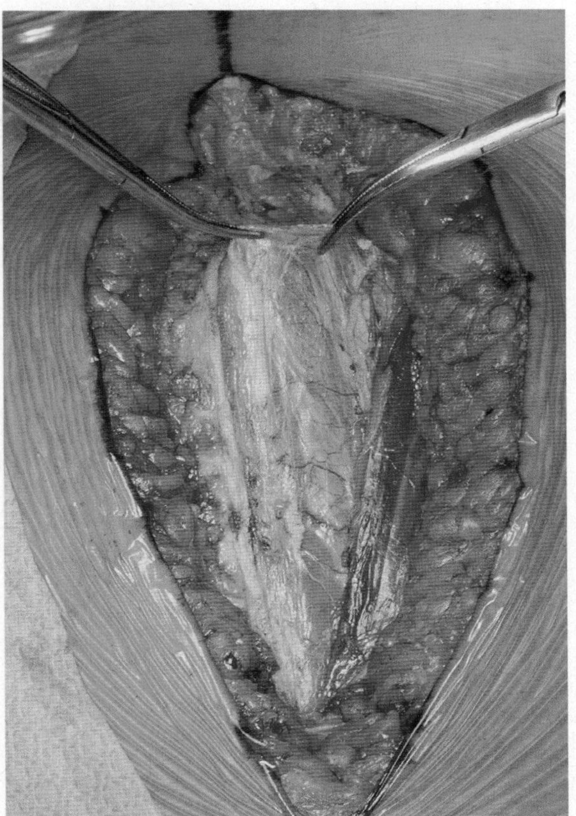

Tech Figure 8.1.9. The peritoneum is grasped and tented up for sharp entry.

Exposure

- Once the peritoneum has been opened, a self-retaining retractor is placed and the target organ is exposed and delivered (Tech Figs. 8.1.10 to 8.1.12). The type of retractor used depends on the type of incision (vertical or transverse) and surgeon preference. When positioning retractors it is important to avoid placing the lateral blades over the femoral nerve as it emerges lateral to the psoas muscle. This can lead to peripheral neuropathy and postoperative difficulty with walking. To ensure safe placement, lift the abdominal wall as the retractor is placed, then check to confirm no bowel has been trapped beneath a blade and that the blade is not pressing on the sidewall of the pelvis (Tech Fig. 8.1.13).
- If pelvic or intra-abdominal adhesions are present, first mobilize the pelvic organs and restore normal anatomy before packing the bowel away from the pelvis. This may require dividing omental, intestinal, or abdominal wall adhesions with either Metzenbaum scissors or radiofrequency energy. Once normal anatomy is restored, use moist laparotomy sponges to pack away small and large bowels, carefully placing the blades of the retractors in such a way that no bowel is strangulated.

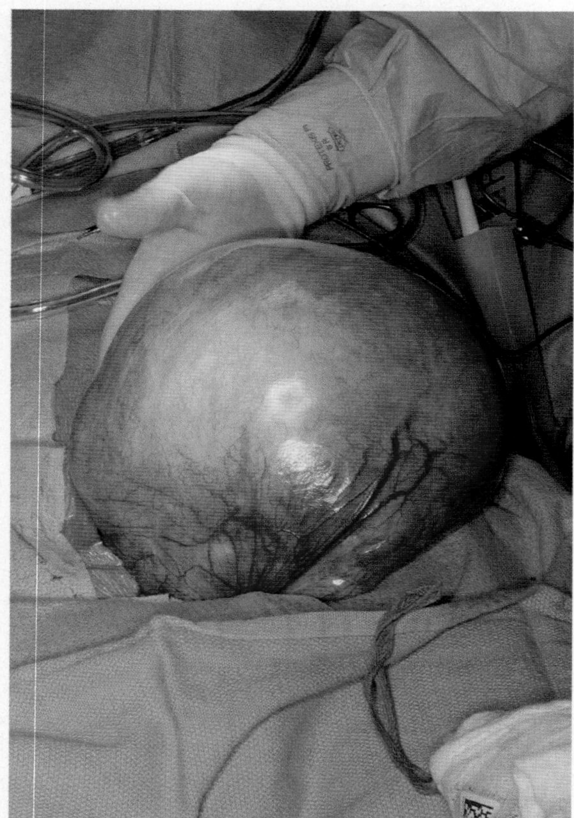

Tech Figure 8.1.10. The uterus is delivered through the incision.

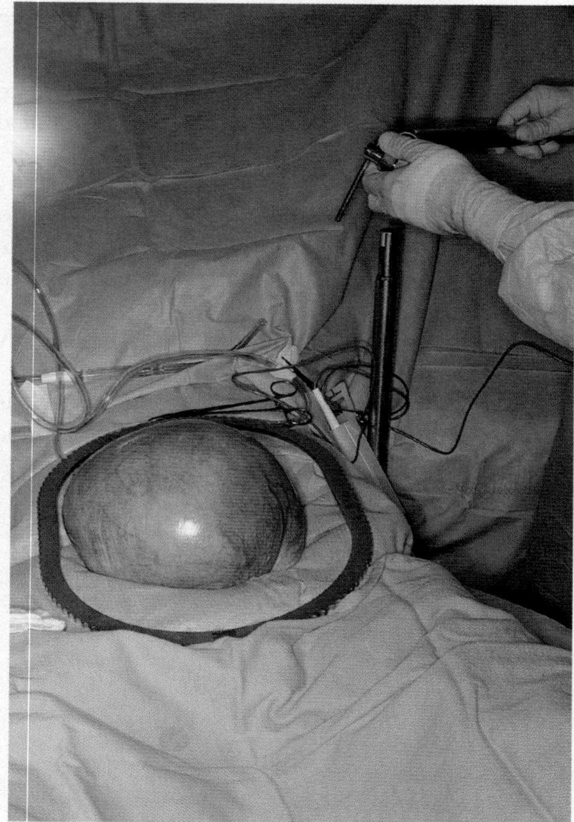

Tech Figure 8.1.11. Bookwalter post and ring.

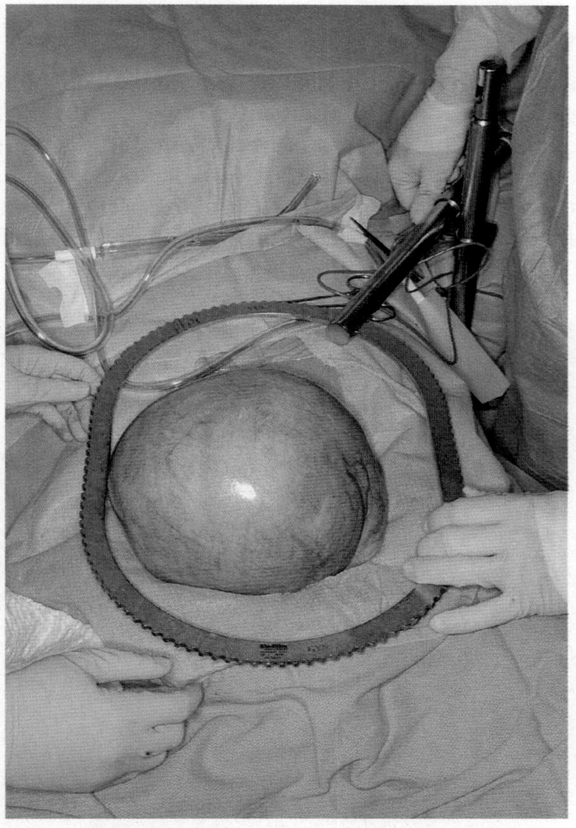

Tech Figure 8.1.12. Bookwalter assembled.

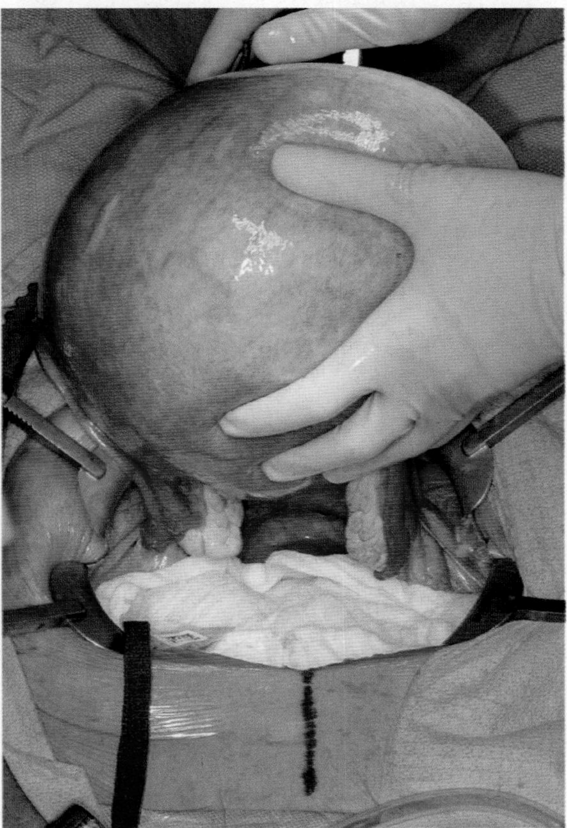

Tech Figure 8.1.13. Bookwalter with side-wall retractors in place.

Broad ligament dissection

- Large Kelly clamps are placed across each uterine cornu including the round ligament to allow easy retraction of the uterus during surgery (Tech Fig. 8.1.14). The round ligament is then clamped at approximately the mid-portion and divided with a monopolar instrument (Tech Fig. 8.1.15). The clamped end is then suture ligated and the clamp removed. If the round ligament is divided too close to the uterus, exposure of the broad ligament becomes limited making the incision of the peritoneum over the broad ligament more difficult.

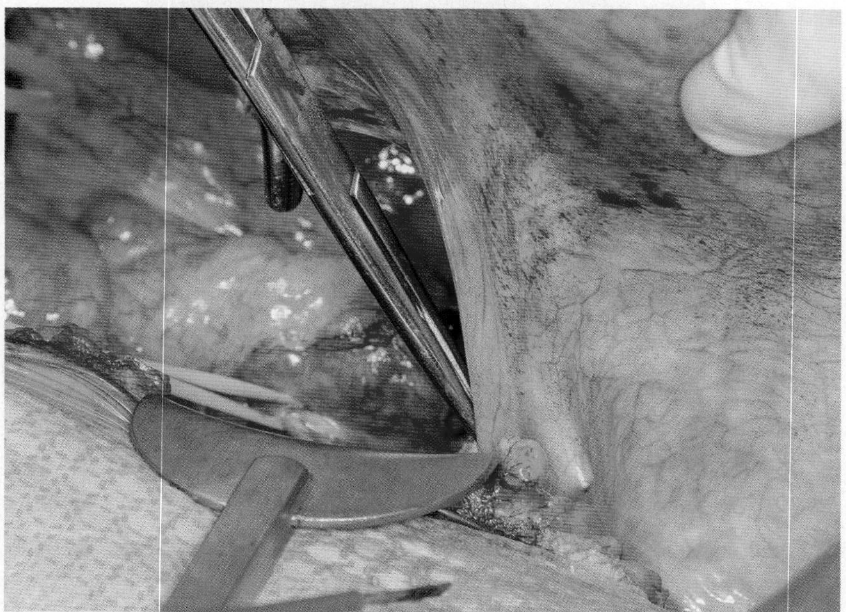

Tech Figure 8.1.14. The round ligament is identified.

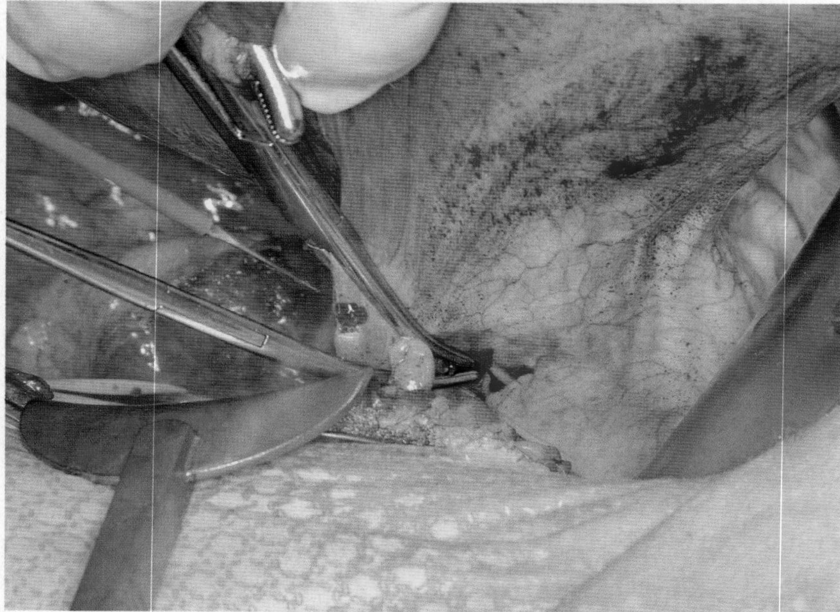

Tech Figure 8.1.15. The round ligament is clamped and divided.

- The anterior and posterior leaves of the broad ligament are incised. Anteriorly, the broad ligament is divided to the level of the uterine artery, then medially along the vesicouterine peritoneum, separating the bladder from the lower uterine segment and underlying vagina (**Tech Figs. 8.1.16** and **8.1.17**). The retroperitoneum is then entered by extending the incision on the posterior leaf of the broad ligament superiorly, remaining lateral to the infundibulopelvic

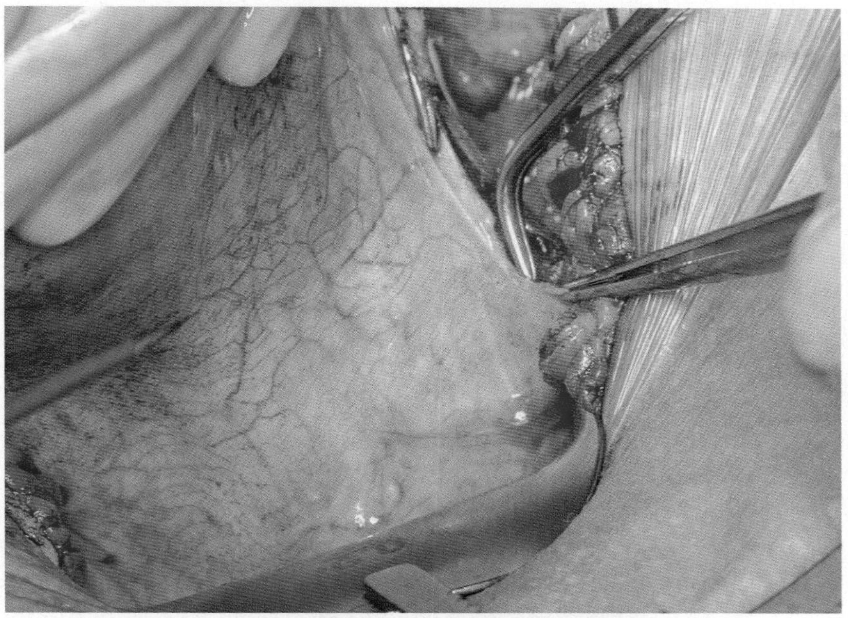

Tech Figure 8.1.16. The vesicouterine peritoneum is incised over the underlying cervix.

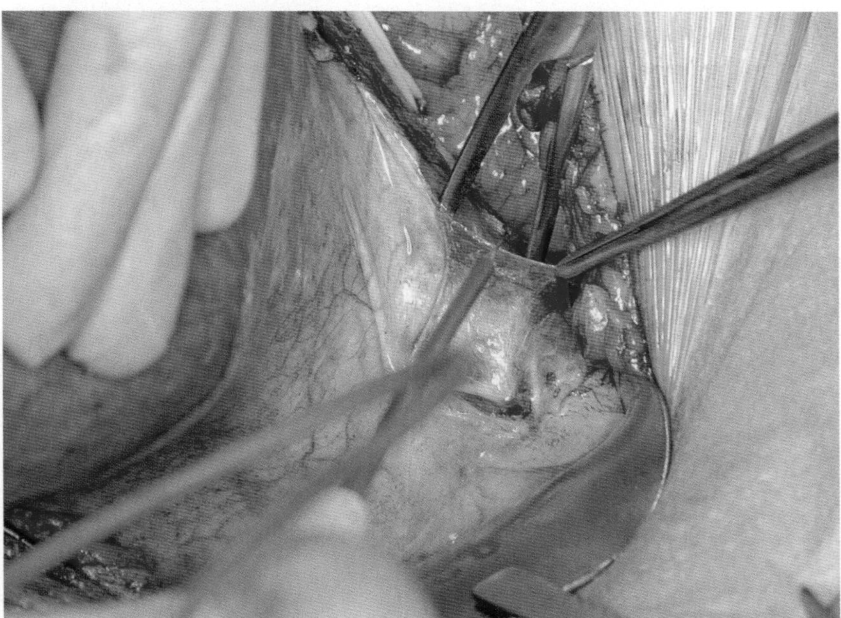

Tech Figure 8.1.17. By incising the vesicouterine peritoneum, the bladder is dissected off the cervix.

ligament (Tech Figs. 8.1.18 and 8.1.19). Blunt dissection with a Yankauer suction tip or a finger clears the loose connective tissue overlying the external iliac artery allowing for identification of the ureter (Tech Figs. 8.1.20 and 8.1.21). By following the external iliac artery superiorly to its bifurcation, the ureter can be identified at its most superficial point crossing into the pelvis over the bifurcation of the internal and external iliac arteries. The ureter can then be traced to the medial leaf of the peritoneum coursing inferior to the infundibulopelvic ligament. Visualization of ureteral peristalsis confirms the ureter's identity.

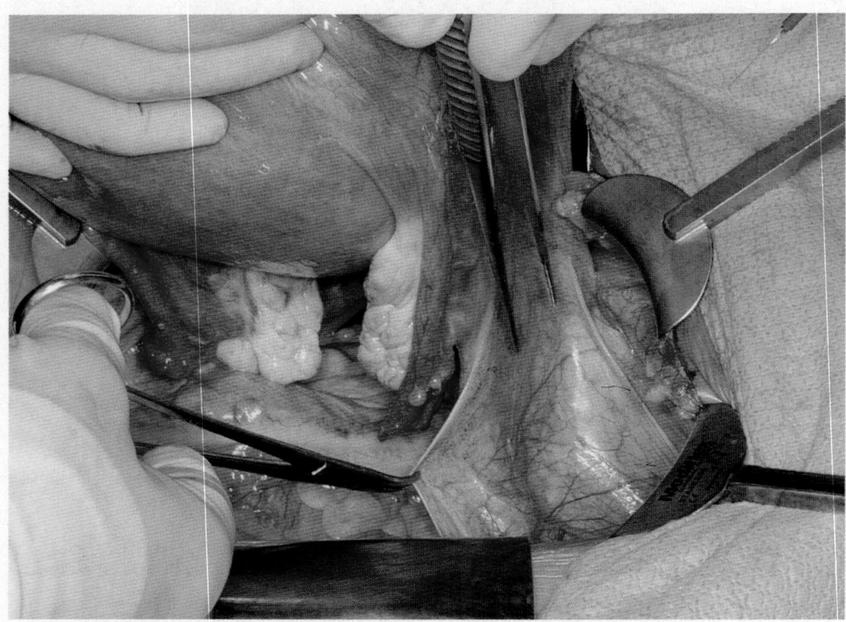

Tech Figure 8.1.18. The posterior leaf of the broad ligament is tented up.

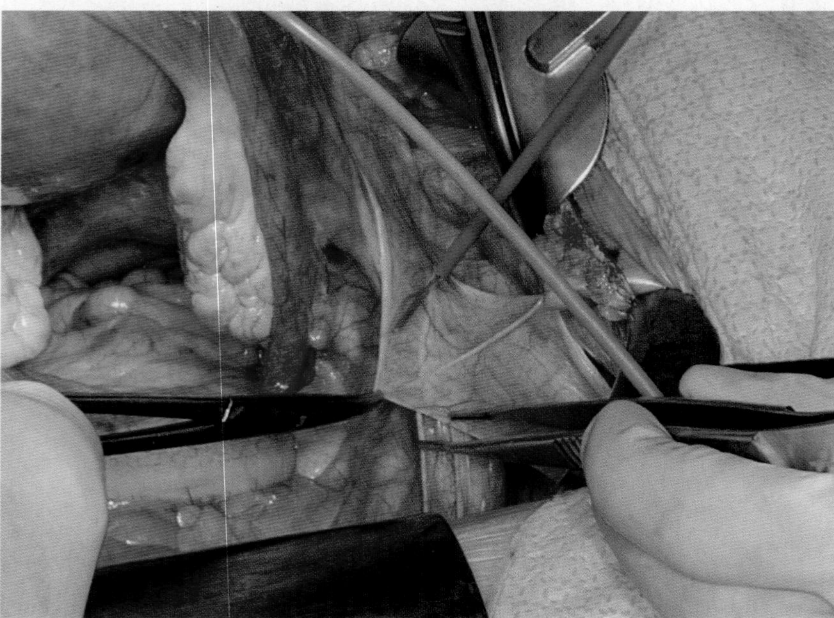

Tech Figure 8.1.19. The posterior leaf of the broad ligament is incised lateral to the gonadal vessels.

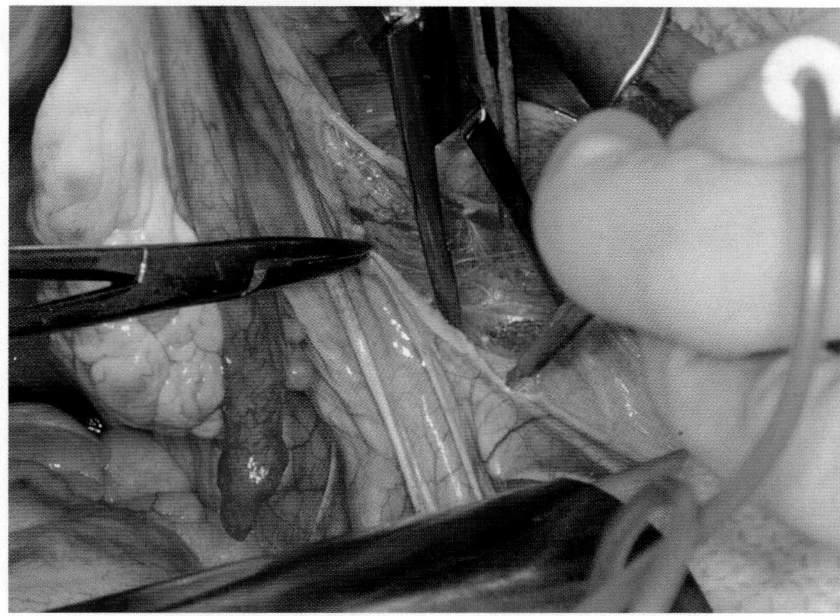

Tech Figure 8.1.20. The peritoneum is extended to better visualize the retroperitoneum.

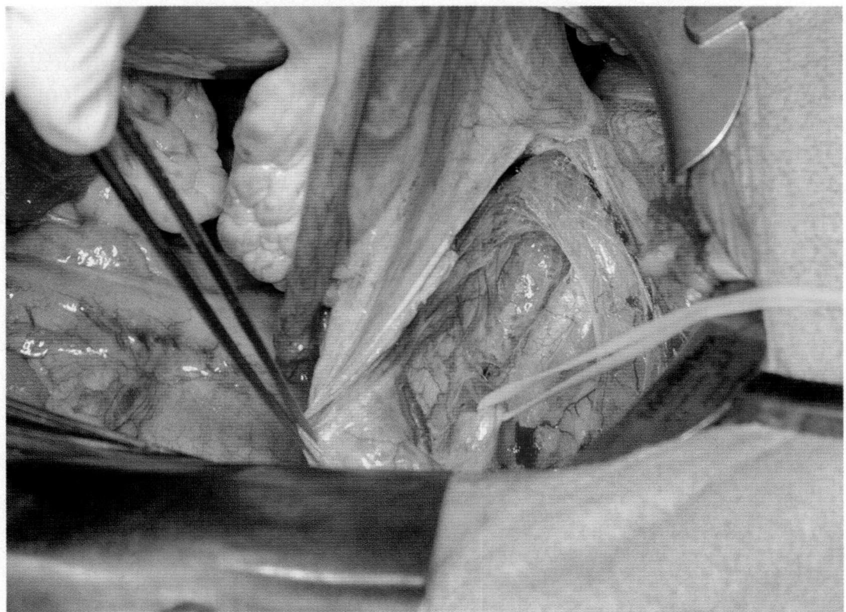

Tech Figure 8.1.21. Vessel loop around the identified ureter.

Adnexal removal

- If the ovaries are to be removed, first identify the ureter, then create a peritoneal window located inferior to the infundibulopelvic ligament, superior to the ureter and lateral to the ovary (**Tech Fig. 8.1.22**). This is accomplished by dissecting the vessels away from the ureter and clamping the intervening tissue with two curved clamps. The vessels are then transected and suture ligated first with a free tie followed by a suture ligature placed just medial to the free tie. This technique prevents hematoma formation. The underlying medial leaf of the broad ligament is then skeletonized up to the utero-ovarian ligament.

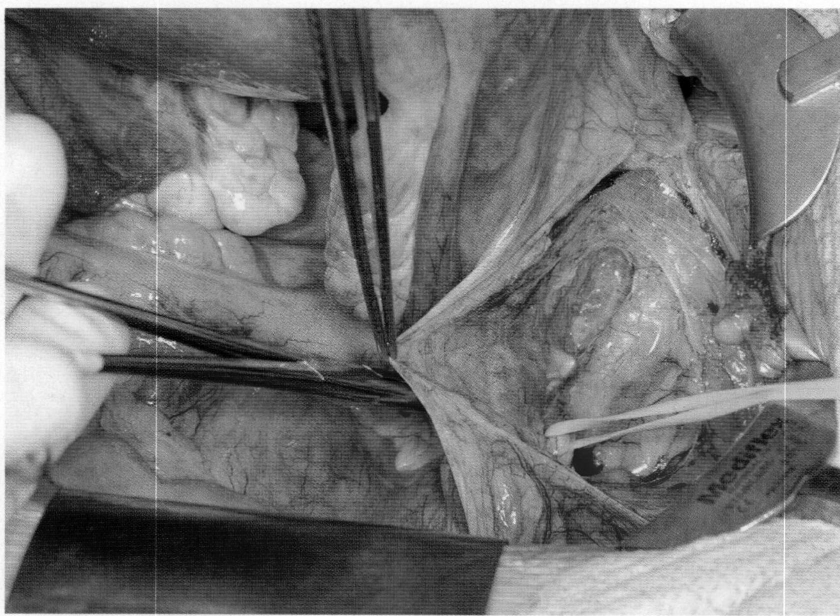

Tech Figure 8.1.22. Formation of peritoneal window between gonadal vessels and the ureter.

Conservation of ovaries and tubes

- If the ovaries are to be conserved, identify the ureter, and then create a peritoneal window in the posterior leaf of the broad ligament located under the utero-ovarian ligament and fallopian tube. Clamp the utero-ovarian with two clamps (the large Kelly clamp placed on the cornua initially may be adjusted to ensure complete occlusion of the utero-ovarian vessels at the uterine cornua, the second clamp used is generally a Heaney clamp), incise and ligate with a free tie followed by a suture ligature placed medially to the free tie (**Tech Figs. 8.1.23** to **8.1.26**). See **Tech Figure 8.1.27** for technique differentiation of adnexal conservation versus adnexal excision.

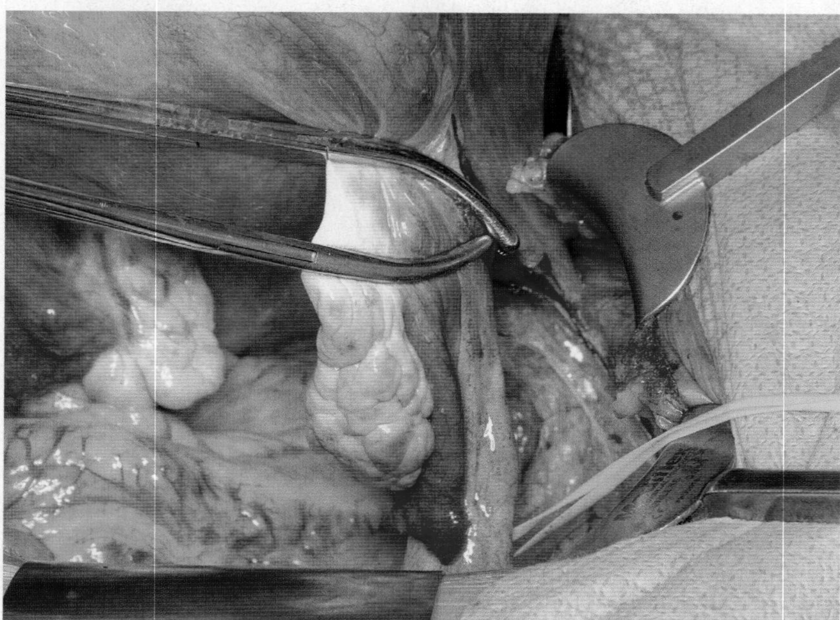

Tech Figure 8.1.23. Haney clamps on the utero-ovarian ligament.

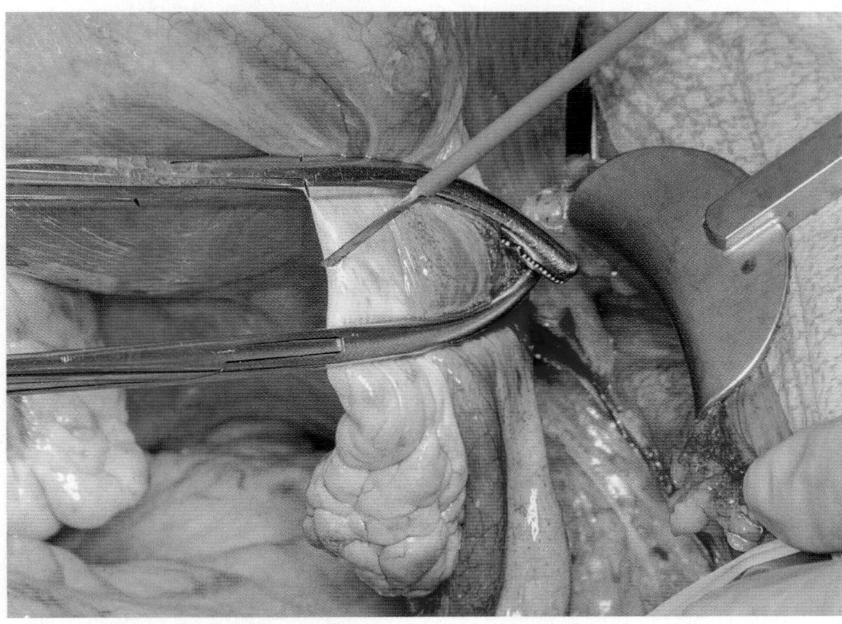

Tech Figure 8.1.24. Division of the utero-ovarian ligament.

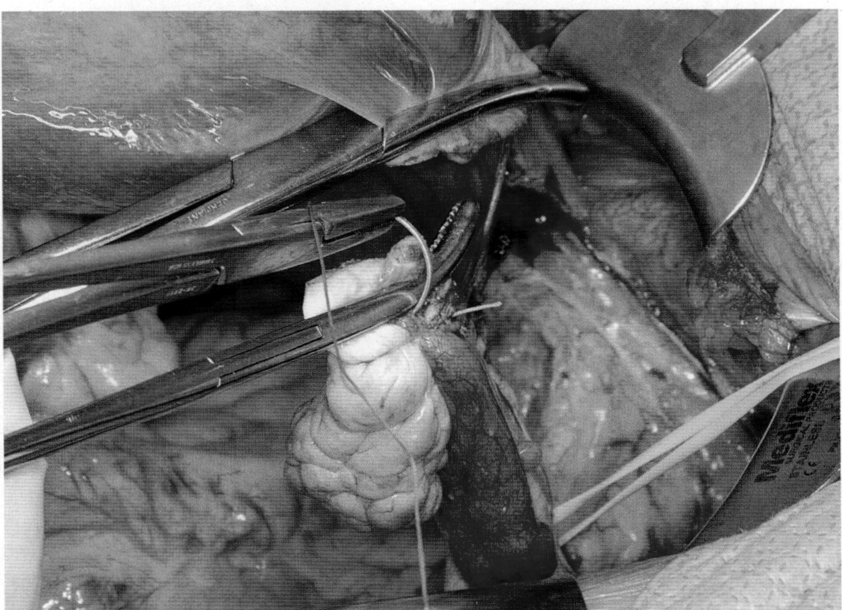

Tech Figure 8.1.25. The utero-ovarian ligament is suture ligated.

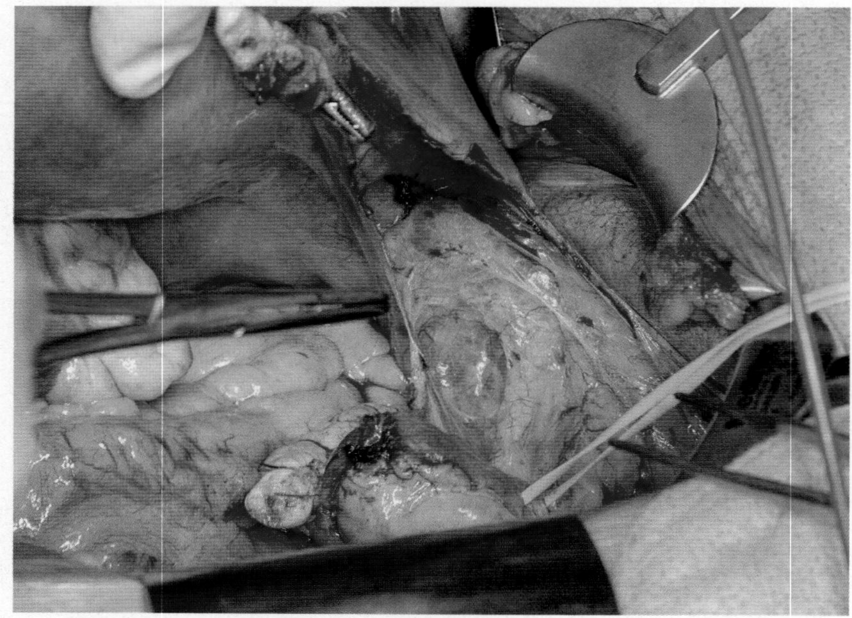

Tech Figure 8.1.26. The utero-ovarian pedicle is released once hemostatic.

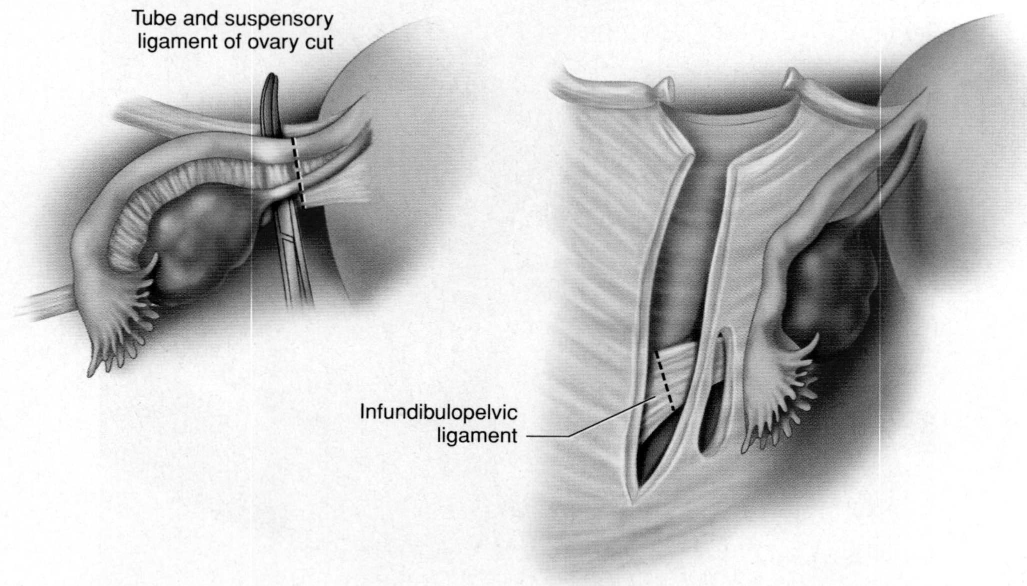

Tech Figure 8.1.27. Technique for adnexal conservation versus oophorectomy at the time of abdominal hysterectomy.

Uterine artery ligation

- Prior to ligating the uterine artery, it is imperative to dissect both the bladder and rectum away from the uterus. By dissecting the bladder off the lower uterine segment, the ureter is concomitantly lateralized, reducing the risk for ureteral injury during uterine artery ligation. This is accomplished by incising the vesicouterine peritoneum and identifying the avascular plane between the bladder and the lower uterine segment (Tech Fig. 8.1.16). Once this plane is entered, gently dissect the bladder away using small amounts of monopolar energy with blunt dissection or sharply with the Metzenbaum scissors (Tech Fig. 8.1.17).
- If the rectum requires mobilization from the posterior cervix, identify a similarly avascular plane between the rectum and vagina. This plane can be found by incising the posterior peritoneum between the uterosacral ligaments just beneath the cervix. Dissecting this plane mobilizes the rectum away from the posterior vagina and cervix.
- Identify and skeletonize the uterine vessels using a monopolar instrument to dissect away any loose connective tissue overlying the vessels. Place a curved clamp perpendicular to the uterine artery at the junction of the cervix and lower uterine segment. The tip of the clamp should rest directly adjacent to the cervix (Tech Fig. 8.1.28). Place a clamp medial to the curved clamp to prevent bleeding from the uterus (Tech Fig. 8.1.29). Finally, cut and ligate the uterine artery (Tech Figs. 8.1.30 to 8.1.32).
  - For an *extrafascial technique,* the cardinal ligament and any remaining broad ligament are divided by placing straight clamps medial to the uterine vascular pedicle and parallel to the cervix, incising with a scalpel, or radiofrequency electrical energy, and suture ligating these

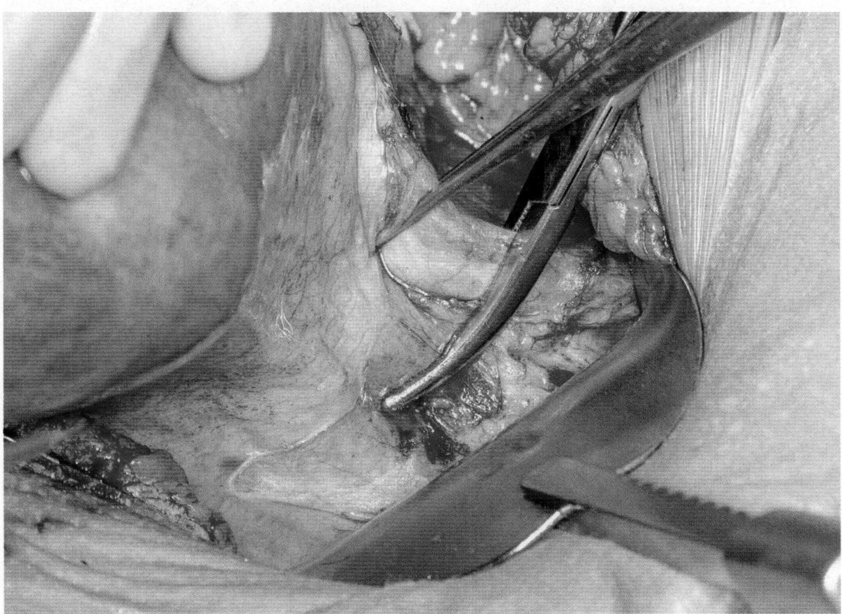

Tech Figure 8.1.28. The utero-ovarian pedicle is released once hemostatic.

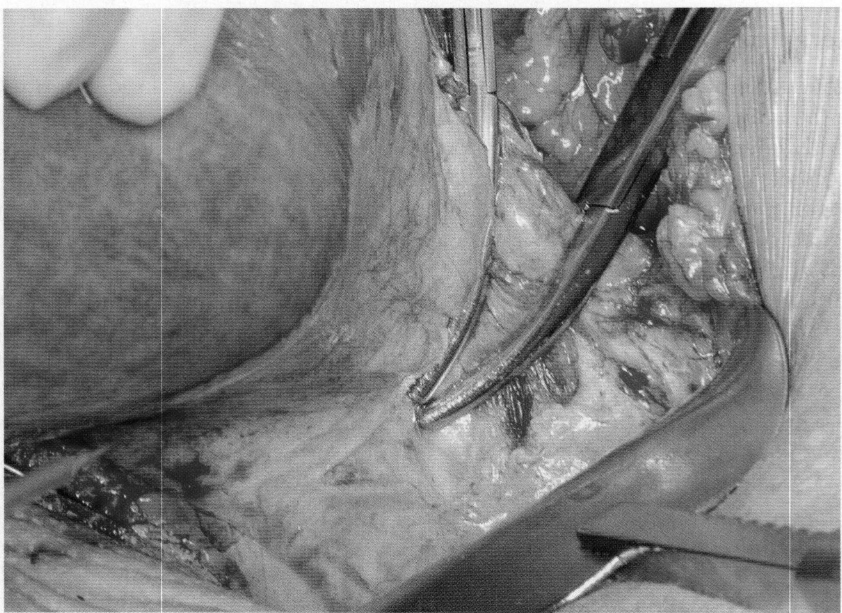

Tech Figure 8.1.29. The uterine artery is clamped at the level of the internal os.

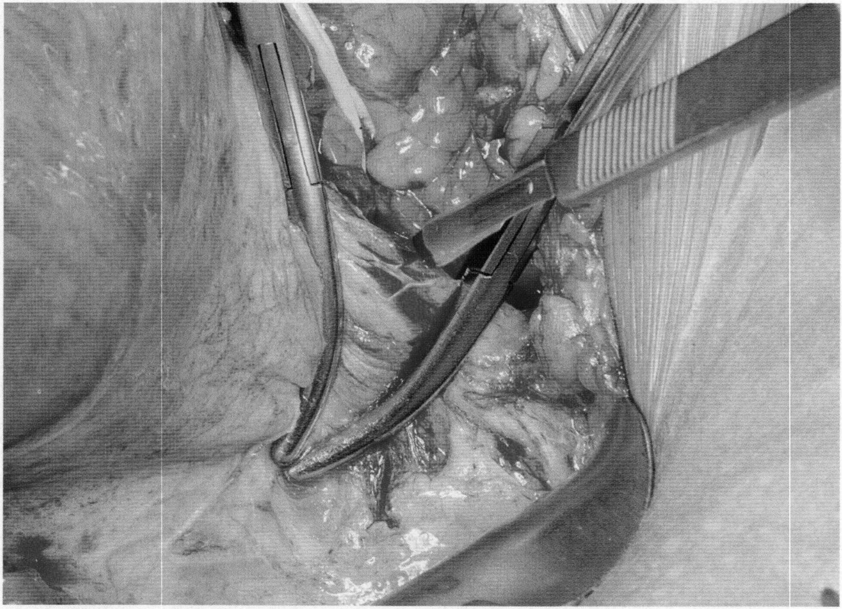

Tech Figure 8.1.30. The uterine artery is cut.

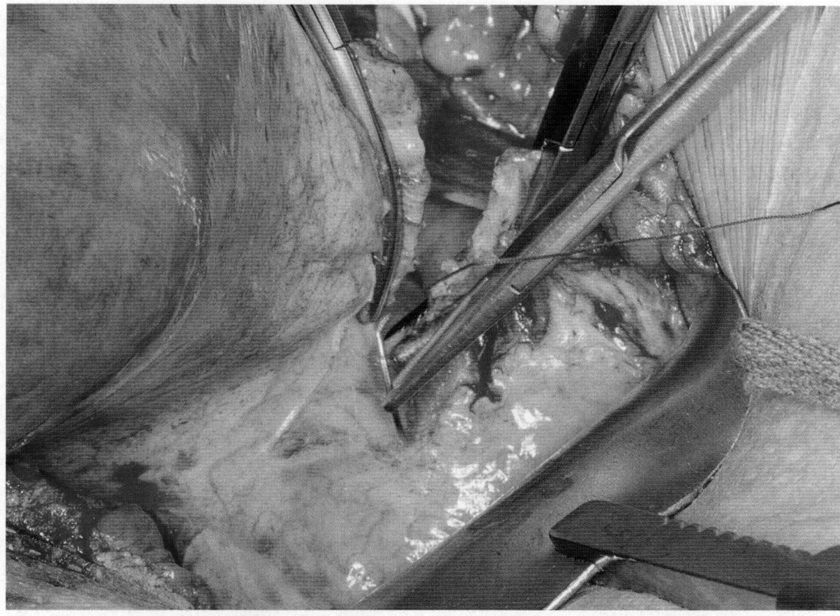

Tech Figure 8.1.31. The cut uterine artery is suture-ligated.

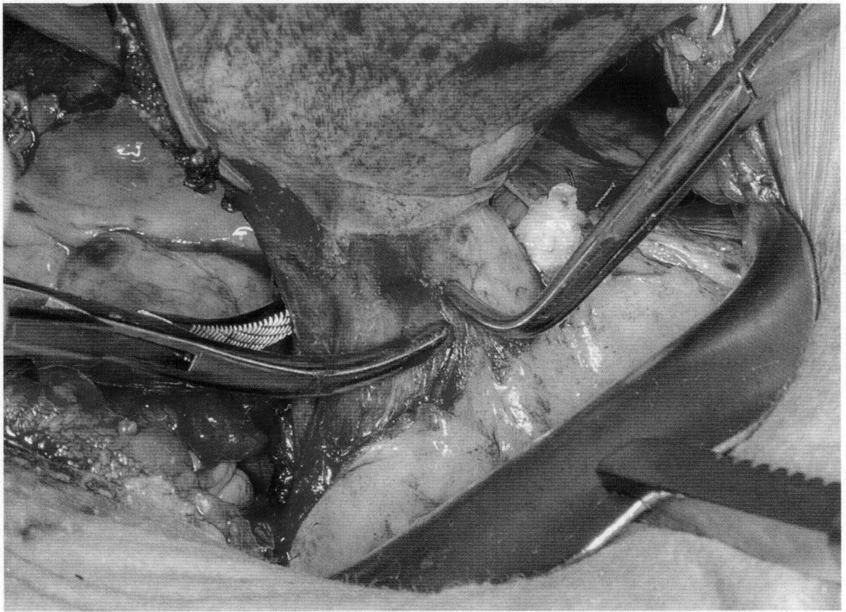

Tech Figure 8.1.32. The contralateral uterine artery is clamped, cut and suture-ligated.

pedicles until the end of the cervix is reached (Tech Figs. 8.1.33 to 8.1.36). Colpotomy can then be made either by placing curved clamps across the vagina just beneath the cervix. Be careful to preserve as much vagina as possible, then amputate the cervix from the vagina using Jorgenson scissors (Tech Figs. 8.1.37 to 8.1.39). Another technique is to place a sponge stick in the vagina pushing anteriorly in order to delineate the anterior vaginal apex. Using a monopolar instrument, incise the vagina where the vaginal sponge stick is demarcated and until the sponge is identified. Continue this incision circumferentially around the cervix with an active electrode or with clamps placed along the vaginal–cervical junction and incise with Mayo scissors (Tech Fig. 8.1.40). Deliver the specimen through the abdominal incision and carefully inspect the tissue to ensure the entirety of the cervix has been removed.

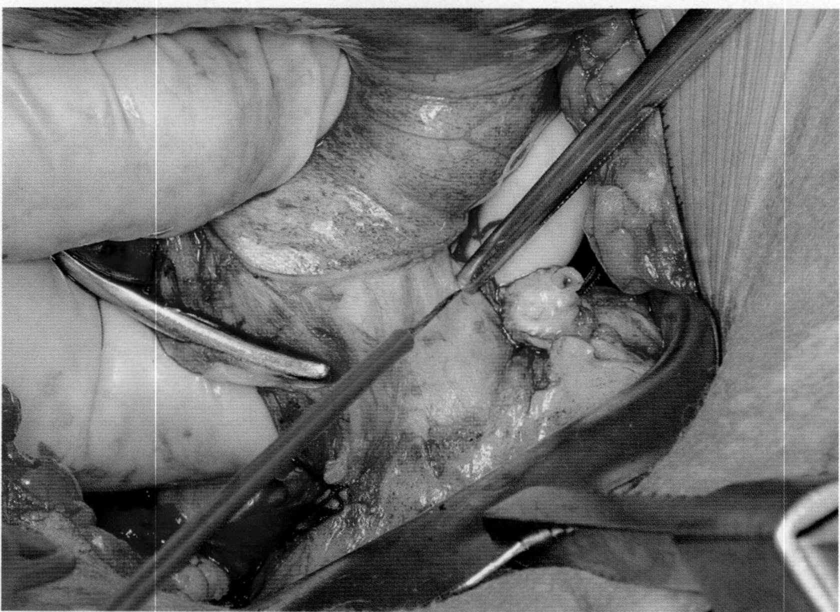

Tech Figure 8.1.33. In this particular case, the uterus is amputated from the cervix before completing the hysterectomy for better visualization.

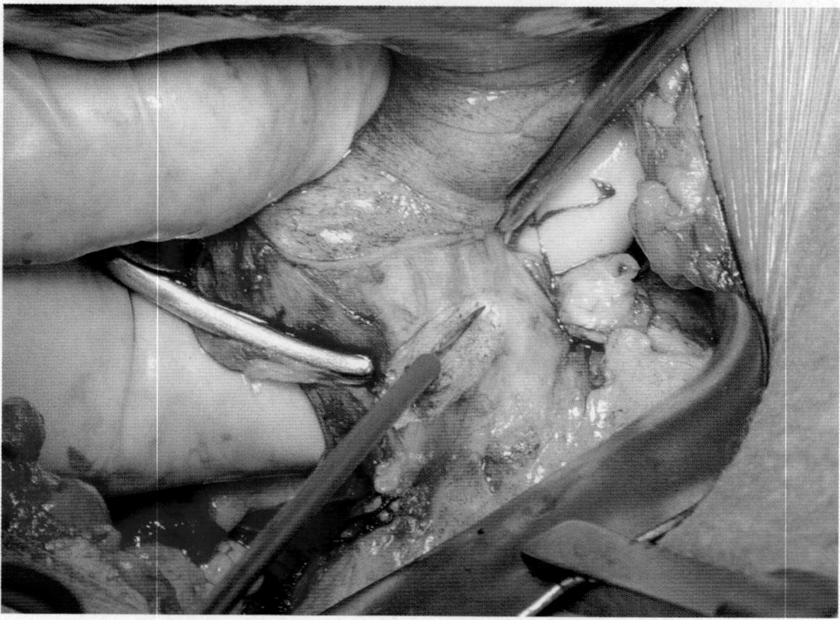

Tech Figure 8.1.34. The uterus is amputated from the cervix using radiofrequency electrical energy.

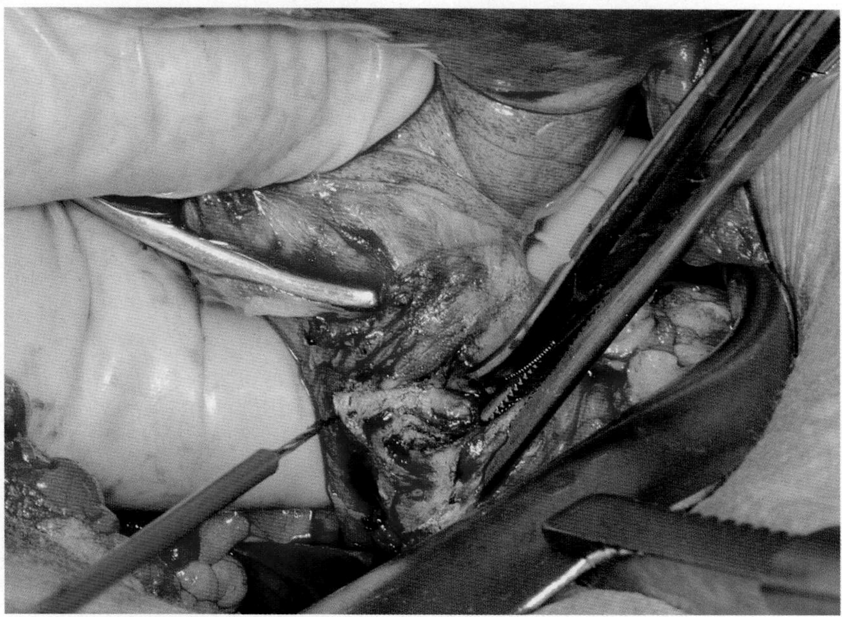

Tech Figure 8.1.35. The cervical stump is grasped with a clamp.

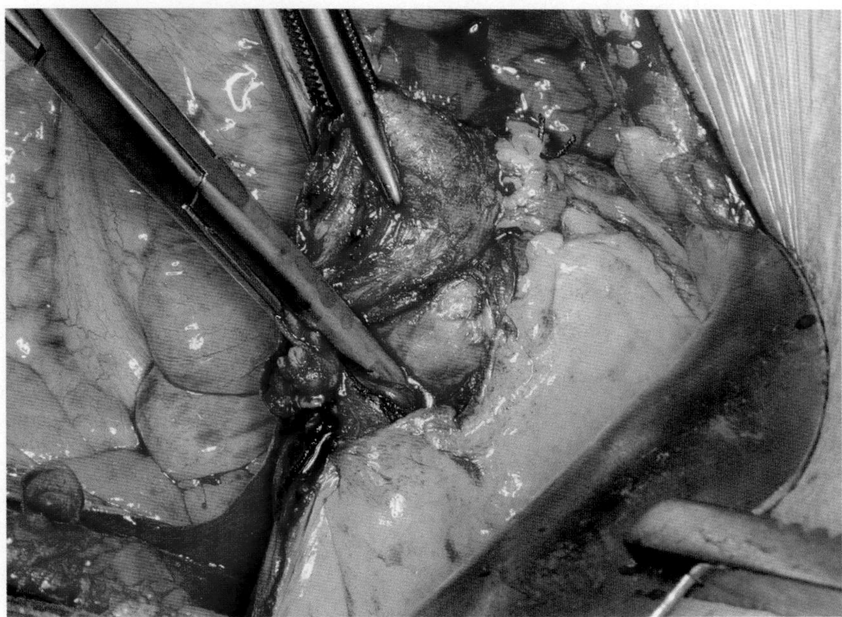

Tech Figure 8.1.36. The cardinal ligament is clamped with a straight clamp, cut, and suture-ligated.

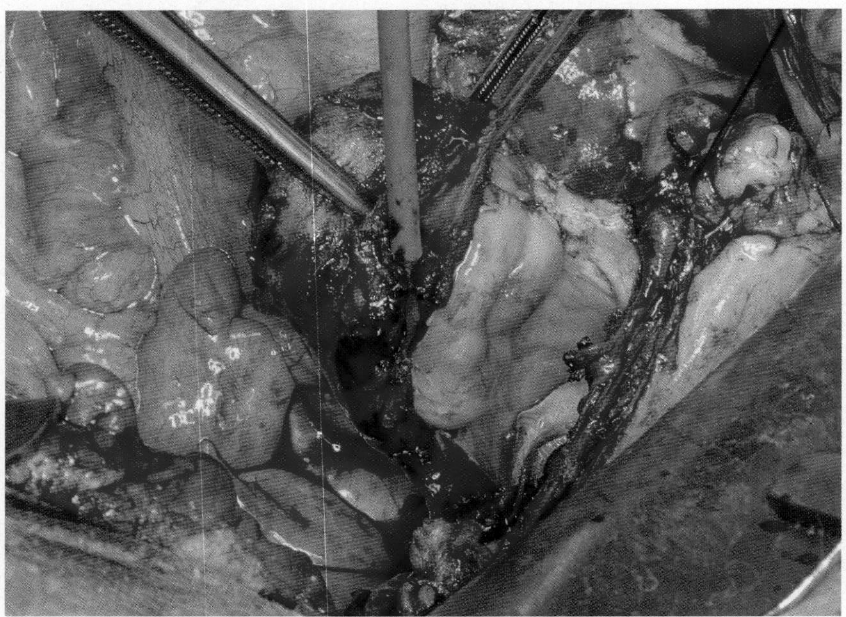

Tech Figure 8.1.37. The anterior vagina is incised, exposing the cervix.

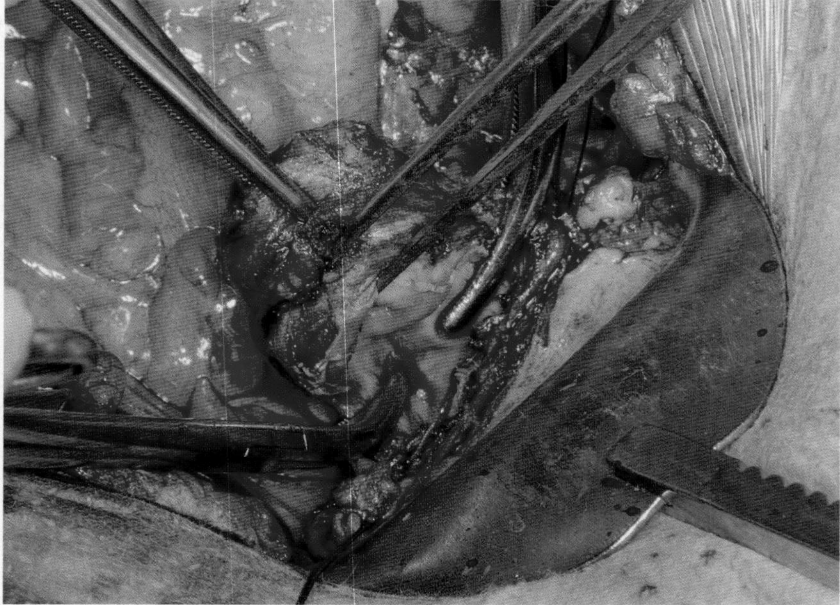

Tech Figure 8.1.38. Curved clamps are placed on the posterior vagina.

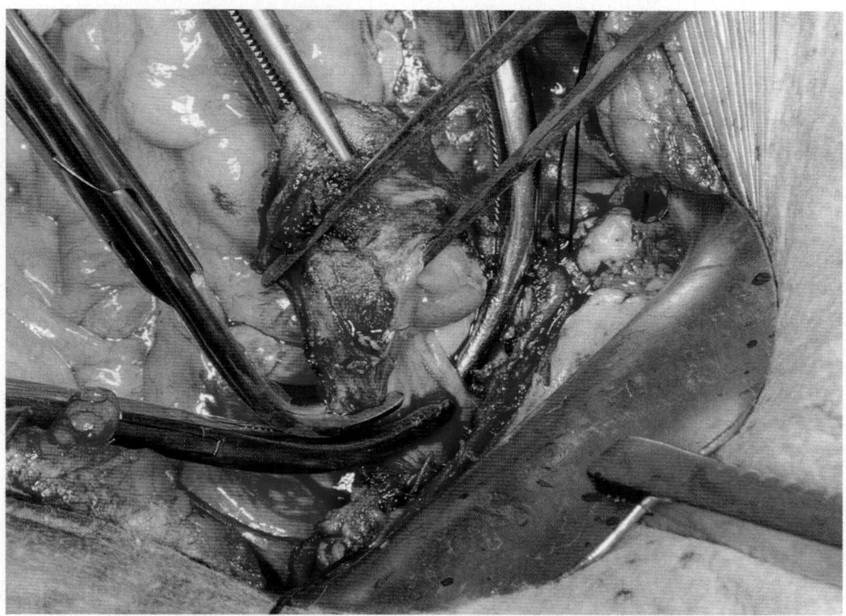

Tech Figure 8.1.39. Jorgensen scissors are used to incise the posterior vagina and amputate the cervix.

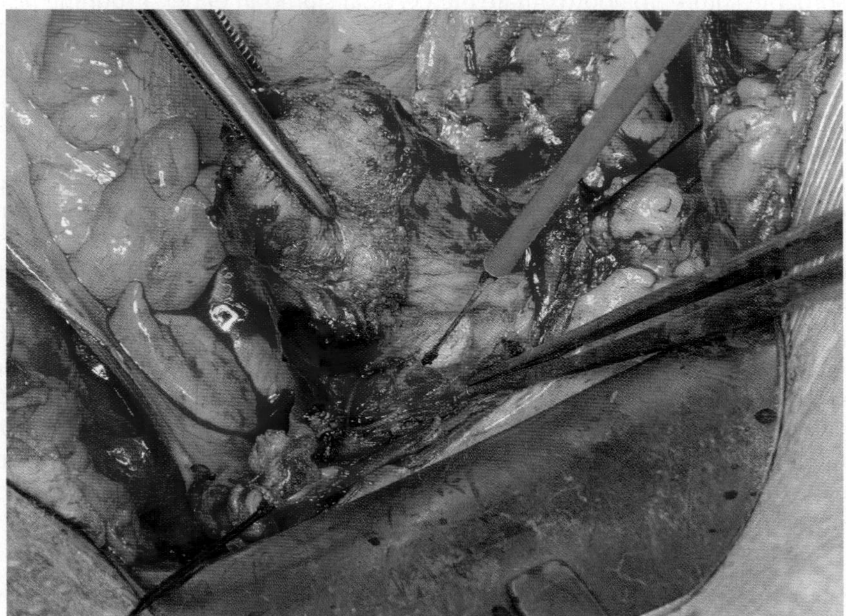

Tech Figure 8.1.40. Radiofrequency electrical energy is used to make a colpotomy.

- An *intrafascial hysterectomy* is performed in theory to preserve the neurovascular supply at the cervicovaginal junction by maintaining the pubovesicocervical fascia. This technique differs from an extrafascial hysterectomy after the uterine artery has been ligated (see **Tech Fig. 8.1.41**). Make transverse incisions on the anterior and posterior surfaces of the cervix, below the level of the uterine vasculature. Then, bluntly dissect the pubovesicocervical fascia off the lower uterine segment and cervix (i.e., with a gauze-covered finger). If the incision is made too deeply into the cervix, the loose fascial plane can be easily missed and cause unnecessary bleeding. Place a curved clamp inside the fascia on each side of the uterus to incorporate the uterosacral ligaments and upper vagina just below the cervix. Incise the vagina with Mayo scissors and amputate the uterus and cervix.

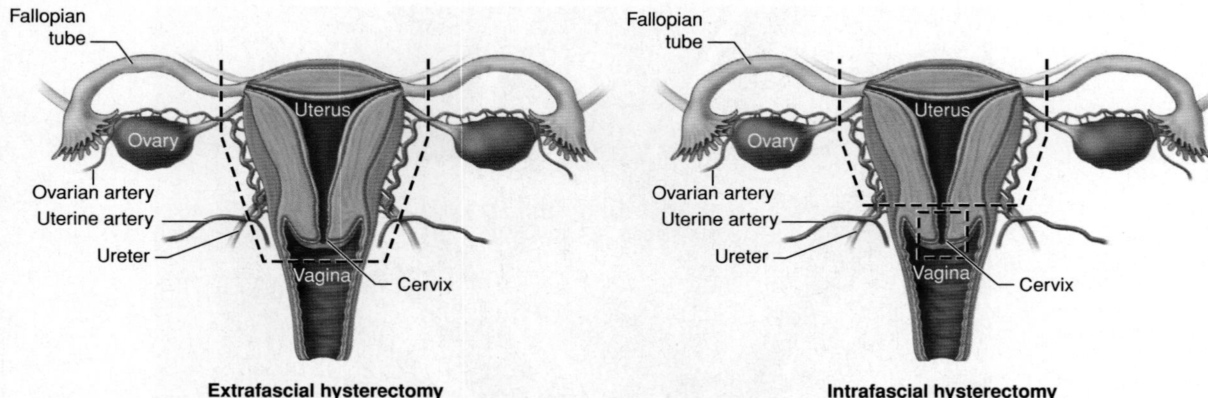

Tech Figure 8.1.41. Extrafascial versus intrafascial hysterectomy technique.

Supracervical hysterectomy

- In order to preserve the cervix, transect the cardinal and broad ligaments midway between the level of the internal and external cervical ostia. Then, amputate the cervix with a scalpel or a monopolar instrument. To avoid continued cyclical bleeding from retained endometrial tissue, use an electrocautery loop or radiofrequency energy to resect or fulgurate the endocervix.[7] Use a large absorbable suture, to approximate the cervical stump in either a running fashion or with interrupted figure-of-eight sutures.

Vaginal cuff closure

- Place Kocher clamps on the anterior and posterior aspects of the vaginal cuff. Using large absorbable suture, secure both angles with figure-of-eight stitches being careful to incorporate full thickness vagina with vaginal mucosa in each stitch. If curved clamps are used to incise the vagina, then the clamps at each angle can be used to facilitate angle stitch placement. Once the angles are secured, place interrupted figure-of-eight stitches between the angles to close the vaginal cuff and to achieve hemostasis.
- The association between hysterectomy and pelvic organ prolapse is controversial; however, many experts agree that the vaginal apex should be suspended at the time of hysterectomy. This can be accomplished either by performing an intrafascial hysterectomy or by incorporating the uterosacral ligaments in the vaginal cuff closure, specifically while placing the angle stitches.[8] Unfortunately, there is no data to support either method. Therefore, the decision to perform an apical suspension and the technique are largely based on surgeon preference.

Abdominal closure

- Thoroughly irrigate the pelvis with warm saline or Ringer's lactate solution. Confirm hemostasis of all pedicles and inspect the bladder and ureters. For a vertical incision, it is not required to close the peritoneum. Approximate the fascia with permanent suture in a running unlocked fashion. Fascial closure of a Pfannenstiel or Maylard incision may be performed using large delayed absorbable suture. A Cherney incision requires a more tailored closure in order to provide additional support for the approximated musculature. Close the peritoneum using a running absorbable stitch. Transfix the ends of the rectus tendons to the inferior portion of the lower flap of the rectus sheath with five or six interrupted delayed-absorbable or permanent sutures in a horizontal mattress configuration. To avoid osteomyelitis, do not suture the rectus muscles to the periosteum of the symphysis pubis.

PEARLS AND PITFALLS

- To avoid ureteral injury, open the peritoneum and identify the ureter along the medial leaf inferior to the gonadal vessels.
- Retroperitoneal dissection is easiest with a blunt instrument such as the Yankauer suction tip.
- The urinary bladder should be dissected off the cervicovaginal junction prior to ligation of the uterine arteries.
- To help identify the cervicovaginal junction, insert a sponge stick (4 × 4 cm sponge folded into a ringed forceps) into the vagina applying pressure in a caudal and anterior direction.
- If excessive bleeding is encountered, a clamp should never be placed blindly which may cause inadvertent injury. Instead, hold pressure with a finger or sponge and identify key structures prior to vessel ligation.
- Use the 0-vicryl tie on the specimen side of the IP ligament to secure the ovaries to the Kelly clamp on the uterine cornua for better exposure.
- In order to optimize exposure, large uteri with benign disease can be removed in a supracervical fashion, followed by removal of the cervix secondarily.
- Placing the patient in a small degree of Trendelenburg helps to clear the pelvis of bowel and improve exposure.
- Prior to terminating the procedure, inspect all vascular pedicles and the vaginal cuff to assess for hemostasis.
- If delineation of the urinary bladder proves difficult, the bladder can be back-filled with sterile milk or methylene blue which will identify any defects.
- Use sterile water to irrigate instead of saline for clear visualization of bleeding vessels.

POSTOPERATIVE CARE

- The average length of hospital stay after abdominal hysterectomy in the United States is 3 days.[9] Routine postoperative care includes monitoring a patient's fluid and hemodynamic status, pain control, and rehabilitation toward resuming normal diet and activity. Postoperative pain is often initially controlled with intravenous medications such as narcotics and nonsteroidal anti-inflammatory drugs (NSAIDs). Patient-controlled analgesia is also frequently used. Parenteral analgesics may be transitioned to oral medications fairly rapidly, as soon as the same day of surgery or the first postoperative day. An early transition to oral medications should be encouraged to reduce the effects of intravenous narcotics on the bowel.
- Typically, postoperative colonic stasis resolves after 3 days. Evidence does not support the routine use of nasogastric tubes to decrease this interval.[10] Early feeding of a regular diet is recommended which may help stimulate the bowel and decrease the length of hospital stay. Early ambulation, as soon as the night of surgery, is recommended
- Remove the bladder catheter within 24 hours after surgery and as early as the day of surgery. Bladder catheter discontinuation by postoperative day 1 decreases urinary tract infections.[11]
- Upon discharge from the hospital, the patient is encouraged to resume normal activity as quickly as is comfortable with a few exceptions. These include abstaining from sexual intercourse to allow the vaginal cuff to heal and abstaining from heavy lifting greater than 10 pounds to prevent fascial dehiscence for 6 weeks. Unfortunately there is no strong evidence to support these recommended limitations; however, studies implicate vaginal intercourse as the most common inciting event in vaginal cuff dehiscence.[12] The patient should be seen within 2 to 4 weeks postoperatively by her physician for a gentle vaginal and abdominal examination to ensure her incisions are healing well.

OUTCOMES

- The outcomes of abdominal hysterectomy are very good. Without complication, most patients fully recover and are pain free within 4 to 6 weeks after surgery. Most women report symptom relief, no change in sexual function, and satisfaction with the procedure. Complication rates are low, and the rate of unintended major surgical procedures such as operative injury to intra-abdominal organs requiring repair or return to the operating room within 8 weeks postoperatively is approximately 0.3% to 0.7%.[13]

COMPLICATIONS

- The most common major complications after abdominal hysterectomy are hemorrhage, urinary tract injury, and bowel injury.[13] Hemorrhage complicates approximately 2% of abdominal hysterectomies, with an average blood loss of 300 to 400 mL.[13] Careful intraoperative inspection of pedicles before closure may help prevent this complication. Diligent attention to a patient's postoperative hemodynamic status, including vital signs and oliguria, is necessary to identify excessive bleeding early and to reduce the patient's risk for long-term sequelae. Depending on the source of bleeding, the approach may differ in evaluation and treatment. When the patient is stable and hemorrhage of any kind is suspected, CT imaging of the abdomen and pelvis with intravenous contrast provides the best way to identify active intra-abdominal hemorrhage. Stable patients with intraperitoneal hematoma can be managed expectantly or with radiographic embolization of the hypogastric vessels. Clotting parameters should be checked and any coagulopathy should be treated to expedite bleeding resolution. In contrast, an unstable patient with a surgical abdomen should return to the operating room as quickly as possible for surgical exploration. Profuse vaginal bleeding may resolve with an examination under anesthesia and additional vaginal cuff suture placement at the site of bleeding.

- Suspected intraoperative urinary tract injury must be evaluated and repaired if present. A postoperative ureteral injury may be asymptomatic or may present as flank or groin pain, fever, or prolonged ileus. The incidence of ureteral injury after total abdominal hysterectomy is 0.4 of 1,000 and the incidence of bladder injury is less than 1%.[13] Ureteral injury most commonly occurs while ligating the ovarian vessels or the uterine artery. Urinary bladder injury occurs most commonly during bladder dissection off the lower uterine segment, cervix, and upper vagina. Therefore, identification of the ureter through retroperitoneal dissection and careful dissection of the vesicouterine peritoneum to push the bladder away from the cervix thus displacing the ureter laterally is essential to reduce the risk of urinary tract injury.
- Bowel injuries primarily occur during adhesiolysis or upon entering the abdominal cavity and have a reported incidence of approximately 0.2% to 1%.[13] Superficial serosal defects do not require repair; however, injuries involving the muscularis or the mucosa require primary repair either with direct closure or resection/anastomosis depending upon the size of the injury. Small injuries to the bowel do not require postoperative dietary restrictions or a nasogastric tube. The risk of small bowel obstruction after abdominal hysterectomy is 13.6/1,000 and presents most commonly with abdominal distention, abdominal pain, vomiting, and an inability to pass flatus.[13] Abdominal films can confirm the diagnosis. The majority of small bowel obstructions resolve with conservative management that includes nasogastric tube placement and parenteral hydration. Persistent obstruction despite these measures may require surgical correction.
- Other complications of abdominal hysterectomy include infection, thromboembolic disease, and vaginal cuff dehiscence. Routine prophylactic antibiotics reduces postoperative infection overall; however, despite their administration, a low rate of urinary tract (4%), wound (3%), vaginal (0.2%), and intra-abdominal (0.1%) infections remains.[14] Subcutaneous or intra-abdominal abscesses may require drainage by either re-opening the abdominal incision and applying packing, or by placing percutaneous drains (Fig. 8.1.3). For women receiving thromboembolic prophylaxis for abdominal hysterectomy, the rate of VTE is 0.2%.[14] A postoperative patient who develops localized tenderness, asymmetric swelling in an extremity, dyspnea, pleuritic pain, tachypnea, or tachycardia should be evaluated for pulmonary embolism and deep VTE and treated accordingly. Vaginal cuff dehiscence is a rare complication that can become a surgical emergency if bowel eviscerates and becomes incarcerated. The risk of vaginal cuff dehiscence after abdominal hysterectomy is approximately 0.12%.[13] A woman may present with abdominal pain, profuse vaginal discharge, pelvic or vaginal pressure, or protrusion of bowel from the vagina. A simple dehiscence may be repaired vaginally; however, in the case of evisceration the bowel must be carefully inspected for damage which requires abdominal exploration.

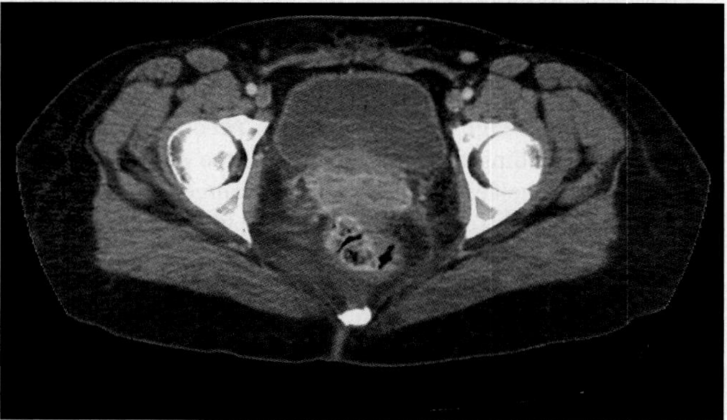

Figure 8.1.3. Pelvic abscess after hysterectomy.

KEY REFERENCES

1. Hendrix SL, Schimp V, Martin J, Singh A, Kruger M, McNeeley SG. The legendary superior strength of Pfannenstiel incision: a myth? *Am J Obstet Gynecol.* 2000;182:1446–1451.
2. Jacoby VL, Autry A, Jacobson G, Domush R, Nakagawa S, Jacoby A. Nationwide use of laparoscopic hysterectomy compared with abdominal and vaginal approaches. *Obstet Gynecol.* 2009;114:1041–1048.
3. Morelli M, Venturella R, Mocciaro R, et al. Prophylactic salpingectomy in premenopausal low-risk women for ovarian cancer: primum non nocere. *Gynecol Oncol.* 2013;129:448–451.
4. Committee on Practice Bulletins—Gynecology, American College of Obstetricians and Gynecologists. ACOG Practice Bulletin No. 84: prevention of deep vein thrombosis and pulmonary embolism. *Obstet Gynecol.* 2007;110:429–440.
5. Gould MK, Garcia DA, Wren SM, et al; American College of Chest Physicians. Prevention of VTE in nonorthopedic surgical patients: antithrombotic therapy and prevention of thrombosis, 9th ed, American college of Chest Physicians Evidence-Based Clinical Practice Guidelines. *Chest.* 2012;141(2 Suppl):e227S–e277S.
6. ACOG Committee on Practice Bulletins—Gynecology. ACOG Practice Bulletin No. 104: antibiotic prophylaxis for gynecologic procedures. *Obstet Gynecol.* 2009;113(5):1180–1189.
7. Kilkku P, Grönroos M, Rauramo L. Supravaginal uterine amputation with perioperative electrocoagulation of endocervical mucosa: description of the method. *Acta Obstet Gynecol Scand.* 1985;64:175–177.
8. Thakar R, Sultan AH. Hysterectomy and pelvic organ dysfunction. *Best Pract Res Clin Obstet Gynaecol.* 2005;19:403–418.
9. Wu JM, Wechter ME, Geller EJ, Nguyen TV, Visco AG. Hysterectomy rates in the United States, 2003. *Obstet Gynecol.* 2007;110:1091–1095.
10. Charoenkwan K, Phillipson G, Vutyavanich T. Early versus delayed (traditional) oral fluids and food for reducing complications after major abdominal gynaecologic surgery. *Cochrane Database Syst Rev.* 2007;CD004508.
11. Phipps S, Lim YN, McClinton S, Barry C, Rane A, N'Dow J. Short term urinary catheter policies following urogenital surgery in adults. *Cochrane Database Syst Rev.* 2006;CD004374.
12. Hur HC, Guido RS, Mansuria SM, Hacker MR, Sanfilippo JS, Lee TT. Incidence and patient characteristics of vaginal cuff dehiscence after different modes of hysterectomies. *J Minim Invasive Gynecol.* 2007;14:311–317.
13. Maresh MJ, Metcalfe MA, McPherson K, et al. The VALUE national hysterectomy study: description of the patients and their surgery. *BJOG.* 2002;109:302–312.
14. Mäkinen J, Johansson J, Tomás C, et al. Morbidity of 10 110 hysterectomies by type of approach. *Hum Reprod.* 2001;16:1473–1478.

Chapter 8.2 Conventional Laparoscopic Hysterectomy Including Laparoscopic Supracervical Hysterectomy

Stephen E. Zimberg, Michael L. Sprague, Katrin S. Arnolds

GENERAL PRINCIPLES

Definition

Hysterectomy is the most common nonobstetric operation performed in the United States with 602,457 procedures performed in 2003 alone.[1] It is also the most common surgical procedure performed on women in Western countries, with 23.3% of women aged 18 years or older undergoing the procedure.[2] The primary indication listed for hysterectomy are fibroids (31%), uterine prolapse (14.5%), endometriosis (11%), abnormal uterine bleeding (14%), and cancers of the genital tract (10%).[3] Cohen revisited this using the 2009 United States Nationwide Inpatient Sample and found a decrease in the total number of hysterectomies performed, 479,814, in women 18 years of age or greater,[4] with 86.6% performed for benign indications. Note that the decrease in numbers does not necessarily reflect a drop in the actual number of hysterectomies performed as this and the previous studies looked primarily at inpatient statistics and does not reflect the shift to the outpatient performance of these procedures. In fact, Loring et al.,[5] looking at a large retrospective review of hysterectomies performed between 2004 and 2012, noting that, in 2004, 2 of 194 laparoscopic hysterectomies were performed in an outpatient setting, whereas, by 2012, 85% (293/344) were performed as outpatient procedures. Still, the study is instructive in that 56% were completed abdominally, 20.4% were performed laparoscopically, 18.8% done vaginally, and 4.5% performed with robot assistance. Furthermore, Wright et al.[6] documented a change in the performance of hysterectomy for benign indications with the introduction of the robot between 2007 and 2010. In his study, there were 40% abdominal, 30.5% laparoscopic, 9.5% robot-assisted, and 19.9% vaginal showing that robotic and conventional laparoscopic approaches continue to decrease the numbers of abdominal procedures, although 40% or more are still done as an open laparotomy.

The access to laparoscopic minimally invasive hysterectomy also appears to be related to patient socioeconomic status and geographic location. Patel et al.[7] studied a retrospective cohort of 32,436 patients from the 2010 Healthcare Cost and Utilization Project and noted 32% of the patients underwent laparoscopic hysterectomy (LH) compared to 67% abdominal hysterectomy. Stratifying this, women most likely to undergo LH were less than 35, Caucasian, and privately insured. Geographically in the United States, women in the Northeast were far more likely to have an LH compared to the Midwest and South. Our urban hospitals were more likely than rural, and teaching hospitals more likely than nonteaching, to offer LH with government-owned hospitals least likely to offer LH.

The goal of this chapter is to give the reader the tools to advance from the performance of hysterectomy by laparotomy to a laparoscopic, minimally invasive approach for most procedures.

Anatomic Considerations

Minimally invasive hysterectomy includes total laparoscopic hysterectomy (TLH), laparoscopic supracervical hysterectomy (LSH), robotic-assisted hysterectomy (RAH), and laparoscopic-assisted vaginal hysterectomy (LAVH). The basic technique for the laparoscopic portion of all of the subgroups is similar and will be described below as either the TLH or LSH.

There are few contraindications for the TLH approach because this technique can be used in both benign and malignant conditions. Additionally, most large uteri can be efficiently addressed using conventional laparoscopic techniques by an experienced surgical team. Kovac[8] outlined three basic technical issues to determine the route of hysterectomy for benign disease as they are the difficulties that make most gynecologists apprehensive:

1. Adequacy of the vaginal passageway (e.g., virginity, orthopedic restrictions to the lithotomy position, and a narrow vagina of <2 fingerbreadths, especially at the apex of the vagina)
2. The size of the uterus (e.g., leiomyomata)
3. Potential, severe, extrauterine risk factors suggestive of serious pelvic disease (e.g., endometriosis, adnexal pathology, and adhesions)

Though Kovac originally described an algorithm of obstacles for the performance of vaginal hysterectomy, the use of conventional laparoscopy circumvents these obstacles and allows for a minimally invasive solution for each issue.

Particular consideration must also be paid to obesity in the performance of laparoscopic surgery. This affects up to 36.5% of Europeans and more than 39.5% of American patients. Guraslan and colleagues[9] completed a retrospective review of 153 patients undergoing TLH stratified by BMI. The rate of conversion to laparotomy (9.8%), blood loss, total complications (5.9%), and length of stay did not vary between the groups and they concluded that LH was safe and feasible in the obese and morbidly obese population. This was echoed by Mathews[10] though they noted potential issues with increased abdominal pressure and Trendelenburg positioning resulting in increased airway pressure and end-tidal CO_2, in obese versus nonobese patients. Increased BMI did not appear to be associated with differences in blood loss, duration of surgery, length of stay, or complication rates.

Additionally, a relative contraindication to laparoscopy was thought to be the presence of a ventriculoperitoneal shunt. Cobianchi and colleagues[11] examined this in a case series and literature review. They concluded that the current generation valves were unlikely to cause issues with gas leakage under 80 mm Hg, which is well below that of the current standard insufflation pressures of 10 to 15 mm Hg. A possible exception is laparoscopy immediately following a newly implanted shunt for both adults and children.

IMAGING AND OTHER DIAGNOSTICS

Gynecologic diagnostic centers use pelvic ultrasound as the first-line imaging technique for evaluation of gynecologic complaints such as pelvic pain, abnormal uterine bleeding, and pelvic masses. This has been the primary imaging modality of uterine evaluation, showing the number and extent of fibroids, presence of endometrial disease, and presence and characterization of adnexal masses. With the controversies surrounding power morcellation and undetected malignancy, diffusion-weighted MRI and diffusion tensor imaging have been shown to accurately diagnose preoperatively endometrial, myometrial, and cervical malignancies with great accuracy,[12] though tissue diagnosis is the gold standard. In the absence of this, traditional MRI is a reasonable diagnostic tool for use in larger uteri prior to hysterectomy, particularly in the perimenopausal age range when malignancy is more common. Blood tumor markers, most notably CA125, have been used but with limited success. CA125 is elevated with uterine tumors, dependent on size, adenomyosis, and other inflammatory conditions in the abdomen, making it of limited diagnostic use. The combination of MRI and serum fractionated LDH may have a role for planning the surgical approach in suspicious myometrial lesions.

PREOPERATIVE PLANNING

Proper preoperative assessment will facilitate an efficient procedure. Patients for which hysterectomy is being considered should have a recent pap smear and an endometrial biopsy, as clinically indicated, to rule out cancerous or precancerous processes. Imaging, as suggested above, should be performed to document uterine and adnexal pathology.

Decisions must be made with the patients regarding hysterectomy type and approach. The mode of surgical approach is decided between total abdominal hysterectomy (TAH), transvaginal hysterectomy (TVH), or LH, and the type of hysterectomy is determined between LSH and TLH. Decisions must be made as to whether to remove or to keep the cervix in particular. Although ACOG guidelines continue to recommend vaginal hysterectomy in most cases, recent studies question that approach. Allam et al.[13] completed a randomized controlled trial which found that although TLH had a longer operating time, there was less blood loss, fewer complications, and less postoperative pain than with TAH or VH. Similarly, Pokkinen et al.[14] noted reduced need for analgesics in LH compared with vaginal hysterectomy.

Though supracervical hysterectomy has been performed as long as total hysterectomy, there are no studies that conclusively define the optimal procedure. Nesbitt-Hawes[15] concluded that, given the currently available evidence, all forms of hysterectomy should be offered to women requiring hysterectomy. She noted that it could not be stated that LSH prevents long-term pelvic organ prolapse, offer improved sexual function, or reduce operative risk, though it does provide faster return to work. In a recent study from Italy, however, Saccardi et al.[16] noted women in their LSH group reported a greater ease of recovery of sexual function as opposed to TLH.

Complicating the decision-making on the type of hysterectomy is the effect of TLH and LSH on ovarian reserve. Yuan and colleagues[17] looked at ovarian reserve in patients undergoing total versus supracervical hysterectomy by assessing anti-müllerian hormone. Their data show serum AMH levels decreased significantly at 4 months posthysterectomy in patients in their 30s and 40s, with a much greater decrease in patients having a TLH over those with LSH. These data suggest that LSH is better than TLH in preserving ovarian function, and need to be considered when discussing with your patient.

SURGICAL MANAGEMENT

Positioning and Approach

The patient is first placed in dorsal lithotomy position with laparoscopic leg cradles such as Allen stirrups. This allows the legs to be cushioned and allows for access to the perineum, with flexion of the knees and hips to avoid neuromuscular injury.[18] Intermittent compression devices are also placed on the calves at this time. As basic as it sounds, having an operating room table with ability to achieve adequate patient Trendelenburg position is of paramount importance (Fig. 8.2.1). Trendelenburg is often 35 degrees or greater to allow the intestine to migrate cephalad, thereby exposing the pelvic anatomy.

Securing the patient safely on the table is often a challenge, particularly with obese patients. We have been placing the patient directly on an egg crate mattress secured to the operating table as described by Klauschie and coworkers (Fig. 8.2.2).[19] This allows for the use of Trendelenburg with minimal slippage and has the advantage of working even with the morbidly obese patient without extra straps or shoulder braces that can predispose to neurologic and other injuries in longer procedures. One particular axiom is that the larger the patient, the greater the Trendelenburg angle that is required for adequate visualization. Steep Trendelenburg position is not without consequences; however, ocular complications, alopecia, as well as nerve injury have been reported.[20] Gould et al.[21] reported the use of less Trendelenburg angle in a blinded trial which lowered the angle from 40 to 28 degrees, and found no difference in the operative times for pelvic surgery among 16 different surgeons.

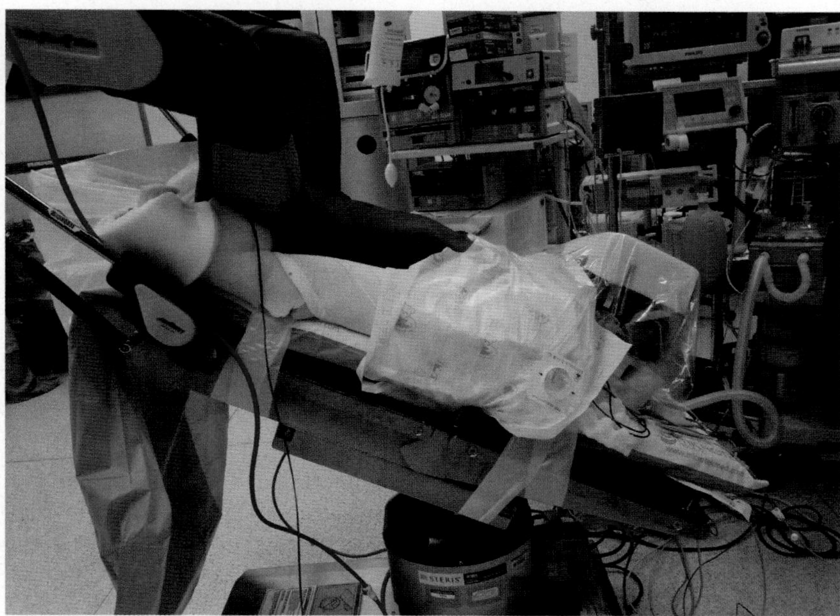

Figure 8.2.1. Placement of patient in Trendelenburg position.

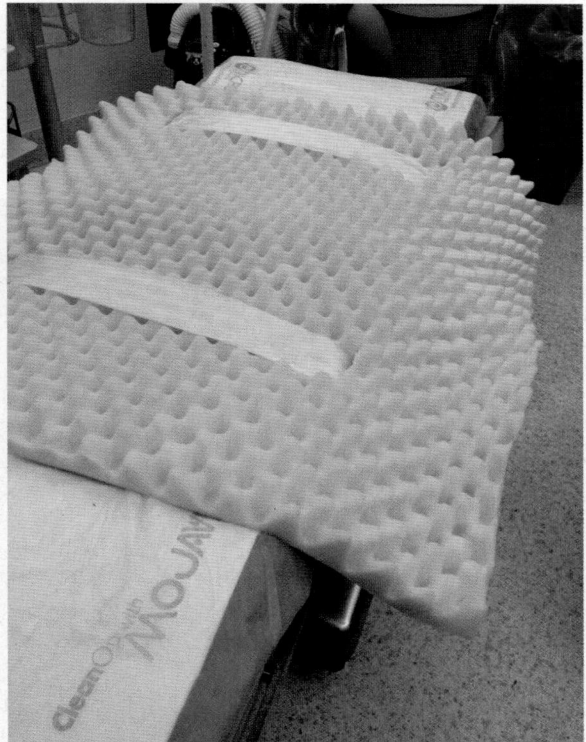

Figure 8.2.2. Securing the egg crate mattress to operating table.

Procedures and Techniques

Total laparoscopic hysterectomy

Step 1: Placement of uterine manipulator and bladder catheter

Before instrumentation of the patient, standard prophylactic antibiotics and DVT prophylaxis are administered. The Caprini (ACCP) score guidelines account for the type of surgery, obesity, previous VTE, and other complicating factors such as malignancy to determine need and dosing.[22] Antibiotic prophylaxis and VTE prophylaxis should be based on BMI (and volume of distribution), not ideal weight.

A standard Foley catheter is placed to drain the bladder during the procedure. One can consider the use of a dual port (three-way) catheter to allow filling and draining of the bladder when significant lower uterine segment and bladder adhesions are anticipated or when encountered. This allows for rapid installation of saline to delineate the borders of the bladder and prevent incidental cystectomy. The surgeon can use blue dye if a cystotomy is encountered to assess the water tightness of closure.

A uterine manipulator with a pericervical cup is placed to allow for greater movement of the uterus with fewer ports to achieve the desired angles at which to operate. For both TLH and LSH, we use the V-Care uterine manipulator (ConMed Endosurgery, Utica, NY) (Tech Fig. 8.2.1). Other manipulators are available and may work equally well for these procedures. The cervix is grasped with a single-tooth tenaculum and dilated to 21 French. The manipulator is introduced and the balloon inflated. For the TLH, the cup of the manipulator is sewn onto the cervix to assist in tissue removal. For the supracervical procedures, the manipulator is placed without suturing.

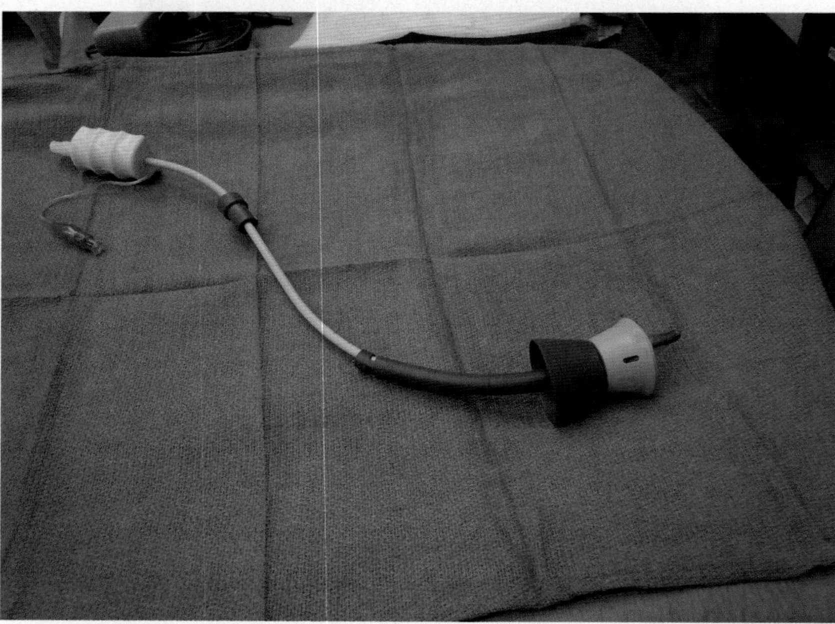

Tech Figure 8.2.1. V-Care uterine manipulator.

Van den Haak and colleagues[23] recently reviewed 25 articles covering 10 uterine manipulators. Interestingly, they found that though convenient, definitive documentation of efficacy and safety was scant. Their review did not find the "optimal" manipulator. There has also been speculation that dilatation of the cervix and placement of any manipulator may upstage an undiagnosed uterine endometrial carcinoma. Iavazzo and Gkegkes[24] recently reported "the assumption that uterine manipulators can induce intra-operative dissemination of tumor cells is suggested to be a derivative of common sense. The existence of cases with positive peritoneal cytology after uterine manipulation cannot be determined with certainty, and whether manipulators result in metastasis at peritoneum or disease recurrence." In cases where it is impossible to place a manipulator, use of a standard infant nasal suction bulb or bulb top of an Asepto syringe in the vagina will often delineate the vaginal edges (Tech Fig. 8.2.2).

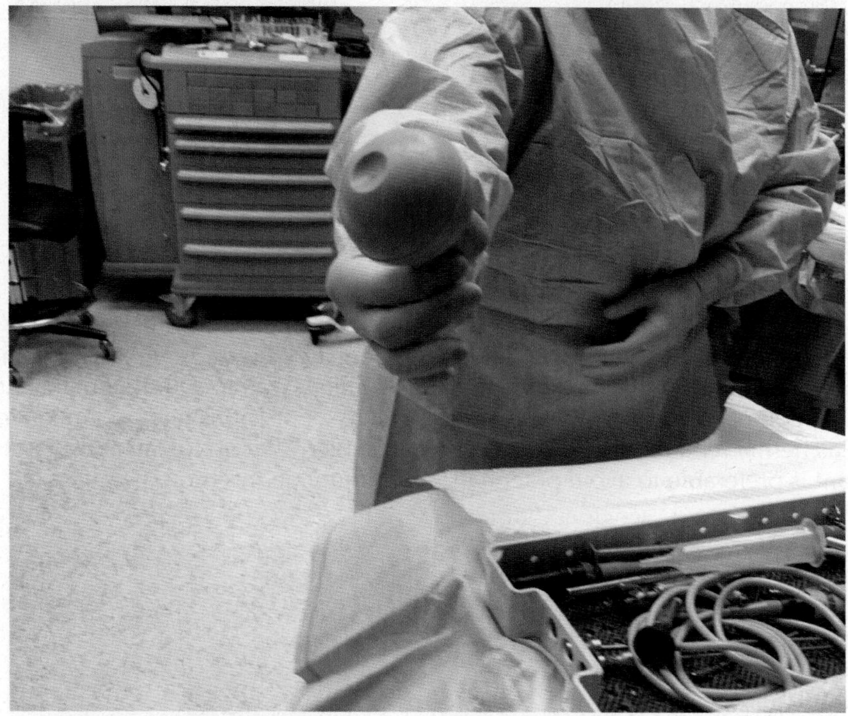

Tech Figure 8.2.2. Use of the bulb top of an Asepto bulb syringe. The bulb portion goes in the vagina first up against the cervix.

Step 2: Placement of primary trocar

Our approach to initial trocar placement is predicated on factors including uterine size and type of previous abdominal surgery. For uteri 16 weeks pregnancy size or less, we place the camera port at the umbilicus (Tech Fig. 8.2.3). This is a 5-mm port for most patients, though 10-mm ports should be considered in more obese patients to prevent damage to the instruments and camera from torque. The angle of port insertion at the umbilicus should be 45 degrees for normal BMI patients and more toward a 90-degree angle with increasing obesity due to the position of the umbilicus in relation to the aortic bifurcation. We employ the direct optical insertion technique under direct vision rather than a blind Veress needle insertion. Tinelli et al.[25] reported no statistically significant difference in complications between direct insertion and Veress needle, suggesting that the visual entry systems offer statistical advantage in terms of time savings and reduced minor vascular and bowel injuries. The key concept is not to be "wed to the umbilicus" or Veress needle.

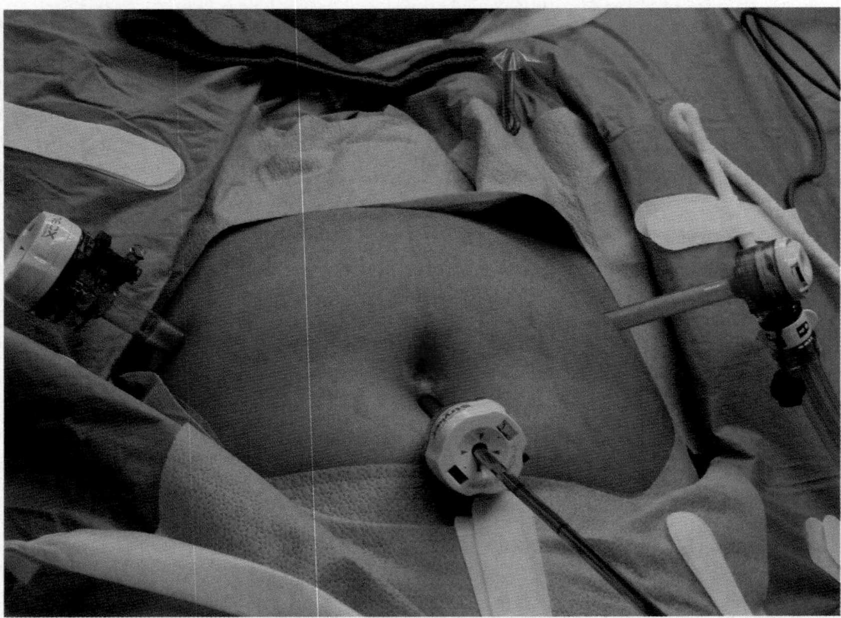

Tech Figure 8.2.3. Standard camera port placement for uteri 16 weeks or less.

When the uterus is greater than 16 weeks size, then the camera port is placed above the umbilicus in the midline up to a level several centimeters below the lower costal margin (Tech Fig. 8.2.4). These should be placed at 90-degree angle to the abdominal wall to avoid tunneling and will give greater visualization of the pelvis. When there is a history of previous mid-abdominal or umbilical surgery such as hernia repair with mesh or colorectal surgery, the use of Palmer's point in the left upper quadrant is preferable to avoid potential bowel injury on insertion.

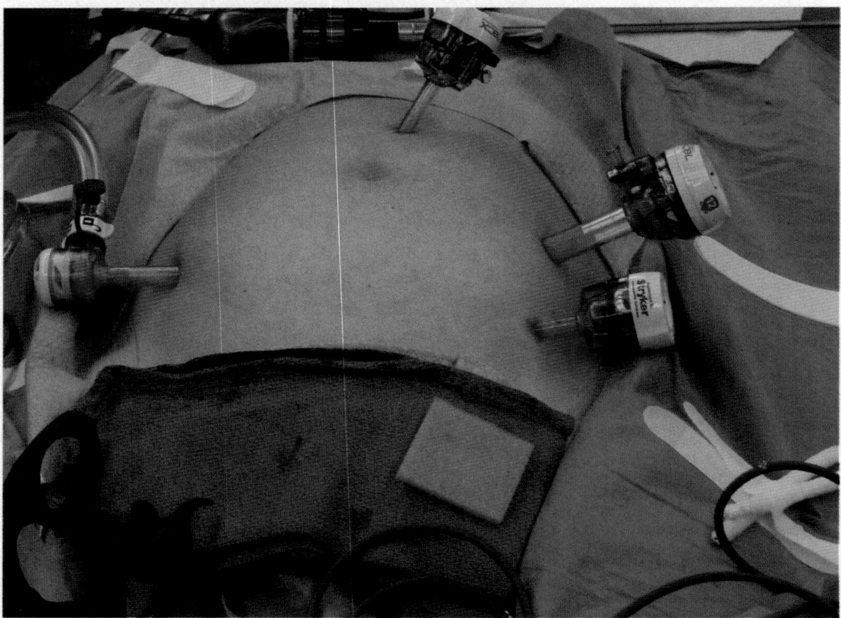

Tech Figure 8.2.4. Port placement for larger uteri with camera above the umbilicus in the midline.

Step 3: Placement of secondary trocars

Once the patient is placed in Trendelenburg position, the abdomen is insufflated with CO_2 to a final pressure of 12 to 15 mm Hg, and the secondary ports are placed under direct vision. If the operating surgeon is on the patient's right side, then a 10-mm trocar is placed in the right lower quadrant above the anterior superior iliac spine (ASIS). The safe distances from the midline to avoid internal epigastric artery injury are 6 cm from the midline at the level of the ASIS and 9 cm off the midline at the level of the umbilicus.[26] The exact placement depends on the size of the uterus as this port will migrate cephalad as the uterus enlarges. The second 5-mm trocar will be placed on the right side approximately 10 cm above the 10-mm trocar. The third 5-mm trocar is placed on the patient's left side at approximately the same level as the right-sided port. If the surgeon is operating from the patient's left side, then the port locations are reversed. For morbidly obese patients, consideration should be given to using all 10-mm ports to allow use of instruments with greater diameter and avoid damage to instruments due to torque.

Step 4: Instrumentation for optimal visualization

The insufflation tubing is placed on one of the lateral ports to decrease lens fogging. Efficient evacuation of smoke and water vapor from lysed tissue is essential for good visualization. We employ the AirSeal (Tech Fig. 8.2.5) insufflator (Surgiquest, Millford, CT, USA) which allows heated insufflation with CO_2 and smoke evacuation from a single port (either 5 to 10 mm). Additionally, the device is calibrated to maintain a steady, preset pneumoperitoneum, even when the vaginal cuff is open, which is an advantage in TLH and obese patients.

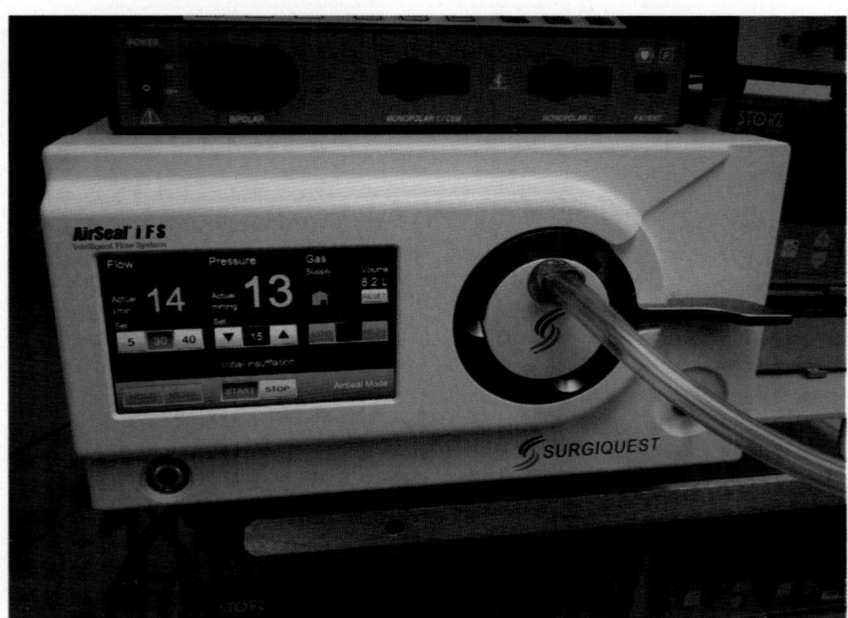

Tech Figure 8.2.5. AirSeal insufflation device.

The general instrumentation used is in the standard laparoscopy sets available in most operating rooms. Soft bowel graspers, Maryland graspers, and single- and double-toothed tenaculums are the primary instruments for manipulation of tissue and bowel. Electrosurgical devices are used to coagulate blood vessels and cut tissue. We commonly use an ultrasonic device for dissection, vessel sealing, and tissue division, as one instrument can be used for most steps (Tech Fig. 8.2.6). Advanced bipolar devices (such as LigaSure [Covidien, Boulder, CO, USA], EnSeal [Ethicon Endo Surgery, Somerville, NJ, USA], PlasmaKinetic, and others) can also be used.

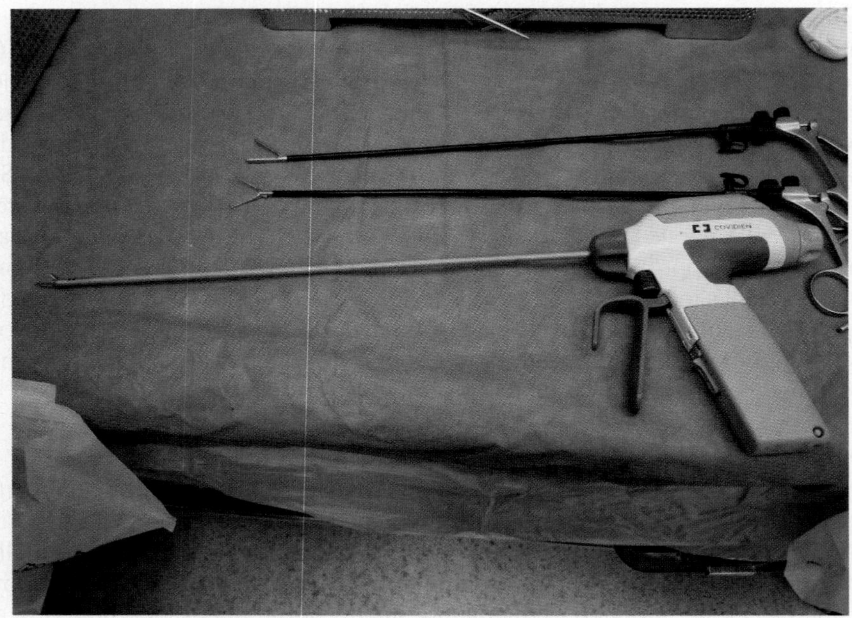

Tech Figure 8.2.6. Ultrasonic energy device.

Standard irrigation sets with power irrigation and suction are used to keep the surgical field clean for dissection. In patients where there is extensive pelvic adhesion or endometriosis, the use of lighted ureteral stents should be considered. Placed at the beginning of the procedure, they offer a way to avoid complications by "lighting the path" **(Tech Fig. 8.2.7)**.

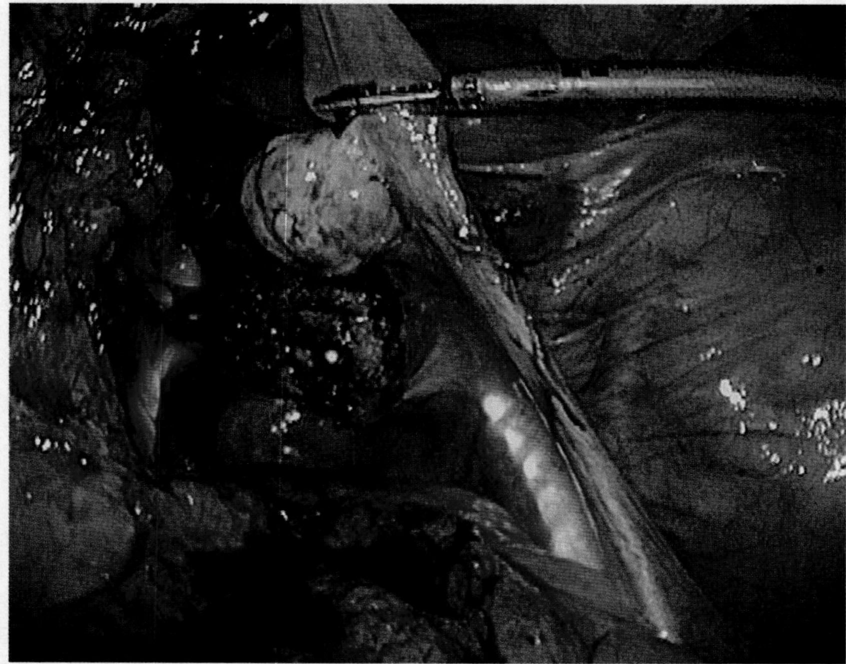

Tech Figure 8.2.7. Use of lighted ureteral stents to help with visualization of the ureters in complex cases.

Step 5: Divide the round ligament, tube, and utero-ovarian ligament

If the ovary is to be removed, the infundibulopelvic ligament is skeletonized, desiccated with bipolar radiofrequency device, and divided (Tech Fig. 8.2.8). The Sonicision ultrasonic device is then used to transect the fallopian tube, round ligament, and utero-ovarian ligament as the first step of the procedure (Tech Fig. 8.2.9).

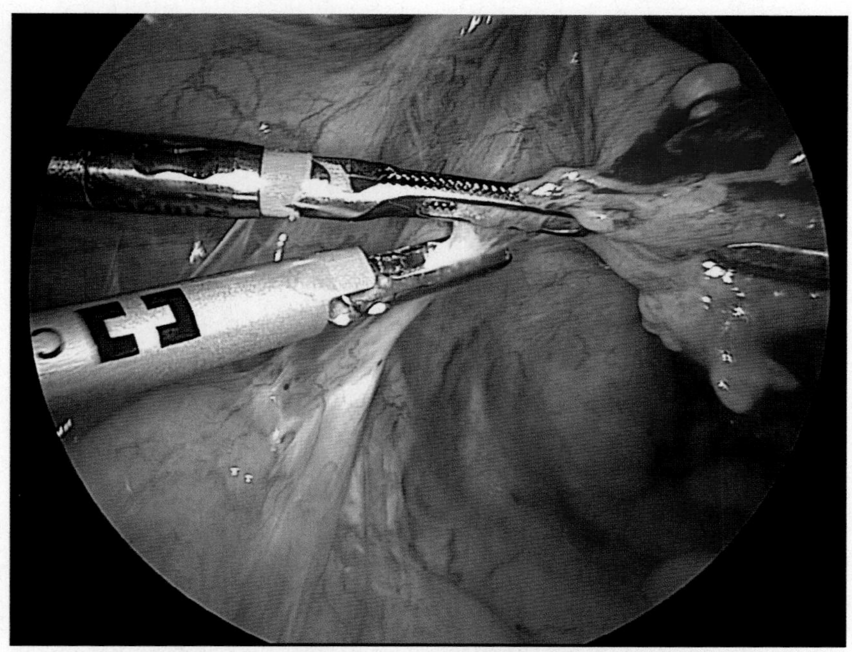

Tech Figure 8.2.8. Inspect the pelvic structures, desiccate and divide the infundibulopelvic ligament.

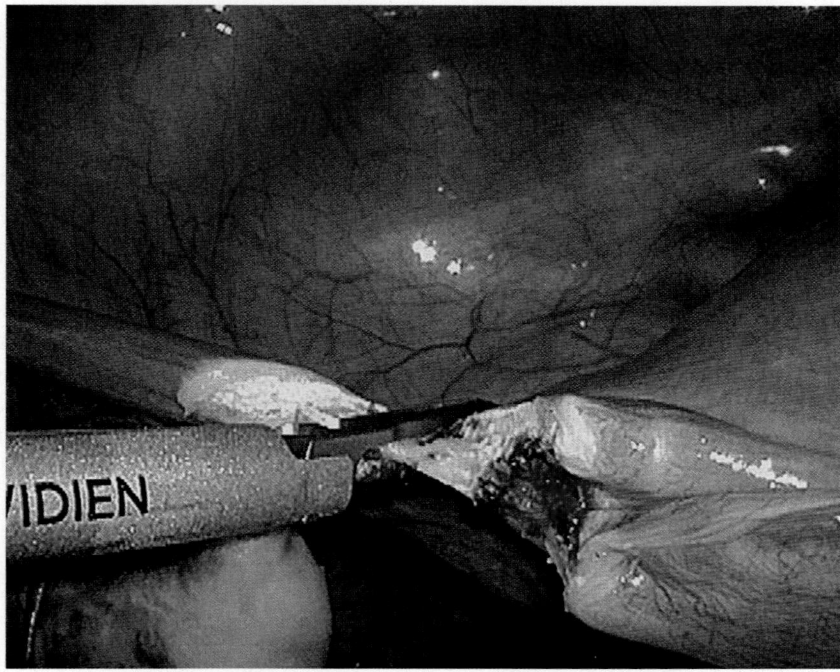

Tech Figure 8.2.9. Transect the fallopian tube, round ligament, and utero-ovarian ligament.

Step 6: Divide the superior portion of the broad ligament

The upper portion of the broad ligament is then incised (**Tech Fig. 8.2.10**) and the bladder flap is developed by opening the anterior leaf and deflecting the bladder caudally. The insufflated CO_2 will help open the leaves of the broad ligament by filling and expanding areolar tissue and sharp dissection will expose the uterine vessels.

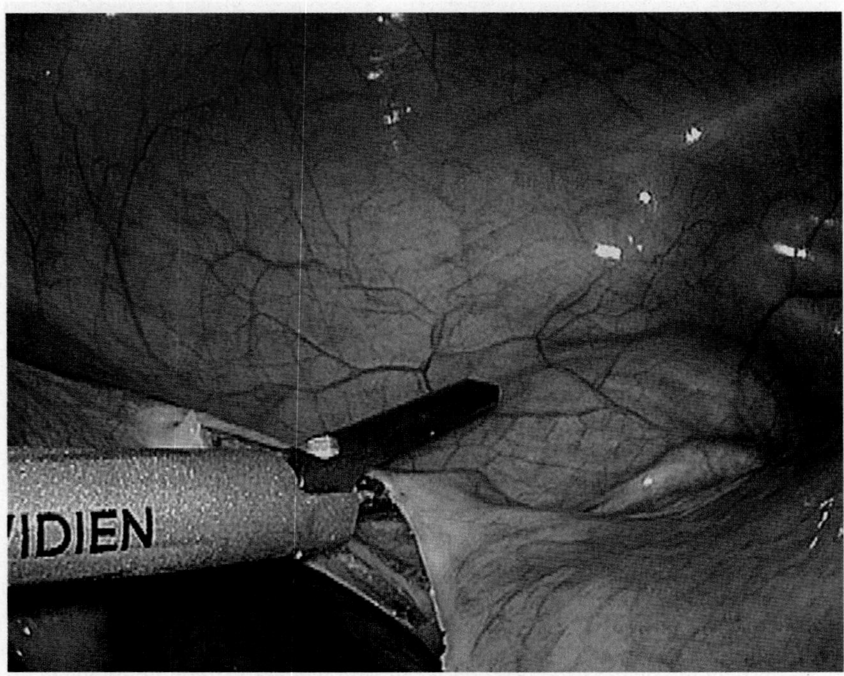

Tech Figure 8.2.10. Divide superior portion of broad ligament.

Step 7: Isolate, divide, and lateralize cardinal ligaments

Once isolated, the uterine artery and veins are desiccated with bipolar radiofrequency device and divided (**Tech Fig. 8.2.11**). Technically, the ultrasonic devices should handle up to 7-mm-diameter vessels which include most uterine arteries encountered, but our experience has been that bipolar cautery is often needed for reliable bleeding control. The vessels are then "lateralized" in a series of "V" motions to move the vessels laterally and over the manipulator cup (**Tech Fig. 8.2.12**). This also moves the ureter laterally and out of the surgical field.

The bladder flap is then further developed over the manipulator cup by sharp and blunt dissection (**Tech Fig. 8.2.13**). This moves the bladder out of the way for the colpotomy. Adhesions in this area are common and sharp dissection is used to remove the bladder from the lower uterine segment and cervix. Injury to the bladder is most common in this location. If it does occur, complete the dissection of the bladder from the cervix with adequate margins prior to repairing the bladder. Use a simple, two-layer closure with 3-0 polydioxanone (PDS-like) or polyglactin (Vicryl-like) suture. Cystoscopy postprocedure is mandatory if this occurs to ensure satisfactory watertight repair.

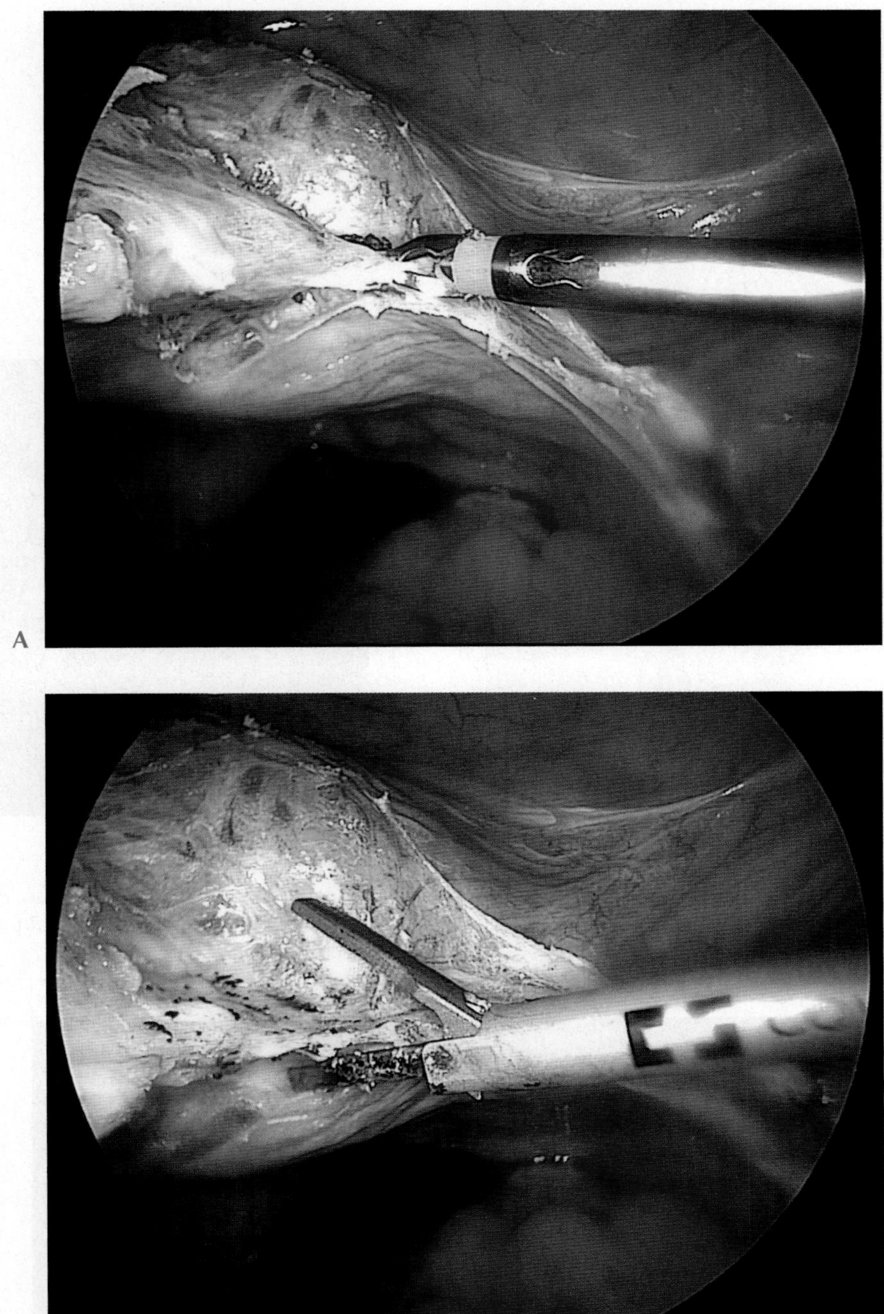

Tech Figure 8.2.11. Desiccate and divide the uterine artery and vein. **A** shows desiccation of the uterine artery and vein with bipolar cautery. **B** shows division of the uterine artery and vein using ultrasonic energy.

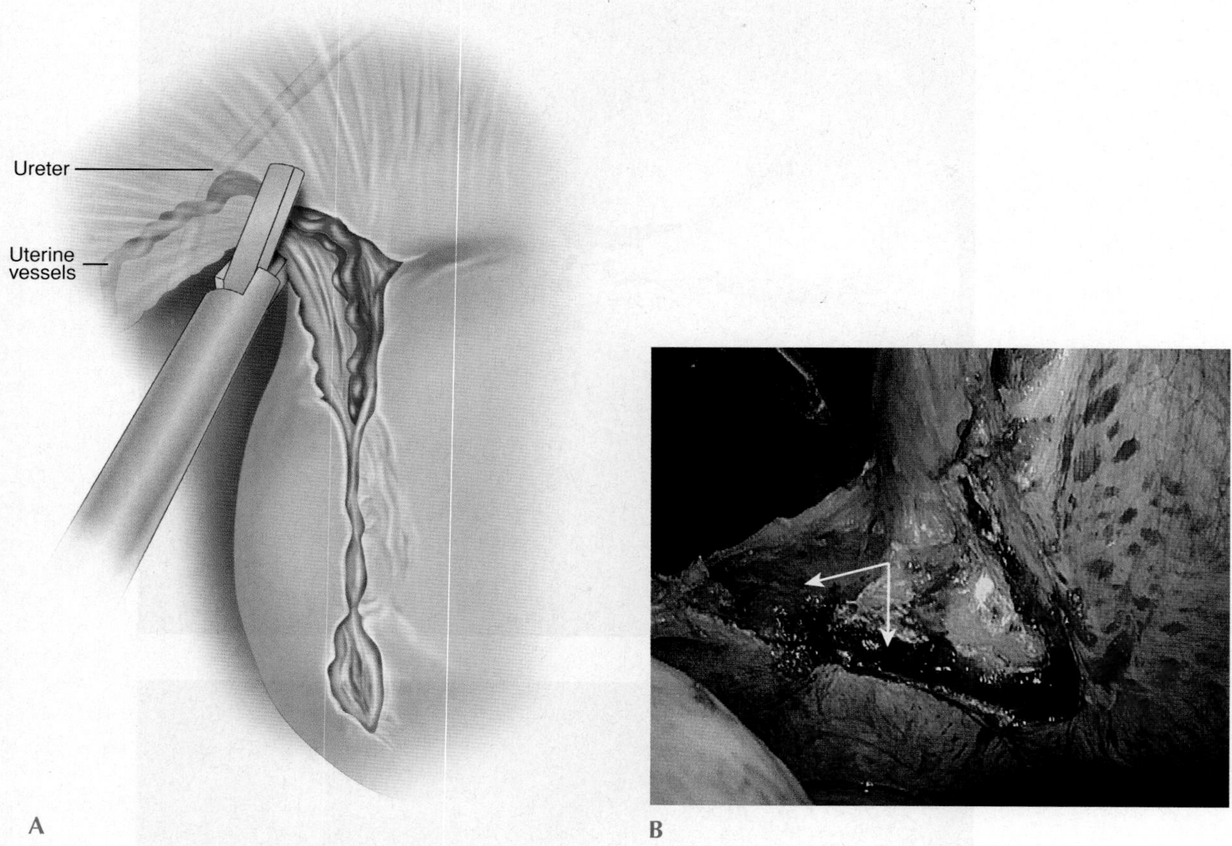

Tech Figure 8.2.12. Lateralize the uterine vessels over the manipulator cup with a "V" technique. A: Artist rendition of placement of energy device to lateralize the vessels over the manipulator cup with a "V" Technique. B: "v" technique lateralizing over the lower uterine segment.

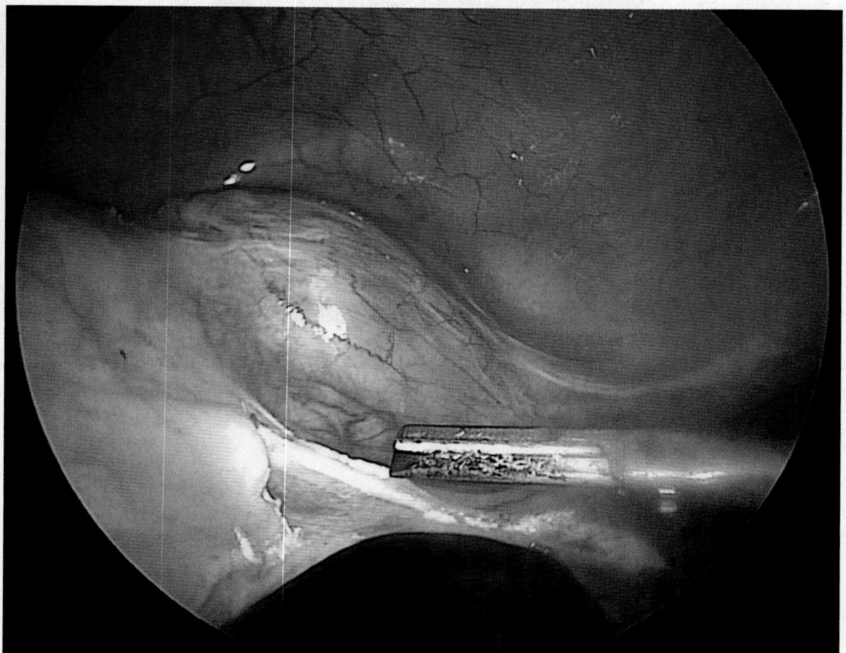

Tech Figure 8.2.13. Expose the vagina over the manipulator cup by deflecting the bladder caudally.

Step 8: Repeat procedure on the contralateral side

Step 9: Colpotomy

Colpotomy proceeds along the manipulator cup from the vaginal attachments over the manipulator cup using ultrasonic energy, or monopolar radiofrequency instrument (Tech Figs. 8.2.14 and 8.2.15). The dissection is occurring over the V-Care cup, Rumi-type manipulator, McCartney Tube, sponge on a sponge-stick, or other device that is being used in the vagina to delineate the fornices. The

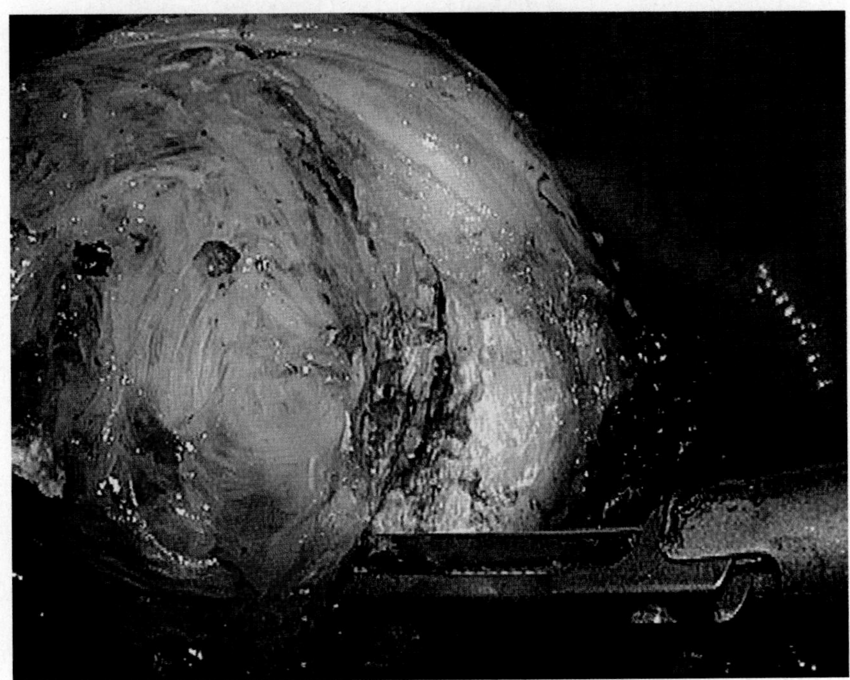

Tech Figure 8.2.14. Dissect the cervix over the manipulator cup.

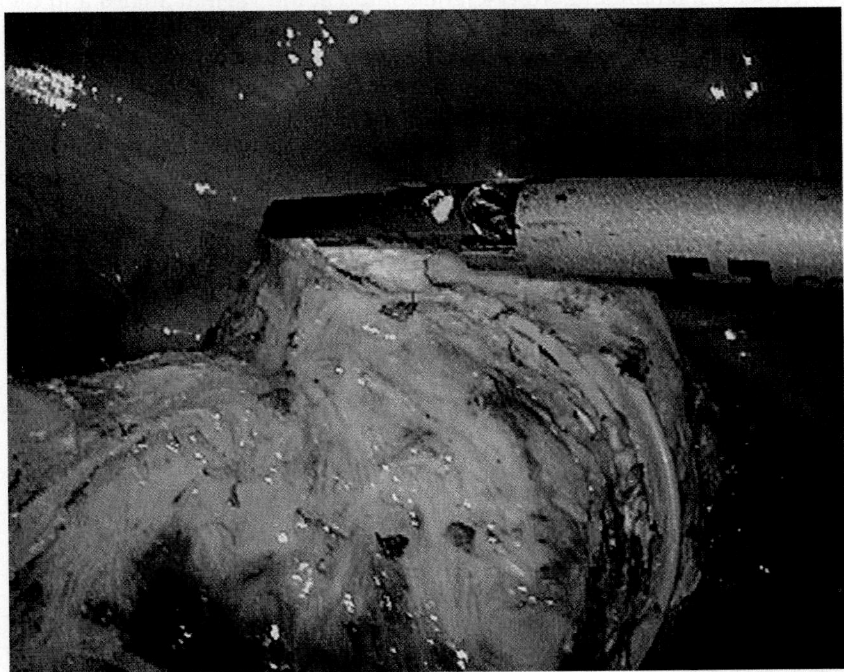

Tech Figure 8.2.15. Remove the cervix from the vagina.

uterus is pulled into the vagina and the fundus can be used to occlude the vagina and maintain pneumoperitoneum (**Tech Fig. 8.2.16**). Alternatively, the uterus can be removed completely and a wet lap pad, wet lap placed in a glove, or similar device can be used to occlude the vagina.

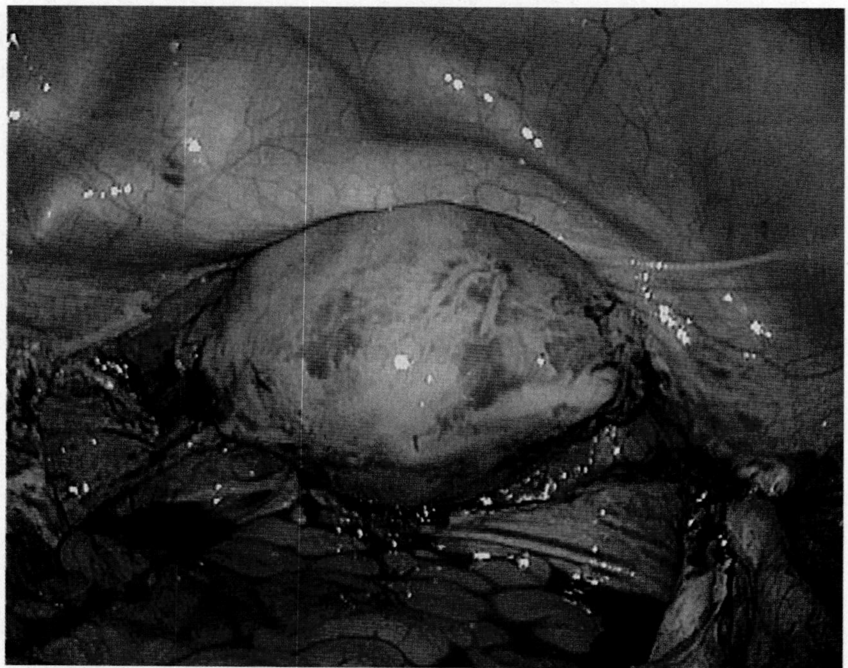

Tech Figure 8.2.16. Pull the uterus into the vagina to hold pneumoperitoneum in smaller specimens.

Step 10: Vaginal cuff closure

Once removed from its vaginal attachments, the pedicles are inspected for bleeding. We have been using a modified Richardson stitch at the vaginal angles, incorporating the uterosacral ligaments as originally described for open hysterectomy by E. H. Richardson in 1929 (**Tech Fig. 8.2.17**).[27] This involves placement of a stitch in a figure-of-eight fashion at the vaginal angles and include the

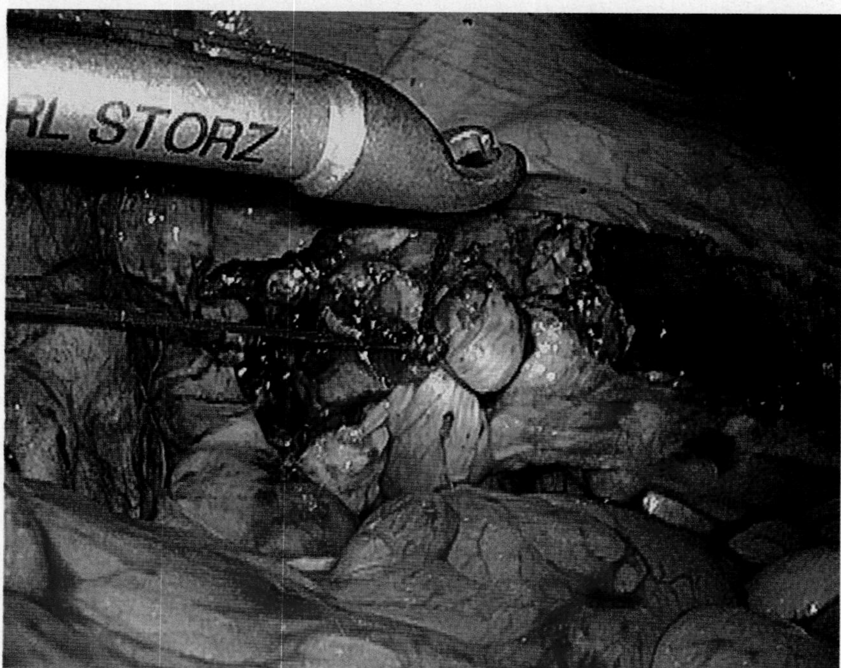

Tech Figure 8.2.17. Modified Richardson stitch.

distal portion of the uterosacral ligament, being careful not to include the vaginal mucosa in this permanent suture material. Care must also be taken not to kink the ureter when placing this stitch as it lies in close proximity. We generally use 0-gauge prolene for this. The remaining portion of the vagina is approximated using absorbable suture in interrupted or figure-of-eight fashion, using 0-gauge polydioxanone or polyglactin (**Tech Figs. 8.2.18** and **8.2.19**). Alternatively, 0-gauge barbed

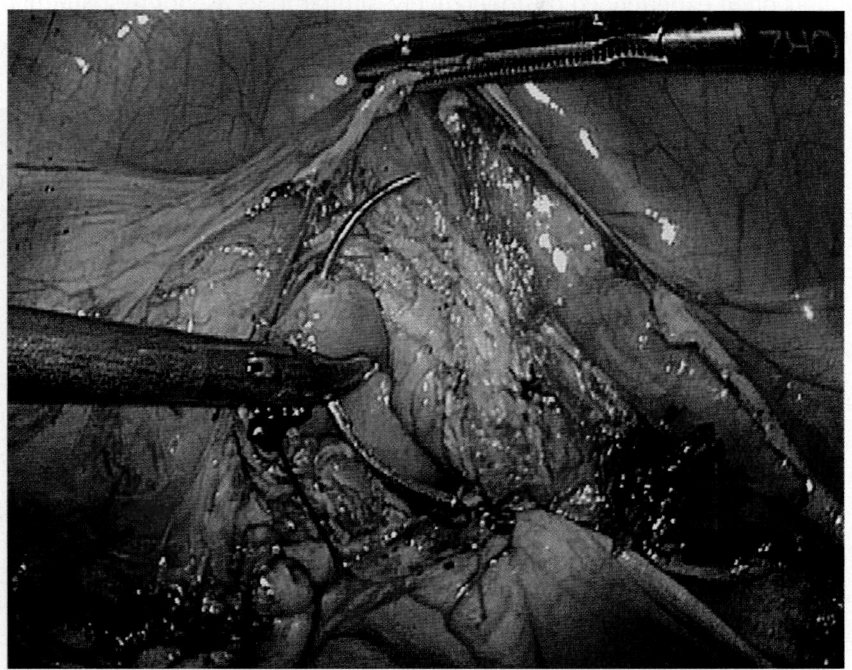

Tech Figure 8.2.18. Colpotomy closure using interrupted absorbable suture.

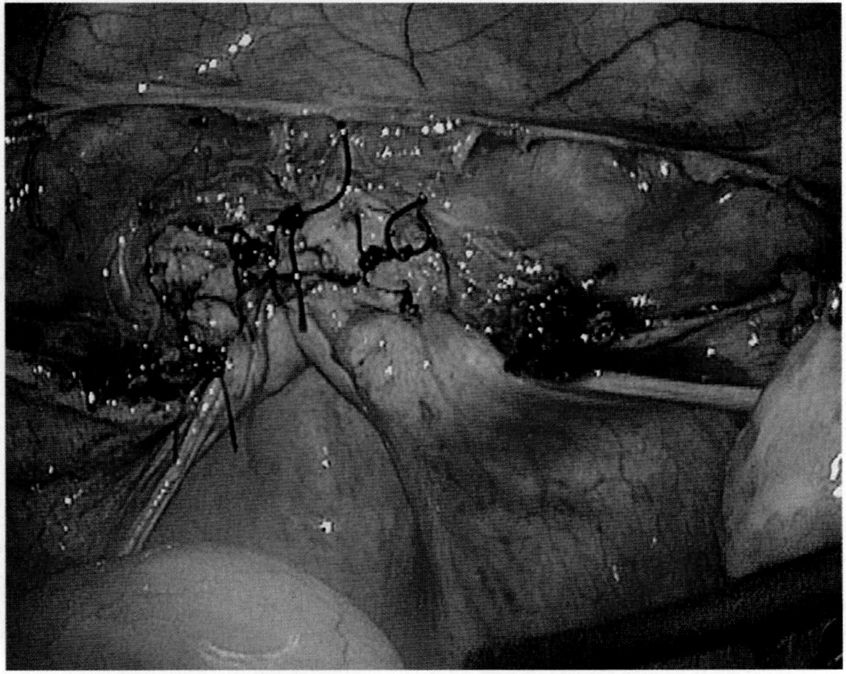

Tech Figure 8.2.19. Finished, interrupted, and suspended vaginal closure.

sutures, such as V-Lock, Quill, or Stratafix can be used for this purpose (Tech Fig. 8.2.20). Care must be taken to get beyond the thermal damage to the cuff in taking the closing bites of vagina. Care must also be taken not to incorporate bladder, minimizing the possibility of postoperative fistula. The finished cuff is well suspended as seen in Tech Figs. 8.2.21 and 8.2.22. To help with pain management postoperatively, we have been using 5 cc of 2% lidocaine jelly intravaginally at the end of the procedure. This can also be used postoperatively in the form of 5 cc of Uroject (prepackaged lidocaine jelly) every 4 to 6 hours which will help with some of the low pelvic pain that these patients often experienced postoperatively, similar to its use for dyspareunia in breast cancer patients.[28]

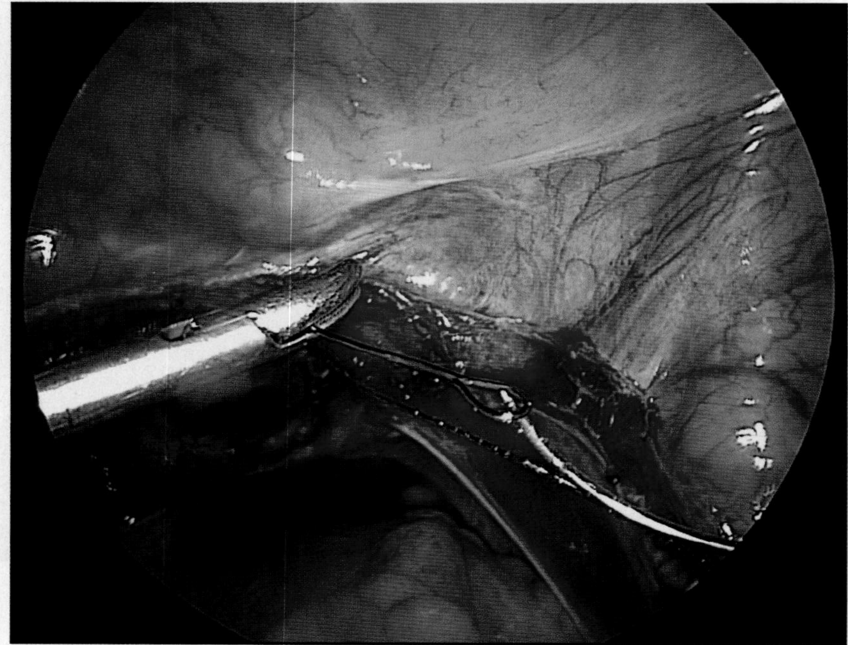
A

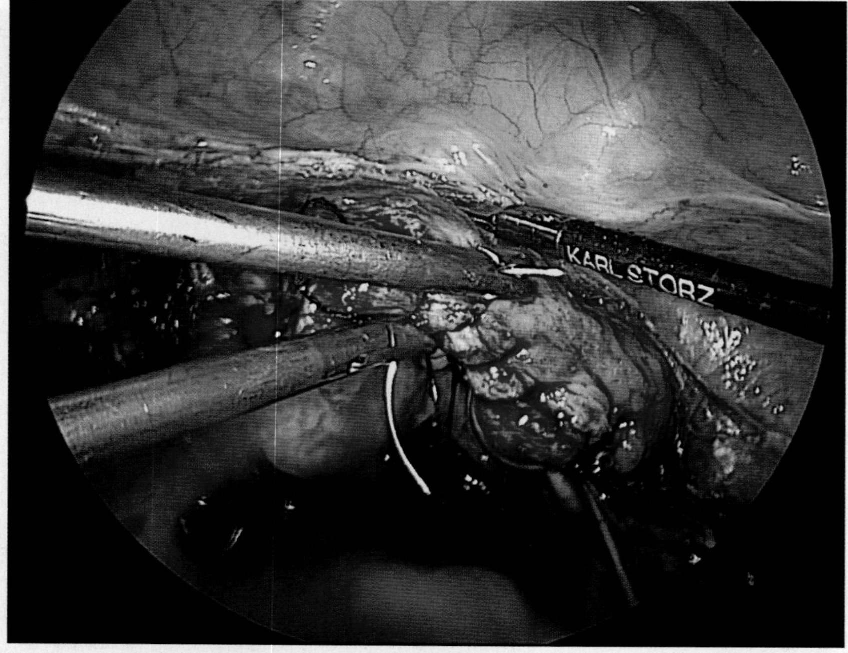

B

Tech Figure 8.2.20. Colpotomy closure using barbed suture. A securing the barbed suture with the looped end of the suture and B 2 layer closure of the vaginal cuff using the barbed suture.

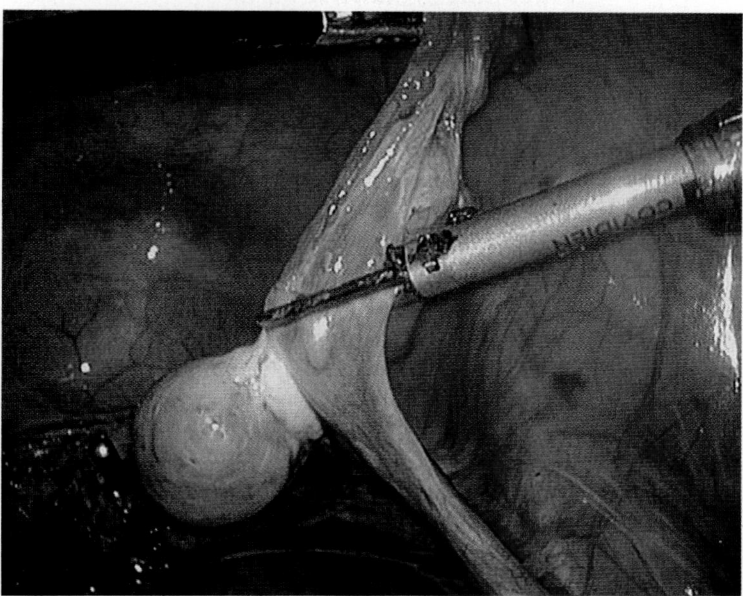

Tech Figure 8.2.21. Prophylactic salpingectomy.

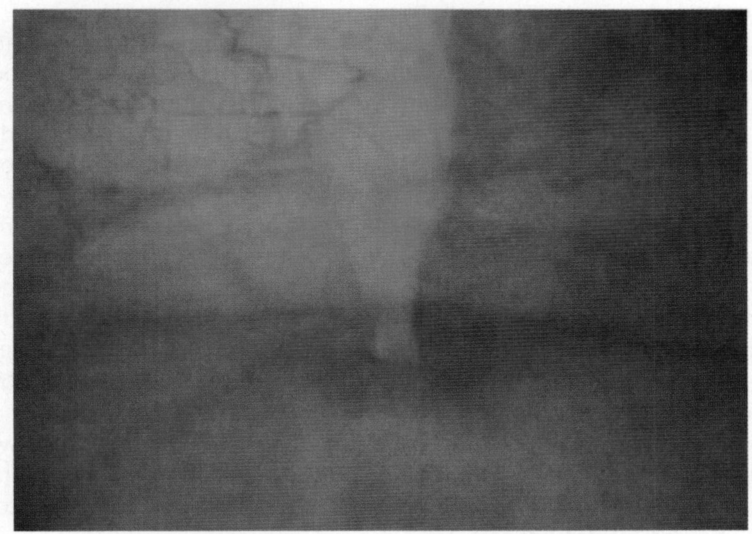

A

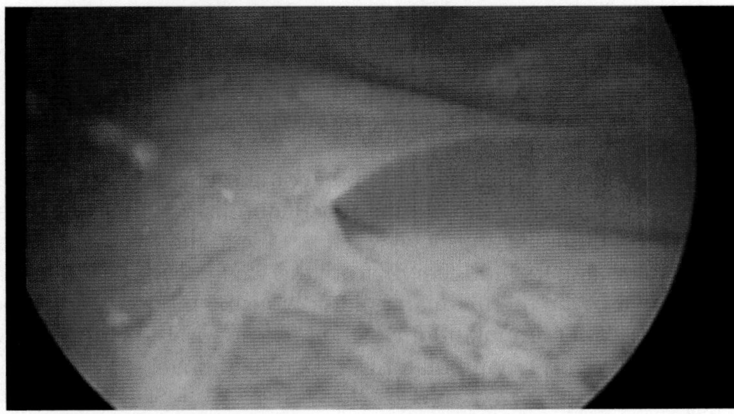

B

Tech Figure 8.2.22. Cystoscopy with fluorescein dye or pyridium. **A** shows Fluorescein dye shooting from theutereteral orifice with a distinctive yellow "highlighter" appearance. **B** shows flow of Pyridium stained urine from the ureter.

Step 11: Handling of the fallopian tubes

If the ovaries are left *in situ,* we have been removing the fallopian tubes prophylactically to decrease the risk of tubal or adnexal malignancy later in life as recently reaffirmed by the National Cancer Institutes.[29] This is done using the same energy sources used for the rest of the hysterectomy, and involves dividing the fimbriated end of the fallopian tube from the ovary and the remaining tube from its mesentery. It is important to take all of the fimbriated ends, as that is the portion associated with malignancy (Tech Fig. 8.2.21). It adds little time and morbidity to the procedure and may confer benefits over our patient's lifetimes.

Step 12: Handling of larger uterine specimens

Uterine specimens greater than 10 to 12 weeks pregnancy size will generally not fit through the vagina without significant tearing and may be impossible to remove via that route due to large fibroids or patient body habitus. For many specimens, vaginal morcellation can be accomplished in the standard fashion using coring or bivalve techniques to achieve specimen extraction. Because of concerns about power morcellation, some practitioners are placing the uterus in a containment bag before vaginal morcellation to theoretically decrease risk, though the efficacy of their use vaginally has not been proven.

Alternatively, specimens can be removed through a small 4- to 5-cm mini-lap Pfannenstiel incision, made suprapubically, or by extending the umbilical incision. This will be described below under the section on Extracting the Uterine Corpus.

Step 13: Cystoscopy

It has been our practice to undertake cystoscopic examination in every patient after a TLH, or complicated supracervical hysterectomy prior to leaving the operating room. Though the literature on the value of this is not clear, we have found the practice invaluable. A standard cystoscope setup is used with either a 30- or 70-degree cystoscope. The bladder is usually filled with normal saline and the walls of the bladder examined for injury or defect, specifically a through-and-through stitch from the cuff closure or possible electrical injury. The ureters are inspected for urine flow. Traditionally we used indigo carmine dye to aide in observing urine flow from ureters, but this is no longer available. We have been using pyridium 200 mg, by mouth prior to the procedure, or fluorescein dye (1 cc) at the time of the procedure to evaluate the ureteral jets (Tech Fig. 8.2.22). Alternatively, one can fill the bladder with 10% dextrose and observe the jets as the difference in viscosity is readily apparent. This simple, 5-minute procedure, can, by identifying GU injuries, decrease postoperative complications. Identification of issues at this juncture allows for immediate repair rather than delayed recognition.

In cases where cystoscopy setups are not available, the bladder can be filled with saline from the abdominal irrigator set and the 5-mm hysteroscope placed through the urethra for bladder evaluation. This gives the same information without having to open a formal cystoscopy set which may be an issue in some institutions.

Laparoscopic supracervical hysterectomy

Step 1: See steps 1 to 8 of total laparoscopic hysterectomy in Procedure and Techniques section

To accomplish the LSH, Steps 1 through 8 of the preceding section are accomplished (see also Surgical Management, p. 112). Once the uterine vasculature is occluded, the uterus is amputated from the cervix at the level of the isthmus (Tech Fig. 8.2.23). In the case of supracervical hysterectomy, we have been cauterizing the endocervix from the vaginal side at the beginning of the procedure, prior to placement of the uterine manipulator by using monopolar cautery as well as from above with bipolar cautery after amputation. We then use a reusable Hulka tenaculum or V-Care (ConMed EndoSurgery, Utica, NY) manipulator as described above.

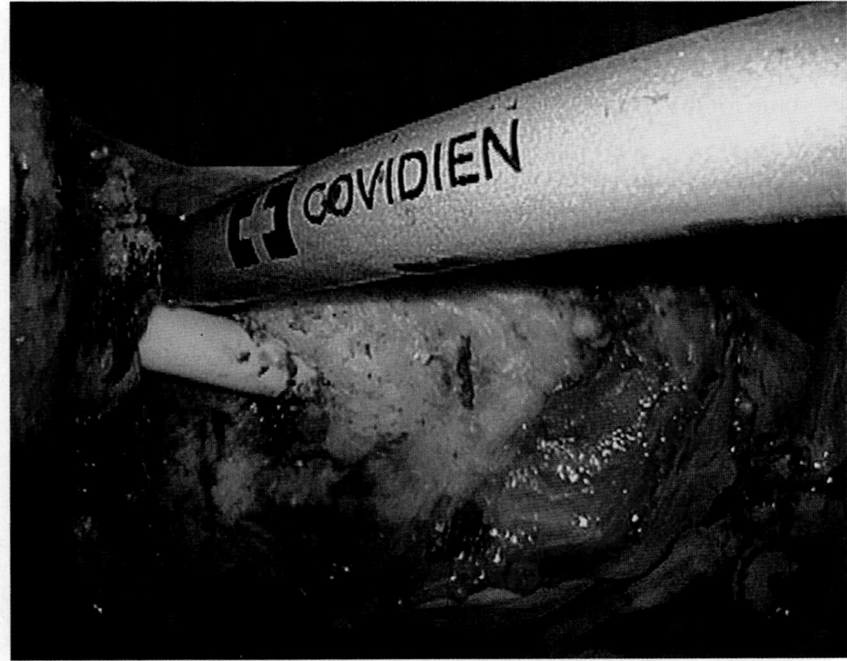

A

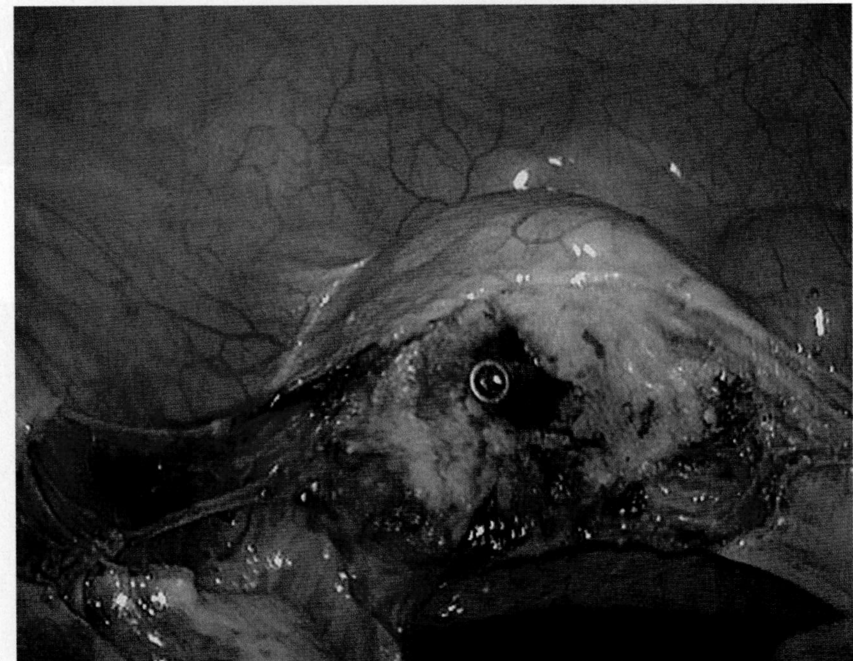

B

Tech Figure 8.2.23. Amputation of the uterus at the level of the isthmus with V-Care manipulator in place. **A** shows removal of the lower uterine segment from the cervix using ultrasonic energy. **B** shows the appearance of the cervix after uterine removal with the top of the V-care manipulator visible.

Step 2: Amputation of the uterine cervix

The uterus is amputated from the cervix using an ultrasonic energy device at the level of the internal os (see Tech Fig. 8.2.23). Alternatively, monopolar energy in the form of scissors, hook, or wire loop can be used for this purpose. Once this is performed, the endocervix is cauterized from the abdominal side using a reusable bipolar instrument to lessen the chance of cyclic bleeding (**Tech Fig. 8.2.24**). The combination of cautery of the endocervix with monopolar cautery from the vaginal side and this step of cautery with bipolar energy from the abdominal side has dropped our cyclic bleeding rate to approximately 2% and will be discussed below. Most remaining spotting postoperatively can be treated in the office by the use of silver nitrate applied to the endocervix. The cervix is then closed abdominally using a single stitch of 0-gauge absorbable suture such as polyglycan, a step that prevents the leakage of peritoneal fluid from the open cervical os which can be troublesome for the patient (Tech Fig. 8.2.25).

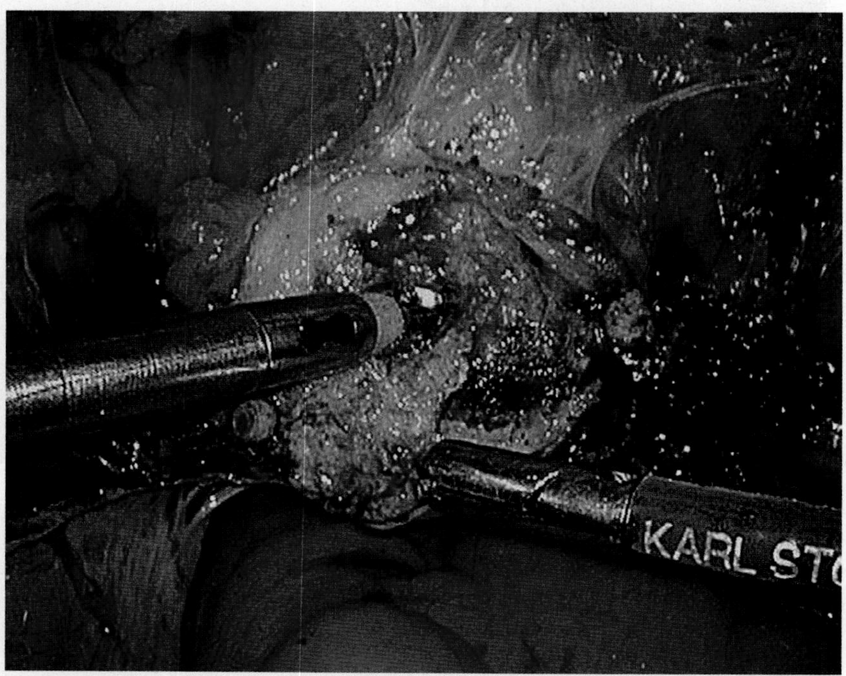

Tech Figure 8.2.24. Cautery of the endocervix with bipolar energy.

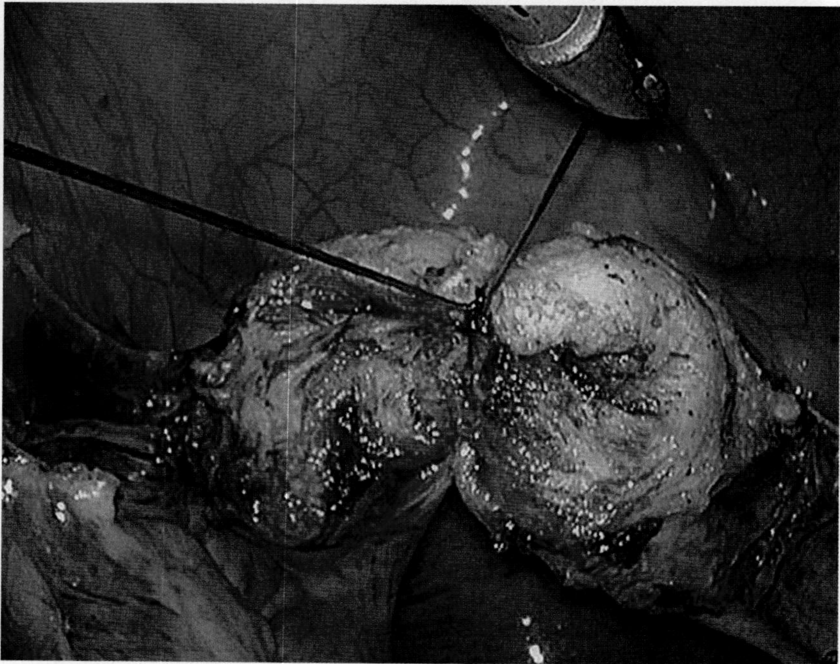

Tech Figure 8.2.25. Closure of the cervix with polyglycan suture.

Step 3: Extraction of the uterine corpus

Prior to the FDA Black Box warning on the use of power morcellators in 2014, all specimens would have been handled by use of a power mechanical morcellator placed through one of the port sites. We had been using the lower quadrant port sites for this purpose to enhance visualization and make it easier to track loose fragments. Though not currently available in many institutions due to the FDA warning, some practitioners continue to use power morcellators by morcellating the uterus in a specimen bag to minimize the spread of aerosolized tissue. Current data is unclear as to whether or not this is efficacious.

What we have been doing to remove the retained supracervical specimen is utilize some form of mini-laparotomy with a self-retaining wound retractor in the suprapubic area with a 4- to 5-cm incision or use the umbilicus with a 2.5-cm extension.

For the suprapubic incision (Tech Fig. 8.2.26), a 4- to 5-cm incision is made above the pubis in the midline much as one would plan a Pfannenstiel incision. Bovie monopolar cautery is then used to open the subcutaneous fat and open the fascia. The peritoneal cavity is then entered with the insufflation gas still on to keep the bowel out of the way and facilitates insertion of the retractor. A GelPort retractor is placed through the incision (Tech Fig. 8.2.27). Once this is in place, the gas is turned off, and the specimen is drawn into the incision and externally morcellated with a series of "C" incisions which will elongate the specimen and allow it to be systematically removed from the cavity (see Tech Figs. 8.2.28 and 8.2.29, **Video 8.2.1**). We have been able to remove specimens greater than 3,000 g in this manner (Tech Fig. 8.2.30). It is unclear as of this writing whether the use of bag actually adds safety to the procedure. The use of the GelPort allows for re-insufflation after

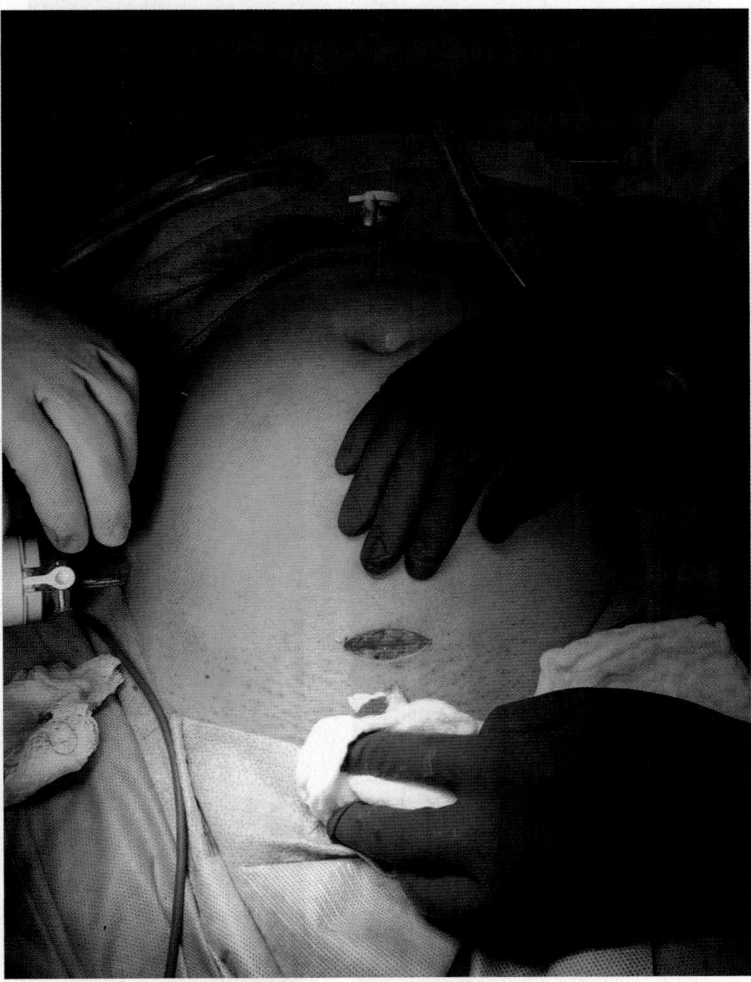

Tech Figure 8.2.26. 4-cm mini-lap Pfannenstiel incision.

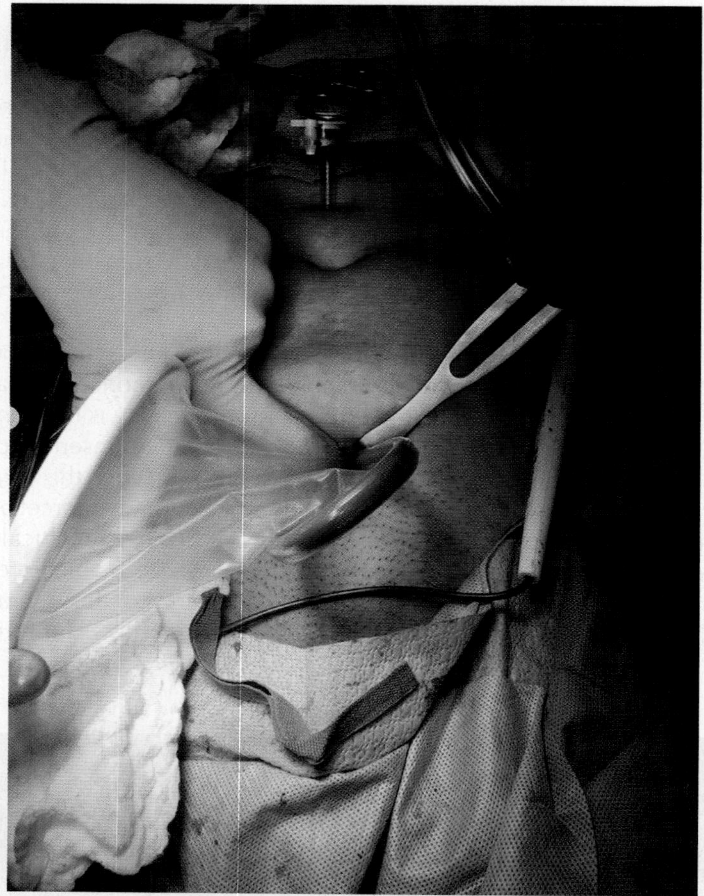

Tech Figure 8.2.27. Placement of GelPort self-retaining retractor.

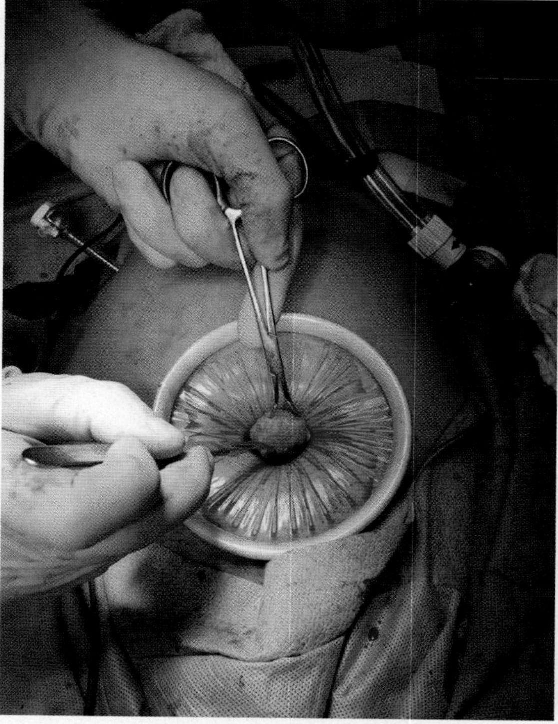

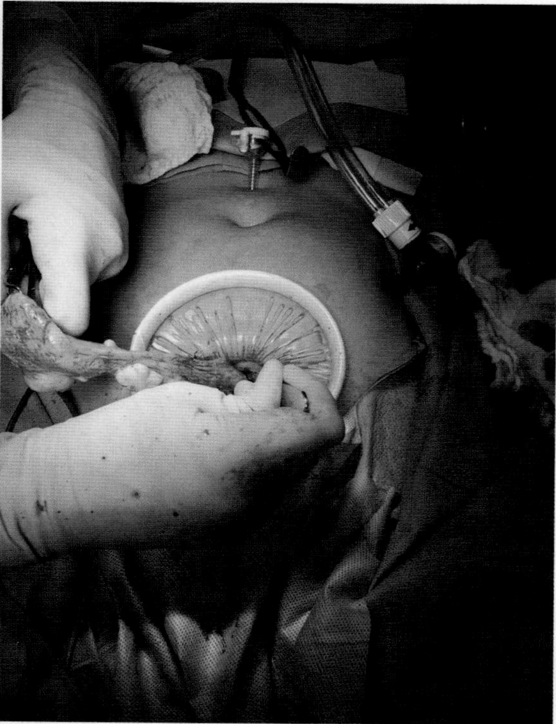

Tech Figure 8.2.28. A: Bring specimen into retractor and start morcellating. **B:** Uterine specimen removed by external morcellation.

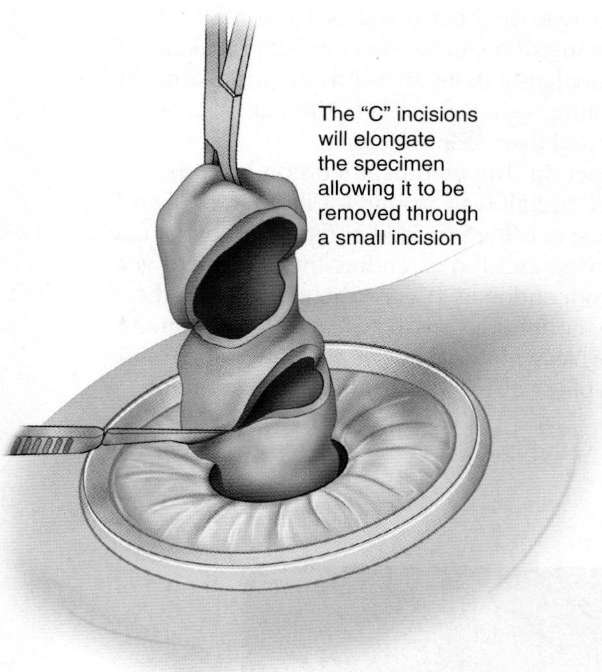

A

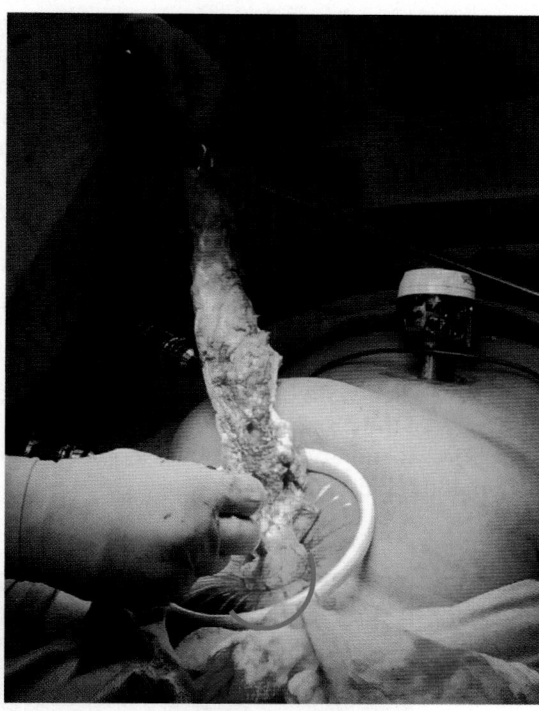

B

Tech Figure 8.2.29. Uterine specimen being removed with a "C" technique of external uterine morcellation. **A:** artist rendition of uterine specimen being removed with a "C" technique of external morcellation and **B:** "C" technique to remove large specimens.

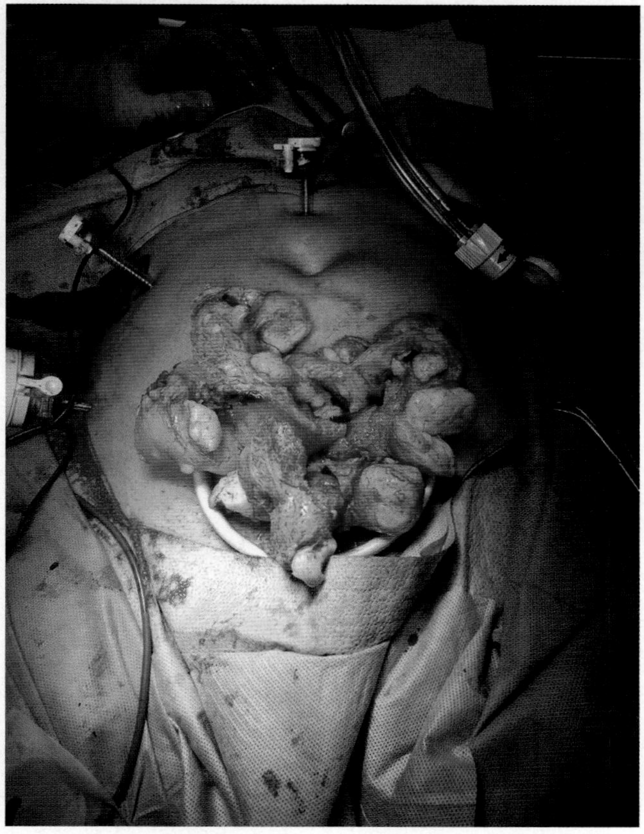

Tech Figure 8.2.30. Removal of large volume of tissue through mini-lap incision.

specimen removal to affect a washout of the peritoneal cavity or check pedicles. Closure of the mini-laparotomy is done in the standard fashion and the incision can be injected with local analgesics or liposomal lidocaine (Experal) which will impart analgesia to the incisions for approximately 72 hours, allowing for performance in the outpatient setting (**Tech Fig. 8.2.31**). Alternatively, one can just close the mini-Pfannenstiel in standard fashion and then re-insufflate.

The umbilicus may also be a reasonable site for extraction. The umbilical incision is made around the top or bottom of the umbilicus and extended to half way around (or through the central portion of the umbilicus if it is large enough). The fascia is then incised and the peritoneal cavity opened. The fascia can be extended by use of an omega incision extending the tails out to get more space. This allows placement of a 12-mm or 15-mm endobag to draw the uterus up to the incision and keep it contained near the incision. Again, continuous small "C" incisions are made in the specimen to remove it through the small incision. As with the GelPort, the GelPOINT Mini (Applied Medical) can be used in the umbilicus (or anyplace else) to re-insufflate and continue other parts of the procedure if necessary.

As in the section on Total Laparoscopic Hysterectomy, the fallopian tubes are removed to lower ovarian and tubal cancer risk.

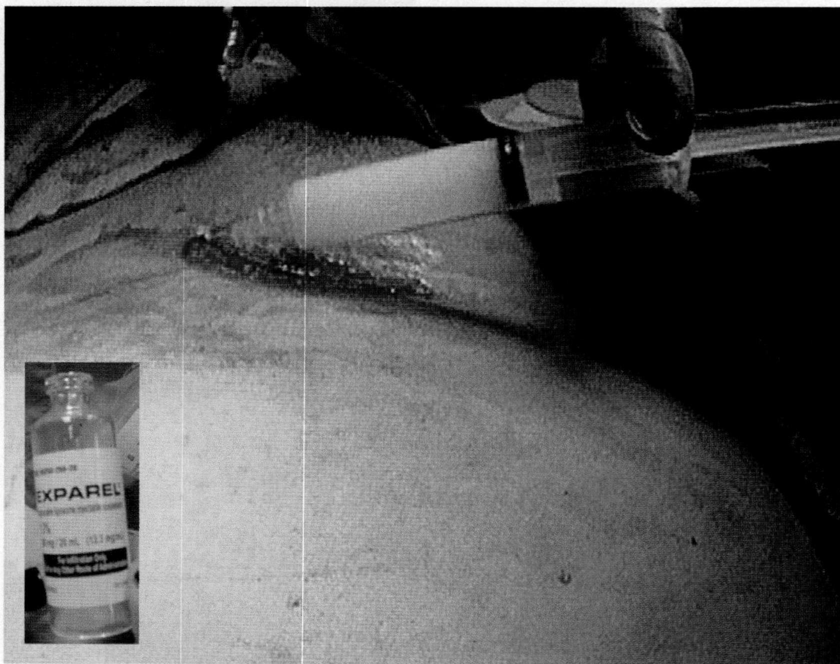

Tech Figure 8.2.31. Inject 4-cm incision with Exparel or other analgesic and close.

PEARLS AND PITFALLS

- If **the uterus greater than 14** to **16 weeks size,** place camera trocar above the umbilicus or left upper quadrant.
- If there are **suspected adhesions,** place primary camera trocar above the umbilicus or left upper quadrant.
- If the **bladder is adhesed to lower uterine segment,** use three-way Foley catheter and fill the bladder with saline or methylene-blue-dyed fluid to delineate the bladder margins.
- If there is **cyclic spotting/bleeding post LSH,** cauterize cervix from the vaginal side and abdominal side.
- If the **patient is obese,** use egg crate mattress on operating table to minimize movement and place camera above umbilicus to maximize visualization. Use of AirSeal insufflation device to aid in visualization and maintain pneumoperitoneum.
- Use lighted ureteral stents to visualize the ureters and allow for safe dissection if there is **dense low pelvic adhesion or endometriosis.**
- Use a bulb syringe top in the vagina or infant suction if the **uterine manipulator cannot be used to delineate the vaginal fornices.**
- If there is **low pelvic pain postprocedure,** use lidocaine jelly 2% in the vaginal mucosa at the end of the procedure and postoperatively to help with the vaginal pain.
- If there is **need for cystoscopy and equipment is not available,** instill saline from irrigator into the bladder and use 5-mm laparoscope as a cystoscope.

POSTOPERATIVE CARE

In the absence of bladder or ureteral injury, or history of previous urinary retention with surgery, the urinary catheter is removed in the operating room and the patient undergoes standard postoperative care. Once the patient's postoperative pain and nausea is controlled with PO meds, and she passes a voiding trial, the patient is discharged from the PACU with instructions for postoperative evaluation in 2 weeks. For patients unable to urinate, which is an occasional issue secondary to dissection, anesthesia, or concomitant procedures, a bladder scan is performed to confirm there is urinary retention and that the patient is not just dry from lack of fluid. A catheter is left in for 2 days and is removed in the office after a bladder challenge to avoid overdistention and damage. A standard hemoglobin and hematocrit are checked prior to discharge. The patient is discharged with narcotic analgesics, nonsteroidal analgesics, and stool softeners; and in the case of TLH, vaginal lidocaine jelly, as previously described.

A large part of successful transition from the postoperative unit to home is predicated on management of preoperative expectations so that the patient and her family know she is being discharged on the day of surgery and what her limitations might be. With the patient in an outpatient setting, they are encouraged to achieve early ambulation prior to leaving. We have also found that the use of an abdominal binder is helpful when ambulating in the postoperative period as this gives support to the patient's core. Early ambulation is key in rapid recovery and minimizing complications.

OUTCOMES

Both LSH and TLH are minimally invasive alternatives for hysterectomy. Re-operation rates are equivalent in the two procedures with no differences in intraoperative and postoperative complications, with a trend toward lower complications in the LSH group.[30] A method-specific procedure, sometimes necessitated after an LSH, was trachelectomy for either bleeding or malignancy, and occurs in about 2.7% of patients, and repair of vaginal cuff dehiscence after TLH which occurred in approximately 0.7% of patients. Einarsson and colleagues[31] did a prospective quality-of-life (QOL) evaluation in total versus LSH patients using validated QOL questionnaires. LSH appears to provide greater improvement in short-term QOL compared with TLH. No significant differences were noted in postoperative pain or return to normal daily activities. Mastering both techniques will allow for continued conversion to minimally invasive alternatives for most gynecologic procedures and should be in all gynecologic surgeon's armamentarium.

COMPLICATIONS

As with any procedure, complications related to laparoscopy by itself, and complications related to the type of surgery may occur. Bojahr et al.[32] published data on 1,706 consecutive LSH patients in 2006. The mean uterine weight was 226 g with mean operative time of 91 minutes. Fifty-two percent had previous laparotomy. Of the 1,706 procedures, there were 14 patients that were converted to laparotomy due to size and immobility, and one for adhesions. There were two bladder injuries and one ureter injury in an 818-g uterus. Overall, there was a 1.2% postoperative complication rate including infection and bleeding. Kafy et al.[33] also reported on 1,792 patients comparing complications between abdominal, vaginal, and LH. The overall morbidity was 6.1% with one bowel injury in the laparoscopic and abdominal hysterectomy groups, and one ureter injury in the abdominal hysterectomy group. Vaginal hysterectomy was associated with more urinary retention and hematoma formation. Conversion rates were 1.7% in the laparoscopic group and 0.4% in the vaginal hysterectomy group. Re-operation rate was 0.4% in the abdominal group with overall morbidity being low in all groups and no reported mortality. In a 2014 Korean study, Kim et al.[34] looked at an 11-year trend in surgical complications between abdominal hysterectomy, multi-port LH, and single-port hysterectomy. Major complications such as bladder, ureteral, and bowel injury were most common in multi-port hysterectomy, with vaginal cuff dehiscence making up almost half the complications in all groups. The total number of complications was mostly in the multi-port hysterectomy group with the single port having the least complications. Overall, there was a 5.3% complication rate in the abdominal group, an 8.7% rate in the multi-port hysterectomy group, and 2.4% in the single-port group, showing that LH is achievable with low morbidity in most groups observed.

Laparoscopic removal of large uteri represents a particular challenge, whether total or supracervical. Alpern [35] completed a retrospective analysis of Kaiser Permanente's experience of 446 consecutive cases over 500 g. The mean uterine weight was 786 g (500 to 4,500). Life-threatening complications occurred in 0.7% of cases and required re-operation in 0.45% of cases. There were six cystotomies, and 92.8% of the cases were discharged on postoperative day 0 with a 1.1% re-admission rate. There was no association between perioperative complication morbidity and patient/surgical characteristics. Uccella, in the following year, reported on a series of 71 TLH cases with uteri greater than 1 kg as well as a literature review.[36] The median weight was 1,120 g (1,000 to 2,860) and there was a 4.2% (three patients) conversion rate to open surgery, two for dense adhesions, and one because of inability to place a uterine manipulator. The median operative time was 2 hours and median blood loss was 200 mL. There were two perioperative complications; one with vaginal bleeding 10 days postoperatively managed conservatively and one with vaginal cuff hematoma, also managed conservatively showing that larger uteri can indeed be handled efficiently and safely in a minimally invasive fashion.

TLH has a unique complication in the form of vaginal cuff dehiscence postoperatively. This can happen from several days to years after surgery and is usually brought on by vaginal intercourse. It is a matter of debate as to whether this is secondary to the suturing technique or use of energy to the cuff, particularly with monopolar energy. In a 2012 Italian study, Uccella[37] completed a multi-institutional analysis of 12,398 patients who underwent hysterectomy for both benign and malignant diseases, and looked at the rate of cuff dehiscence with the various closure types. TLH was associated with the highest number of cuff separations 23 (0.64%) versus 6 vaginal (0.13%). Laparoscopic suturing of the vaginal cuff had the highest separation rate at 0.86% over transvaginal suturing at 0.24%. Reducing the monopolar current from 60 to 50 W did not alter the rates. Blikkendaal[38], in a retrospective cohort Dutch study, compared techniques of laparoscopic cuff closure; looking at incidence of dehiscence with transvaginal interrupted, laparoscopic interrupted, or laparoscopic running suture with conventional or bidirectional barbed suture. Their data did not show superiority of one technique over any other. Fuchs-Weizman and colleagues[39] performed a retrospective analysis of 2,382 TLH between 2009 and 2011. She reported 23 (0.96%) cuff dehiscences and 4 had recurrent dehiscence. The type of energy, mode of closure, and suture material did not differ between groups. Women with more extensive procedures were at higher risk and continuous suturing of the cuff was a probably superior to interrupted suturing in their study.

LSH has three unique complications associated with it that are procedure specific. The first is continued cyclic bleeding since the cervix is left *in situ,* likely due to retained endometrial type tissue in the endocervical canal. Nouri[40] recently published a meta-analysis on the subject revealing that there are varying rates of postoperative cyclic bleeding in premenopausal women, depending on the method used to prevent bleeding. There was a 16.2% rate if nothing was done (up to 24%). Excision of the endocervix was still associated with high levels of bleeding (14%), and the best results came from bipolar electrocoagulation of the endocervix which dropped the level to 2.6% on average. All cyclic bleeding postoperatively was looked at regardless of age, BMI, presence of endometriosis or adenomyosis, and history of previous cesarean delivery. Similarly, we have found that monopolar cautery of the endocervix from the vagina prior to the hysterectomy, followed by bipolar coagulation of the endocervix after uterine amputation has decreased the rate of cyclic postoperative bleeding at Cleveland Clinic. Much of this can be further reduced by the use of silver nitrate in the cervical os in the office for refractory cases with trachelectomy being necessary for very few.

Prior to 2014, power morcellation had been used to remove uterine tissue and fibroids for LSH and larger TLH that could not be removed vaginally. Issues associated with the power morcellators were iatrogenic spread of endometriosis and myomatosis, as well as possible upstaging of undiagnosed carcinoma or sarcomas of the uterus and tubes. Due to concerns about possible spread of undiagnosed carcinoma of the endometrium or uterine sarcoma, the FDA issued a Black Box warning on power morcellators in 2014 and we are no longer using them for tissue management. Descriptions of how to remove larger uteri and supracervical specimens are described in detail under Step 3 of Laparoscopic Supracervical Hysterectomy in the Procedures and Techniques section.

KEY REFERENCES

1. Wu JM, Wechter ME, Geller EJ, Nguyen TV, Visco AG. Hysterectomy rates in the United States, 2003. *Obstet Gynecol.* 2007;110:1091–1095.
2. Merrill RM. Hysterectomy surveillance in the United States, 1997 through 2005. *Med Sci Monit.* 2008;14:CR24–CR31.
3. US Department of Health and Human Services Centers for Disease Control and Prevention National Center for Health Statistics. Health, United States 2006 with chart book on trends in the health of Americans. Table 99. Hyattsville, MD: National Center for Health Statistics Health; 2006.
4. Cohen SL, Vitonis AF, Einarsson JI. Updated hysterectomy surveillance and factors associated with minimally invasive hysterectomy. *JSLS.* 2014;18(3):e2014.00096.
5. Loring M, Morris SN, Isaacson KB. Minimally invasive specialists and the rates of laparoscopic hysterectomy. *JSLS.* 2015;19(1):e2014.00221.
6. Wright JD, Ananth CV, Lewin SN, et al. Robotically assisted vs laparoscopic hysterectomy among women with benign gynecologic disease. *JAMA.* 2013;309(7):689–698.
7. Patel PR, Lee J, Rodriguez AM, et al. Disparities in use of laparoscopic hysterectomies: a nationwide analysis. *J Minim Invasive Gynecol.* 2014;21(2):223–227.
8. Kovac, SR. Route of hysterectomy: an evidence-based approach. *Clin Obstet Gynecol.* 2014;57(1):58–71.
9. Guraslan H, Senturk MB, Dogan K, Guraslan B, Babouglu F, Yasar L. Total laparoscopic hysterectomy in obese and morbidly obese women. *Gynecol Obstet Invest.* 2015;79:184–188.

10. Matthews KJ, Brock E, Cohen SA, Chelmow D. Hysterectomy in obese patients: special considerations. *Clin Obstet Gynecol.* 2014;57(1):106–114.
11. Cobianchi L, Dominioni T, Filisetti C, et al. Ventriculoperitoneal shunt and the need to remove a gallbladder: time to definitely overcome the feeling that laparoscopic surgery is contraindicated. *Ann Med Surg (Lond).* 2014;3(3):65–67.
12. Kara Bozkurt D, Bozkurt M, Nazli MA, Mutlu IN, Kilickesmez O. Diffusion-weighted and diffusion-tensor imaging of normal and diseased uterus. *World J Radiol.* 2015;7(7) 149–156.
13. Allam IS, Makled AK, Gomaa IA, El Bishry GM, Bayoumy HA, Ali DF. Total Laparoscopic hysterectomy, vaginal hysterectomy, and total abdominal hysterectomy using electrosurgical bipolar sealing technique: a randomized controlled trial. *Arch Gynecol Obstet.* 2015;291:1341–1345.
14. Pokkinen SM, Kalliomaki ML, Yli-Hankala A, Nieminen K. Less postoperative pain after laparoscopic hysterectomy than after vaginal hysterectomy. *Arch Gynecol Obstet.* 2015;292:149–154.
15. Nesbitt-Hawes EM, Maley PE, Won HR, et al. Laparoscopic subtotal hysterectomy: evidence and techniques. *J Minim Invasive Gynecol.* 2013;20:424–434.
16. Saccardi C, Gizzo S, Noventa M, et al. Subtotal versus total laparoscopic hysterectomy: could women sexual function recovery overcome the surgical outcomes in pre-operatory decision making? *Arch Gynecol Obstet.* 2015;291:1321–1326.
17. Yuan H, Wang C, Wang D, Wang Y. Comparing the effect of laparoscopic supracervical and total hysterectomy for uterine fibroids on ovarian reserve by assessing serum anti-Mullerian hormone levels: a prospective cohort study. *J Minim Invasive Gynecol.* 2015;22: 637–641.
18. Agostini J, Goasquen N, Mosnier H. Patient positioning in laparoscopic surgery: tricks and tips. *J Visc Surg.* 2010;147:e227–232.
19. Klauschie J, Wechter ME, Jacob K, et al. Use of anti-skid material and patient-positioning to prevent patient shifting during robotic-assisted gynecologic procedures. *J Minim Invasive Gynecol.* 2010;17: 504–507.
20. Wen T, Deibert CM, Siringo FS, Spencer BA. Positioning-related complications of minimally invasive radical prostatectomies. *J Endourol.* 2014;28(6):660–667.
21. Gould C, Cull T, Wu YX, Osmundsen B. Blinded measure of Trendelenburg angle in pelvic robotic surgery. *J Minim Invasive Gynecol.* 2012;19(4):465–468.
22. Caprini JA. Risk assessment as a guide for the prevention of the many faces of venous thromboembolism. *Am J Surg.* 2010;199(1 Suppl): S3–10.
23. van den Haak L, Alleblas C, Neiboer TE, Rhemrev JP, Jansen FW. Efficacy and safety of uterine manipulators in laparoscopic surgery: a review. *Arch Gynecol Obstet.* 2015;292:1003–1011.
24. Iavazzo C, Gkegkes JD. The role of uterine manipulators in endometrial cancer recurrence after laparoscopic or robotic procedures. *Arch Gynecol Obstet.* 2013;288:1003–1009.
25. Tinelli A, Malvasi A, Istre O, Keckstein J, Stark M, Mettler L. Abdominal access in gynaecological laparoscopy: a comparison between direct optical and blind closed access by Verres needle. *Eur J Obstet Gynecol Reprod Biol.* 2010;148(2):191–194.
26. Joy P, Simon B, Prithishkumar IJ, Isaac B. Topography of inferior epigastric artery relevant to laparoscopy: a CT angiographic study. *Surg Radiol Anat.* 2016;38:279–283.
27. Richardson EH. A simplified technique for abdominal panhysterectomy. *Surg Gynaecol Obstet.* 1929;48:248–251.
28. Goetsch MF, Lim JY, Caughey AB. A practical solution for dyspareunia in breast cancer survivors: a randomized controlled trial. *J Clin Oncol.* 2015;33:3394–3400.
29. Falconer H, Yin L, Gronberg H, Altman D. Ovarian cancer risk after salpingectomy: a nationwide population-based study. *J Natl Cancer Inst.* 2015;107(2):pii: dju410.
30. Boosz A, Lermann J, Mehlhorn G, et al. Comparison of re-operation rates and complication rates after total laparoscopic hysterectomy (TLH) and laparoscopy-assisted supracervical hysterectomy (LASH). *Eur J Obstet Gyne Repro Biol.* 2011;158:269–273.
31. Einarsson JI, Suzuki Y, Vellinga TT, et al. Prospective evaluation of quality of live in total versus supracervical laparoscopic hysterectomy. *J Minim Invasive Gynecol.* 2011;18:617–621.
32. Bojahr B, Raatz D, Schonleber G, Abri C, Ohlinger R. Perioperative complication rate in 1706 patients after a standardized laparoscopic supracervical hysterectomy technique. *J Minim Invasive Gynecol.* 2006; 13:183–189.
33. Kafy S, Huang JY, Al-Sunaidi M, Wiener D, Tulandi T. Audit of morbidity and mortality rates of 1792 hysterectomies. *J Minim Invasive Gynecol.* 2006;13:55–59.
34. Kim SM, Park EK, Jeung IC, Kim CJ, Lee YS. Abdominal, multi-port and single-port total laparoscopic hysterectomy: eleven-year trend comparison of surgical outcomes complications of 936 cases. *Arch Gynecol Obstet.* 2015;291:1313–1339.
35. Alperin M, Kivnick S, Poon KY. Outpatient laparoscopic hysterectomy for large uteri. *J Minim Invasive Gynecol.* 2012;19:689–694.
36. Uccella S, Cromi A, Serati M, Casarin J, Sturla D, Ghezzi F. Laparoscopic Hysterectomy in case of uteri weighing >1 kilogram: a series of 71 cases and review of the literature. *JMIG.* 2014;21:460–465.
37. Uccella S, Ceccaroni M, Cromi A, et al. Vaginal cuff dehiscence in a series of 12,398 hysterectomies: effect of different types of colpotomy and vaginal closure. *Obstet Gynecol.* 2012;120:516–523.
38. Blikkendaal MD, Twijnstra AR, Pacquee SC, et al. Vaginal cuff dehiscence in laparoscopic hysterectomy: influence of various suturing methods of the vaginal vault. *Gynecol Surg.* 2012;9:393–400.
39. Fuchs Weizman N, Einarsson JI, Wang KC, Vitonis AF, Cohen SL. Vaginal cuff dehiscence: risk factors and associated morbidities. *JSLS.* 2015;19(2):e2013.00351.
40. Nouri K, Demmel M, Greilberger U, et al. Prospective cohort study and meta-analysis of cyclic bleeding after laparoscopic supracervical hysterectomy. *Int J Gynaecol Obstet.* 2013;122:124–127.

Chapter 8.3 Single Port Total Laparoscopic Hysterectomy

Chad M. Michener

GENERAL PRINCIPLES

Definition

- Single-port laparoscopic (SPL) surgery has also been termed single-incision laparoscopic surgery (SILS) and laparoendoscopic single-site (LESS) surgery.
- SPL hysterectomy is performed through a single incision, most commonly placed through the umbilicus.
- The incision can vary in size and location depending on the need for intra-abdominal palpation and/or specimen extraction.
- SPL hysterectomy may apply to either standard laparoscopic or a robotic single-port approach.

Nonoperative Management

- Nonoperative management of conditions that may require hysterectomy (e.g., abnormal uterine bleeding, leiomyoma, endometriosis, chronic pelvic pain, preinvasive and invasive diseases of the uterus and cervix). Consider:
  - Hormonal therapy (e.g., oral or intramuscular progesterone)
  - Progesterone-releasing intrauterine devices
  - Uterine fibroid embolization
  - Hysteroscopic resection of leiomyoma
  - Endometrial ablation
  - Cervical conization (for cervical dysplasias)
  - Radiation therapy (for cervical and uterine malignancies)
  - Total vaginal hysterectomy (which is less invasive)
  - Total abdominal hysterectomy (for very large uteri that would have to be morcellated)

IMAGING AND OTHER DIAGNOSTICS

- Imaging will depend on the indication for hysterectomy. However, pelvic ultrasonography, saline infusion sonography, or pelvic magnetic resonance imaging (MRI) will often be performed for patients considering hysterectomy for abnormal uterine bleeding and leiomyoma.
- Diagnostic and operative hysteroscopy should be used to rule out endometrial pathology that can be treated by simple hysteroscopic resection or ablation.
- Low-grade endometrial cancers do not need pelvic imaging as a group, but imaging should be individualized based on physical examination and risk of metastasis. High-grade endometrial cancers should have computed tomography (CT) of the abdomen and pelvis and either chest radiograph of CT of the chest.
- Presumed early-stage cervical cancers should have pelvic MRI to rule out large tumors or deep cervical wall invasion and a positron emission tomography (PET) scan should be considered to rule out obvious regional and distant metastases.

PREOPERATIVE PLANNING

- Consideration should be made for route of specimen removal (vaginal or abdominal) and discussed with the patient.
- Prior surgical history is important to consider in deciding on placement of the incision.
  - Patients with prior mesh placement in the umbilicus may require supraumbilical incision.
  - If an ostomy is needed (for endometriosis or locally invasive endometrial carcinoma), the stoma site can be used as the SPL access site.

SURGICAL MANAGEMENT

- Proper equipment is essential for the procedure.
  - *Visualization:* A 30-degree or flexible-tip laparoscope will aid in avoiding instrument alignment that can cause a loss-of-depth perception. Alternatively, a 30-degreee bariatric length laparoscope will help get the assistants and surgeons hands further apart.
  - *Access:* Multiple commercially available ports are available that allow two to three instruments to be used along with a camera at one time.
  - *Triangulation:* Articulating instruments can help with triangulation, but are not mandatory.
  - *External instrument clashing:* Use of different length instruments (e.g., a bariatric grasper and standard length vessel sealing device) can help limit external instrument clashing.
  - *Suturing:* Use of the Endo Stitch device (Ethicon Endo-surgery, Cincinnati, OH) allows for easier suturing in SPL.
    - Intracorporeal knot tying techniques can be learned which helps with this task.
- Preoperative work-up is the same as for standard and robotic-assisted laparoscopy.

Positioning

- Patient is placed on the operating table on a beanbag (Fig. 8.3.1A) or a foam pad (Fig. 8.3.1B) with buttocks extended an inch or two off of the bed.
- Additional intravenous lines and arterial lines can be placed as needed.
- Arms should be tucked and padded at the patient's sides.
  - Arm trays can be used if the arms extend beyond the bed.
  - The regular arm boards can also be used as an alternative if they are also locked against the operating table.
- A pad or a blanket should be placed over the patient's chest and either 3″ cloth tape or a chest strap should be used to maintain position in steep Trendelenburg (Fig. 8.3.1C).
- See Figure 8.3.2A–C.

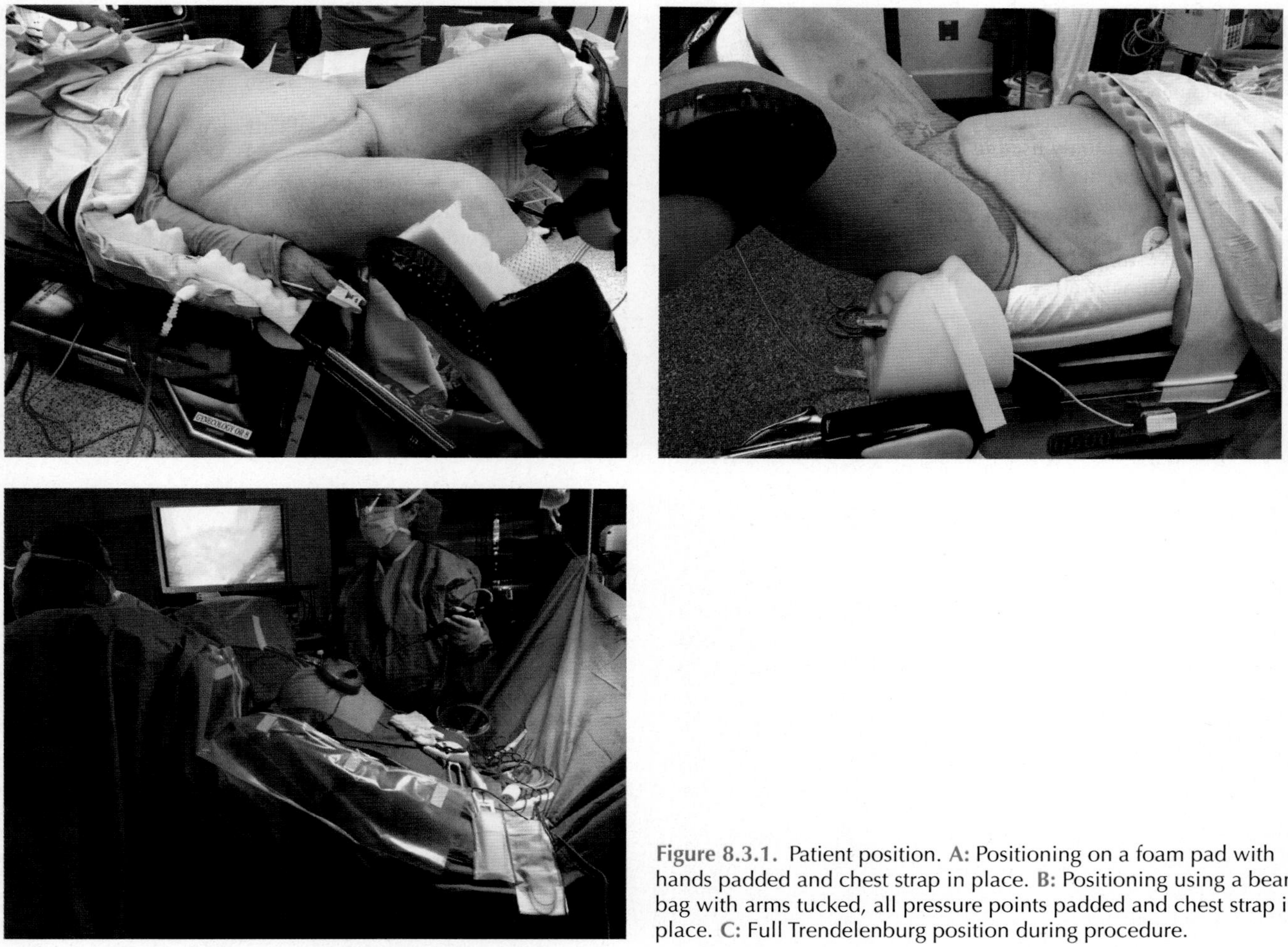

A B C

Figure 8.3.1. Patient position. A: Positioning on a foam pad with hands padded and chest strap in place. B: Positioning using a bean bag with arms tucked, all pressure points padded and chest strap in place. C: Full Trendelenburg position during procedure.

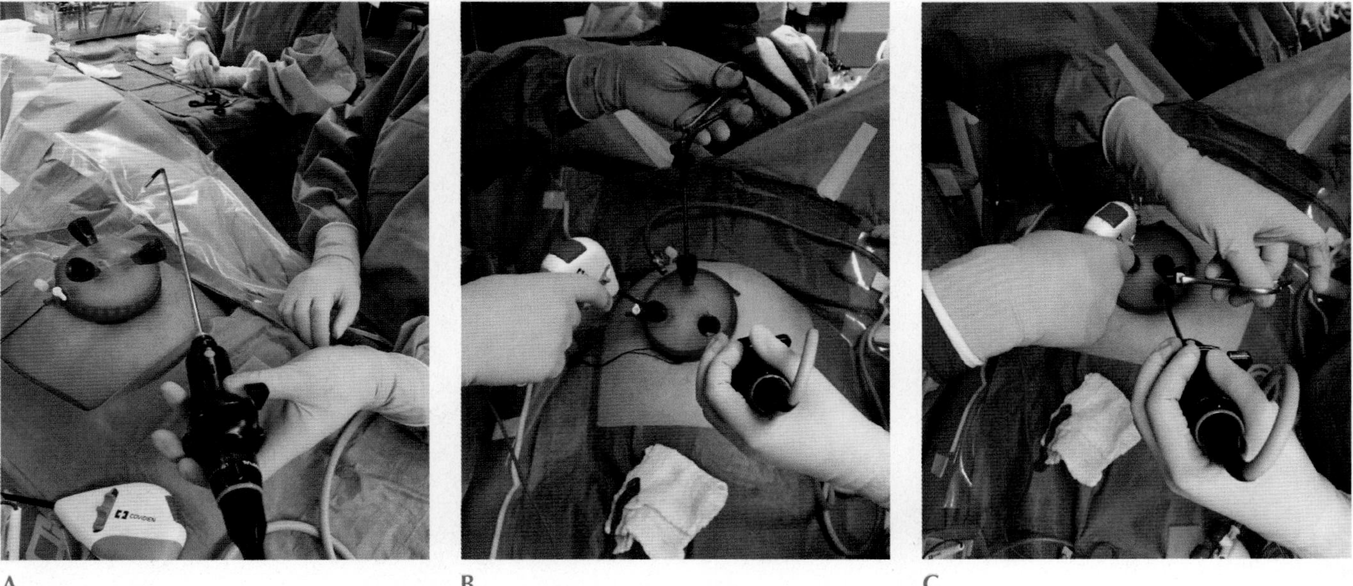

Figure 8.3.2. Flexible laparoscope and hand positioning straight instrumentation. A: The flexible laparoscope allows you to "see around corners." B: Position of hands working on the right side of the pelvis. C: "Crossing over" with left hand during left-sided pelvic dissection.

Approach

- Typical approach uses the umbilicus as the entry point into the abdomen.
  - Infraumbilical, transumbilical, and Omega incisions are the most commonly used incisions.
- Alternative sites can be used if there is history of umbilical surgery or mesh.
  - In patients with prior abdominoplasty or myocutaneous flap harvesting, the umbilicus is in its native location on the abdominal wall, but may have underlying mesh associated with it.
  - An ostomy site can be used for access if ostomy is planned for advanced cancer or endometriosis.
- Closure of the vaginal cuff may be performed laparoscopically or transvaginally.
  - The lowest risk of vaginal cuff dehiscence was noted with transvaginal closure in some studies[1]:
    - TLH laparoscopic suturing 0.86%
    - TLH vaginal suturing 0.3%
    - Abdominal hysterectomy 0.21%
    - Vaginal hysterectomy 0.18%

Procedures and Techniques (Video 8.3)

Anesthesia and positioning

- Following general anesthesia, the patient is placed in the low lithotomy position with arms tucked and padded at the sides and a strap placed across the patient's chest.
- Tolerance of steep Trendelenburg position can be tested prior to prepping the patient.

Prepping and draping

- Vagina, perineum, and abdomen are sterilely prepared and the patient draped.

Antibiotics and bladder drainage

- The appropriate intravenous antibiotics are given and a Foley catheter is inserted into the bladder.

Manipulation of the uterus

The uterine manipulator is placed (if being used). In endometrial cancer or hyperplasia consider cauterizing fallopian tubes laparoscopically prior to placement of manipulator.

Local anesthesia

We use 0.25% or 0.5% bupivacaine injected circumferentially around the umbilicus for local anesthesia prior to making the incision (Tech Fig. 8.3.1A).

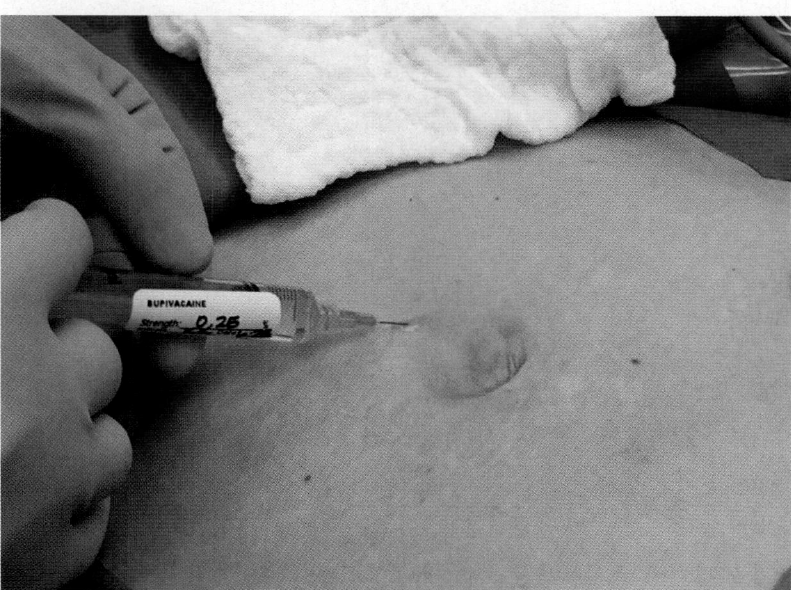

A

Tech Figure 8.3.1. Abdominal access and port placement with the GelPOINT®. **A:** An "umbilical block" using 6 to 10 mL of bupivacaine. *(continued)*

Abdominal incision

- Typical transumbilical abdominal entry is carried out by grasping the edges of the umbilicus at 3 and 9 o'clock with Allis clamps (Tech Fig. 8.3.1B), incising the umbilicus ~1.5 cm in the midline through its base (Tech Fig. 8.3.1C), replacing the Allis clamps just below the skin at the base of the umbilicus and everting the umbilical skin outward, incising the fascia with curved Mayo scissors, grasping the peritoneum with hemostats and entering the peritoneum sharply. The peritoneum and fascia are the extended with electrocautery.

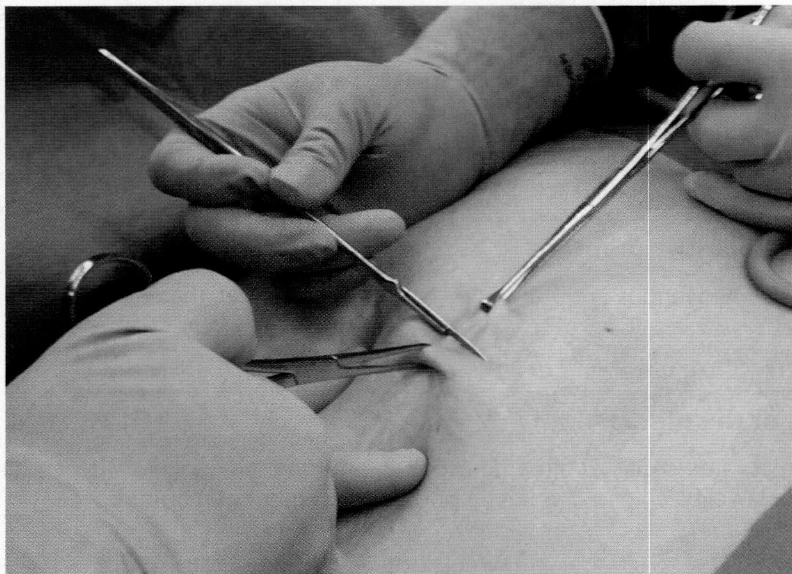

B

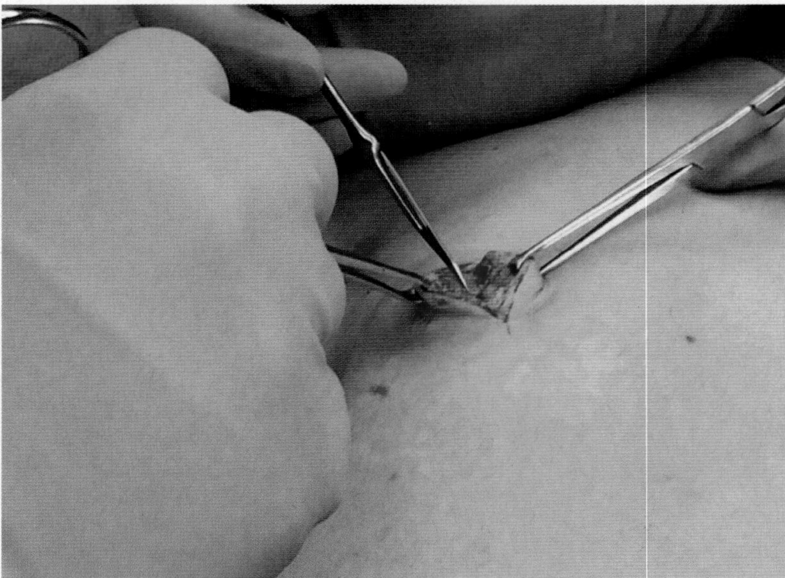

C

Tech Figure 8.3.1. (*continued*) **B:** Grasp the umbilicus at 3 and 9 o'clock with Allis clamps. **C:** Incise the skin 1.5 to 2 cm across the edges and trough the base of the umbilicus, then grasp and transect the fascia, then the peritoneum to 1.5 to 2 cm. (*continued*)

Abdominal access device placement

- The single-port access device is placed (Tech Fig. 8.3.1D–I).

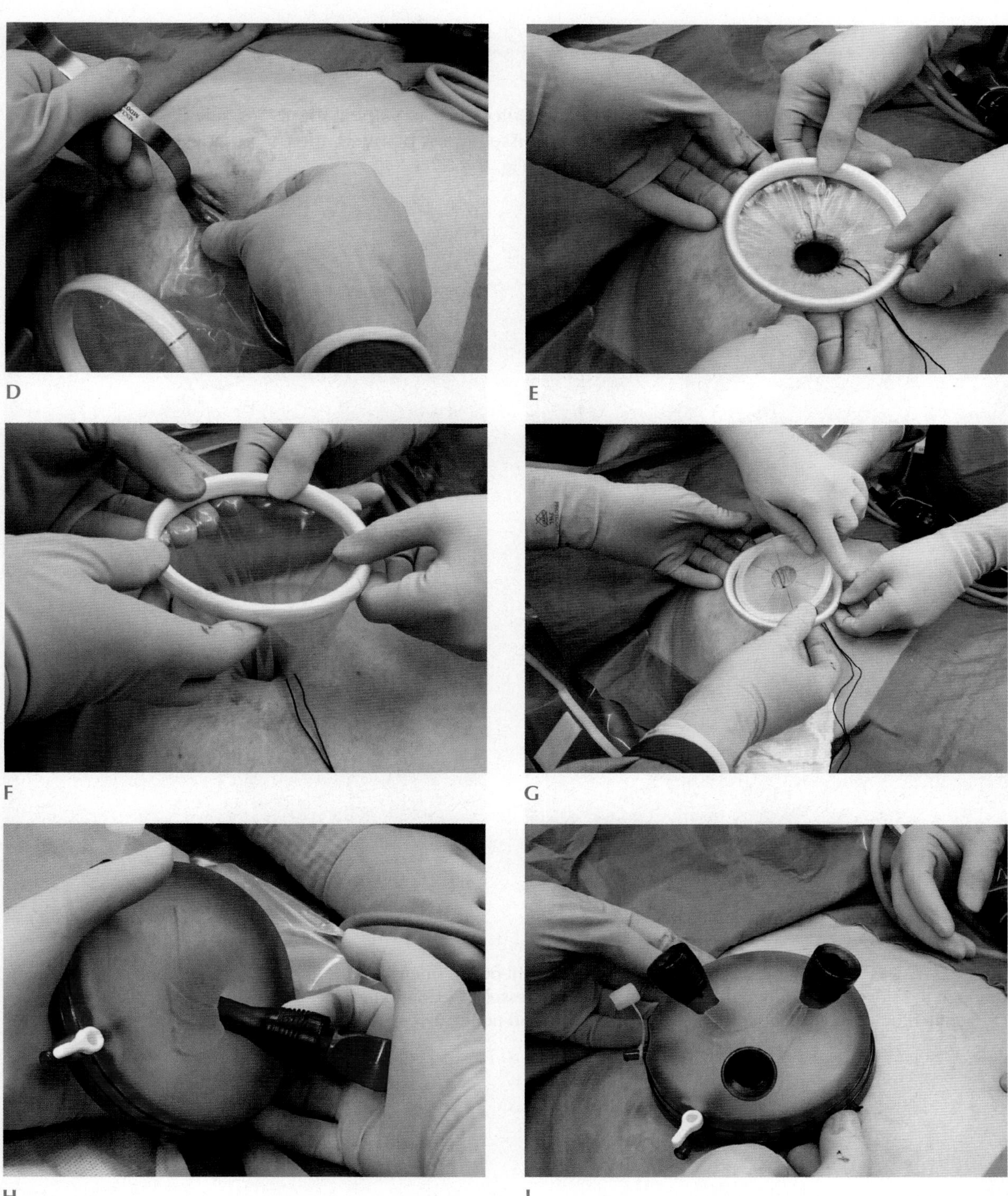

Tech Figure 8.3.1. (*continued*) D: Place an s-retractor to assist with placement of the ring of the retractor sleeve. E: Roll outer ring of the sleeve inward to tighten. F: This will expand the incision and protect the wound. G: Place the instrument shield. H: Place three to four trocars through the gel starting wide and aiming each to center of gel. I: Placement of the gel cap onto the ring.

Abdominal survey and pelvic washings

Methodical abdominal and pelvic survey should be carried out to identify any additional pathology. Pelvic washings should be obtained for cases done for high-grade endometrial cancer and re-staging of ovarian cancer, if indicated.

Pelvic sidewall anatomy and access

- Pelvic sidewall anatomy can be identified transperitoneally in some patients (Tech Fig. 8.3.2A). However, in other patients, or if retroperitoneal dissection is planned, the pelvic sidewall is opened and anatomic structures identified (Tech Fig. 8.3.2B–E).

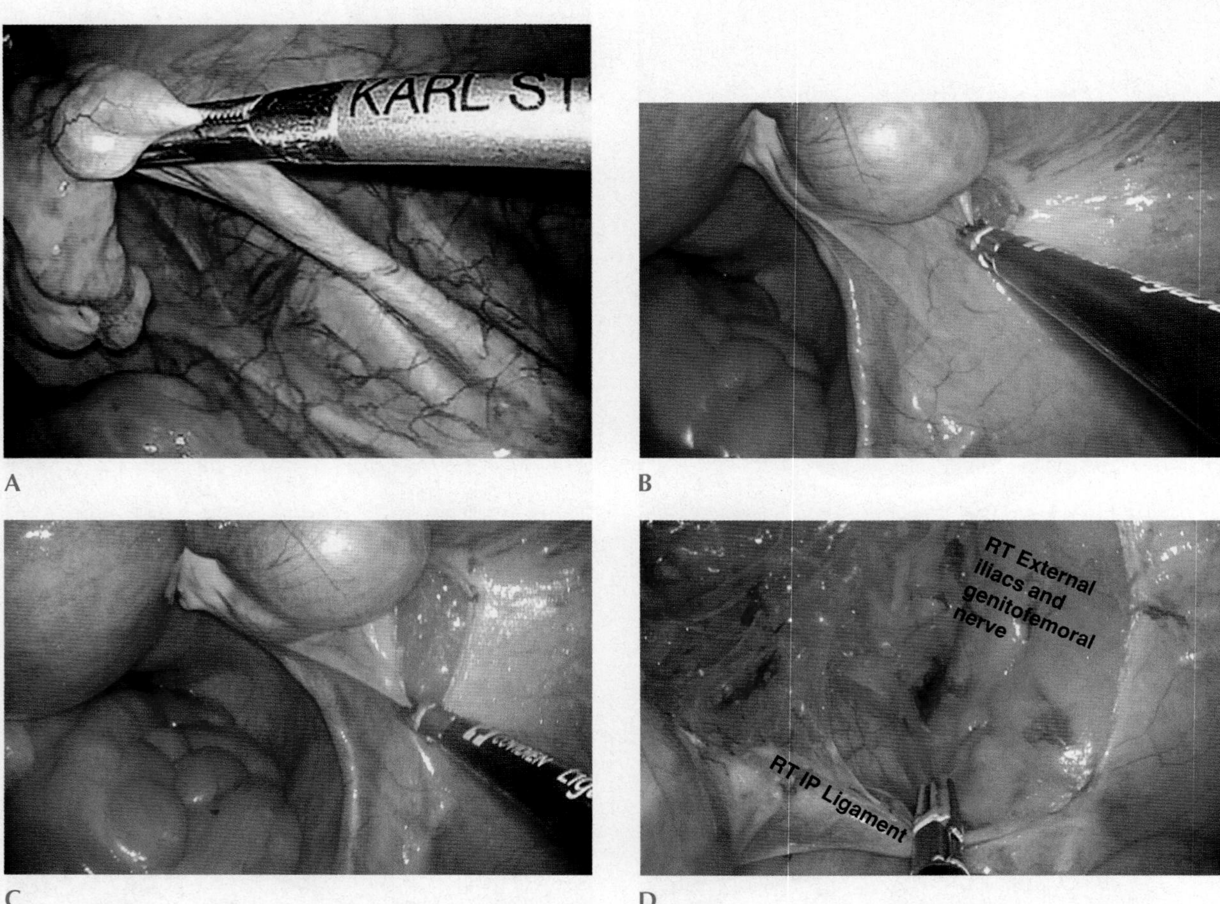

Tech Figure 8.3.2. Laparoscopic pelvic anatomy and right pelvic sidewall dissection. A: Transperitoneal anatomy. B: Open the sidewall peritoneum lateral to the gonadal vessels. C: Continued opening of sidewall peritoneum. D: Gentle blunt and sharp dissection to expose vessels and ureter. (*continued*)

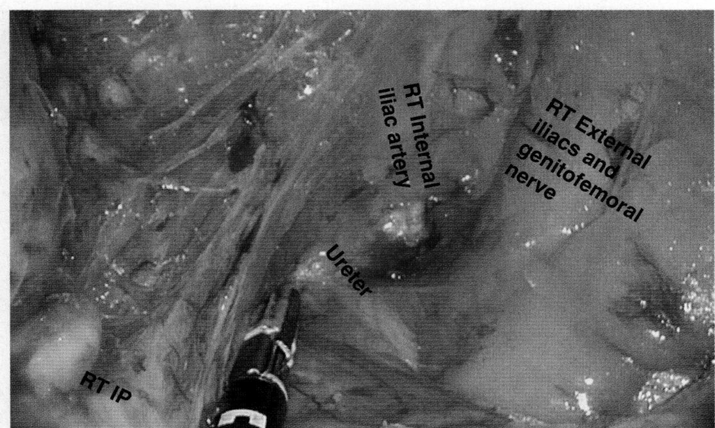

Tech Figure 8.3.2. (*continued*) **E:** Retroperitoneal anatomy with labels.

Takedown of the adnexal ligaments and bladder flap

- The infundibulopevic ligaments are skeletonized, cauterized, and transected (**Tech Fig. 8.3.3A**). A vessel sealing device is used for each pedicle. The round ligaments are cauterized and incised (**Tech Fig. 8.3.3B**). The bladder flap is created from lateral to medial and then taken down along the anterior vaginal wall (**Tech Fig. 8.3.3C–D**).

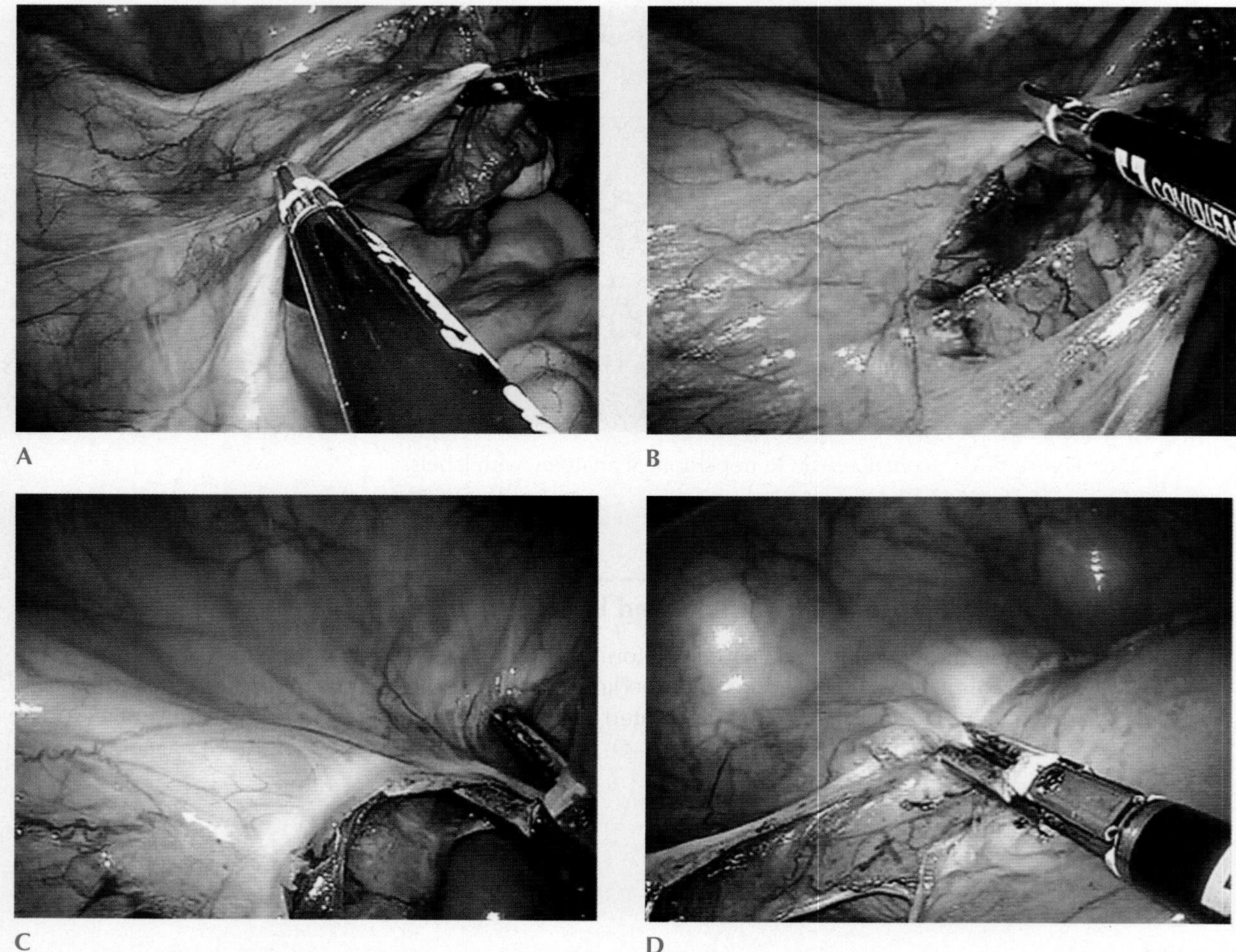

Tech Figure 8.3.3. Left sidewall and bladder flap dissection and control of uterine vessels. A: Left infundibulopelvic ligament is cauterized and transected. B: Left round ligament transection. C: Start of left bladder flap dissection. D: Bladder flap dissection continued medially at level of colpotomy cup. (*continued*)

Uterine vessels and cardinal ligaments

- Uterine arteries are skeletonized, then taken down with the vessel sealing device.
  - We place a seal for back bleeding, then take the uterine artery with another seal inferior to this (Tech Fig. 8.3.3E,F).
- Cardinal ligaments are taken down in successive bites, each inside of the last until the vessels are taken down below the cervicovaginal junction or lateral to the colpotomy ring (Tech Fig. 8.3.3G–I).

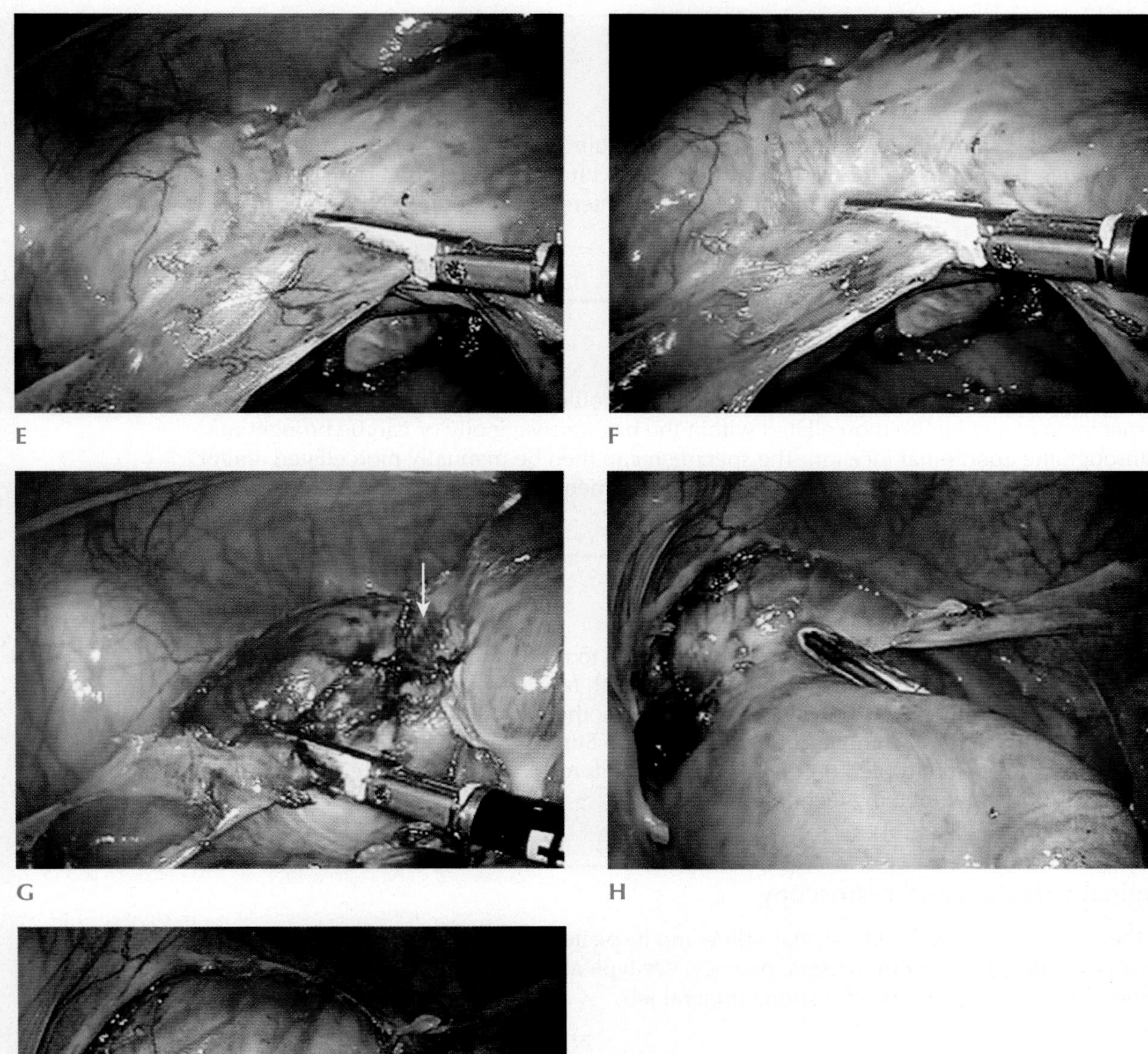

E F G H I

Tech Figure 8.3.3. (*continued*) E: Medial and cephalad left lower uterine segment transected to control back bleeding. F: Dessicate and transect right uterine artery. G: Dessication of cardinal ligaments and vessels being taken down below colpotomy ring (*arrow*). H: Dessication and transect of right uterine artery. I: Back bleeding bite along right lower uterine segment with transection of right cardinal ligament.

Colpotomy is performed

- Circumferential colpotomy is performed.
  - See Tech Fig. 8.3.4A–D.
  - This can be performed with monopolar energy, ultrasonic shears, or a laparoscopic scalpel. I prefer the monopolar hook, typically starting with the posterior portion of the colpotomy first (Tech Fig. 8.3.4A,B) and then moving circumferentially around to the anterior colpotomy (Tech Fig. 8.3.4C,D).

Specimen extraction

- Most uteri can be removed transvaginally.
- If the uterus is too large for vaginal extraction, it should be placed in a specimen bag. The specimen can either be morcellated within the bag transvaginally or can be brought out through the abdominal incision. The specimen can then be manually morcellated and/or the incision extended enough to remove the specimen intact within the specimen bag.

Cuff closure

- See Tech Fig. 8.3.4.
- Transvaginal—we currently use this technique due to reports suggesting that there is a lower risk of vaginal cuff dehiscence when compared with laparoscopic closure. Typically, five to six figure-of-eight sutures of 0-polyglycolic acid (or another absorbable) suture are used.
- Laparoscopic—closure simplest utilizing and Endo Stitch device with either a running 2-0 barbed suture or interrupted 0-polyglycolic acid suture can be used with either extracorporeal or intracorporeal knot tying techniques.

Vaginal irrigation and cystoscopy

- The vagina is irrigated with normal saline and inspected for bleeding or tears. Cystoscopy can be utilized to confirm ureteral patency. We typically inject 25 mg of fluorescein dye intravenously then observe for strong ureteral jets.

Laparoscopic irrigation, inspection and closure

- The pelvis is irrigated with saline, lactated ringers, or sterile water (Tech Fig. 8.3.4E,F).
- All sites of dissection are inspected for hemostasis.
- Instruments and access port are removed and the pneumoperitoneum is expressed.
- We close the fascia with interrupted 0-polyglycolic acid suture.
  - We use delayed absorbable suture for cases where the incision was extended or when chemotherapy or radiation will be given.
  - We use permanent suture if there was previous or current umbilical hernia.

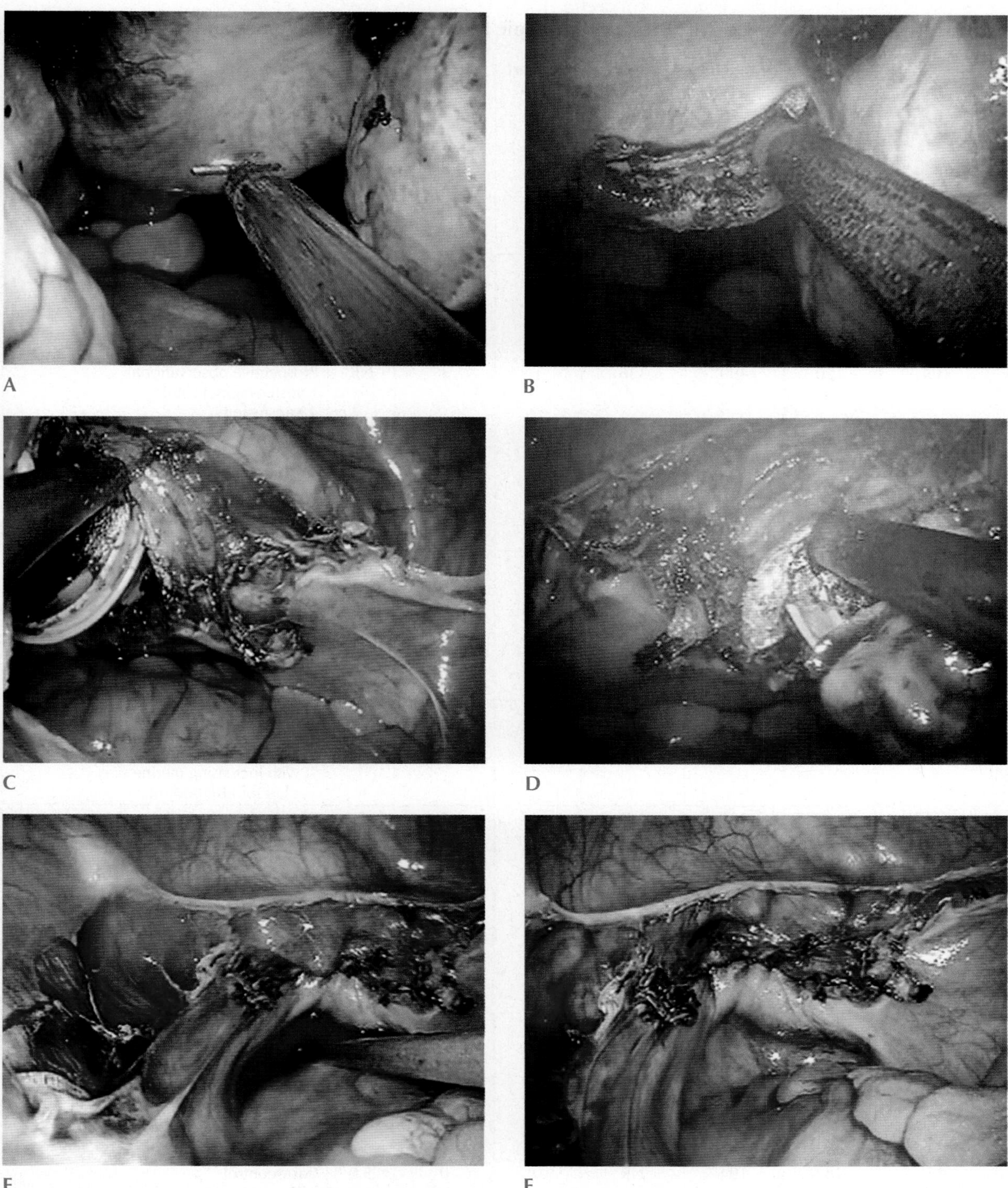

Tech Figure 8.3.4. Colpotomy and closure. A: Start posterior colpotomy with monopolar hook. B: Continued circumferential colpotomy to right side. C: Left anterolateral colpotomy. D: Completion of anterior colpotomy on colpotomy ring. E: After transvaginal cuff closure, pelvis is copiously irrigated and hemostasis ensured. F: Final cuff appearance and pelvic inspection.

Table 8.3.1 Selected Reports of Single-Port Total Laparoscopic Hysterectomy—Outcomes and Complications

Author (year)	*n*	Op Time (min)	Median EBL (mL)	Uterine Weight (g)	Convert Xlap	Convert Multi-port	LOS (days)	Notes and Complications in SPL
Jung (2010)	30	100	100	167	0	1	3	Retrospective REVIEW of SPL No major complications
Yim (3) (2010)	52	117	100	162	0	0	3.4	Retrospective REVIEW of SPL vs. S-TLH Lower EBL, shorter LOS, SPL had lower pain scores immediate postop, but not at 6, 24, or 48 hrs 1 umbilical drainage
Jung (4) (2011)	30	89	45	173	0	4	3	RCT of SPL vs. S-TLH similar op times, but higher analgesic use in SPL despite similar pain scores 1 ureter injury 1 transfusion
Park (2011)	105	120	400	336	1	3	NR	Prospective observational 1 vesicovaginal fistula 4 transfusions
Fanfani (6) (2012)	30	105	30	105	0	1	1	Retrospective matched case-control Comparing SPL vs. S-TLH vs. mini-laparoscopic hysterectomy Longer op time than both Less pain than S-TLH 1 EBL >500 mL
Li (2012)	52	130	158	NA	0	1	6	RCT comparing SPL vs. S-TLH Increased op time (19 min) with higher patient satisfaction scores
Fagotti (2013)	38	107	30	NR	0	0	NR	Retrospective case-control of SPL vs. robotic single-site hysterectomy SPL had lower EBL and more patients with 1 d LOS
Song (2013)	21	110	200	600	1	4	4	Retrospective review of SPL with uterine weight >500 g Increased op time and EBL correlated with increasing uterine size. 1 × lap for EBL 800 mL
Park (2013)	274 (total hyster-ectomy only)	103	340	NR	1	5	3	Prospective, single surgeon 1 vaginal bleed 1 vaginal abscess 1 rectal injury 1 vesicovaginal fistula 2 umbilical hernia 1 vaginal dehiscence 2 bladder injury 1 ureter injury 33 transfusions
Kim (2014)	50	91	198	355	0	2	3	Case-control SP-TLH vs. SP-LAVH. Shorter OR time (16 min) and lower pain scores at 24 and 36 hrs for SP-TLH 1 vaginal dehiscence 1 vaginal bleeding 1 cystotomy
Park (2014)	37	183	194	NR	0	0	5.0	Case-control All endometrial cancer 100% had pelvic LND 18.9% had para-aortic LND 1 bladder injury
Lee (2015)	25	137	100	642	0	0	3	Retrospective case-control of SPL vs. S-TLH for uterine wt. >500 g Shorter LOS than S-TLH No difference in pain scores at 6/24, or 48 hrs 1 ureter injury

SPL, single-port total laparoscopic hysterectomy; S-TLH, standard-total laparoscopic hysterectomy; SP-LAVH, single-port laparoscopic-assisted vaginal hysterectomy; EBL, estimated blood loss; Xlap, laparotomy; LOS, length of stay; LND, lymph node dissection.

PEARLS AND PITFALLS

✖ External instrument clashing
○ Use flexible instruments.
○ Turn the handle of the grasper upside down to gain additional distance between hands.
○ Use a bariatric length 30-degree or flexible-tip laparoscope.
○ Use bariatric-length grasper can be used with standard length vessel sealing devices.
✖ Difficulty seeing around the uterus
○ To see the left side of the uterus, place the tip of the flexible camera near the left sidewall and flex the tip back to the right. To see the right side of the uterus, place the camera over the fundus and get a "birds-eye" view of the dissection.
✖ Difficulty suturing
○ Use of the Endo Stitch device will help get around the absence of angulation to the vagina.
○ Flexible graspers or flexible Endo Stitch device can also help to overcome external instrument clashing during suturing.
✖ Difficulty progressing safely with surgery
○ Add an additional trocar if necessary.
○ Practice in the laboratory with a box trainer starting with ports farther apart, gradually moving them closer together until the distance is similar to single-port device.

POSTOPERATIVE CARE

- Postoperative care is similar to standard laparoscopic hysterectomy with Foley to gravity drainage at least 6 to 8 hours postop. Aggressive use of nonnarcotic analgesics such as acetaminophen and ketorolac can minimize opioid requirements. Activity and diet are advanced as tolerated in the immediate postoperative period. The majority of patients can be discharged home on postoperative day 1, even with incisions that were extended for specimen extraction or hand-assist procedures.
- Typical recovery time is 4 weeks. The major complaint at the postoperative visit is persistent fatigue.
- We instruct patients to avoid: driving for 2 weeks, lifting more than 10 pounds for 4 weeks, and placing anything in the vagina for 6 weeks.

OUTCOMES

- Data comparing single-port total laparoscopic or single-port laparoscopic-assisted vaginal hysterectomy have been reported as case reports to as many as 274 hysterectomies in one series.[2] SPL has been shown to be similar to standard multi-port laparoscopic cohort in terms of intraoperative and postoperative complications, length of hospital stay, estimated blood loss, and blood transfusion rates (**Table 8.3.1**). Operative times for the single-port approach for hysterectomy appears to be approximately 8 minutes longer in one meta-analysis.[3] Although a decrease in postoperative pain has been one of the purported benefits of single-port laparoscopic surgery, data have been mixed in randomized controlled trials.[4–7]

COMPLICATIONS

- The most common complications are similar to that of laparoscopic hysterectomy. Urinary tract infection and port site cellulitis are the most common infectious complications that we have seen. Injury to visceral organs is similar to that of standard laparoscopic hysterectomy. The complication that is likely to have a higher risk in single-port laparoscopic hysterectomy is umbilical hernia which occurs in 0% to 2.4% of patients.[8] We have minimized this complication with attention to closure technique using fascial closure alone with interrupted absorbable figure-of-eight sutures for low-risk women and nonabsorbable sutures for patients at higher risk for hernia (prior umbilical hernia, obesity, steroid use, and need for chemotherapy or radiation).

KEY REFERENCES

1. Uccella S, Ceccaroni M, Cromi A, et al. Vaginal cuff dehiscence in a series of 12,398 hysterectomies: effect of different types of colpotomy and vaginal closure. *Obstet Gynecol.* 2012;120(3):516–523.
2. Park JY, Kim TJ, Kang HJ, et al. Laparoendoscopic single site (LESS) surgery in benign gynecology: perioperative and late complications of 515 cases. *Eur J Obstet Gynecol Reprod Biol.* 2013;167(2):215–218.
3. Murji A, Patel VI, Leyland N, Choi M. Single-incision laparoscopy in gynecologic surgery: a systematic review and meta-analysis. *Obstet Gynecol.* 2013;121(4):819–828.
4. Yim GW, Jung YW, Paek J, et al. Transumbilical single-port access versus conventional total laparoscopic hysterectomy: surgical outcomes. *Am J Obstet Gynecol.* 2010;203:26.e1–e6.
5. Jung YW, Lee M, Yim GW, et al. A randomized prospective study of single-port and four-port approaches for hysterectomy in terms of postoperative pain. *Surg Endosc.* 2011;25(8):2462–2469.
6. Eom JM, Choi JS, Choi WJ, Kim YH, Lee JH. Does single-port laparoscopic surgery reduce postoperative pain in women with benign gynecologic disease? *J Laparoendosc Adv Surg Tech A.* 2013;23(12):999–1005.
7. Fanfani F, Fagotti A, Rossitto C, et al. Laparoscopic, minilaparoscopic and single-port hysterectomy: perioperative outcomes. *Surg Endosc.* 2012;26(12):3592–3596.
8. Gunderson CC, Knight J, Ybanez-Morano J, et al. The risk of umbilical hernia and other complications with laparoendoscopic single-site surgery. *J Minim Invasive Gynecol.* 2012;19(1):40–45.

Chapter 8.4

Robotically Assisted Hysterectomy

Habibeh Ladan Gitiforooz

GENERAL PRINCIPLES

Definition

- Robotic hysterectomy is a highly effective, minimally invasive approach to removing the uterus in patients with a variety of uterine conditions. Robotic approach can be very effective for morbidly obese patients and for large fibroids weighing more than 500 g. It can also be a very effective tool for patients with multiple pelvic surgeries and severe adhesions.

Differential Diagnosis

- Sarcoma, leiomyosarcoma, large fibroid uterus, fibroma, endometrial stromal sarcoma, adenomyosis, and endometrial carcinoma.

Anatomic Considerations

- A large, wide, uterus can be difficult to manipulate and this can limit visibility.
- The blood supply to a wide cervix can be very close to the ureters.
- Lifting the uterus to incise the uterosacral ligament posteriorly can be challenging.
- The ureters can be closer to the uterosacral ligament than usual.

Nonoperative Management

- Conservative, nonoperative management can be designed depending on the patient's symptoms.
- Heavy menstrual bleeding, bulk and pressure symptoms, and mild hydronephrosis may respond well to uterine artery embolization.
- Heavy bleeding may respond to oral contraceptive pills, progestins, or an IUD.

IMAGING AND OTHER DIAGNOSTICS

- See Figures 8.4.1 to 8.4.6.

PREOPERATIVE PLANNING

- Pap and HPV testing must be up-to-date in all cases.
- An up-to-date, in office, endometrial biopsy is a very important part of evaluation. Some studies suggest that more than 50% of sarcoma can be diagnosed by an office endometrial biopsy.
- Early evaluation of hemoglobin and bleeding.
- Gonadotropin releasing hormone and IV or oral iron therapy can prevent unnecessary blood transfusions.
- An examination under anesthesia is performed to assess the height and width of the uterus to plan the position of the midline port (Fig. 8.4.7).
- Cystoscopy is indicated in all cases. Administer intraoperative fluorescein or use dextrose 10% as the distending hysteroscopic fluid to evaluate ureteral integrity.
- Oral/nasal gastric tubes are important to avoid injury to a distended stomach.

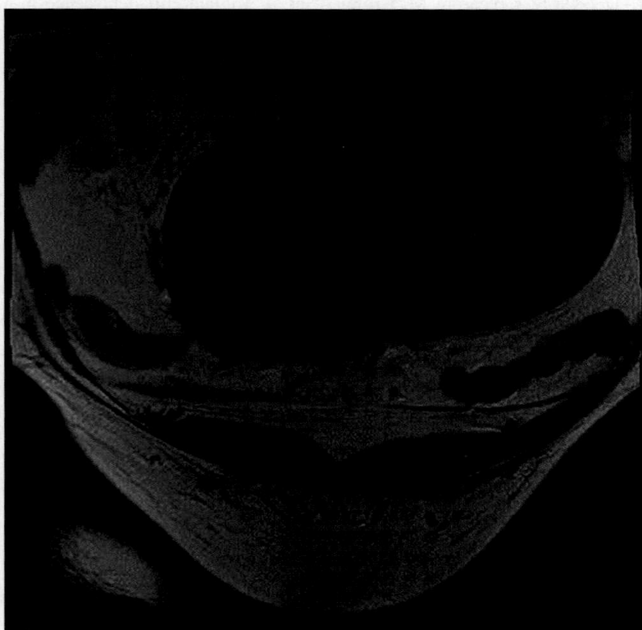

Figure 8.4.1. MRI 3 large midline fibroids.

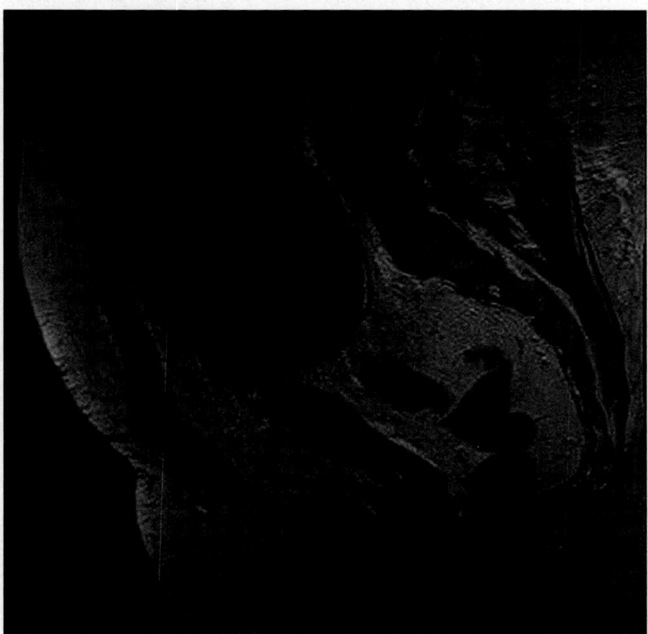

Figure 8.4.2. MRI-2 large midline mass of fibroids above umbilicus.

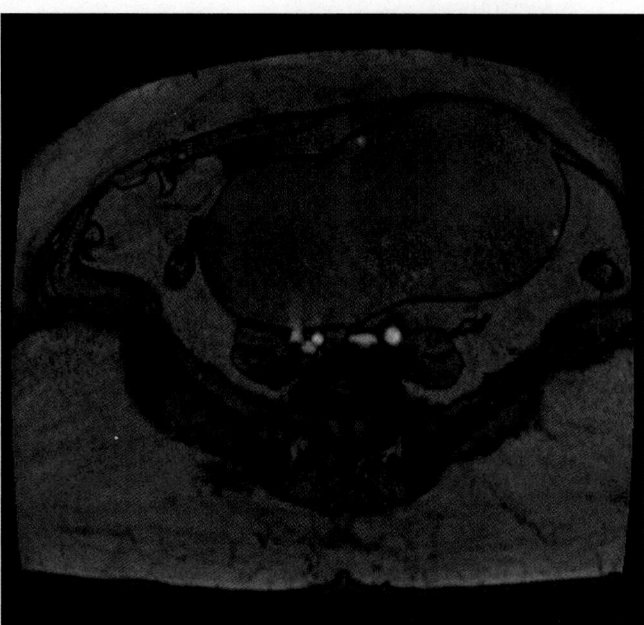

Figure 8.4.3. MRI 1 bilobed fibroid.

SURGICAL MANAGEMENT

- Indication of using the robotic approach may include:
  - patients with endometriosis and previous surgery with adhesions (Fig. 8.4.8),
  - other pelvic surgeries such as history of colon resection or multiple cesarean sections (see Fig. 8.4.8),

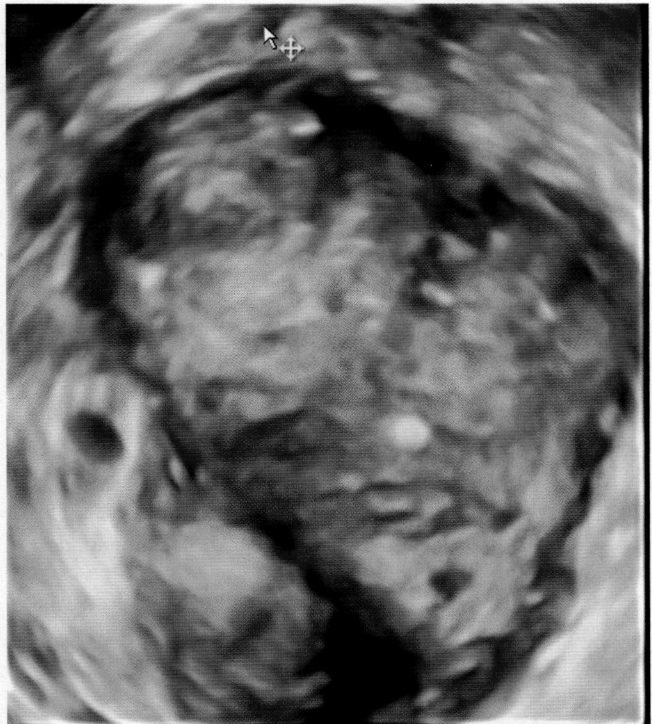

Figure 8.4.4. 3D ultrasound picture of fibroid uterus.

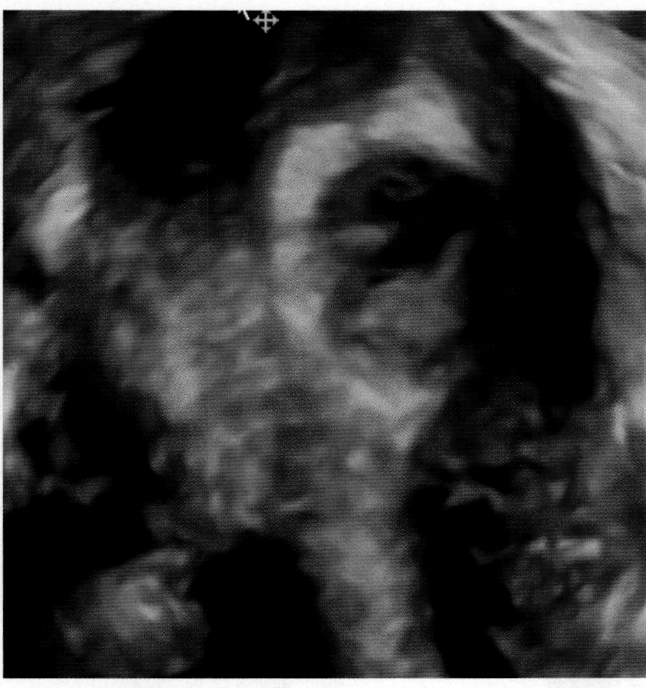

Figure 8.4.5. Degenerative fibroids.

  - patients with a history of failed myomectomy and uterine artery embolization.

Positioning

- Proper chest wrap is important to prevent obese patients from moving up the operating table in Trendelenburg position. Keeping in mind ventilation, IV lines, and the blood pressure cuff and pulse oximeter (Fig. 8.4.9).
- Perineal access to the uterus is an important part of operative positioning for manipulation and morcellation (Fig. 8.4.10).

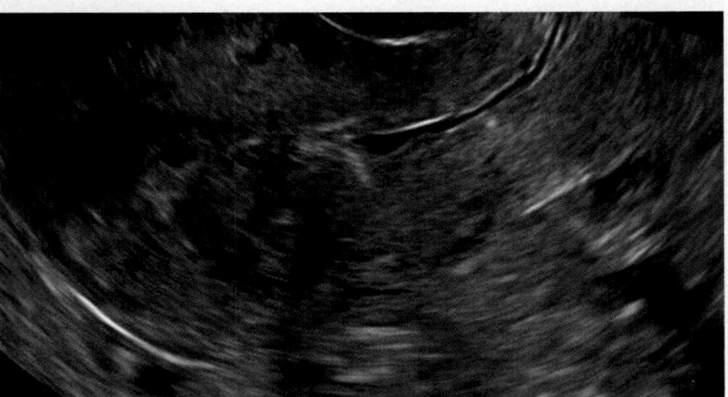

Figure 8.4.6. SIS picture showing 4 cm fibroid. The majority of the fibroid is located within the muscularis and is not approachable through the endometrium.

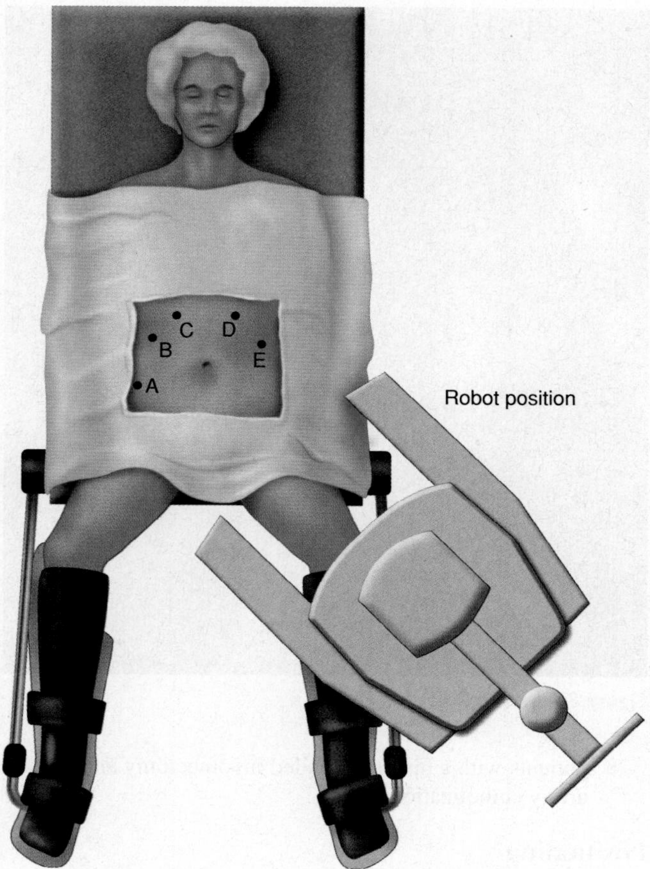

Figure 8.4.7. EUA is performed to assess and plan the position of parts.

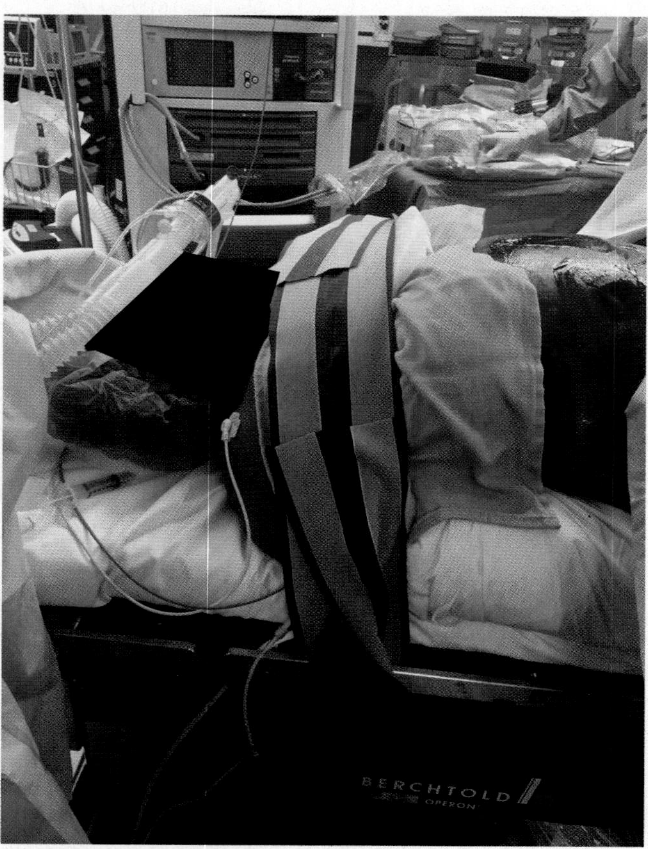

Figure 8.4.9. Wrap the chest to the operating table to prevent patients from sliding when placed in Trendelenburg position.

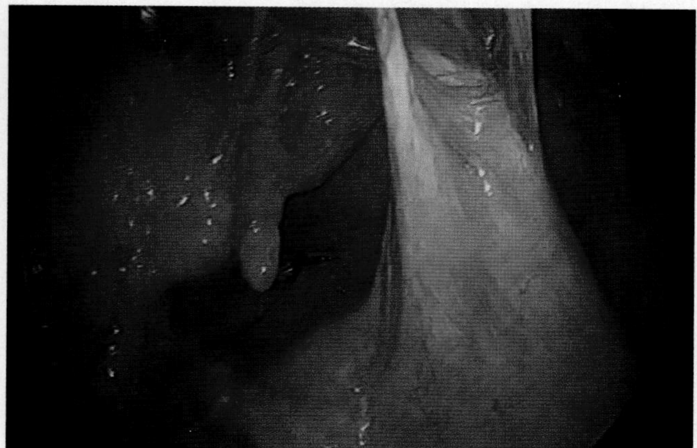

Figure 8.4.8. This patient had four cesarean sections. Note the bladder and uterine adhesions to the anterior abdominal wall.

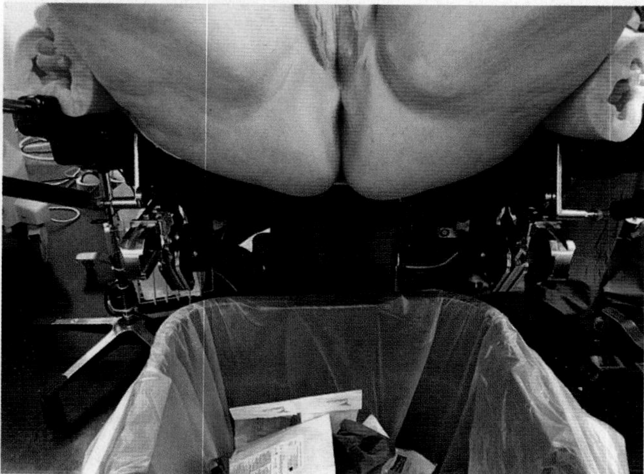

Figure 8.4.10. Perineal access to retrieve large specimens and move the uterine manipulator freely.

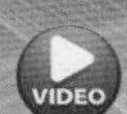

Procedures and Techniques (Video 8.4)

Port placement

- The first step is usually the midline 12-mm trocar placement. This trocar has to be longer if the patient is morbidly obese. This will allow for easy docking of the camera port and free movement of the camera arm (Tech Fig. 8.4.1). It has to be placed supraumbilically and preferably 10 cm away from the fundus of the uterus (Tech Fig. 8.4.2). To reduce the risk of stomach injuries with high trocar placement, it is important to ensure an empty and collapsed stomach. If the patient has a midline, upper abdominal incision or abdominal wall mesh with hernia repair, the left upper quadrant can be the safest entry to the peritoneal cavity (Tech Figs. 8.4.3 and 8.4.4).
- Place two 8-mm robotic trocars after insufflation of the abdomen and when the patient is in the steep Trendelenburg position.
- Care should be taken to keep enough space from the midline trocar and the right sided 8-mm trocar to give free range of movement to the right-side arm. This setup will avoid collision of the robotic arms (Tech Fig. 8.4.5). The right lower quadrant 12-mm port position is important. The movement of a heavy uterus from side to side and anterior to posterior can be helped with a tenaculum from this port. The tenaculum is more useful for a large uterus than the uterine manipulator.
- Tunneling of trocars in obese patients can cause collision of the robotic arms.

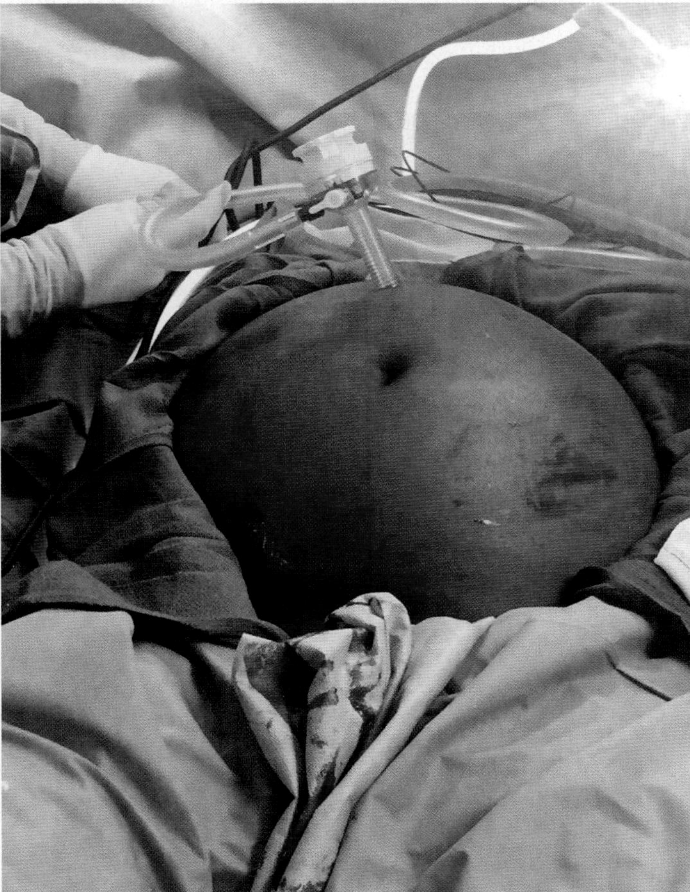

Tech Figure 8.4.1. Use a long trocar in an obese patient. This allows for easy docking of the camera port.

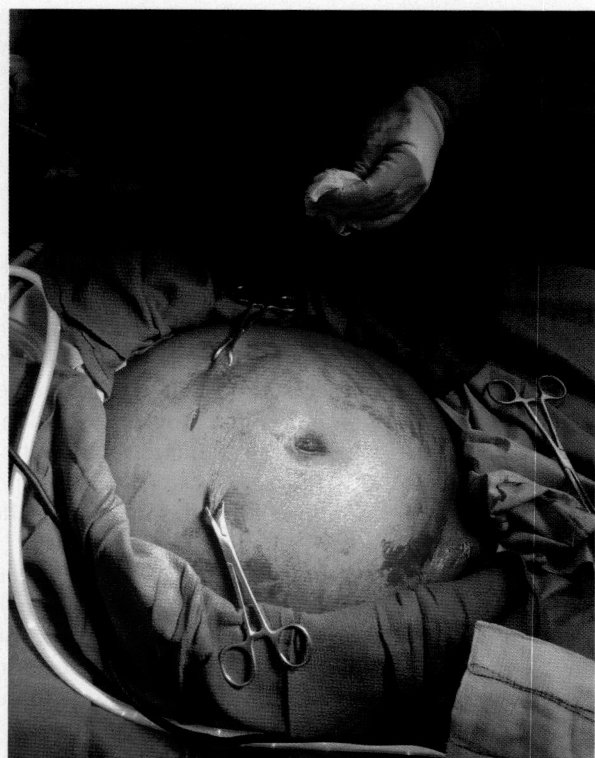

Tech Figure 8.4.2. A supraumbilical 12 mm trocar should be placed 10 cm away from the uterine fundus if possible.

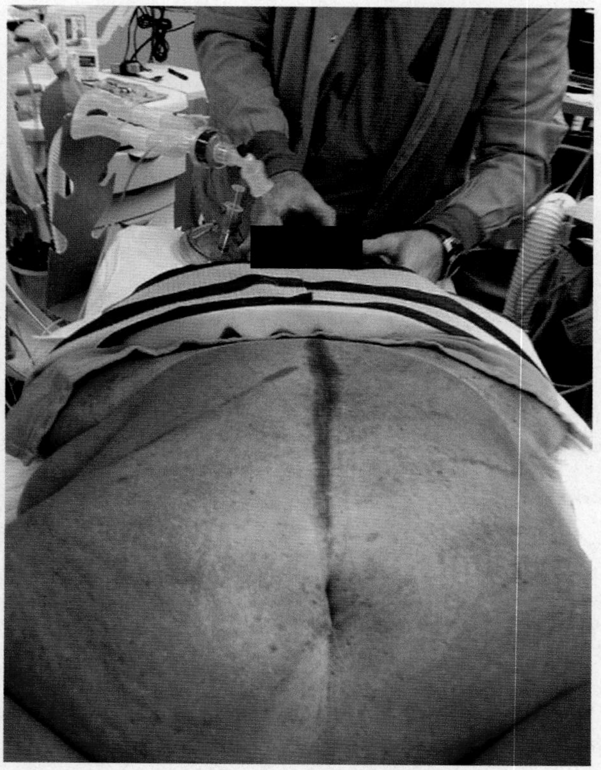

Tech Figure 8.4.3. In an obese patient with a history of a midline upper abdominal incision a left upper quadrant entry may be the safest entry.

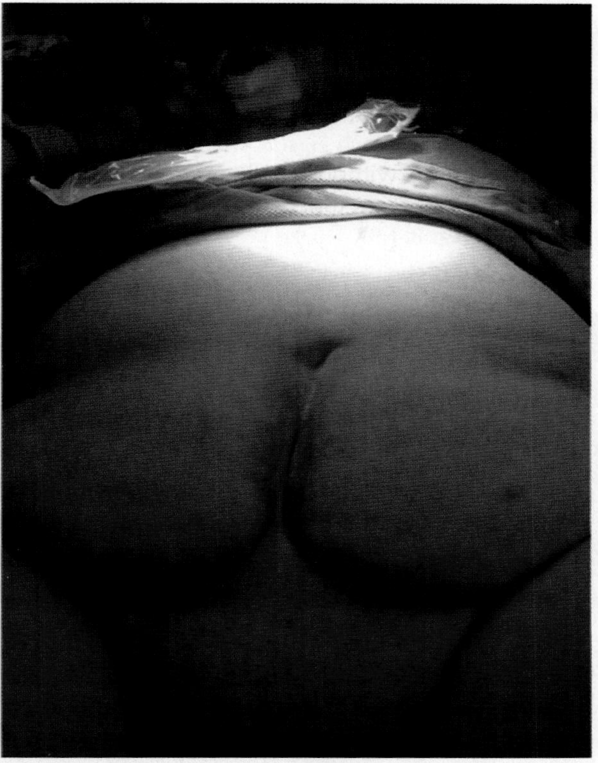

Tech Figure 8.4.4. Abdominal wall mesh with hernia repair in an obese patient.

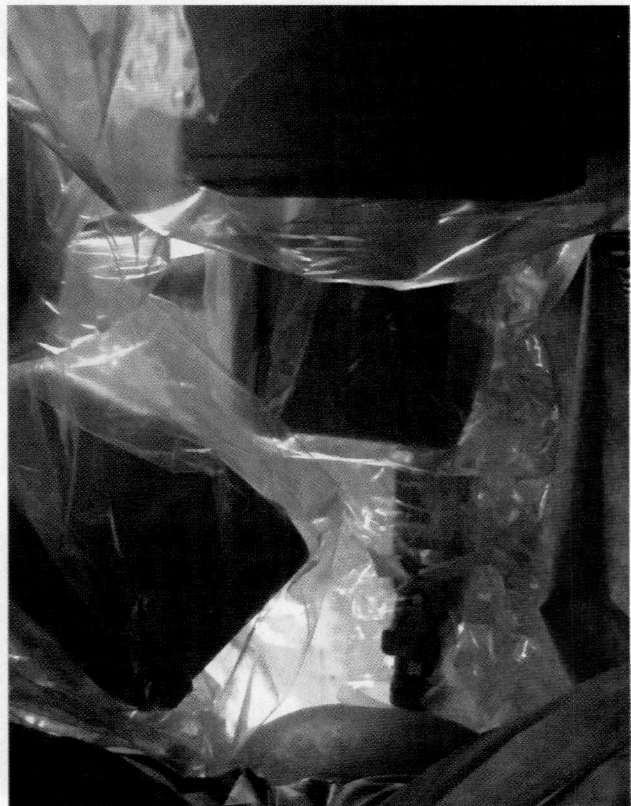

Tech Figure 8.4.5. Keep enough space between the midline trocar and the right sided trocar to avoid arm collision.

Vessel sealer

- It is very important to keep hemostasis well controlled, especially with a large uterus.
- Seal the uterine vessels of both the right and left sides before incising as there can be a great deal of back bleeding from the uterus (Tech Figs. 8.4.6 and 8.4.7).
- Stay as close as possible to the uterus without digging into it (Tech Fig. 8.4.8).
- Large blood vessels between the fallopian tube, ovarian ligament, and round ligament may exist. Seal them patiently (Tech Fig. 8.4.9).

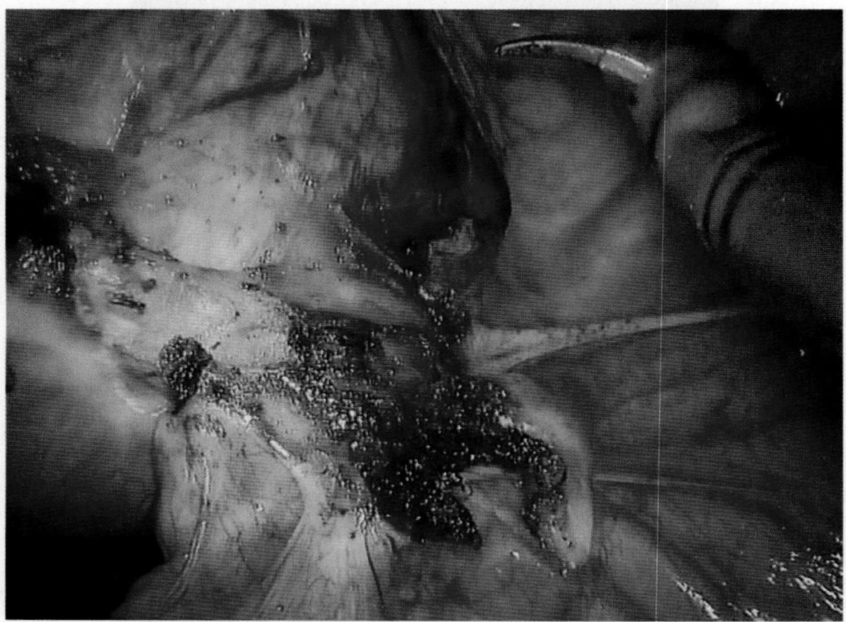

Tech Figure 8.4.6. Seal the vessels on both sides before incising to prevent back bleeding.

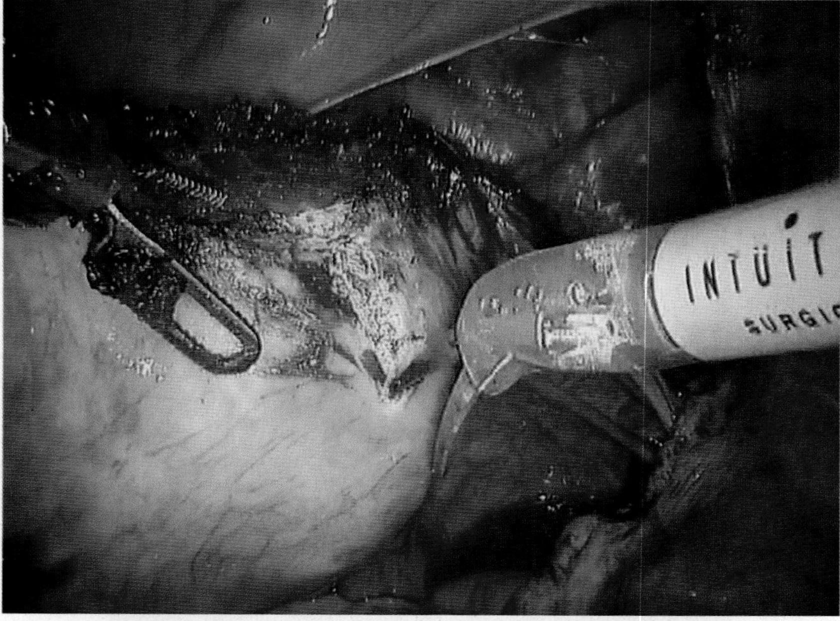

Tech Figure 8.4.7. Stay as close to uterus without digging into it.

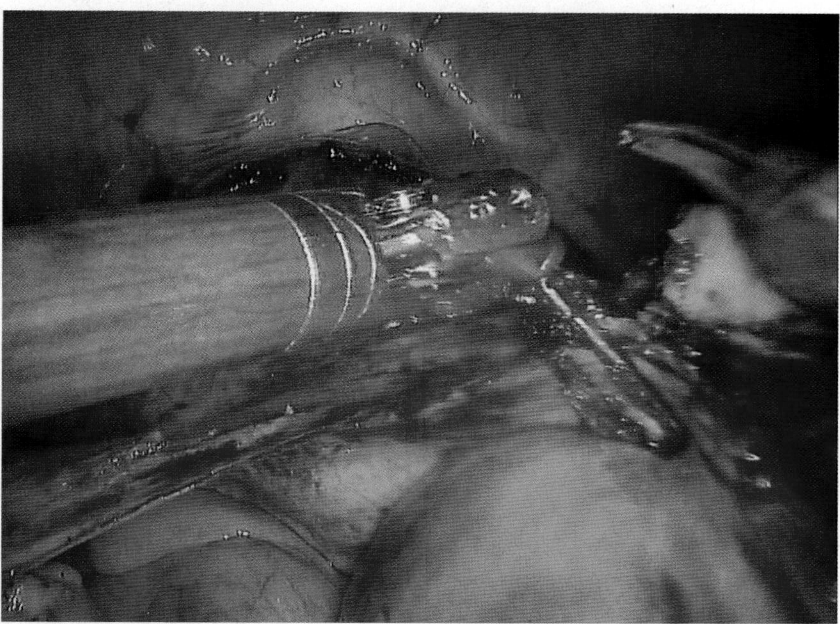

Tech Figure 8.4.8. Incise the parametria without entering the myometrium to decrease bleeding.

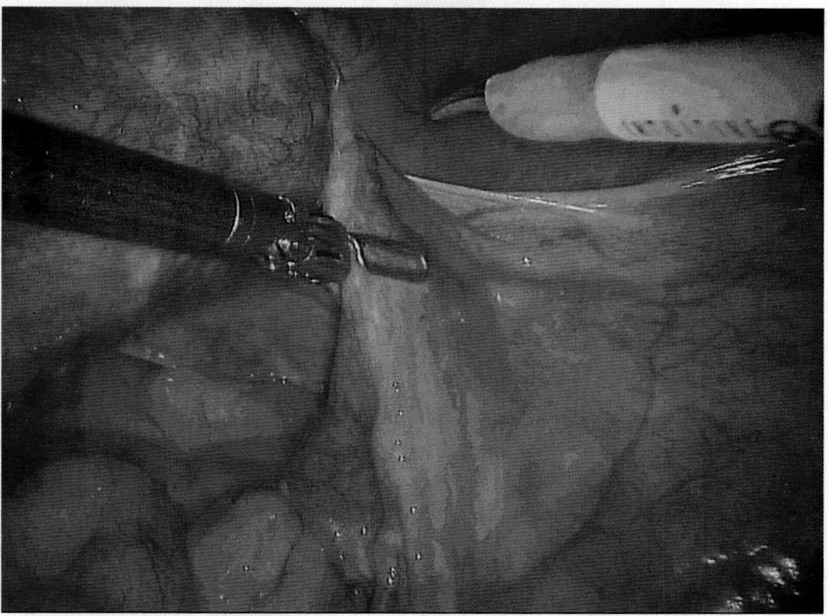

Tech Figure 8.4.9. Coagulate large blood vessels between the ovarian and round ligaments.

Manipulation of the uterus

- When using the uterine manipulator try to stay on one side. Go all the way down to the vaginal fornix and seal all the blood supply before changing to the opposite side. This will help save time and prevent the manipulator from breaking.
- The assistant can move the uterus from side to side with the help of a tenaculum. It is better to seal the vessels before using the tenaculum to prevent extra bleeding.

Separation of cervical vaginal junction

- Increase the abdominal CO_2 pressure and CO_2 flow; this will help keep the CO_2 pressure up during colpotomy. This step must be performed quickly in obese patients as ventilation may be a problem.
- In the case of a large uterus, it is easier to perform colpotomy on the posterior aspect first.
- Lifting a heavy uterus will be harder after an incision is made on the cervicovaginal junction.

Evacuation of the specimen

- Using a Lahey clamp, pull the specimen into the vagina. Then protect the vaginal wall with a weighted speculum posteriorly. Use side retractors and a large blade to excise large fragments (**Tech Figs. 8.4.10** and **8.4.11**). The specimen can be placed in a large bag laparoscopically. Then, deliver the neck of the bag from the vagina and excise the specimen in the bag. This step will add to operative time.

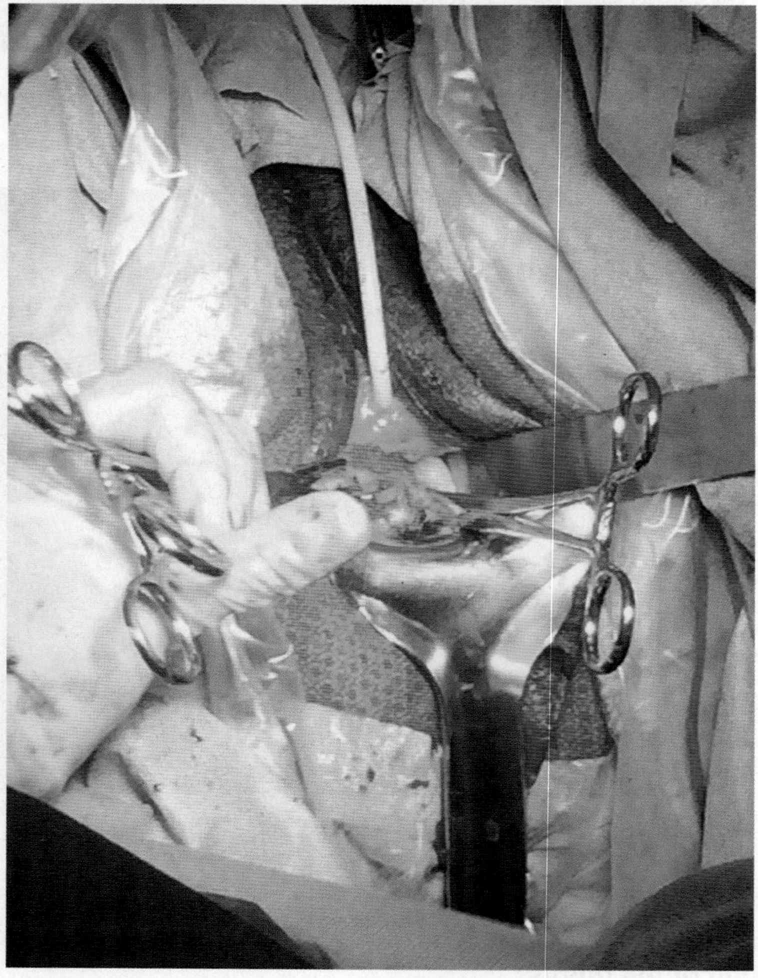

Tech Figure 8.4.10. Using a Lahey clamp, deliver the specimen into the vagina and use a large blade to excise the specimen.

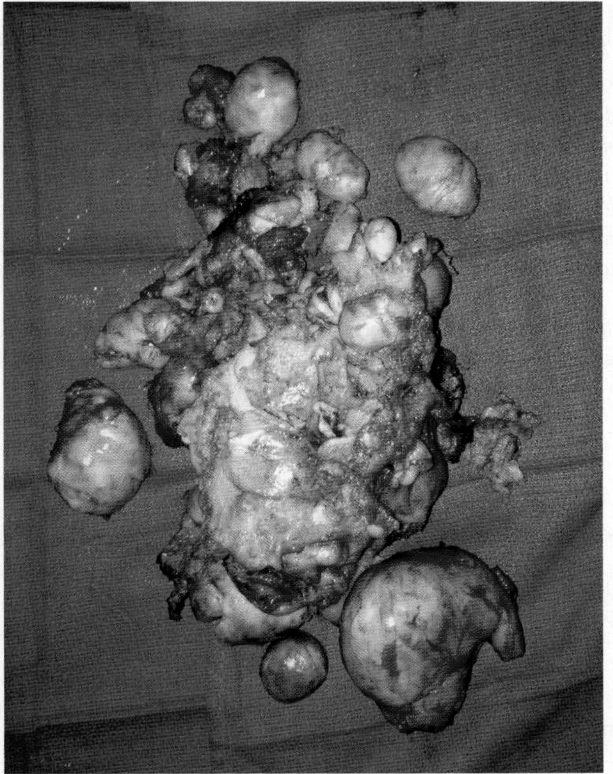

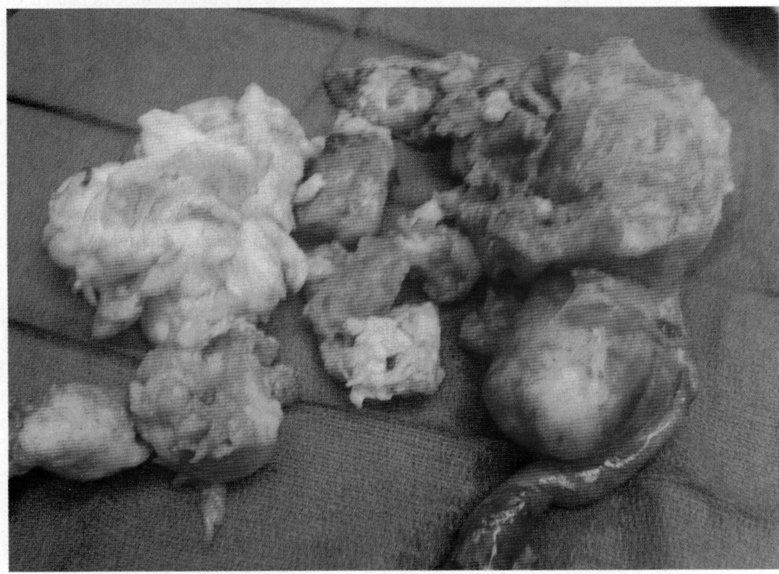

Tech Figure 8.4.11. Large pieces can be excised with large blade.

Port closure

- Fascial closure is indicated for a port site of 10 mm or larger to prevent hernia formation.
- Inject local anesthetic to all port sites at the end of surgery. This helps with postoperative pain management.

PEARLS AND PITFALLS

- ○ Use a long, midline trocar in obese patients.
- ✖ Short trocars may be dislodged during the surgery and cause air leaks, poor visibility, and tissue trauma.
- ○ Right sided robotic port placement is very important. Improper site selection will lead to limited right sided instrument utility and robotic camera arm collision.
- ○ Tunneling of the trocars in obese patients can be prevented by proper 90 degree port placement.
- ○ Unnecessary movement of the uterine manipulator should be avoided.
- ✖ The uterine manipulator can break or become loose. This limits the ability to complete a minimally invasive surgery.
- ○ Using interrupted sutures for vaginal closure will help drain any bleeding and prevent blood collection.

POSTOPERATIVE CARE

- The majority of robotic hysterectomies may be performed as outpatient surgery.
- Postoperative analgesia may include narcotic pain relief.
- Scopolamine patch for 24 hours to prevent postoperative nausea.

OUTCOMES

- The potential and risk of occult malignancy in reproductive-age women is extremely low.

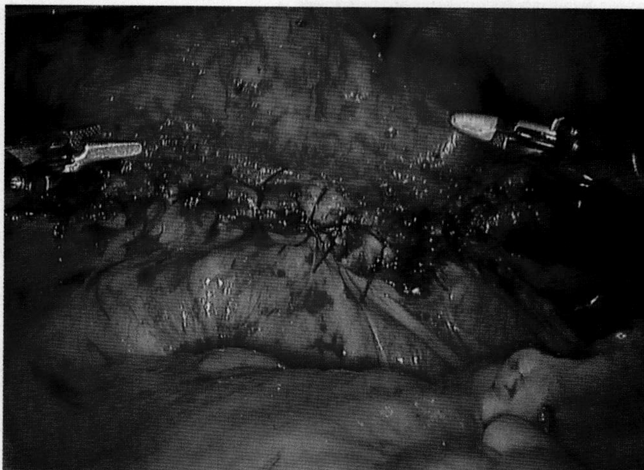

Figure 8.4.11. Vaginal cuff closure with interrupted figure of eight sutures can prevent cuff dehiscence.

- Preoperative endometrial biopsy can identify the malignancy in two-thirds of sarcoma.
- Vaginal cuff dehiscence can be prevented by proper technique (Fig. 8.4.11).

COMPLICATIONS

- Ureter injury may be recognized with routine cystoscopy.
- Thermal spread ureteral injury can take up to two weeks to become apparent.
- Thermal bowel injury can happen, especially with a larger uterus, as part of the operative field is much higher and closer to the bowel.

KEY READINGS

Gallo T, Kashani S, Patel DA, Elsawhi K, Silasi DA, Azodi M. Robotic-assisted laparoscopic hysterectomy: outcomes in obese and morbidly obese patients. *JSLS.* 2012;16:421–427.

Goodrich SK, Knight J. Uterine sarcoma: ability of preoperative evaluation to identify malignancy and correct histology. *Gynecol Oncol.* 2015;137(Suppl 1):97–98.

Payne TN, Dauterive FR. A comparison of total laparoscopic hysterectomy to robotically assisted hysterectomy: surgical outcomes in a community practice. *J Minim Invasive Gynecol.* 2008;15(3):286–291.

Ricci S, Angarita A, Cholakian D, et al. Preoperative patient stratification results in low rates of occult uterine malignancy in women undergoing uterine surgery and morcellation. *Gynecol Oncol.* 2015;137(Suppl 1):11–12.

Chapter 8.5

Vaginal Hysterectomy

Cecile A. Unger

GENERAL PRINCIPLES

Definition

- Total vaginal hysterectomy is an operation that can be performed when removal of the uterus is indicated in cases of either benign disease or carcinoma *in situ* of the cervix.
- Vaginal hysterectomy is most often performed in cases of pelvic pain, abnormal uterine bleeding, or uterovaginal prolapse.

PREOPERATIVE PLANNING

- The preoperative health assessment for any hysterectomy includes a complete history and physical examination. There is no routinely recommended imaging, cardiopulmonary testing, or laboratory tests. This type of testing is ordered for patients based on their medical comorbidities. Many hospitals have their own requirements for preoperative assessments, which are often based on the patient's age in combination with their medical comorbidities and frailty.
- A normal Papanicolaou (Pap) smear should be documented before hysterectomy. In patients who are at risk for endometrial cancer, endometrial sampling should also be obtained. If cancer or an adnexal mass or cyst is suspected, a transvaginal ultrasound is necessary.
- Careful review of a patient's medication list is important before performing a hysterectomy. Because of the increased risk of bleeding due their antiplatelet effects, all nonsteroidal anti-inflammatory drugs and aspirin should be stopped at least 7 days before surgery. Multivitamins containing vitamin E should also be discontinued 10 to 14 days before surgery. Because of the increased risk of venous thromboembolic events, oral contraceptive pills and hormone replacement therapies should ideally be stopped 4 to 6 weeks before surgery. This may be challenging in women who are on hormone therapies for abnormal bleeding, but cessation should be considered.
- Before proceeding with hysterectomy, assessment of a patient's risk for intra- or postoperative anemia and need for autologous blood products is necessary. This is especially important for patients with abnormal uterine bleeding and baseline anemia. These patients should also be evaluated for preoperative iron supplementation or transfusion.
- Informed consent should be obtained in the office. Patients should be well informed of the risks and benefits of the procedure, as well as the alternatives to hysterectomy. Most importantly, confirmation of completion of childbearing must be done.
- Prior to surgery, a pregnancy test is necessary in all patients of reproductive age.
- Hysterectomy is a clean-contaminated procedure, and prophylactic intravenous antibiotics should be ordered, to be administered within 60 minutes of incision time. First- or second-generation cephalosporins are first-line antibiotics.
- All patients undergoing hysterectomy are considered "moderate risk" and require venous thromboembolism prophylaxis. In most patients, either low-dose unfractionated heparin, low–molecular-weight heparin, or intermittent pneumatic compression devices are recommended. In higher-risk patients, dual prophylaxis, and in some cases, postoperative prophylaxis may be necessary.
- Route of hysterectomy is dependent on the following factors: vaginal caliber and accessibility to the uterus, uterine size and shape, uterine mobility, cancer and extrauterine disease, surgeon skillset, available support facilities, and surgeon and patient preference.
- A thorough bimanual examination is necessary prior to deciding on route of hysterectomy. Care should be taken to note the following factors to help determine the degree of difficulty that will be present in performing the procedure: the size, mobility, and descent of the uterus; the size and shape of the bony pelvis (a pubic arch of less than 90 degrees may preclude a vaginal hysterectomy whereas a wide angle will facilitate the approach); the caliber of the introitus and the vagina.

SURGICAL MANAGEMENT

- According to the American College of Obstetricians and Gynecologists (ACOG),[1] vaginal hysterectomy is the safest and most cost-effective method to remove the uterus for noncancerous reasons. In general, based on current data, vaginal hysterectomy is associated with better outcomes and fewer complications.
- There are few absolute contraindications to the vaginal approach for hysterectomy; however, there are factors that generally preclude this approach, including (1) the suspicion of malignancy; (2) the presence of known extrauterine disease or adnexal disease; (3) a narrow pubic arch (<90 degrees); (4) a narrow vagina (narrower than 2 fingerbreadths, especially at the apex); and (5) a fixed, immobile uterus. In the absence of one of these factors, vaginal hysterectomy should be the approach of choice whenever feasible given its well-documented advantages.
- There are some conditions and patient-specific characteristics that can make vaginal hysterectomy technically challenging. These factors are not contraindications to vaginal hysterectomy, but should be identified preoperatively and anticipated at the time of surgery.
- These conditions include the enlarged or undescended uterus, previous cesarean sections, and uterine prolapse. These factors should be taken into consideration during surgical planning, and while they may make the procedure more challenging, can be overcome with a few helpful pearls that we will review in this chapter.

Positioning

- Patients are positioned in dorsal lithotomy position using either candy cane stirrups (Fig. 8.5.1), or yellow fin stirrups (Fig. 8.5.2). Patients should be positioned so that the edge of the buttocks is at the edge of the surgical table. Care is taken

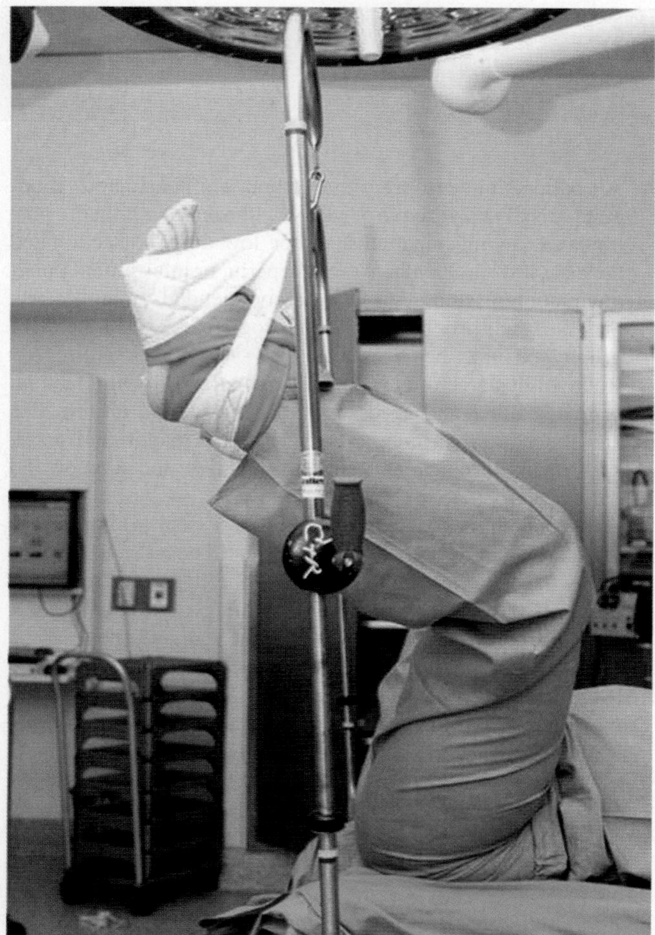

Figure 8.5.1. Dorsal lithotomy positioning using candy cane stirrups.

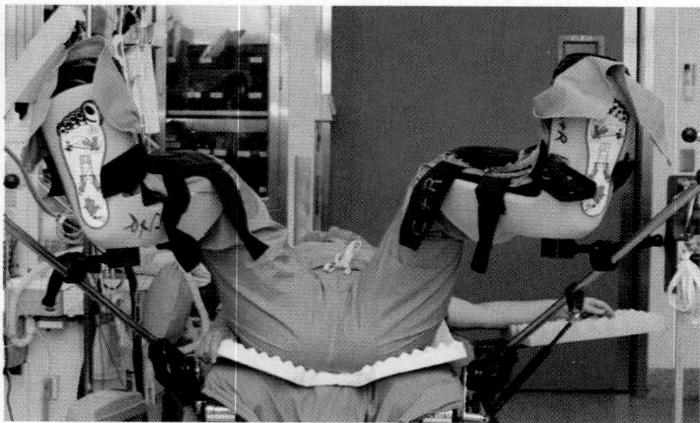

Figure 8.5.2. Dorsal lithotomy positioning using yellowfin stirrups.

not to hyperflex or extend the legs in order to avoid postoperative neuropathies. Foam can be used to pad the bony prominences of the limbs, and also to fill dead space in the stirrups. The arms can be left out at the sides, and are positioned in anatomic position with care taken to not hyperextend the limbs to avoid brachial plexus injuries.

Approach

- The procedure is performed transvaginally.

Suture ligation of the uterosacral ligaments

- Many providers enter the anterior cul-de-sac before ligating the uterosacral pedicles. We believe that suture ligation of the uterosacral ligaments prior to anterior entry facilitates descent of the uterine specimen, making it easier to identify the vesicouterine reflection, and decreasing the risk of injury to the bladder at the time of anterior entry.
- The cervix is placed on upward and lateral retraction using the tenacula. A curved Heaney clamp is placed in the posterior cul-de-sac with one blade underneath the uterosacral ligament and the opposite blade over the uterosacral ligament (**Tech Fig. 8.5.7**). In order to prevent possible ureteral injury, it is important to place the clamp along the uterine cervix so that some tissue of the cervix is included in this clamp.
- A curved Mayo scissor is used to transect the pedicle and a No. 0 polyglactin suture is used to tie off of the pedicle before releasing the clamp. A Heaney fixation stitch of No. 0 polyglactin is used for all pedicles (**Tech Figs. 8.5.8** and **8.5.9**). The uterosacral ligaments are suture ligated bilaterally using this method.
- If there is oozing of blood at the posterior vaginal cuff, the posterior peritoneum can be reefed to the vaginal epithelium between the uterosacral pedicles using a No. 2-0 or 0 polyglactin suture in a running locked fashion.

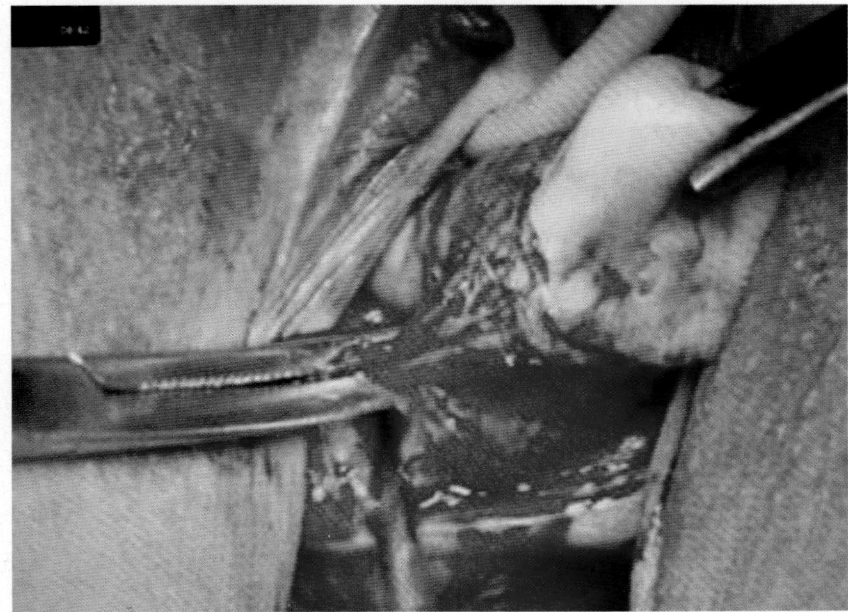

Tech Figure 8.5.7. Clamping of the right uterosacral ligament.

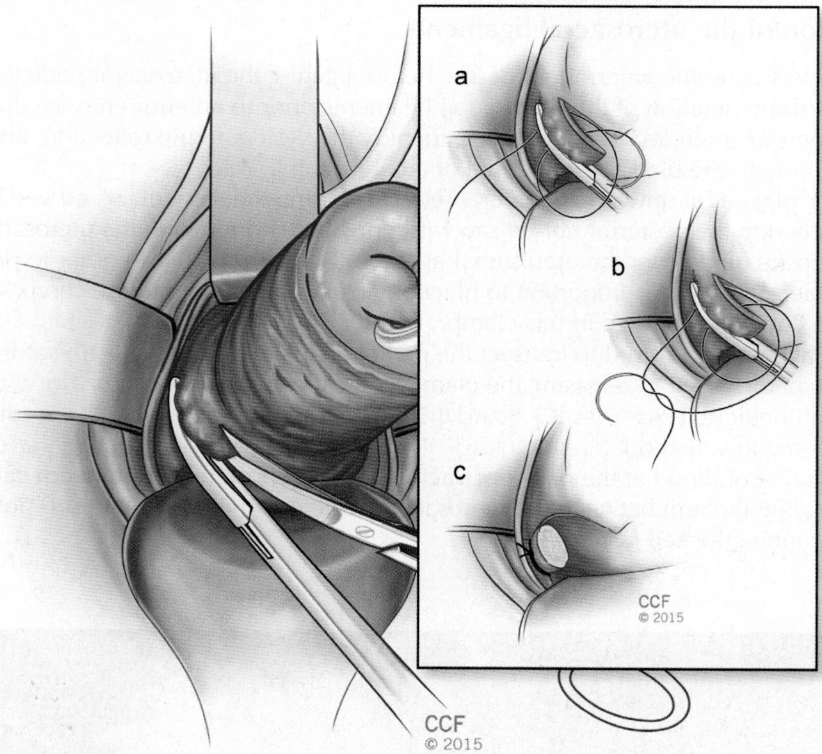

Tech Figure 8.5.8. Clamping, transection, and suture ligation of the uterosacral ligament. Reprinted with permission, Cleveland Clinic Center for Medical Art & Photography © 2015, all rights reserved.

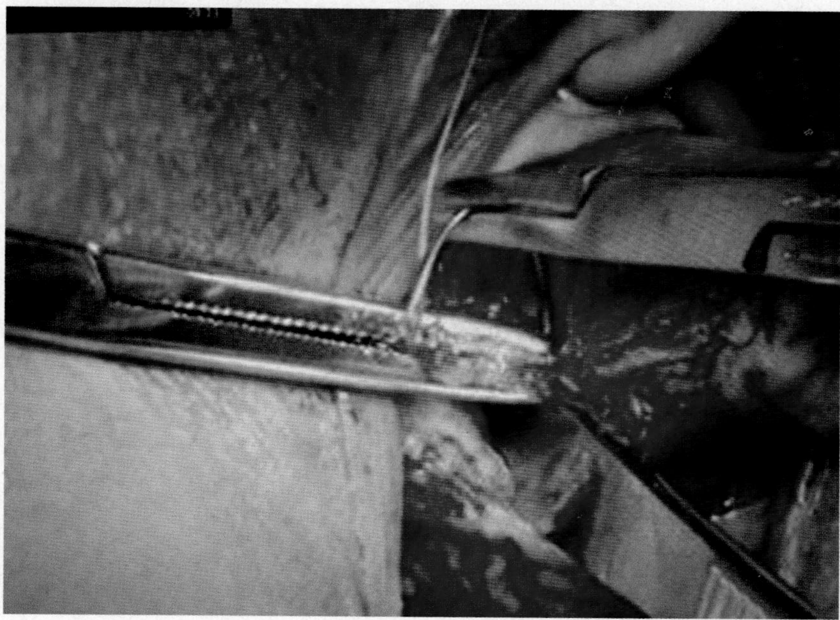

Tech Figure 8.5.9. Suture ligation of the right uterosacral ligament.

Entry into the anterior cul-de-sac

- Downward traction is applied to the cervix and the anterior vaginal epithelium and underlying bladder are dissected off of the cervix and lower uterine segment.
- A right-angle retractor is placed under the vaginal epithelium and is used to elevate the bladder to help facilitate dissection (**Tech Fig. 8.5.10**).
- Anterior dissection is carried all the way to the vesicouterine peritoneal reflection. This is considered by many to be one of the most challenging steps of the vaginal hysterectomy. However, if dissection is not carried up to the vesicouterine fold, entry into the anterior cul-de-sac will be very challenging, and there is an increased risk of injury to the bladder. The right-angle retractor can then be placed underneath the bladder to better visualize the vesicouterine fold, which appears like a thin white transverse line across the lower uterine segment.
- With downward traction on the cervix, the vesicouterine fold is tented upwards with pickup forceps and it is entered using the curved Mayo scissors (**Tech Figs. 8.5.11** and **8.5.12**).
- A finger is immediately placed in the incised hole and explored to ensure that there is no injury to the bladder. The bladder can be identified by palpating the bulb of the Foley catheter. A right-angle retractor is then placed beneath the finger and passed into the anterior cul-de-sac (**Tech Figs. 8.5.13** and **8.5.14**).

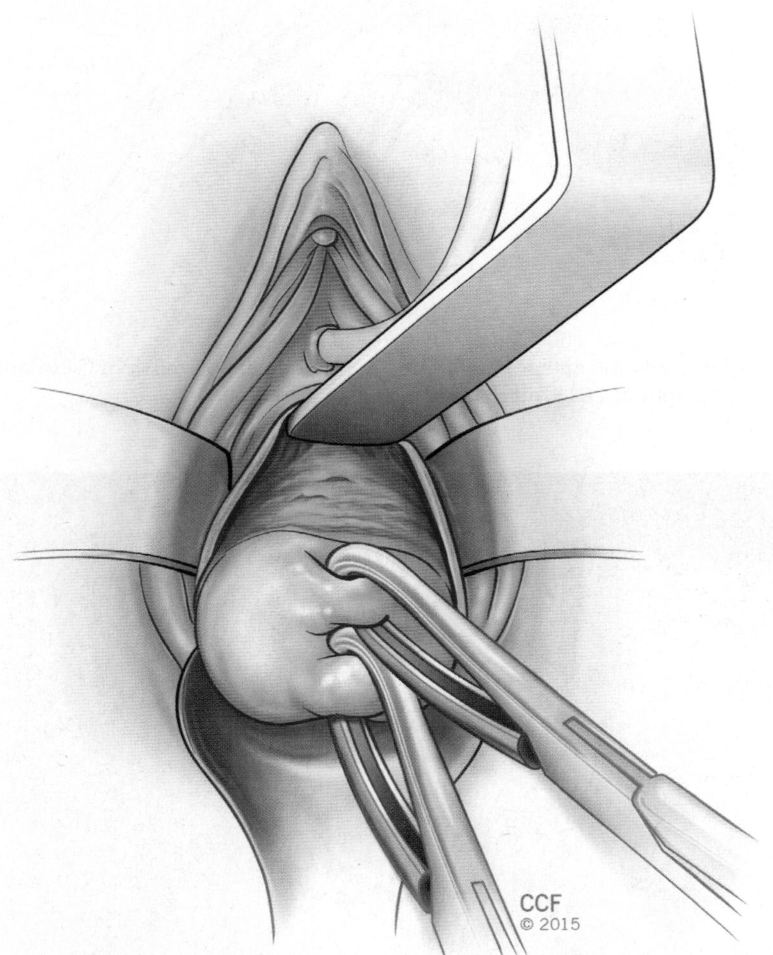

Tech Figure 8.5.10. Dissection of the bladder off of the anterior cervix. Reprinted with permission, Cleveland Clinic Center for Medical Art & Photography © 2015, all rights reserved.

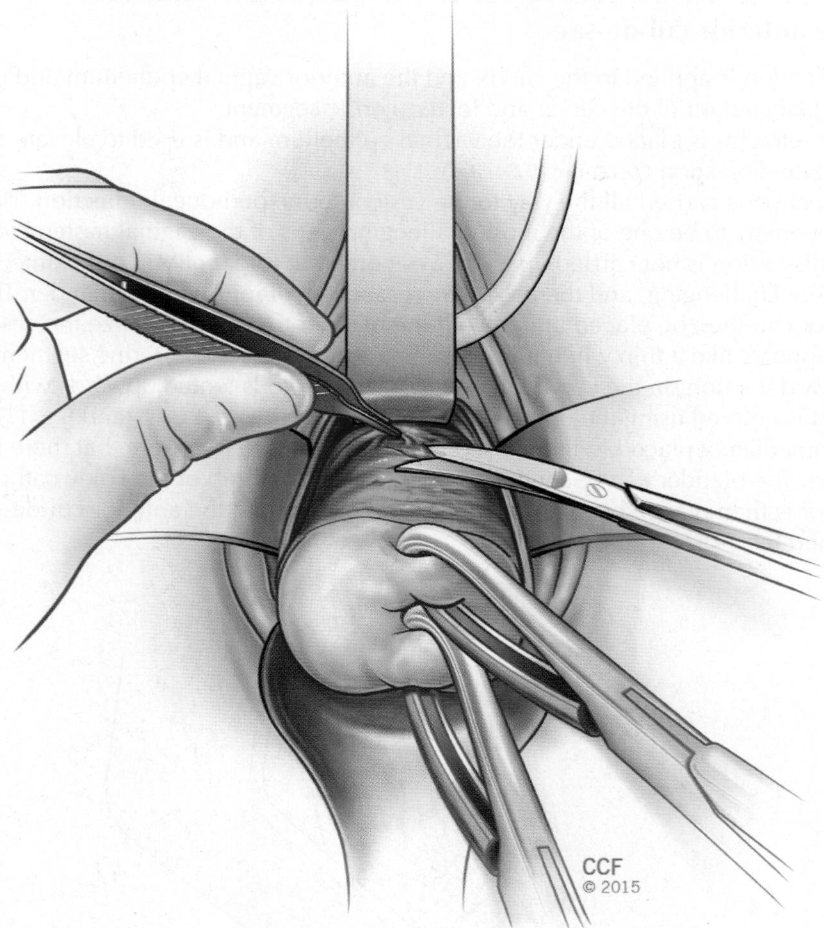

Tech Figure 8.5.11. Entry into the anterior cul-de-sac. Reprinted with permission, Cleveland Clinic Center for Medical Art & Photography © 2015, all rights reserved.

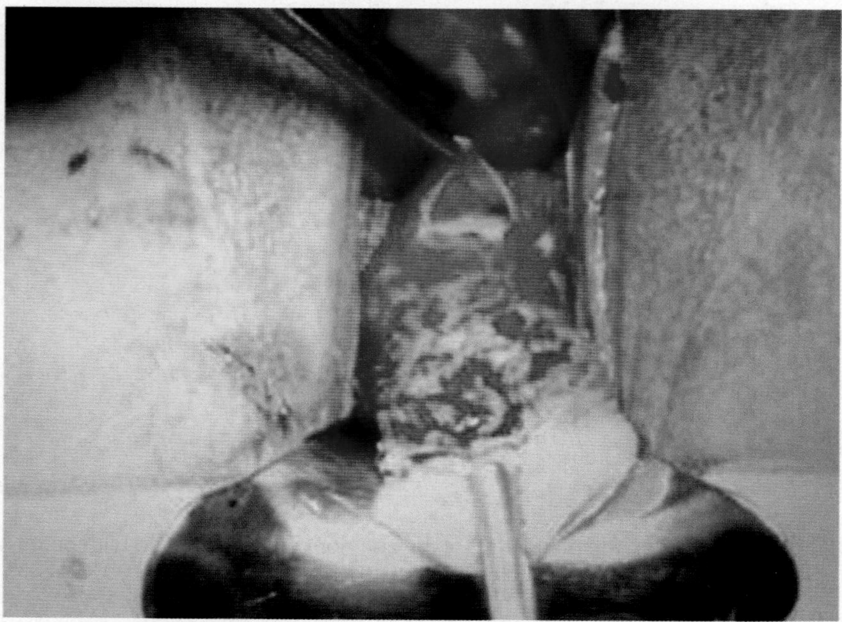

Tech Figure 8.5.12. Entry into the anterior cul-de-sac.

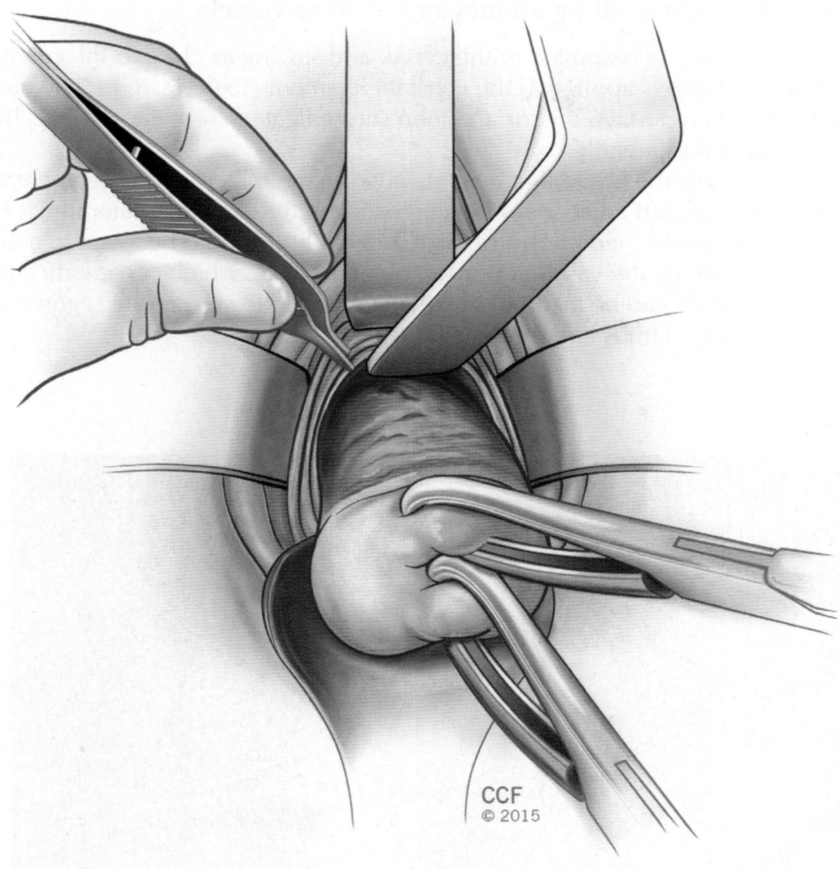

Tech Figure 8.5.13. Placement of a right-angle retractor into the anterior cul-de-sac. Reprinted with permission, Cleveland Clinic Center for Medical Art & Photography © 2015, all rights reserved.

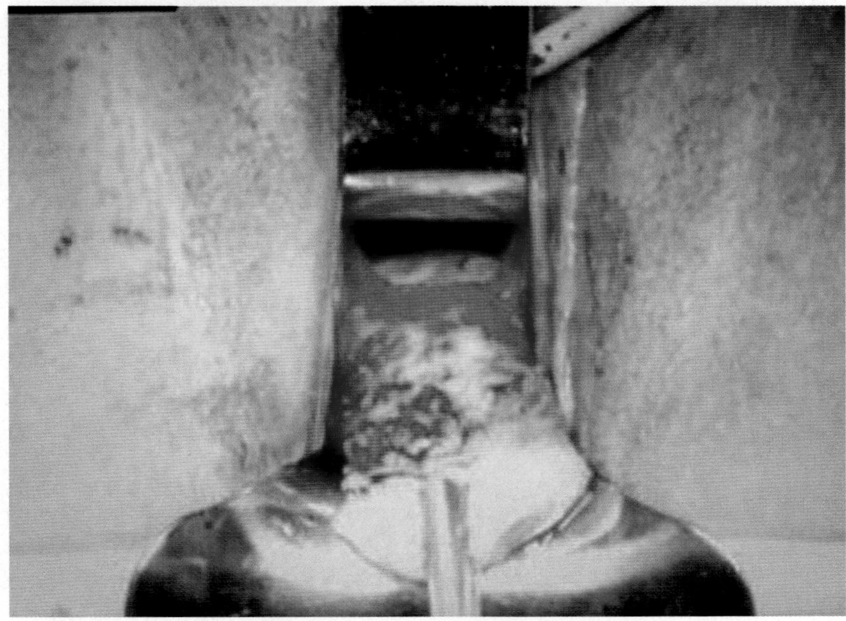

Tech Figure 8.5.14. Placement of a right-angle retractor into the anterior cul-de-sac. Reprinted with permission, Cleveland Clinic Center for Medical Art & Photography © 2015, all rights reserved.

Suture ligation of the cardinal ligaments and uterine vessels

- Upward and lateral traction is applied to the cervix and staying as close to the cervix as possible, a Heaney clamp is applied to the cardinal ligament (Tech Fig. 8.5.15), which is transected with the curved Mayo scissor and then suture ligated (Tech Fig. 8.5.16). This procedure is performed bilaterally.
- The remaining portion of the broad ligament attached to the lower uterine segment containing the uterine artery is clamped adjacent to the cervix and suture ligated bilaterally. A Heaney fixation suture can be performed on this pedicle, but caution should be taken to avoid placing the needle directly through the vascular portion of the pedicle, which can create a hematoma. In addition, great care should be taken to hug the cervix and lower uterine segment to avoid lateral placement of the clamps and possible injury to the ureters.

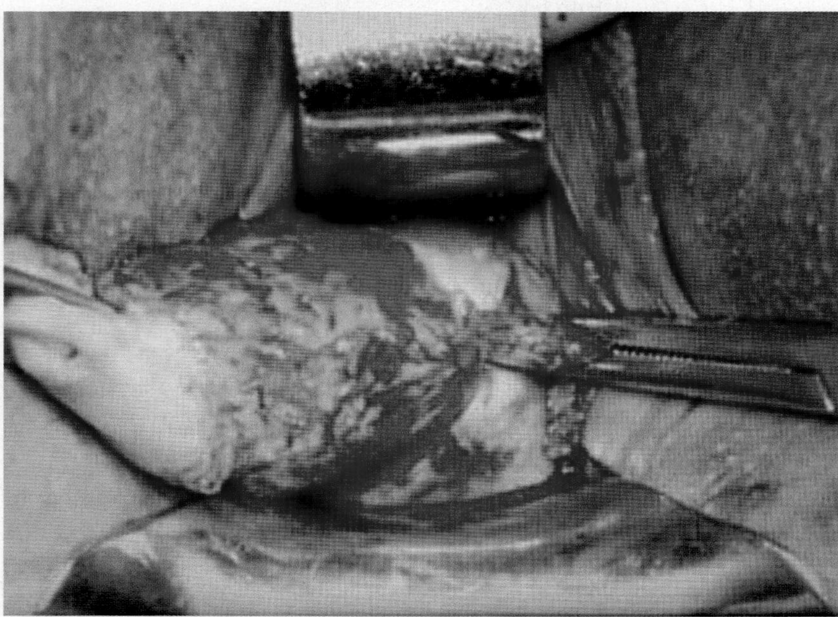

Tech Figure 8.5.15. Clamping of the left cardinal ligament.

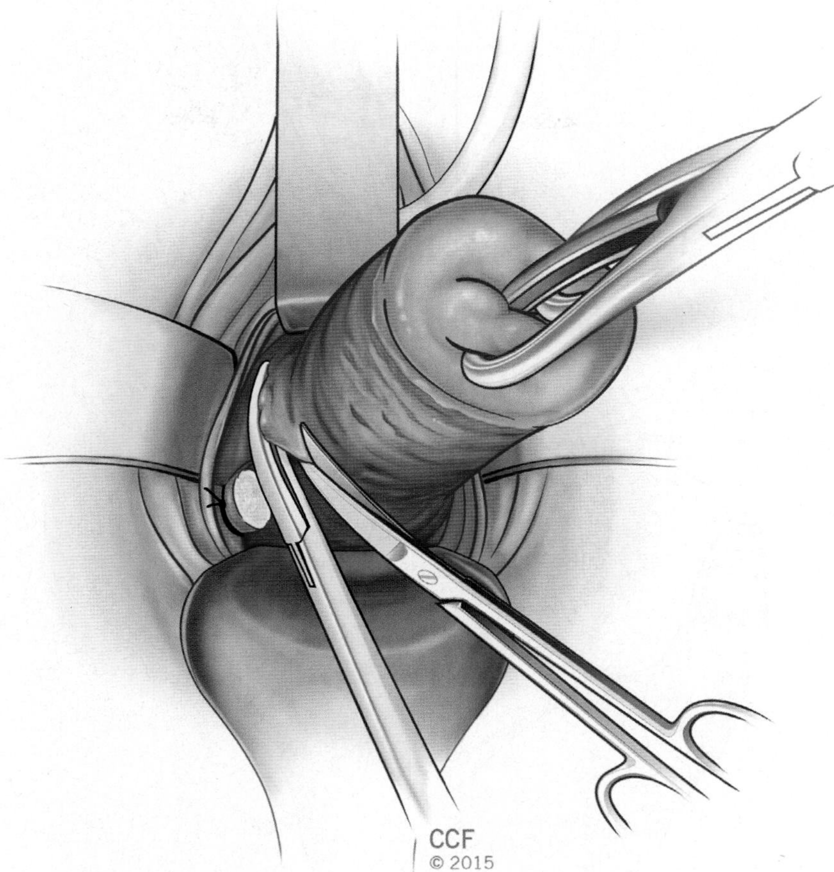

Tech Figure 8.5.16. Clamping, transection, and suture ligation of the cardinal ligament. Reprinted with permission, Cleveland Clinic Center for Medical Art & Photography © 2015, all rights reserved.

Suture ligation of the utero-ovarian pedicles

- Once all of the pedicles are suture ligated, and the cornua of the uterus are reached, the cervix is retracted upwards and tenacula or towel clamps are sequentially placed in a "hand over hand" fashion on the uterine segment until the fundus of the uterus can be delivered posteriorly (Tech Figs. 8.5.17 and 8.5.18).
- Caution should be taken in applying too much traction at this stage of the procedure, as the remaining utero-ovarian pedicles can easily be avulsed.
- A finger is placed under the utero-ovarian pedicle and round ligament and a Heaney clamp is then passed along the path of the finger and used to clamp the pedicle. A second Heaney clamp is then placed alongside the first, and the pedicle is double suture ligated (Tech Figs. 8.5.19 to 8.5.21).
- The uterus and cervix are then removed from the peritoneal cavity and can be passed off the surgical field.

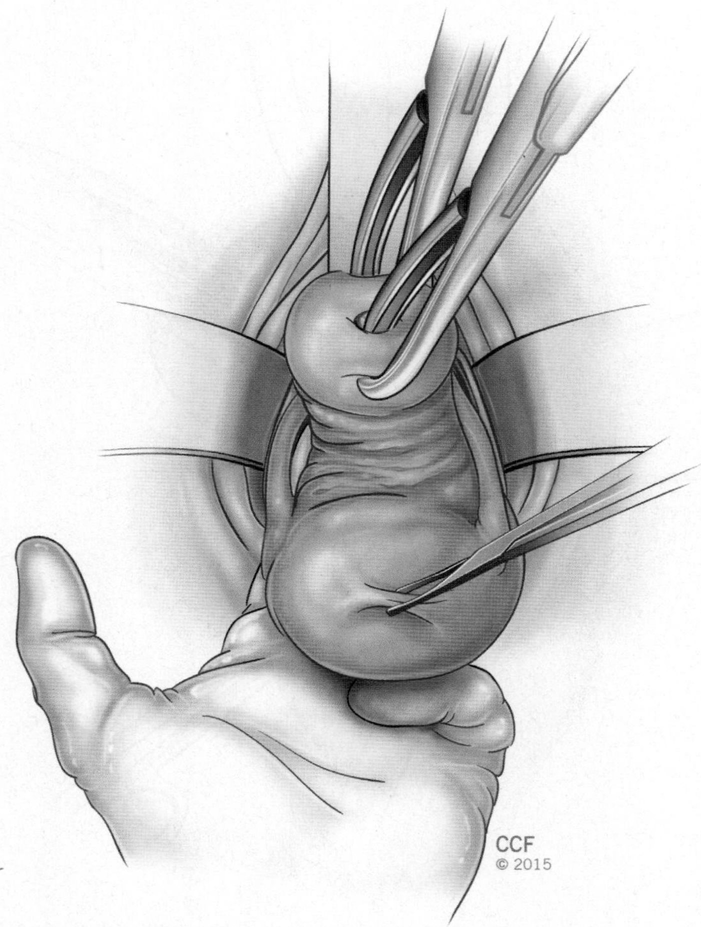

Tech Figure 8.5.17. Fundus of the uterus delivered posteriorly. Reprinted with permission, Cleveland Clinic Center for Medical Art & Photography © 2015, all rights reserved.

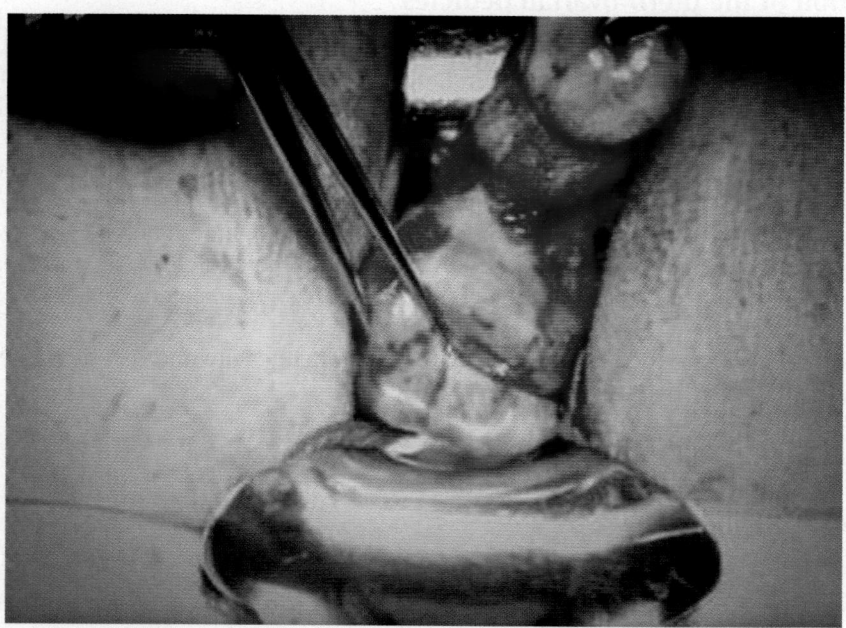

Tech Figure 8.5.18. Fundus of the uterus delivered posteriorly.

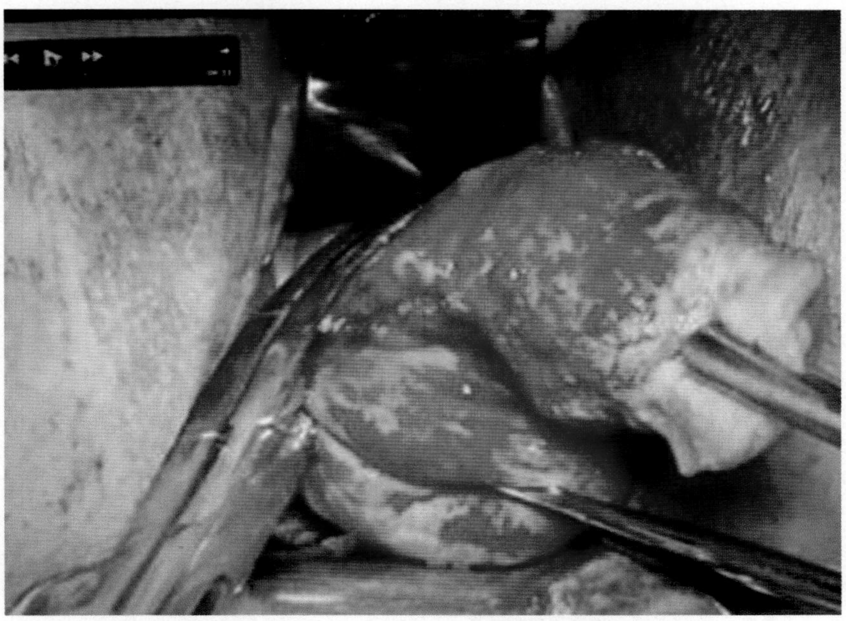

Tech Figure 8.5.19. Right utero-ovarian ligament clamped.

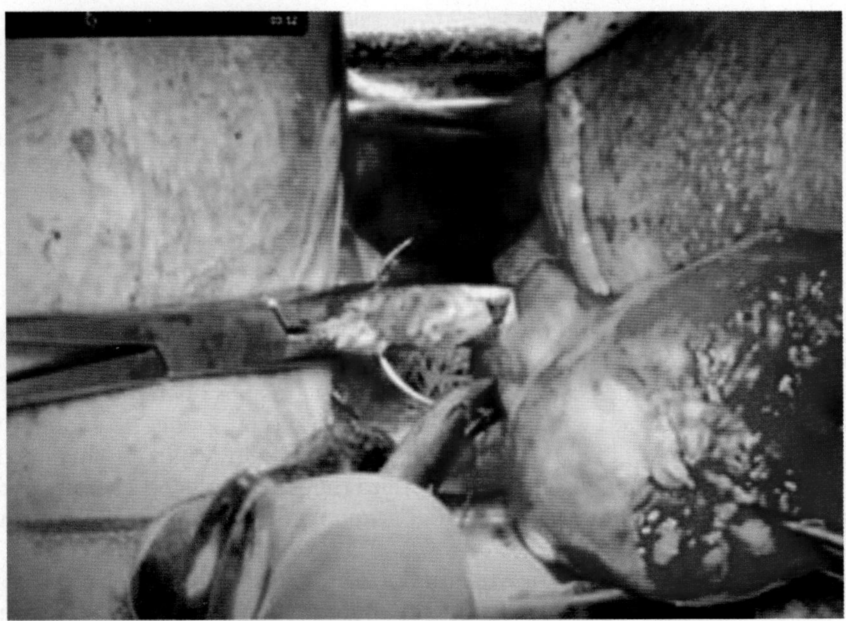

Tech Figure 8.5.20. Right utero-ovarian ligament suture ligated.

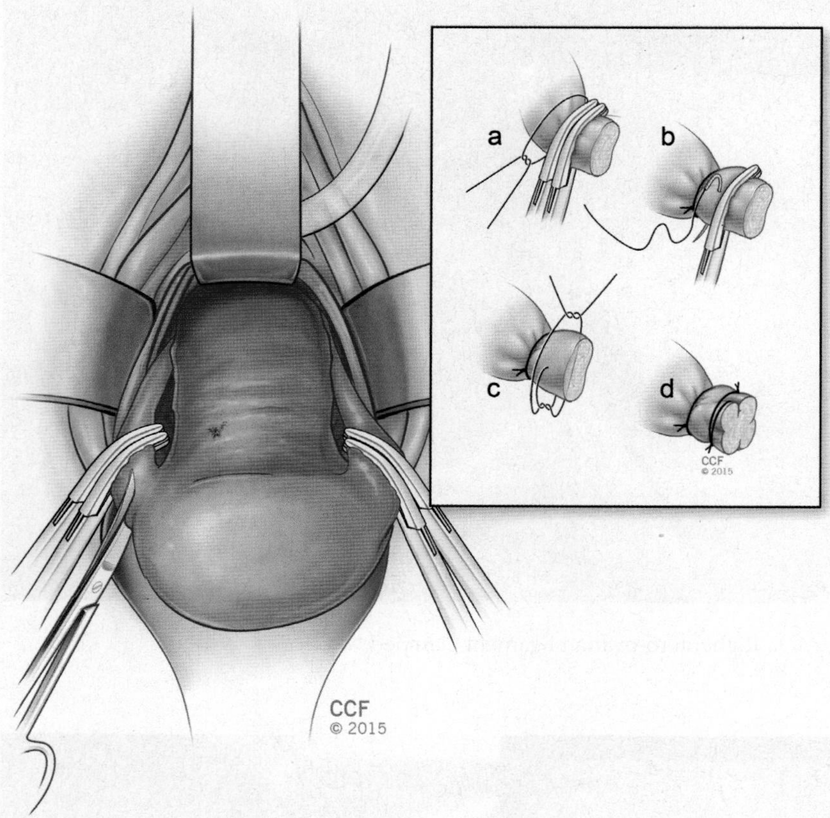

Tech Figure 8.5.21. Clamping, transection, and suture ligation of the utero-ovarian ligaments. Reprinted with permission, Cleveland Clinic Center for Medical Art & Photography © 2015, all rights reserved.

Salpingo-oophorectomy

- Removal of the fallopian tubes and ovaries is not always performed at the time of vaginal hysterectomy, but is sometimes indicated. There are two techniques commonly used to perform this procedure. Both techniques can be done once the uterus has been removed.
- First, the small bowel is packed with a tagged moist laparotomy sponge. A sponge stick can also be used, but can sometimes get in the way of the operative field. Vaginal retractors are placed at 12 and 6 o'clock to facilitate visualization. A third retractor is placed at either 3 or 9 o'clock, depending on which ovary is the target, in order to retract the contralateral ovary and tube out of the way.
- The first technique involves placing downward traction on the fallopian tube and ovary using an Allis or Babcock clamp in order to identify the infundibulopelvic ligament. Once this is done, one or two Heaney clamps are passed around the ovarian blood supply and the pedicle is transected. This pedicle is then ligated using a free tie followed by a suture. In some cases, a vessel sealing device such as the Ligasure (Valleylab, Boulder, CO) can be used to ligate and seal the pedicle.
- A second technique can be used to isolate the ovarian blood supply by dissecting between the round ligament and the infundibulopelvic ligament. This technique can be done once the uterus is removed, but it can also be done with one side of the uterus separated from the adnexa, and the other remaining attached via the utero-ovarian ligament, which is what we will describe in this section. The technique is similar to what is usually done abdominally to perform an oophorectomy, but requires a good grasp of anatomy when it is performed transvaginally. The round ligament is clamped, cut, and suture ligated, and the pedicle is retracted laterally. The broad ligament and mesosalpinx are then sharply dissected laterally and cephalad until

the infundibulopelvic ligament is isolated and the ovarian vessels can be clamped close to the ovary using a Heaney or long Kelly clamp. These are cut and suture ligated. Of note, the Bovie cautery can be used to open the round ligament and perform the dissection of the mesosalpinx. This is sometimes helpful in maintaining hemostasis as these tissues are often very delicate and friable. With this in mind, gentle handling of the tissues is very important. Once the infundibulopelvic ligament pedicle is ligated, the specimen (containing the uterus and cervix and one of the fallopian tubes and ovaries) can be passed off. With exposure and isolation of the contralateral round ligament, the contralateral ovary is removed in the same manner.

Closure of the vaginal cuff

- The vaginal cuff is sutured with either a running locked stitch or with figure-of-eight stitches using No. 0 or 2-0 polyglactin suture. To maintain vaginal length, a transverse closure is usually preferable (Tech Fig. 8.5.22).

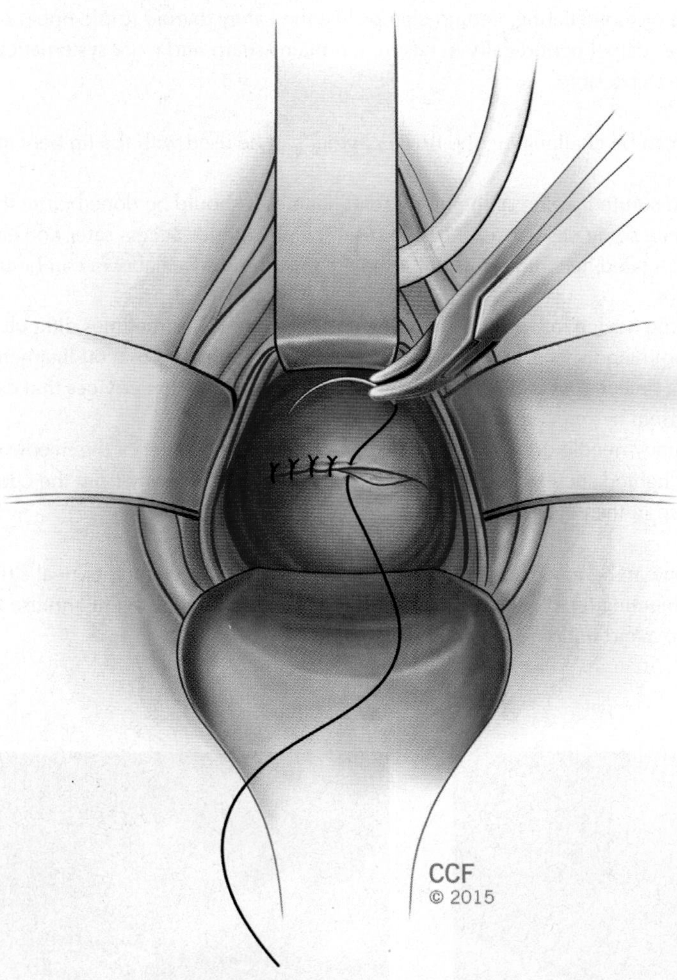

Tech Figure 8.5.22. Transverse closure of the vaginal cuff. Reprinted with permission, Cleveland Clinic Center for Medical Art & Photography © 2015, all rights reserved.

PEARLS AND PITFALLS[2,3]

✖ Obese patients

○ Position the patient properly to maximize access. The buttocks should be positioned well beyond the edge of the operating table; this brings the operating field closer to the surgeon and makes it easier to use long-handled retractors posteriorly.

○ Adequate surgical assistance is important; if possible, use two surgical assistants, one on each side. Candy cane stirrups should be used to allow better access for the assistants.

○ Minimize Trendelenburg position as it will cause the patient to slide up the bed and make posterior entry more difficult.

✖ Enlarged uterus (fibroid uterus)

○ The hysterectomy is performed in the standard fashion. Once the uterine pedicles are ligated, one of the following techniques can be used to remove the specimen and gain access to the remaining pedicles: bivalving or hemisection (Fig. 8.5.3), intramyometrial coring (Fig. 8.5.4), wedge morcellation, myomectomy (Fig. 8.5.5).

○ When using the above techniques, be sure to keep the serosa of the uterus intact to maintain orientation. Orient your scalpel blade so that you are always cutting toward the center of the specimen. Use traction–countertraction while coring or morcellating; certain clamps like the Lahey thyroid (triple hook) clamp can be useful. Be sure to replace the scalpel periodically to ensure it remains sharp and work systematically to remove as much of the central tissue as possible.

✖ Lack of uterine descent

○ The initial cervical incision can be challenging; the Bovie cautery can be used with the tip bent at 45 degrees to make the incision easier.

○ The posterior colpotomy and suture ligation of the uterosacral ligaments should be done before the anterior colpotomy in order to facilitate some descensus of the uterus, making anterior access safer and easier.

○ Once the uterine vessels are ligated, techniques used for the enlarged uterus (see above) can be used to further access the remaining pedicles.

○ Consider using a vessel sealing device rather than clamping and suturing. It is sometimes difficult to place sutures in a tight, poorly illuminated space, so using a vessel sealer above the uterosacral ligaments is sometimes helpful. Choose a device that is shaped like a Heaney clamp. There are devices that exist that are specifically made for vaginal hysterectomy.

○ If suturing, always use a Heaney needle driver, with the suture loaded in the center of the needle curve.

○ Use a disposable fiber-optic lighted suction irrigator to retract redundant tissue away from the course of the needle when suturing high up in the pelvis.

✖ Narrow vaginal opening

○ A small mediolateral incision can be made starting just above the hymen through the perineal structures. To reduce blood loss, start by injecting local anesthetic with a dilute vasoconstricting agent and use the Bovie cautery to make the incision; avoid injury to the anus and rectum.

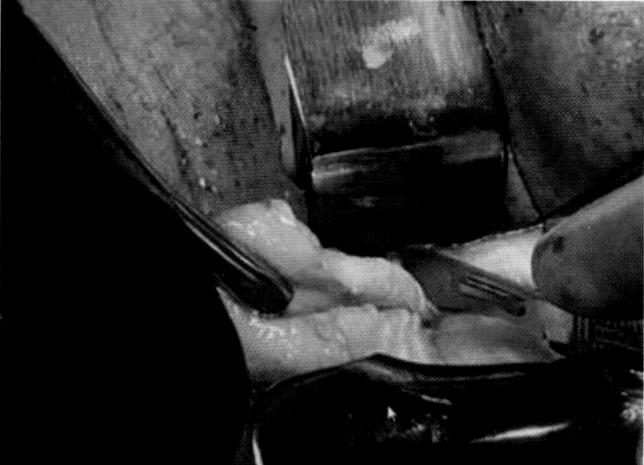

Figure 8.5.3. Bivalving the cervix and uterus.

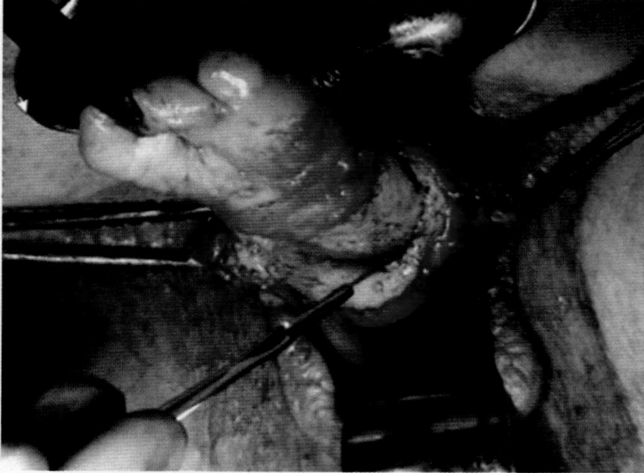

Figure 8.5.4. Intramyometrial coring.

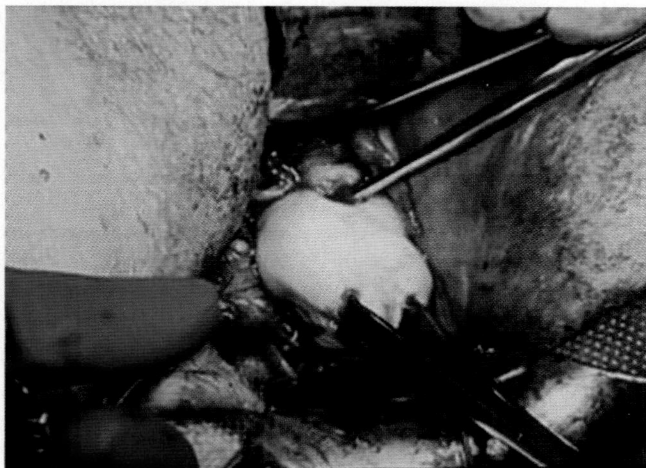

Figure 8.5.5. Myomectomy.

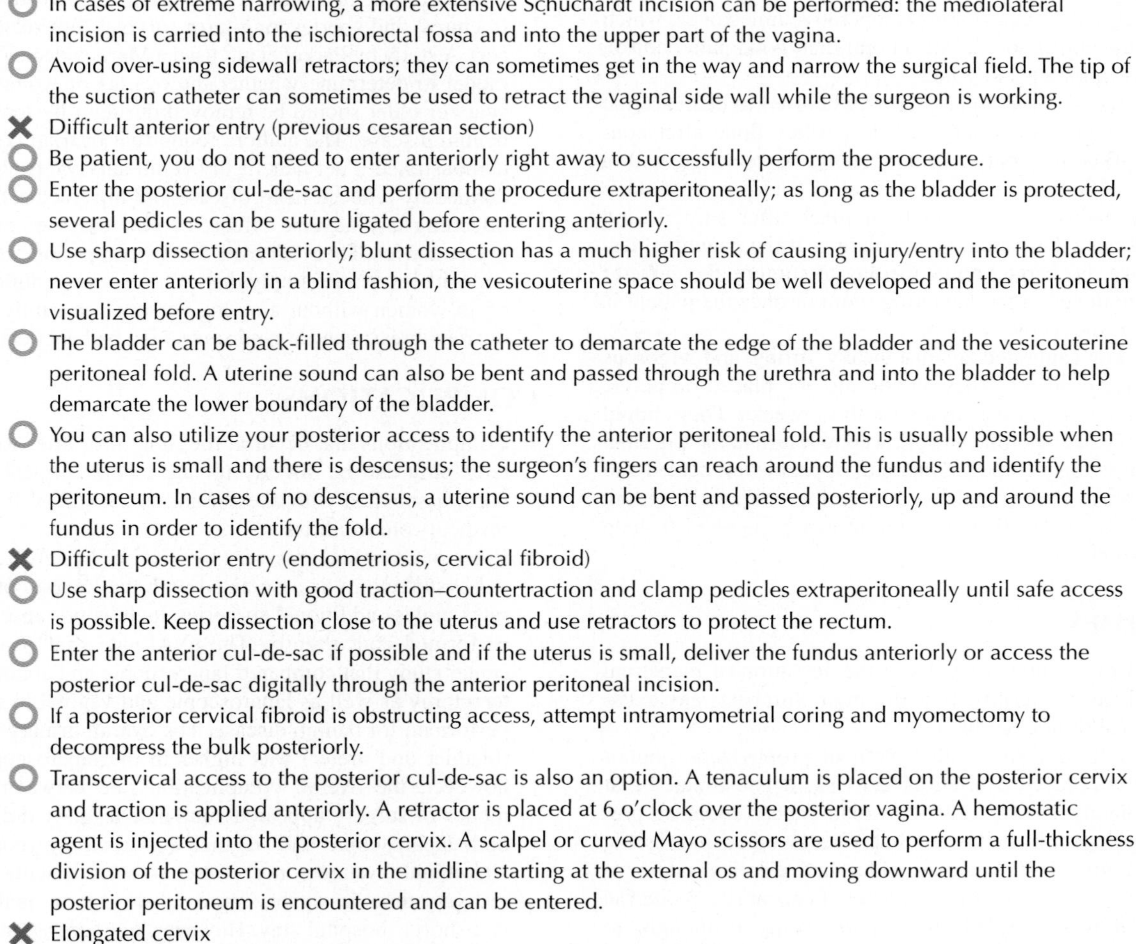

- In cases of extreme narrowing, a more extensive Schuchardt incision can be performed: the mediolateral incision is carried into the ischiorectal fossa and into the upper part of the vagina.
- Avoid over-using sidewall retractors; they can sometimes get in the way and narrow the surgical field. The tip of the suction catheter can sometimes be used to retract the vaginal side wall while the surgeon is working.

✗ Difficult anterior entry (previous cesarean section)

- Be patient, you do not need to enter anteriorly right away to successfully perform the procedure.
- Enter the posterior cul-de-sac and perform the procedure extraperitoneally; as long as the bladder is protected, several pedicles can be suture ligated before entering anteriorly.
- Use sharp dissection anteriorly; blunt dissection has a much higher risk of causing injury/entry into the bladder; never enter anteriorly in a blind fashion, the vesicouterine space should be well developed and the peritoneum visualized before entry.
- The bladder can be back-filled through the catheter to demarcate the edge of the bladder and the vesicouterine peritoneal fold. A uterine sound can also be bent and passed through the urethra and into the bladder to help demarcate the lower boundary of the bladder.
- You can also utilize your posterior access to identify the anterior peritoneal fold. This is usually possible when the uterus is small and there is descensus; the surgeon's fingers can reach around the fundus and identify the peritoneum. In cases of no descensus, a uterine sound can be bent and passed posteriorly, up and around the fundus in order to identify the fold.

✗ Difficult posterior entry (endometriosis, cervical fibroid)

- Use sharp dissection with good traction–countertraction and clamp pedicles extraperitoneally until safe access is possible. Keep dissection close to the uterus and use retractors to protect the rectum.
- Enter the anterior cul-de-sac if possible and if the uterus is small, deliver the fundus anteriorly or access the posterior cul-de-sac digitally through the anterior peritoneal incision.
- If a posterior cervical fibroid is obstructing access, attempt intramyometrial coring and myomectomy to decompress the bulk posteriorly.
- Transcervical access to the posterior cul-de-sac is also an option. A tenaculum is placed on the posterior cervix and traction is applied anteriorly. A retractor is placed at 6 o'clock over the posterior vagina. A hemostatic agent is injected into the posterior cervix. A scalpel or curved Mayo scissors are used to perform a full-thickness division of the posterior cervix in the midline starting at the external os and moving downward until the posterior peritoneum is encountered and can be entered.

✗ Elongated cervix

- The biggest challenge in these cases is usually anterior and posterior entries.
- Careful examination under anesthesia is necessary. Identification of the area of transition between the cervix and fundus at the lower uterine segment is important. The anterior peritoneal fold is usually located at or above this location. The posterior peritoneal fold is usually more distal. Identification of the distal edge of the bladder is also important. Sometimes, a vaginal crease is seen. If this is not the case, backfill of the bladder can be done to identify the demarcation line. A rectal examination can be done to identify the distal demarcation of the

rectum. Once the distal edges of the rectum and bladder are noted, the circumferential cervical incision can be made, high enough to avoid extensive dissection on the cervix, but low enough to avoid injury to viscera.

- The above-mentioned techniques can also be used to help gain access into the anterior and posterior cul-de-sacs.

✖ Uterovaginal prolapse

- The biggest challenge with prolapse is that there is often distortion of the anatomy.
- The bladder reflection is often very distal on the cervix. Therefore, the initial cervical incision should be made distally, with care taken to not amputate the cervix.
- In cases of severe prolapse, the bladder trigone is often everted which displaces the ureteral orifices distally, so that they are close to the distal bladder reflection. Careful dissection of the bladder off of the cervix is key.
- The posterior cul-de-sac is often easier to enter in prolapse cases because it lies behind the upper half or so of the posterior vaginal wall while the distal rectum lies behind it. The posterior peritoneal incision can be used to access the anterior peritoneum as described by the techniques above. This can be helpful in avoiding bladder and ureteral injuries.

POSTOPERATIVE CARE

- Patients may be discharged from the hospital the same day of surgery or after overnight observation depending upon how quickly they meet their postoperative milestones, which include the ability to tolerate an oral diet, good pain control, ability to ambulate and void.
- In some cases, vaginal packing may be used to decrease the risk of hematoma formation. This is often done after concurrent prolapse repairs. Packing must be removed within 24 hours of surgery and before a trial of void is performed.
- A Foley catheter may be left in place after surgery and removed once the patient is ambulating. If the patient is destined to be discharged home the day of surgery, the catheter may be removed in the operating room or once the patient is brought to the recovery room.
- Patients are cautioned against heavy lifting and vigorous activity for 6 weeks. They should also be placed on pelvic rest with nothing in the vagina for those weeks. They should be examined at that time and allowed to return to their normal activities as long as the vaginal cuff appears well healed and intact. In cases of granulation tissue formation or bleeding from the vaginal cuff, silver nitrate can be applied to help with healing.

OUTCOMES

- Removal of the uterus results in the cessation of menstrual flow and causes sterility. In addition, it eliminates any existing cervical or uterine disease.
- The most significant health benefit of prophylactic oophorectomy is reduced ovarian cancer risk. It is estimated that approximately 1,000 cases of ovarian cancer could be prevented each year in the United States if all women undergoing hysterectomy at 40 years or older had elective salpingo-oophorectomy performed.[4] The level of cancer risk reduction associated with prophylactic oophorectomy is thought to range from 80% to 95%.
- While there is well-documented significant reduction in the risk of breast cancer in women with known hereditary breast cancer syndromes such as BRCA, it is unclear what the benefit is for nonhereditary breast cancers.
- Unlike the gradual decline in hormonal function seen with natural menopause that occurs over years, surgical menopause results in an abrupt cessation of all ovarian hormone production. It is important to give thoughtful consideration to this when counseling pre- or perimenopausal women about prophylactic oophorectomy at the time of vaginal hysterectomy. Studies show that premature menopause is associated with an increased risk of cognitive impairment, heart disease, bone fractures, and shorter long-term survival (not related to cancer). A study by Parker et al.[5] used a Markov decision-analysis model to determine whether the ovaries of women aged 40 years or older should be removed during a hysterectomy for benign disease. The authors found that ovarian conservation demonstrated a net benefit in overall survival probability (as defined by reduced heart disease and hip fracture) at age 80, offsetting any adverse effects of new cases of ovarian and breast cancer. Their survival curves comparing women with and without ovaries imply that ovarian conservation up to age 65 in women without a strong personal or family history of ovarian–breast cancer syndromes may be beneficial.

COMPLICATIONS

- Complications that occur at the time of or after vaginal hysterectomy can be directly related to the surgical technique used, associated with anesthesia, or a result of the patient's medical comorbidities.
- Rates of complications vary by route of hysterectomy. Vaginal hysterectomy is associated with the lowest complication rates, unless additional surgeries such as prolapse repair are performed concurrently. The eVALuate trial[6] was a multicenter study that compared laparoscopic and abdominal hysterectomy as well as laparoscopic and vaginal hysterectomy performed for benign disease. The overall urinary injury rate (bladder and ureter) was higher in the laparoscopic group; however, the overall complication rate between the three modes of surgery appeared similar. The study did show that both laparoscopic and vaginal hysterectomy (compared to abdominal hysterectomy) were associated with a quicker recovery time, less pain, improved short-term quality of life, and shorter hospital stay. However, not surprisingly, laparoscopic hysterectomy was associated with longer operating room time and cost.
- Perioperative complications associated with vaginal hysterectomy are rare, but include the following: hemorrhage, hematoma, bowel injury, lower urinary tract injury (ureteral and bladder), infection, abscess, vaginal cuff evisceration, vesicovaginal fistula, complications with anesthesia.
- Bladder injury (cystotomy) can occur in up to 2% of vaginal hysterectomy cases and there are some data that show

that the risk of this type of injury is higher with concurrent prolapse procedures.[7] Previous cesarean section is associated with adhesions between the cervix and bladder and can significantly increase the risk of cystotomy. In these patients, careful dissection is required. Surgeons should consider using mostly sharp technique to dissect the bladder off of the cervix as blunt dissection such as the use of a gloved finger or gauze decreases tactile sensation over the tissues, increasing the risk of entry into the bladder. Immediate recognition and repair of a bladder injury is necessary. Closure should be tension-free, water-tight, and performed in two layers using a No. 2-0 or 3-0 delayed absorbable suture. The bladder is placed to continuous drainage for 7 to 14 days (depending on size and location of the injury). A cystogram of the bladder should be performed prior to catheter removal in cases of large injuries to ensure that there is no leak and that the bladder has been adequately repaired.

- The risk of ureteral injury after vaginal hysterectomy (without concurrent prolapse repair) has been reported to be as high as 0.9%.[7] The distal ureter is the most at risk for injury and the common sites of injury include its passage under the uterine artery as it travels through the cardinal ligament complex to enter the bladder, at the level of the infundibulopelvic ligament, and along the pelvic side wall just above the uterosacral ligament. Ureteral injury is a rare adverse event and can often be detected intraoperatively if proper precautions are taken. Failure to detect an injury can lead to permanent upper urinary tract damage including loss of renal function and complex genitourinary fistula. Intraoperative cystoscopy is an effective method of detecting an intraoperative injury, and we recommend routine cystoscopy after vaginal hysterectomy. Administration of a dye that changes the color of the urine is often useful to visualize ureteral jets at the time of cystoscopy. This is not always necessary, as urine jets can be seen without dye. But if the risk of ureteral injury is high, a dye may be useful to confirm patency. For a long time, intravenous administration of indigo carmine was a safe and commonly used technique to visualize ureteral flow. There has recently been a shortage of this dye, and alternatives have been used. These include intravenous administration of fluorescein, preoperative oral administration of phenazopyridine, and bladder instillation with a hyperosmolar solution such 50% dextrose. In cases where ureteral injury is suspected, intraoperative urology consultation should be obtained. In most cases, the ureteral injury occurs in the distal 4 to 5 cm of the ureter, and this type of injury can usually be repaired with reimplantation of the ureter into the bladder (ureteroneocystostomy). A ureteral stent is usually left in place and the bladder is placed on continuous drainage with a Foley catheter for 10 to 14 days. The stent is removed later and an intravenous urogram is performed to ensure that there is no stenosis, stricture, or fistula at the site of the repair.
- Vesicovaginal fistulae are very rare complications. Patients usually present with early onset constitutional symptoms and eventually develop watery drainage from the vagina 10 to 14 days after surgery. If a fistula tract cannot be visualized on speculum examination or with cystoscopy, a tampon dye test may be performed. This is done by instilling methylene blue dye into the bladder and inserting a tampon inside of the vagina. If the blue dye is noted on the proximal tampon, a bladder fistula is suspected. If there is no dye noted, a uterovaginal fistula should be ruled out, which can also be done with a tampon in the vagina using intravenous indigo carmine or oral phenazopyridine. Alternatively, an intravenous pyelogram or CT urogram can be done to help diagnose a fistula. If the fistula is small, it may heal spontaneously with the bladder to continuous drainage for 6 to 12 weeks. Fistulae that do not heal spontaneously, or are complex or large, will require surgical repair.

KEY REFERENCES

1. ACOG Committee Opinion No. 444: choosing the route of hysterectomy for benign disease. *Obstet Gynecol.* 2009;114(5):1156–1158.
2. Barber MD. Difficult vaginal hysterectomy. In: Walters MD, Barber MD, eds. *Hysterectomy for Benign Disease.* 1st ed. Philadelphia, PA: Elseiver; 2010:136–160.
3. Levy BS. Vaginal hysterectomy: 6 challenges, an arsenal of solutions. *OBG Management.* 2006;18:96–103.
4. Sightler SE, Boike GM, Estape RE, Averette HE. Ovarian cancer in women with prior hysterectomy: a 14-year experience at the University of Miami. *Obstet Gynecol.* 1991;78:681–684.
5. Parker WH, Broder MS, Liu Z, Shoupe D, Farquhar C, Berek JS. Ovarian conservation at the time of hysterectomy for benign disease. *Obstet Gynecol.* 2005;106:219–226.
6. Garry R, Fountain J, Mason S, et al. The eVALuate study: two parallel randomised trials, one comparing laparoscopic with abdominal hysterectomy, the other comparing laparoscopic with vaginal hysterectomy. *BMJ.* 2004;328(7432):129–136.
7. Ibeanu OA, Chesson RR, Echols KT, Nieves M, Busangu F, Nolan TE, et al. Urinary tract injury during hysterectomy based on universal cystoscopy. *Obstet Gynecol.* 2009;113(1):6–10.

Section IV
Cervix

Cervical Conization

Mariam AlHilli

9

GENERAL PRINCIPLES

Description

- Cervical conization refers to surgical excision of a cone-shaped segment of the cervix and surrounding endocervical canal including the squamocolumnar junction.[1]
- The procedure can be performed using cold knife biopsy (cervical conization) or loop electrosurgical excision (LEEP).
- It can be regarded as a diagnostic and therapeutic procedure.
- Cervical conization and LEEP both allow histologic evaluation of the excised tissue, while ablative procedures (cryotherapy or laser) preclude histologic evaluation.

Indications

General Indications

- Excisional therapy with cervical conization or LEEP is the gold standard for treatment of grade 2 and 3 cervical intraepithelial neoplasia (CIN 2-3).
- The advent of highly sensitive and specific screening methods for cervical cancer screening has created a paradigm shift in the diagnosis and management of CIN.
- Cervical conization is generally undertaken in nonpregnant patients of reproductive age with a diagnosis of CIN 2-3, or "young women"[2] with persistent CIN 2 or CIN 3 for 1 year, for treatment purposes and in order to rule out invasive disease.
- A conservative approach in the screening for cervical carcinoma *in situ* has been advocated in recent years, which has minimized the use of invasive diagnostic procedures including cervical conization, particularly in "young women."

Diagnostic Indications

- Lack of complete visualization of transformation zone[3] on colposcopy indicative of an unsatisfactory colposcopic examination of the cervix.
- Lack of consistency between cytologic findings on cervical screening cytology and histologic findings on cervical biopsy.
  - CIN 1 on biopsy preceded by high-grade squamous intraepithelial neoplasia (HSIL) or atypical squamous cells cannot exclude HSIL (ASC-H); (alterative options: co-testing at 12 and 24 months or review of cytology, histology, and colposcopy).
  - Cytology suggests a higher-grade lesion than that found by colposcopic-directed biopsy.
- Persistent positive cytology for dysplasia or persistent high-risk HPV with normal colposcopy:
  - CIN 1 that persists for at least 2 years if continued follow-up is not desired.
- Confirmation of microinvasive squamous cell cervical carcinoma detected on biopsy or suspected on cytology or colposcopy.
  - When cytology, biopsy or endocervical curettage suggests the presence of endocervical glandular lesion.
  - Presence of dysplastic cells within endocervical curettage.

Therapeutic

- Treatment of microinvasive cervical carcinoma[4] where fertility is desired.
  - Treatment with conization is sufficient if margins are negative.
  - Positive margins are highly predictive of recurrent disease and further treatment (repeat conization or hysterectomy) may be indicated.
- Treatment of CIN 2 or CIN 3. Observation is less favored in the following circumstances:
  - Women who do not desire future fertility
  - Inadequate colposcopy
  - Women with recurrent CIN 2 or CIN 3
  - "Young women" with persistent CIN 2 or CIN 3 for 1 year
  - CIN 2 or CIN 3 present within endocervical curettage
  - Worsening colposcopic findings or persistent high-grade cytology for 1 year
- HSIL—"see and treat" option.

Indications in Special Populations

- Women aged 21 to 24 with
  - persistent HSIL for 24 months and no CIN 2 or CIN 3 identified.

---

[1]Transformation zone: the junction between the stratified squamous epithelium of the ectocervix and vagina and the columnar epithelium of the endocervical canal.

[2]Young women: those who, after counseling by their clinicians, consider risk to future pregnancies from treating cervical abnormalities to outweigh the risk of cancer during observation of those abnormalities—no specific age threshold is described.

[3]Transformation zone: the area that lies between the embryologic squamocolumnar junction and the junction present on colposcopy (new squamocolumnar junction). It defines the distal limit of high-grade glandular intraepithelial neopslais, and is invariably the site of origin of the cervical neoplasia.

[4]Microinvasive cervical carcinoma: a lesion that invades below the basement membrane to a depth of 3 mm or less and horizontal spread of less than 7 mm (FIGO stage IA1) or stage IA2: tumor invades to deeper than 3 mm and up to 5 mm with less than 7 mm of horizontal spread.

- persistent CIN 2 or CIN 3 for 24 months after close observation with cytology and colposcopy every 6 months.
- immediate treatment of CIN 2 or CIN 3.
- Pregnant women
  - when strong suspicion for invasive cervical carcinoma based on clinical findings, cytology, or biopsy is present.
  - CIN 2 and CIN 3 are generally managed expectantly with colposcopic examinations every 12 weeks. Repeat biopsy is indicated with the appearance of the lesion worsens or cytology results suggest invasive cancer.
  - endocervical curettage is contraindicated in pregnancy.

IMAGING AND OTHER DIAGNOSTICS

- Prior to cervical conization, a colposcopic evaluation of the cervix is performed to evaluate the extent of disease.
- Colposcopic-guided or direct cervical biopsies of an abnormal ectocervical lesion must be performed.
- An endocervical curettage is an essential component of the evaluation of cervical dysplasia prior to conization, particularly for cervical adenocarcinoma and where atypical glandular cells are detected on cytology.
- The size and shape of cone specimen are determined by patient circumstances and preoperative colposcopic findings.

PREOPERATIVE PLANNING

- Cervical conization is performed under general or regional anesthesia in the operating room for patient comfort and for control of excess bleeding that may accompany the procedure. It is preferred when the lesion is deep within the endocervical canal and where there are no restrictions in the amount of cervical tissue removed.
- LEEP is usually well tolerated with local anesthesia in the office. It is ideal for young, nulliparous women, and those with an obvious ectocervical lesion. It removes less tissue than cervical conization.
- The choice of cervical conization versus LEEP is dependent on several factors including surgeon preference, patient preference, desire for complete excision with minimal thermal effect, and the size and severity of the lesion (refer to Pearls and Pitfalls section).
- Informed consent is needed prior to the procedure.
- Review patient allergies, particularly iodine allergy. If iodine allergy is present, the use of 3% to 5% acetic acid solution is suggested.
- Additional considerations:
  - Anticoagulant usage: Aspirin should be stopped 1 week prior to the procedure and resumed after the procedure. Warfarin should be stopped 5 days prior to the procedure and resumed on the night of surgery. Consult with hematologist for recommendations regarding anticoagulation management in patients with prosthetic heart valves, high-risk thrombophilia, recent venous thromboembolism (within 3 months), and if bridging with low–molecular-weight heparin is required.
  - If a concomitant infection of the genital tract is suspected, delay the procedure until the infection resolves and treats appropriately with antibiotics.
  - A pregnancy test is required in all women of reproductive age where pregnancy may be possible.

SURGICAL MANAGEMENT

- The shape and size of the cone are tailored to the individual situation (Fig. 9.1).
  - A narrow cone is suitable for a lesion deep in the endocervical cancer with a normal ectocervix.
  - A narrow cone is usually needed in postmenopausal women where the squamocolumnar junction moves cephalad into the endocervical canal.

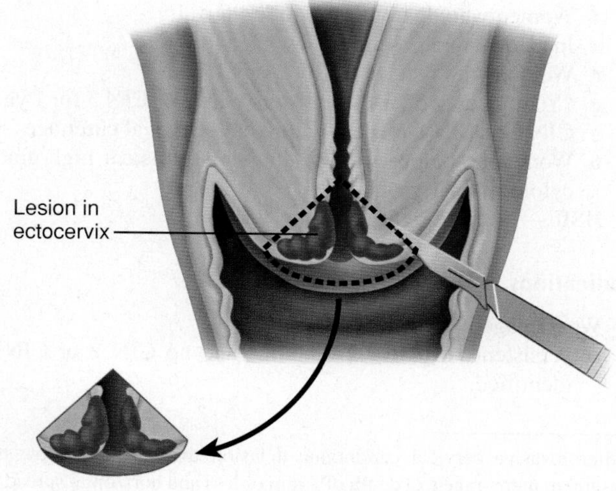

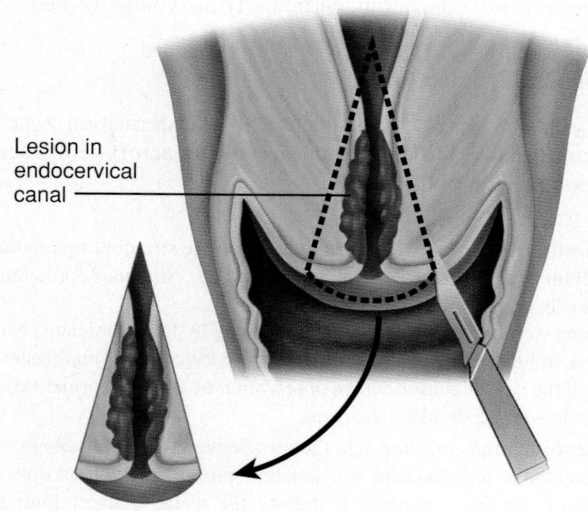

Figure 9.1. A shallow cone with a wide base is performed for lesions located in the ectocervix. A deep cone with a narrow base is performed for lesions in the endocervical canal.

   - If the lesion is large or confined to the ectocervix, a wide cone is performed to obtain clear transformation zone margins.
- The amount of tissue removed generally depends on
   - The location of the squamocolumnar junction: the higher/deeper the squamocolumnar junction, the narrower the cone should be.
   - Endocervical gland involvement.
   - In general, the endocervical portion of the cone/LEEP should be 20 mm wide (10 mm on each side of the cervical canal) and no more than 20 mm deep.

Positioning

- Position the patient in the dorsal lithotomy position using candy cane or Allen's stirrups.

Procedures and Techniques: Cervical Conization (Video 9.1)

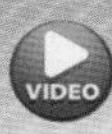

Visualization

- Place a weighted speculum posteriorly and three Deaver retractors to expose the cervix (Tech Fig. 9.1).
- Ensure the entire cervix is well visualized and the vaginal walls are well retracted to prevent injury.

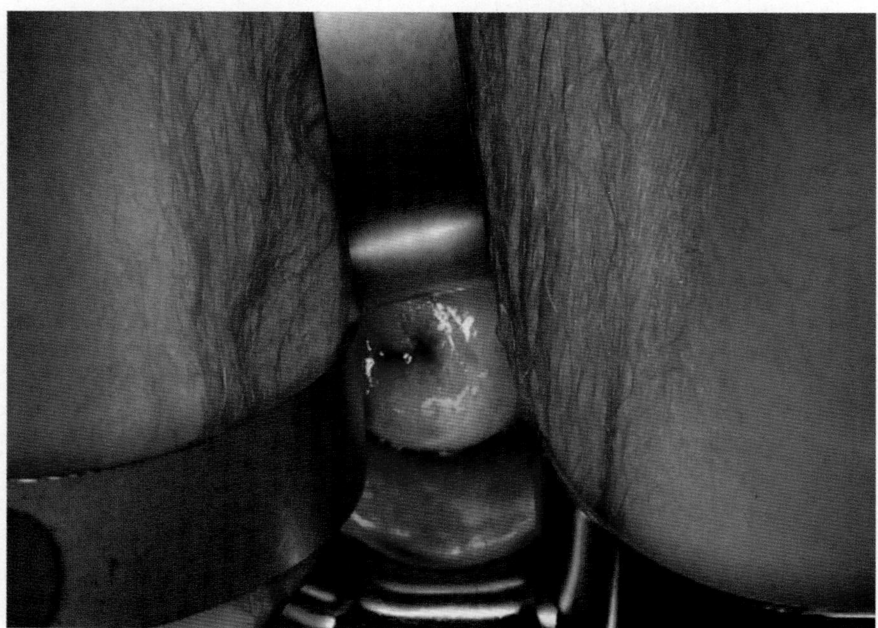

Tech Figure 9.1. Visualization of the cervix with placement of a weighted speculum posteriorly and three Deaver retractors.

Primary hemostasis

- Grasp the cervix laterally at 3 and 9 o'clock with single-tooth tenacula.
- Place stay sutures (hemostatic sutures) at the 3 and 9 o'clock positions of the cervicovaginal junction using 1-0 delayed absorbable suture and remove the tenacula. These sutures are used for traction and hemostasis (Tech Fig. 9.2A).
- Remove the laterally placed Deaver retractors and tag each stay suture with a Kocher clamp. Use stay sutures to stabilize the specimen and to partially occlude the descending branch of the uterine artery (Tech Fig. 9.2B).
- Inject a dilute solution of vasopressin (0.5 mL/100 mL NS [10 units/100 mL]) deep into the four quadrants of the cervix (2, 4, 6, and 8 o'clock positions of the cervix) (5 to 10 cc/quadrant) using an 18-gauge spinal needle. Draw back before injecting to ensure intravascular injection has not occurred. Observe for blanching of the cervical stroma prior to proceeding (Tech Fig. 9.3).

A

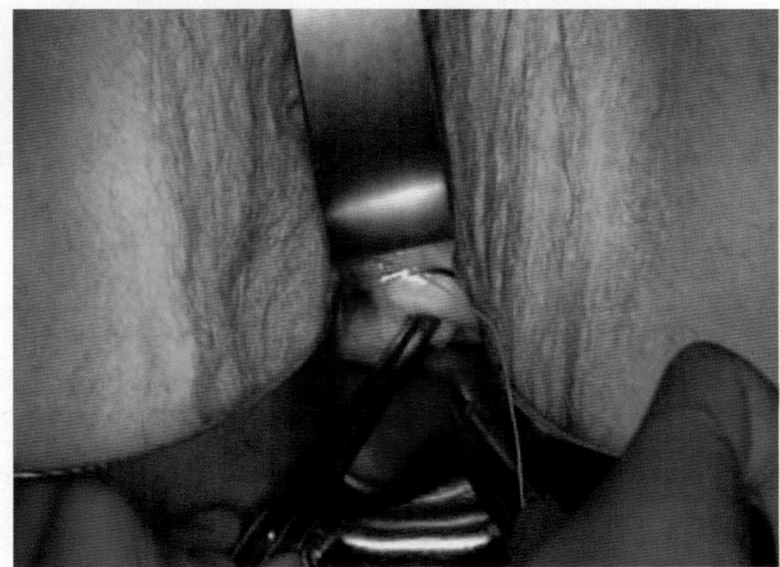

B

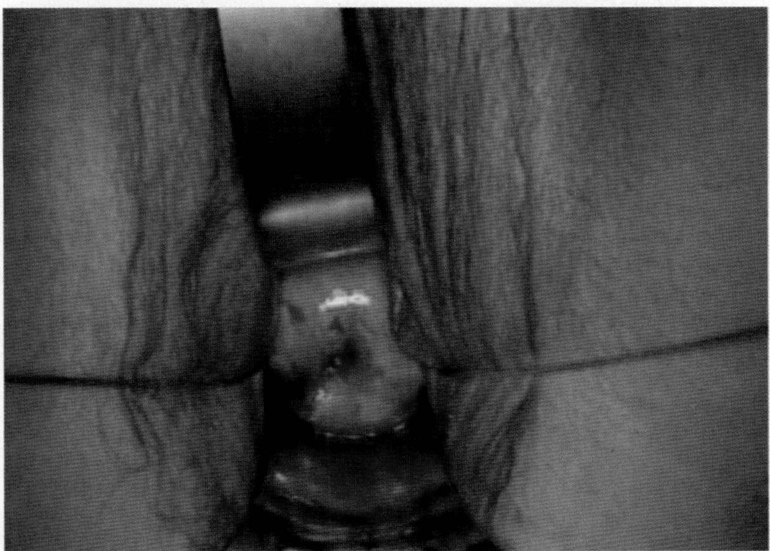

Tech Figure 9.2. A and **B:** Placement of left stay suture lateral to the cervix. Stay sutures are tagged with Kocher clamps and are used to provide traction on the cervix and hemostasis.

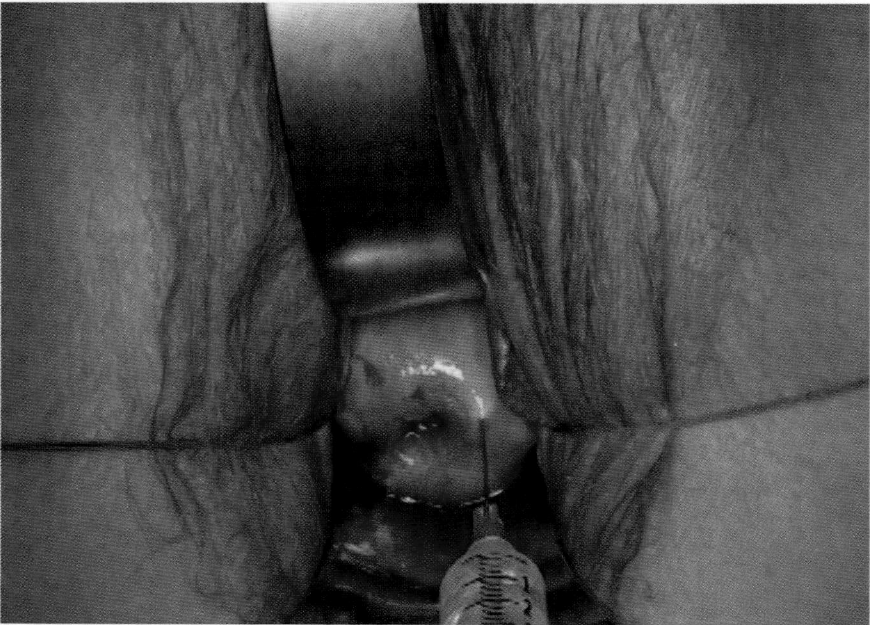

Tech Figure 9.3. Deep injection of cervix with a dilute solution of vasopressin for hemostasis in four quadrants. Blanching of the stroma must be seen.

Preparation

- Bathe the cervix with Lugol's solution to demarcate areas of dysplasia. If the patient has an iodine allergy, use 3% to 5% acetic acid solution instead. Colposcopy may be used as appropriate **(Tech Fig. 9.4)**.
- Use a uterine sound to determine the direction of the endocervical canal and cervical length **(Tech Fig. 9.5)**.

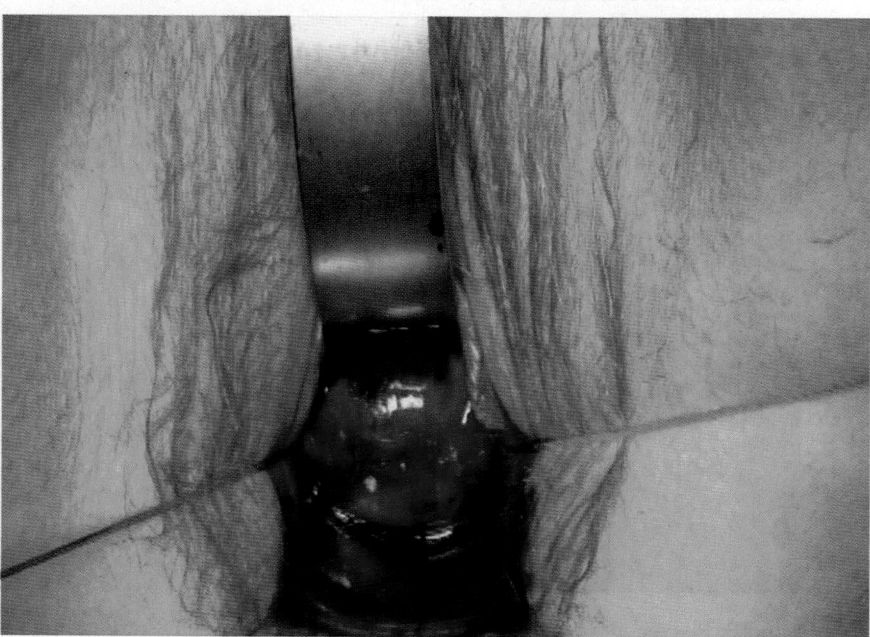

Tech Figure 9.4. The cervix is bathed with Lugol's solution to demarcate areas of dysplasia and identify the transformation zone.

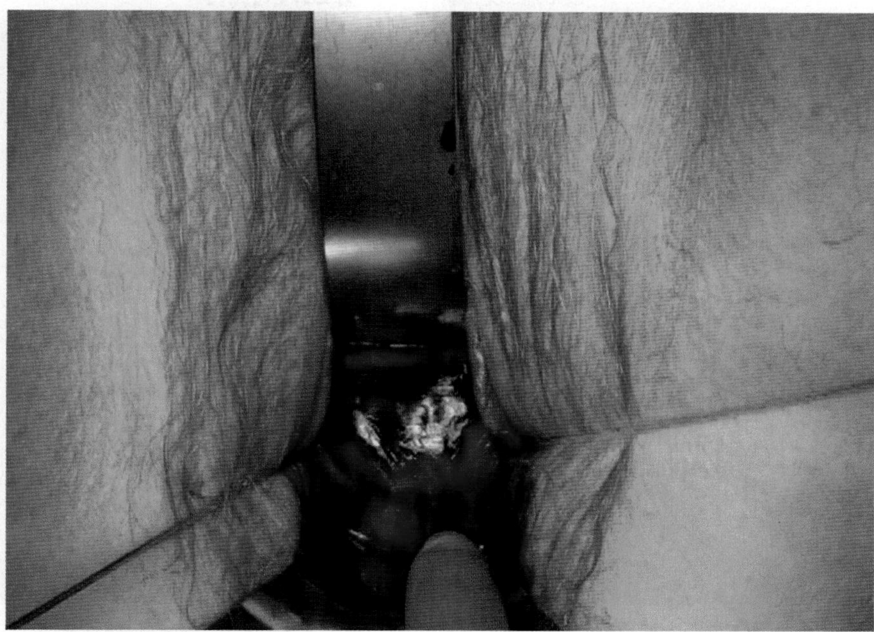

Tech Figure 9.5. The cervix is sounded to identify the length and direction of the cervix.

Excision of cone

- Use a #11 blade to score the cervix making a circumferential clockwise incision starting at 3 o'clock and incorporating the entire transformation zone. Angle the tip of the blade toward the endocervical canal (Tech Fig. 9.6A,B).
- Place a 3-0 silk suture in the cone stroma at 12 o'clock and tie it. Place two additional silk sutures at 4 and 8 o'clock and leave them untied. Tag all three sutures with a Kelly curve clamp and use it to rotate and manipulate the cone. Avoid instruments touching the ectocervix during conization (Tech Fig. 9.7A,B).
- Place traction on the cone using the tagged sutures, and complete the cone resection by re-orienting the blade to remove a wedge of cervical tissue (Tech Fig. 9.8).
- Remove the untied silk sutures and use the tied suture placed at 12 o'clock to orient the specimen (Tech Fig. 9.9).
- Check the adequacy of the cone with a sound and submit the specimen to pathology. Avoid manipulating or touching the ectocervix during the process.

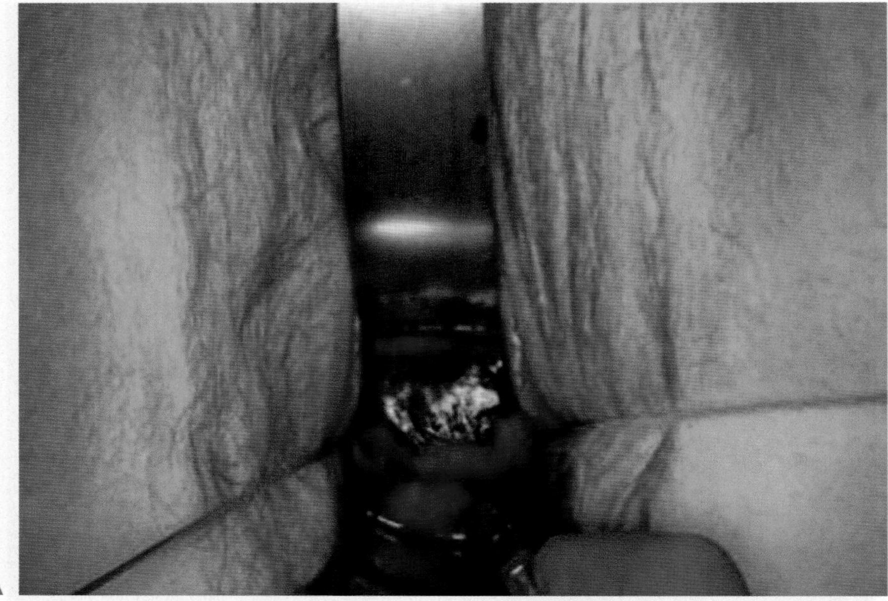

A

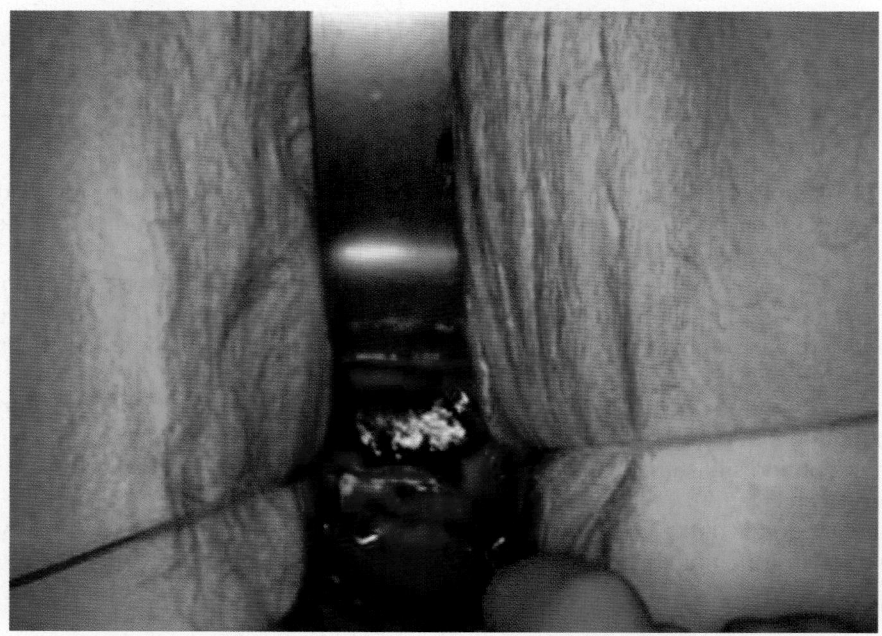

B

Tech Figure 9.6. The cervix is scored with a #11 blade starting at 3 o'clock and going clockwise (**A**) ending at 3 o'clock (**B**).

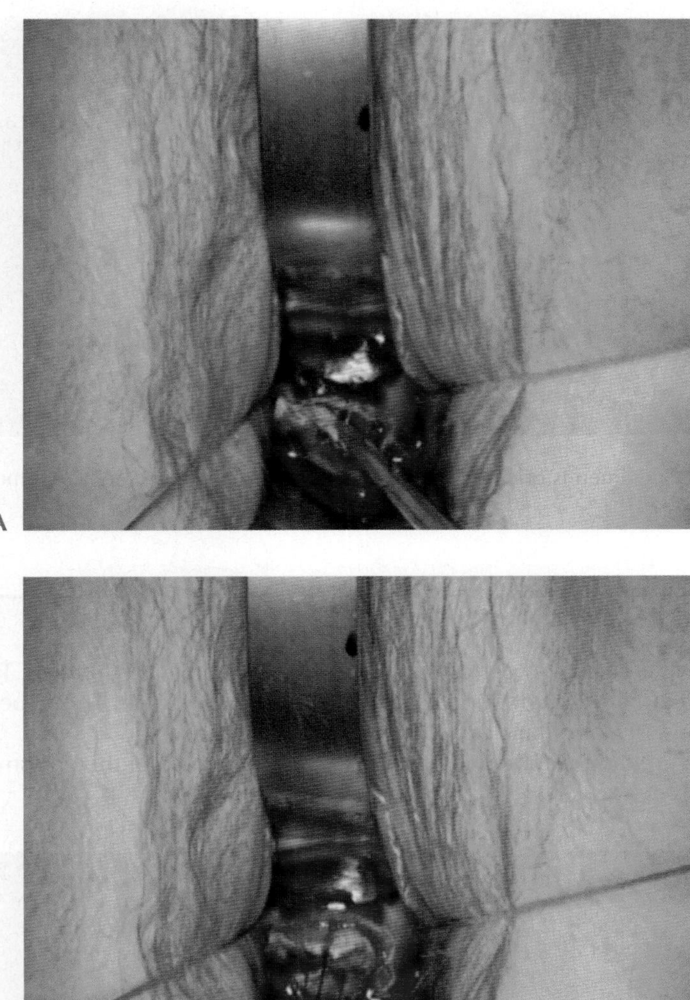

Tech Figure 9.7. **A:** Silk suture is placed at 12 o'clock in the stroma of the cervix avoiding touching or manipulating the ectocervix. This suture is tied. **B:** Two additional silk sutures are placed at 4 and 8 o'clock and are left untied. All three sutures are tagged and used for retraction for the cone.

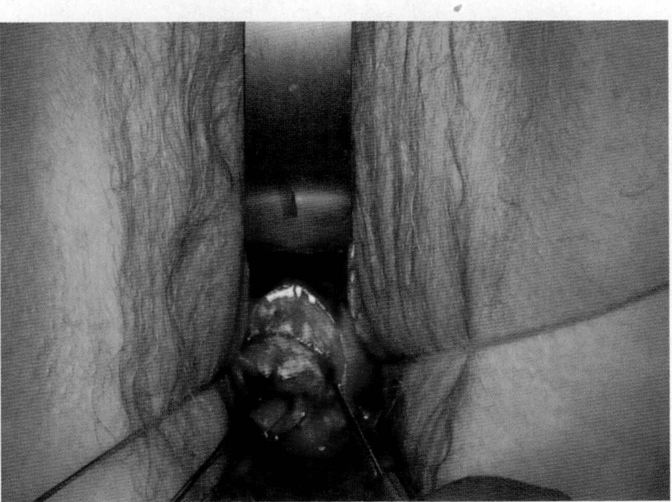

Tech Figure 9.8. The cone is completed by making a deeper incision within the cervical stroma and orienting the blade toward the endocervical canal to remove a wedge of tissue.

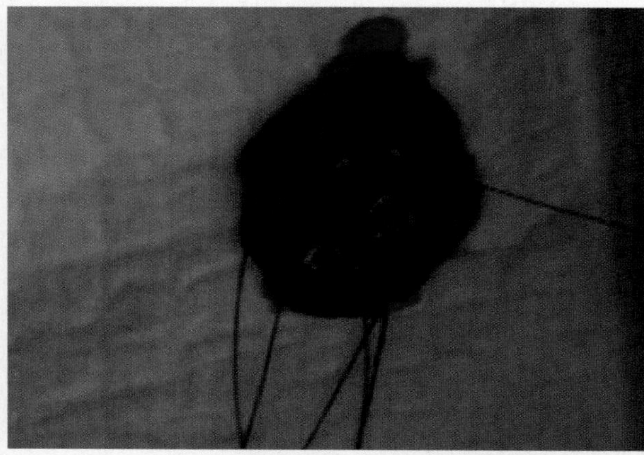

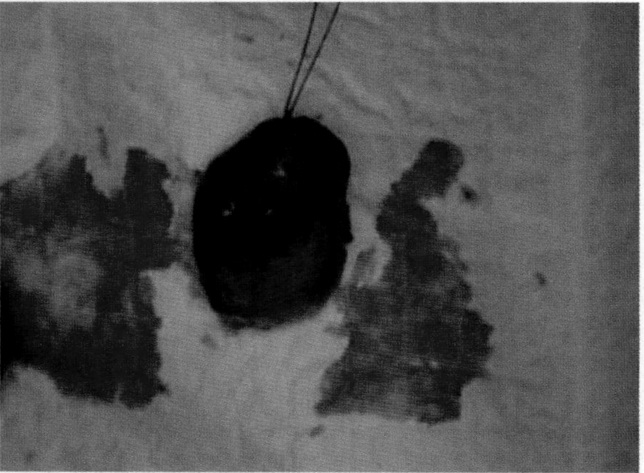

Tech Figure 9.9. The specimen is oriented—the silk sutures at 4 and 8 o'clock are removed and the suture at 12 o'clock is left in place.

Endocervical curettage

- Use an endocervical curette to perform a thorough endocervical curettage. Take caution not to enter the lower uterine segment during the process (Tech Fig. 9.10). This is performed to exclude residual squamous or glandular disease of the endocervical canal.
- An endometrial curettage can be performed to exclude disease of the endometrium.

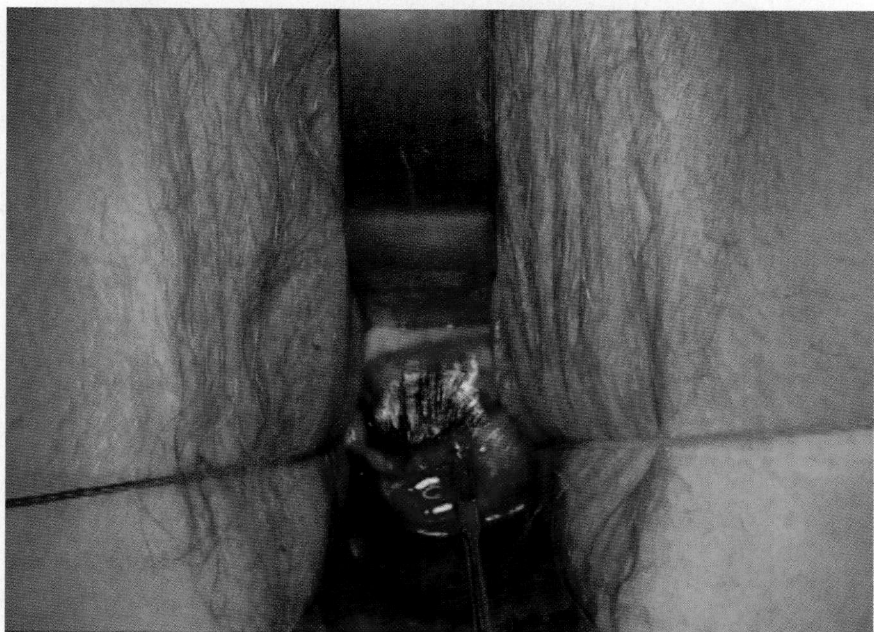

Tech Figure 9.10. Appearance of cervix postconization.

Hemostasis

- Control bleeding using a combination of electrosurgical coagulation (30 W—ball electrode coagulation) and Monsel's (ferric subsulfate) solution (**Tech Fig. 9.11**).
- The cone bed can be sutured with either running absorbable suture or figure-of-eight stiches if excessive bleeding is encountered.
- If hemorrhage is encountered:
  - Inject vasopressin into the cone bed.
  - Place a purse-string suture through the cone bed and tie it. However, this may increase the risk of cervical stenosis.
  - Pack a piece of oxidized cellulose (Surgicel) or thrombin-soaked Gelfoam into the cervical cone bed.
  - Last resort: internal iliac artery embolization or hysterectomy.

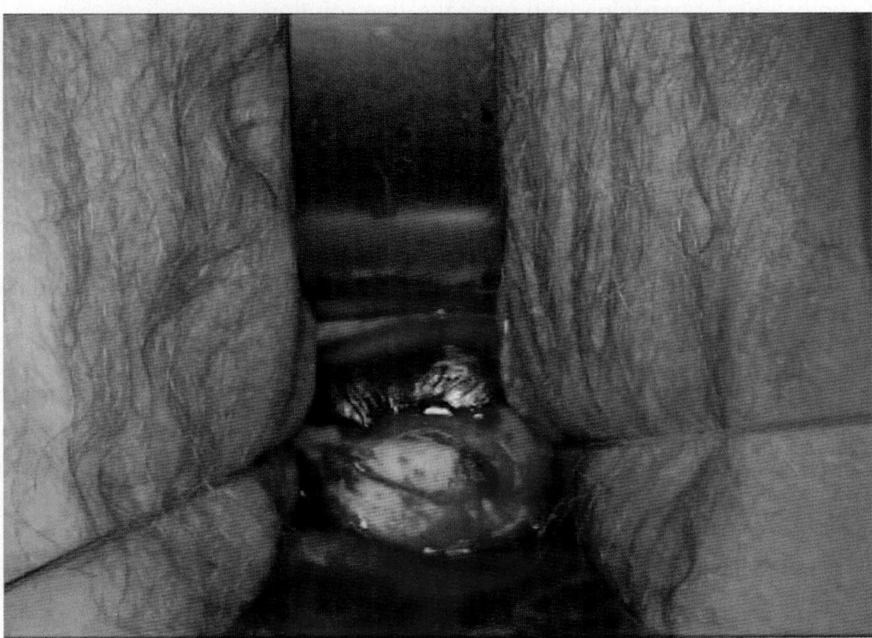

Tech Figure 9.11. An endocervical curettage is performed using a small curette.

Procedures and Techniques: LEEP

Visualization

- Insert a nonconductive nylon or plastic-coated speculum into the vagina and align the cervix.
- Affix an electrical grounding pad on the patient to ensure safety.
- Ensure the entire cervix is well visualized and the vaginal walls are well retracted to prevent injury.

Preparation

- Rinse the cervix and upper vagina with normal saline solution.
- Prepare a solution of vasopressin and lidocaine (20 to 30 mL (0.5 U/mL) vasopressin into 30-mL vial of 1% lidocaine). This serves to provide both local anesthesia and hemostasis.
- Apply 5% acetic acid solution using cotton swabs and inspect the cervix and transformation zone with colposcopy. Apply Lugol's solution to determine the margins of resection.
- Perform colposcopy to evaluate the cervix and determine the location of the transformation zone and the distribution of the lesion.
- Ensure electrosurgical generator is connected and set at 30–40 W (40 cut/40 coag) and a smoke evacuator is connected.
- Select the appropriate shape and size of the loop to be used based on the size and location of the lesion as well as patient characteristics.

Hemostasis and local anesthesia

- Inject 10 cc of 1% vasopressin and 0.5 mL vasopressin at 12, 3, 6, and 9 o'clock deep into the stroma of the cervix and an additional 10 cc superficially at 2, 4, 8, and 10 o'clock.

Excision of cone

- Using cut current and the appropriate tip/loop, resect a cone of cervical tissue. Place the loop 2 mm from the tissue and advance it perpendicularly into the cervix about 2 to 3 mm lateral to the lesion on each side prior to electrosurgical cutting. Aim for approximately 5 to 7 mm depth of tissue. Excessive thermal damage may ensue if resection is too slow. Perform the procedure under colposcopic control.
- Consider performing a second pass (using a square tip loop) in older or postmenopausal patients or when the lesion is large or deep.
- Orient the specimen by cutting through the stroma at 12 o'clock with scissors and submit to pathology.

Endocervical curettage

- Perform an endocervical curettage using both a sharp endocervical curette and a cytobrush.

Hemostasis

- Fulgurate the external edges of the cervix and cone bed with a rollerball tip at 40 W coagulation current.
- Apply Monsel's solution to the cone bed/cervix to maintain hemostasis.
- Consider applying estrogen (Premarin) cream to the cervix.

PEARLS AND PITFALLS

- ○ Cervical conization is recommended over LEEP when margin status is critical for determining residual disease (microinvasive squamous cell carcinoma or adenocarcinoma *in situ*).
- ✕ Excessive cauterization of post cone bed (particularly crater rim) is associated with higher risk of postconization/LEEP cervical stenosis.
- ○ Cervical conization removes more tissue than LEEP and is considered for more severe disease, and that which may extend to the endocervical canal. It generally allows better control of depth of tissue resection.
- ✕ Stay sutures are placed lateral to the cervix at the cervicovaginal junction. They are used to manipulate and stabilize the cone specimen. Placement of sutures unnecessarily in the cone bed is not advised due to the risk of inversion of the cervical canal and burying of residual disease.
- ○ Use of intraoperative colposcopy allows precise evaluation of the amount of tissue needed to be removed and reduces the incidence of positive margins.
- ✕ Avoid touching the ectocervix in order to minimize the effect of artifact on histologic interpretation.
- ○ Fertility is not affected by LEEP or cervical conization.
- ✕ The risk of preterm delivery is increased if the depth of LEEP or cone is greater than 10 mm. The risk of preterm delivery must be balanced against the risk of untreated CIN 2-3.
- ○ Patient is advised that vaginal discharge for up to 3 weeks after the procedure is normal and not unexpected. Similarly minor spotting for 2 weeks postoperatively may occur.
- ✕ Cervical conization is associated with higher rate of extreme prematurity and low birth weight than LEEP. Thus, LEEP is preferred in young nulliparous patients.

POSTOPERATIVE CARE

- Patients are discharged home on the same day.
- Patients are advised to refrain from intercourse, tampon sue, swimming, tub soaking (nothing per vagina) for 28 days.
- Review bleeding precautions. Patients are asked to contact their surgical team in the case of excessive bleeding which consists of soaking a large (maxi) pad in an hour for two consecutive hours.
- Worrisome symptoms to prompt medical attention include:
  - Excessive bleeding (soaking a large pad in a hour × 2 hours)
  - Fever >38.0°C
  - Uterine cramping or pelvic pain
  - Persistent foul smelling discharge.
- Patient is seen in the office in 4 weeks and evaluated for bleeding and cervical stenosis. Evaluation of cervical integrity is done through visual assessment.
- Use of estrogen cream is generally not recommended and has not been shown to reduce the rate of postconization stenosis.

OUTCOMES

- Cervical conization:
  - Increased risk of preterm birth and low birth weight
  - Higher rate of hemorrhage than LEEP
  - Cure rate >95%
- LEEP
  - Increased risk of preterm birth and low birth weight
  - Increased risk of cervical stenosis
  - Risk of unsuspected invasive cancer and high-grade glandular dysplasia 1% to 2%
  - Cure rate >95%
- Positive conization margins:
  - Presence of dysplasia or carcinoma at margins of excisional procedure or endocervical sample is associated with a significantly higher risk of recurrent disease (up to 30%) than uninvolved margins.
    - For CIN 2-3, reassessment with cytology and endocervical curettage 4 to 6 months after the procedure is recommended, and re-excision is optional.
    - For microinvasive cervical carcinoma or adenocarcinoma *in situ*, where future fertility is desired, repeat excision/conization to achieve negative margins is recommended.
    - A hysterectomy may be considered in patients with positive margins who have completed childbearing.

COMPLICATIONS

- Short term:
  - Bleeding
    - Early: within 48 hours of the procedure.
    - Delayed: 10 to 21 days after procedure (5% to 10%)—may be due to erosion of vessel during healing or suture dissolving.
  - Infection: 0.2% to 6.8%
    - Cervicitis—may present with persistent vaginal discharge or bleeding
    - Ascending endometritis—may present with vaginal discharge, bleeding, uterine cramping, abdominal tenderness, or fever
  - Damage to adjacent organs
    - Inadvertent opening of pouch of Douglas
      - A Deaver retractor is placed within the pouch of Douglas to inspect for damage to adjacent organs (bowel or rectum). The vaginal mucosa is then repaired with interrupted 2-0 delayed absorbable suture.

- If the pouch of Douglas (or bladder) is entered with a knife blade, a laparoscopic evaluation (or cystoscopy) is warranted.
  - Uterine perforation
    - If perforation occurs with the use of a blunt object (uterine sound) and the patient is hemodynamically stable, observation is reasonable.
    - If perforation occurs with a sharp object, or perforation of the lateral uterine walls is suspected, laparoscopic evaluation is recommended.
- Long term:
  - Cervical stenosis (0% to 27%): higher risk with increased depth of incision ≥1 to 2 cm (vs. <1 cm) and postmenopausal status.
  - Cervical incompetence—not likely to be clinically significant.
    - Preterm labor: increased risk in women who have undergone more than one conization procedure.
    - Premature delivery
    - Preterm premature rupture of membranes (PPROM)
      - Greater depth of excision is associated with higher rate of preterm delivery and PPROM
      - Increased risk with depth of excision >12 to 15 mm; minimal risk with depth of excision <10 mm or up to 15 mm
  - Miscarriage—second trimester loss
  - Recurrent or persistent CIN—5% to 17%. Higher risk with larger lesions, endocervical gland involvement, positive margins, persistent positive high-risk HPV.

KEY READINGS

American College of Obstetricians and Gynecologists. Practice Bulletin Number 140: management of abnormal cervical cancer screening test results and cervical cancer precursors. 2013;122:1338–1368.

Apgar BS, Kaufman A, Bettcher C, Parker Featherstone E. Gynecology procedures: colposcopy, treatment of cervical intraepithelial neoplasia, and endometrial assessment. *Am Fam Physician.* 2013;87(12):836–843.

Arbyn M, Kyrgiou M, Simoens C, et al. Perinatal mortality and other severe adverse pregnancy outcomes associated with treatment of cervical intraepithelial neoplasia: meta-analysis. *BMJ.* 2008;337:a1284.

Bereck JS, Hacker NF. *Gynecologic Oncology*. 5th ed. Philadelphia, PA: Lippincott Williams and Wilkins; 2010:547.

Bevis KS, Biggio JR. Cervical conization and the risk of preterm delivery. *Am J Obstet Gynecol.* 2011;205(1):19–27.

Castanon A, Landy R, Brocklehurst P, et al. Risk of preterm delivery with increasing depth of excision for cervical intraepithelial neoplasia in England: a nested case control study. *BMJ.* 2014;349:g6223.

Coppleson MZ, et al. *Gyencologic Oncology*. 2nd ed. Vol 1. Philadelphia, PA: Churcill Livingstone; 1992.

Ghaem-Maghami S, Sagi S, Majeed G, Soutter WP. Incomplete excision of cervical intraepithelial neoplasia and risk of treatment failure: a meta-analysis. *Lancet Oncol.* 2007;8(11):985–993.

Krebs HB. Outpatient cervical conization. *Obstet Gynecol.* 1984;63:430–434.

Kyrgiou M, Koliopoulos G, Martin-Hirsch P, Arbyn M, Prendivilee W, Paraskevaidis E. Obstetric outcomes after conservative treatment for intraepithelial or early invasive cervical lesions: systematic review and meta-analysis. *Lancet.* 2006;367(9509):489–498.

Wright TC Jr, Gagnon S, Richart RM, Ferenczy A. Treatment of cervical intraepithelial neoplasia using loop electrosurgical excision procedure. *Obstet Gyneocl.* 1992;79(2):173–178.

Vaginal and Laparoscopic Trachelectomy

Karl Jallad, Robert DeBernardo, Roberto Vargas

10

GENERAL PRINCIPLES

Definition

- A trachelectomy is performed to remove a cervical stump. The stump is the remnant of the uterus following a supracervical hysterectomy.

Differential Diagnosis

- Pelvic mass
- Cervical neoplasia
- Prolapsed fallopian tube
- Gartner duct cyst
- Vaginal polyps
- Vaginal adenosis
- Vaginal endometriosis

IMAGING AND OTHER DIAGNOSTICS

- Patients with abnormal vaginal bleeding require ultrasound imaging. Consider obtaining a CT scan if a pelvic mass is suspected.
- Cervical cancer screening is required preoperatively.

PREOPERATIVE PLANNING

- The route of surgery depends on the indication for trachelectomy, surgeon's experience and comfort, the presence of comorbidities, and the need for concomitant procedures. The preoperative planning for a vaginal trachelectomy begins with a thorough history and physical examination. The surgeon should pay particular attention to the degree of prolapse, the presence of a pelvic mass, adnexal tenderness, and whether the cervix is mobile. A laparoscopic approach should be considered if the patient has unexplained pelvic pain or suspected endometriosis, or if there is an adnexal/pelvic mass requiring removal. Counseling should include the risk of conversion to laparotomy, independent of a minimally invasive approach.
- Confirm the patient's cervical cancer screening is up-to-date.
- Patients with significant medical comorbidities should also undergo preoperative clearance.
- Perform thorough counseling and discuss the risks, benefits, alternative, and different routes of surgery. Obtain a signed, informed consent.

Regardless of the surgical route, a trachelectomy is a clean-contaminated procedure and a prophylactic antibiotic should be administered prior to incision. We commonly use a first- or second-generation cephalosporin.

SURGICAL MANAGEMENT

- The most common indications for trachelectomy are pelvic organ prolapse, pelvic mass, abnormal cytology, bleeding, and pain. Trachelectomy is a relatively safe and effective procedure. Patients should be counseled on the risk of bleeding and injury to the urinary tract or bowel.

Positioning

- Positioning for a vaginal trachelectomy is similar to positioning for a vaginal hysterectomy (see Chapter 8.5, Vaginal Hysterectomy). The patient is placed in the dorsal lithotomy position using candy cane or Allen stirrups. The use of Allen stirrups is preferred in cases where there is a high likelihood of converting to an abdominal procedure or if there is a need for concomitant laparoscopy.
- Positioning for a laparoscopic/robotic trachelectomy is similar to the positioning for a laparoscopic/robotic hysterectomy. The patient is positioned in the dorsal lithotomy position using Allen stirrups with the patient's arms secured to her sides (see chapter on Diagnostic Laparoscopy, Patient Positioning).

Approach

- An abdominal (open, laparoscopic, or robotic) approach is preferred when the patient complains of pelvic pain or endometriosis is suspected. In addition, if a pelvic mass is appreciated on examination or imaging, an abdominal approach is mandatory.
- A vaginal approach is preferred in patients with significant comorbidities, when abdominal exploration is not required or when the trachelectomy is performed due to prolapse.

Procedures and Techniques: Vaginal Trachelectomy (Video 10.1)

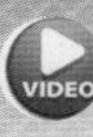

Preparation

- Prepare and drape the patient's vagina, perineum, and lower abdomen.
- Insert a Foley catheter and drain the bladder.

Tenaculum placement

- Place a weighted speculum or retractor in the vagina to expose the cervix.
- Grasp the cervix with a single-tooth or Jacob's tenaculum and gently apply downward traction.
- Circumferentially inject a vasoconstrictor (lidocaine with epinephrine or dilute vasopressin) at the cervicovaginal junction.

Incise the cervicovaginal junction and advance the bladder

- Using a number 10 bladed scalpel or monopolar instrument, circumferentially incise the cervicovaginal junction.
- Using curved Mayo scissors, dissect the vagina and the bladder off the cervix anteriorly and posteriorly.

Enter the posterior cul-de-sac

- Carefully palpate the posterior cul-de-sac.
  - If no adhesions are noted and if entry into the peritoneal cavity is not required, place a Heaney clamp extraperitoneally above the cervical stump bilaterally. Then excise the cervix with a scalpel or Mayo scissors.
  - If entry into the peritoneal cavity is required, deflect the cervix anteriorly, grasp and tent the tissue, and sharply enter the posterior cul-de-sac with Mayo scissors.
    - Then palpate the posterior cul-de-sac to assess for bowel adhesions.

Transect the uterosacral ligaments and enter the anterior peritoneum

- Use a Heaney clamp or a vessel sealing device to clamp and divide the uterosacral ligaments. If a Heaney clamp is used, suture ligate the pedicle with a No. 0 polyglactin 910 (**Tech Fig. 10.1**).

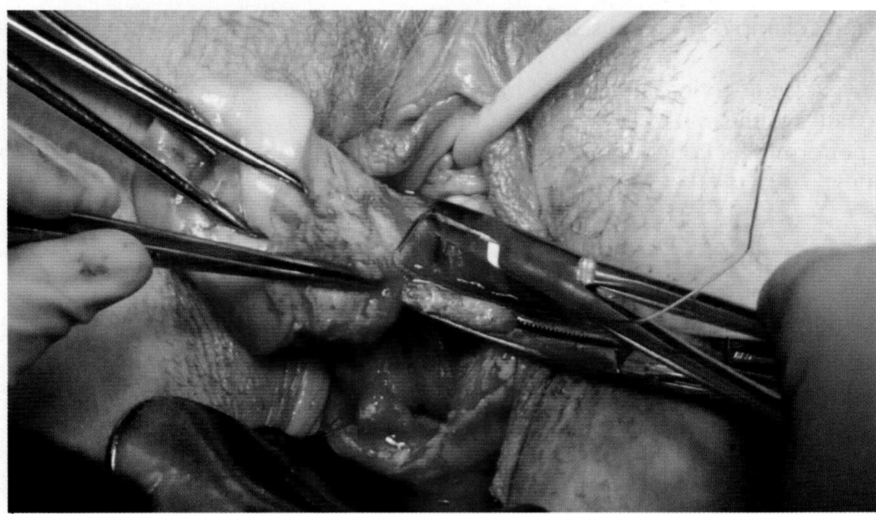

Tech Figure 10.1. The uterosacral ligament has been compressed, transected, and is being suture ligated.

- To decrease bleeding from the posterior incision, we place a running, locked suture using No. 0 polyglactin 910.
- Gently place a moistened and tagged thin, laparotomy sponge in the cavity to sweep the bowels cephalad, away from the field.
- If the surgeon's finger can reach the top of the cervix, and the bladder is not adhered to the cervix, use the surgeon's finger to push anteriorly to delineate the vesicocervical space.
- Use Mayo scissors to dissect the remaining tissue down to the peritoneal layer.
- Then enter the peritoneum sharply and confirm the appropriate space has been accessed (**Tech Fig. 10.2**).

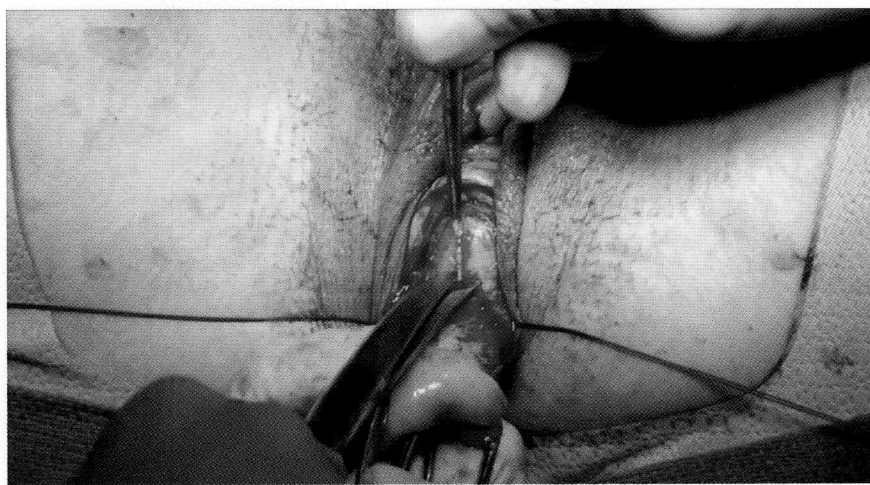

Tech Figure 10.2. Anterior peritoneal entry. After the bladder is advanced anteriorly and superiorly, the vesicocervical peritoneum is entered sharply with Mayo scissors.

- Examine the bladder carefully to confirm no cystotomy has been made.
- Place a right-angle retractor or thin malleable retractor anteriorly to apply gentle pressure on the sponge and to retract the bowel out of the surgical field.

Transect the cardinal ligaments

- Use a Heaney clamp or a vessel sealing device to clamp and divide the remaining cardinal ligaments.
- Deliver the excised cervical stump and inspect for hemostasis. Re-approximate any bleeding or oozing pedicles with simple, interrupted sutures.
- Consider performing a concomitant McCall's suture plication to prevent future prolapse of the vaginal apex.

Closure

- Finally, close the vaginal cuff with No. 0 polyglactin 910 in a continuous or interrupted fashion.
- Perform cystoscopy to assess ureteral patency and bladder integrity.

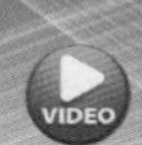

Procedures and Techniques: Laparoscopic Trachelectomy (Video 10.2)

Preparation

- Prep and drape the patient's vagina, perineum, and lower abdomen in a sterile fashion.
- Insert a Foley catheter and drain the bladder.
- Place a vaginal manipulator with an attached cup (i.e., Koh cup) to outline the cervicovaginal junction. Alternatively, a simple vaginal sponge stick may be substituted in the anterior or posterior fornix (**Tech Fig. 10.3**).

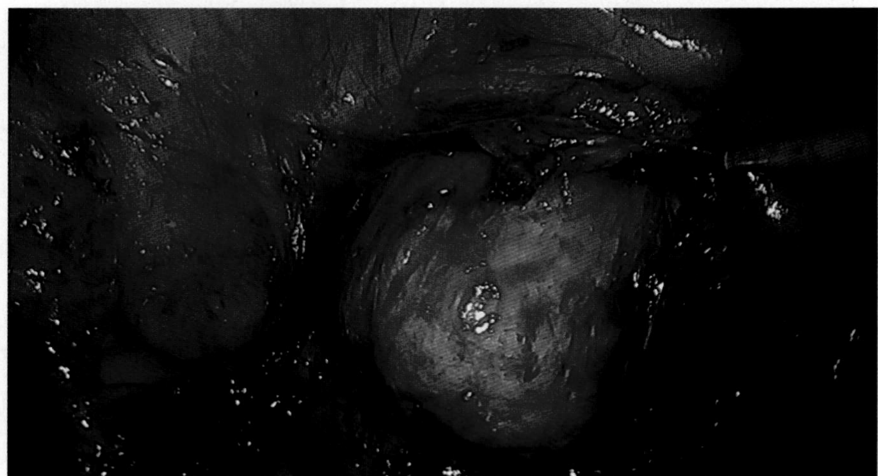

Tech Figure 10.3. Cervical stump. Cephalad traction with a vaginal manipulator will demarcate the cervical stump and cervicovaginal junction. This will also help delineate the vesicocervical peritoneum and rectovaginal space.

Laparoscopic port placement

- Enter the abdomen using the customary laparoscopic entry techniques.
- Place two to three 5-mm trocars in the lower quadrants. Be sure their placement is conducive to triangulation and that the instruments sufficiently reach the cervical stump.

Reflect the vesicocervical peritoneum and create a bladder flap

- Using an active electrode, circumferentially incise the cervicovaginal junction, as delineated by the vaginal cup.
- Apply cephalad traction with the vaginal manipulator and gentle caudal pressure to help develop the bladder flap (**Tech Fig. 10.4**).

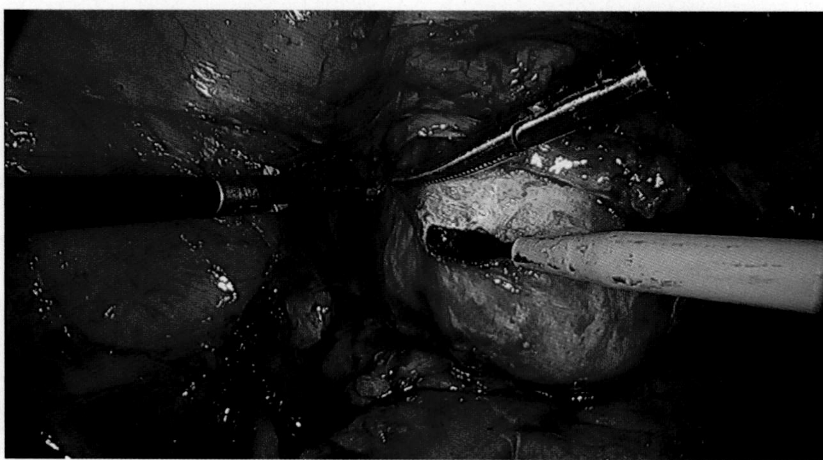

Tech Figure 10.4. Bladder flap. The vesicocervical peritoneum is incised with a monopolar instrument and the bladder is mobilized caudally using blunt and sharp dissection.

Develop the posterior peritoneal space

- Inspect the posterior cul-de-sac to ensure no adhesions exist between the sigmoid colon and the posterior peritoneum.
- If no adhesions are noted, extend the circumferential incision used to create the bladder flap posteriorly. Then mobilize the rectum caudally with gentle pressure.
- If adhesions are noted, perform adhesiolysis with sharp dissection to ensure the rectum is not injured during cervical stump excision.

Transect the uterosacral and cardinal ligaments

- Using advanced radiofrequency (RF) energy, clamp and transect the uterosacral and cardinal ligament complex. Be sure to apply the energy device to remain parallel to the cervix yet medial to the uterine artery pedicles.
- Enter the vaginal mucosa at the level of the cervicovaginal junction, as demarcated by the vaginal cup. Use the RF instrument to make a circumferential colpotomy (Tech Fig. 10.5).
- Re-approximate the vaginal cuff with intracorporeal sutures of No. 0 polyglactin 910 or polydioxanone sutures.
- Perform cystoscopy to assess ureteral patency and to confirm bladder integrity.

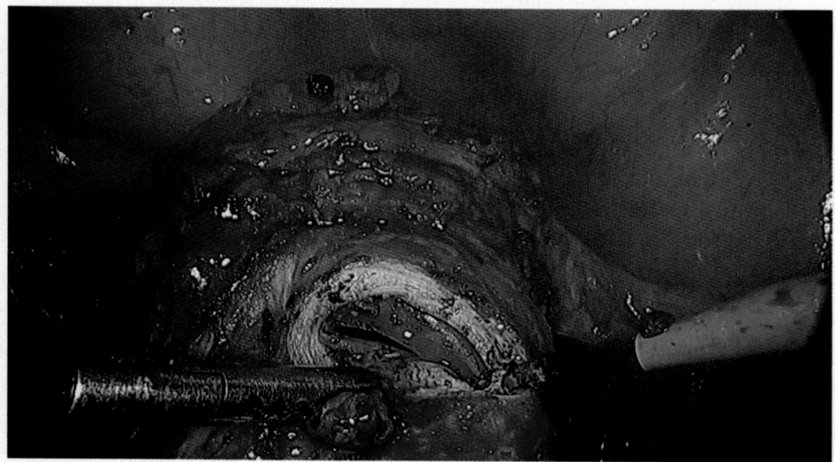

Tech Figure 10.5. Colpotomy. As delineated by the vaginal cup, a colpotomy is created at the cervicovaginal junction.

PEARLS AND PITFALLS—VAGINAL APPROACH

○ Insufficient descensus of the cervix

✖ It is crucial to apply downward traction by pulling on the tenaculum. Once the initial circumferential incision if performed, the surgeon should clamp and cut the uterosacral ligaments to improve descensus of the cervical stump.

○ Difficulty entering the peritoneum

✖ A vaginal trachelectomy can be performed entirely extraperitoneally. The key to success and to minimizing risk of bladder or rectal injury are to dissect and retract the bladder while traction is applied over the cervix.

○ Difficulty with anterior entry

✖ Place a finger through the posterior colpotomy and push anteriorly on the vesicocervical space. This delineates the anterior peritoneum and facilitates entry. Once entry is confirmed, examine the bladder carefully to confirm that no cystotomy has been made.

○ Bowel protruding from vaginal cuff

✖ Place a tagged, radio-opaque, laparotomy sponge in the peritoneal cavity to push the bowel cephalad. Use a right-angle retractor to apply gentle pressure on the sponge and to retract the bowel out of the surgical field.

PEARLS AND PITFALLS—LAPAROSCOPIC APPROACH

○ Unable to visualize stump

✖ It is essential to apply cephalad traction using a vaginal manipulator with a cervical cup (i.e., Koh cup) or with a vaginal sponge stick.

○ Difficulty identifying bladder

✖ Backfill the bladder with saline or dye-containing fluid (i.e., methylene blue) to identify the bladder margins.

POSTOPERATIVE CARE

- Following a vaginal or laparoscopic trachelectomy, the patient can be discharged to home the same day or be admitted overnight for observation.
- Ensure the patient can adequately void prior to discharge home or perform a voiding trial if more complex vaginal reconstruction is concomitantly performed.
- Advise pelvic rest for 4 to 6 weeks and caution the patient against heavy lifting greater than 15 pounds.
- Evaluate the patient in the office during the postoperative period and perform a postoperative pelvic examination to confirm cuff healing and re-approximation.

COMPLICATIONS

- Complications of trachelectomy are low and include:
  - Infection
  - Perioperative bleeding
  - Bowel injury
  - Bladder injury
  - Urinary retention
  - Injury to ureters
  - Cuff cellulitis

KEY READINGS

El-Zohairy MA. Trachelectomy: a review of 15 cases. *J Egypt Natl Canc Inst.* 2010;22(3):185–190.

Hilger WS, Pizarro AR, Magrina JF. Removal of the retained cervical stump. *Am J Obstet Gynecol.* 2005;193(6):2117–2121.

Learman LA, Summitt RL Jr, Varner RE, et al. A randomized comparison of total or supracervical hysterectomy: surgical complications and clinical outcomes. *Obstet Gynecol.* 2003;102(3):453–462.

Nezhat CH, Rogers JD. Robot-assisted laparoscopic trachelectomy after supracervical hysterectomy. *Fertil Steril.* 2008;90(3):850.e1–e3.

Nezhat CH, Nezhat F, Roemisch M, Seidman DS, Nezhat C. Laparoscopic trachelectomy for persistent pelvic pain and endometriosis after supracervical hysterectomy. *Fertil Steril.* 1996;66(6):925–928.

Parkar RB, Hassan MA, Otieno D, Baraza R. Laparoscopic trachelectomy for cervical stump 'carcinoma in situ'. *J Gynecol Endosc Surg.* 2011; 2(1):58–60.

Pasley WW. Trachelectomy: a review of fifty-five cases. *Am J Obstet Gynecol.* 1988;159(3):728–732.

Sheth SS. Vaginal excision of cervical stump. *J Obstet Gynaecol.* 2000; 20(5):523–524.

Section V

Adnexal Surgery

Ovarian Surgery

11

Chapter 11.1 Ovarian Cystectomy

Sharon Sutherland

GENERAL PRINCIPLES

Definition

- An ovarian cyst is a fluid-filled sac located on the surface or within the wall of the ovary. Simple cysts contain serous fluid with no opacities or solid elements, whereas complex cysts contain semisolid or solid elements.

Differential Diagnosis

- Benign ovarian: functional cyst, endometrioma, mature teratoma, serous cystadenoma, mucinous cystadenoma.
- Benign tubal: tubo-ovarian abscess, ectopic pregnancy, hydrosalpinx, paratubal cyst.
- Malignant ovarian: germ cell tumor, sex cord–stromal cell tumor, epithelial carcinoma of ovary or fallopian tube, metastatic tumors.
- Nongynecologic: diverticular or appendiceal abscess or mucocele, bladder or urethral diverticulum, peritoneal inclusion cyst.

Anatomic Considerations

- Major considerations in planning the surgical approach include patient habitus, history of prior abdominal or pelvic surgery, and comorbidities predictive of pelvic adhesive disease and risk of intraoperative injury to adjacent structures.
- Most patients, including those who are morbidly obese, are good candidates for minimally invasive surgery if there is a low suspicion for ovarian malignancy. Laparoscopic ovarian cystectomy with or without robotic assistance has been shown to reduce postoperative morbidity and recovery time compared to laparotomy.

Nonoperative Management

- Asymptomatic simple cysts up to 10 cm in diameter, coupled with a normal CA125 level, may be expectantly managed, even in postmenopausal patients.[1]
- Symptoms that may be related to an ovarian cyst include pelvic or lower back pain, dyspareunia, abdominal distension, and urinary frequency or urgency. For patients with mild symptoms, conservative management may include pelvic rest and over-the-counter analgesics.
- Most functional cysts, including corpus luteum, theca lutein cysts, and ovarian follicular cysts, may have increased vascularity, internal lace-like patterns, multilocular components, or they may be thin walled and unilocular.[2] Fortunately, they usually spontaneously resolve within 3 months. For patients presenting with symptomatic functional cysts, ovulation suppression with combination oral contraceptives may reduce the frequency of functional cysts and associated symptoms; however, oral contraceptives have not been shown to accelerate the resolution of existing functional ovarian cysts.[3]
- For patients with symptomatic, multiple functional cysts due to infertility treatment, ultrasound-guided cyst aspiration may be used to reduce symptoms pending the natural resolution of the cysts.
- Percutaneous drainage of cysts per ultrasound guidance is generally not effective in long-term resolution of nonfunctional cysts, and may be complicated by hemorrhage and injury to adjacent structures.[1]
- The most common benign complex cysts are mature teratomas or dermoid cysts and ovarian endometriomas. For detailed management of an ovarian endometrioma, see Chapter 12.
- In asymptomatic women with ultrasound findings that are pathognomonic for dermoid cysts,[2] expectant management may be offered if there are no other circumstances or signs that indicate risk for malignancy.[4] In a study of women who were expectantly managed, over 75% were followed without need for surgery for a median period of 12.6 months. Ovarian cystectomy was more likely undertaken in younger women, women of increasing parity, past history of ovarian cyst, bilateral ovarian cysts, or larger size of ovarian cyst.[4]
- When there is a high suspicion for malignancy, a careful presurgical evaluation should include an assessment of the patient's genetic risk, imaging studies, and serum tumor markers.
- Ovarian cystectomy is contraindicated if a mass is suspicious for cancer based on transvaginal ultrasound findings, CA125 levels, and/or clinical assessment. For suspected malignancy in women desiring fertility, preoperative or intraoperative consultation with gynecologic oncology as well as with an infertility specialist is recommended to optimize patient's treatment and to preserve fertility when possible.

IMAGING AND OTHER DIAGNOSTICS

- Transvaginal ultrasound is the primary modality for evaluation of ovarian cysts. Management of an asymptomatic cyst is largely based on ultrasound findings, which include the size and echotexture of the ovarian cyst, laterality, and any signs that increase likelihood of malignancy, such as thick (greater than 3 mm) septations, mural nodules, irregular borders, complex internal elements with Doppler flow, and free fluid in the pelvis. Unilocular cysts with thin walls, regular borders, and no internal echoes are very likely to be benign.
- CT and MRI of the pelvis should not be used routinely. They should be reserved for evaluating the pelvis for metastatic disease or to determine the etiology of nonovarian adnexal masses, such as pedunculated leiomyomata.
- Tumor markers: CA125 may be helpful in preoperative evaluation of ovarian cysts particularly in postmenopausal patients. A normal value for CA125 is less than 35 units/mL. CA125 is elevated in 80% of patients with epithelial ovarian cancer but is normal in 50% of patients with ovarian cancer isolated to the ovary. The specificity of CA125 for ovarian malignancy is lower in patients of reproductive age, as CA125 may be elevated in benign conditions such as endometriosis and pelvic infection as well as in nongynecologic inflammatory conditions. The specificity and sensitivity of CA125 are the highest among postmenopausal women with an adnexal mass. Other tumor markers that may be helpful include quantitative beta human chorionic gonadotropin (beta-hCG), lactate dehydrogenase (LDH), and alpha-fetoprotein (AFP). Elevations in these markers may indicate increased risk for germ cell tumors, while elevation in inhibin A and B may indicate increased risk for granulosa cell tumor.
- Cervical cultures: For patients presenting with pelvic pain suspicious for pelvic inflammatory disease, cultures should be collected and empiric antibiotic therapy is recommended per CDC guidelines. Surgical exploration may be necessary in patients with suspected tubo-ovarian abscess who do not improve clinically with conservative management.
- For patients with suspected ectopic pregnancy based on menstrual history, imaging, and laboratory studies, evaluation should be undertaken for possible medical management, with surgical management reserved for those who are unstable or who do not meet criteria for medical management.

PREOPERATIVE PLANNING

- A medical history should include information about menstrual pattern, contraceptive use, pregnancy, and gynecologic conditions including sexually transmitted diseases. A history of gastrointestinal, breast, or other pelvic malignancy may indicate a risk of metastasis to the ovary. Advancing age and menopausal status increase the risk of malignancy in women with adnexal masses.[1]
- A surgical history should include specific detail about prior abdominal and/or pelvic surgeries as well as anesthesia complications or concerns.
- A family history should include specific detail about gynecologic, urologic, breast, and gastrointestinal cancers, and referral to medical genetics should be considered if there is suspicion that patient may be at risk for heritable cancers.
- Prior to surgery, the patient should be counseled:
  - About nonoperative as well as operative treatments for her clinical situation. In general, ovarian cystectomy should not be first-line treatment for women of reproductive age with functional cysts unless there is suspicion for ovarian torsion or the patient has failed conservative management.
  - About the risks of surgery, which include anesthesia complications, hemorrhage and need for blood products, infection, intraoperative injury to gastrointestinal, genitourinary, vascular and neural structures, and unplanned oophorectomy and/or salpingectomy with potential impact on fertility.
  - Conversion to laparotomy may be needed to complete the procedure safely, and its effect on her postoperative course.
  - Incorrect laterality assigned in imaging reports occurs; therefore, the patient should be consented about this possibility and for removal of the affected adnexal cyst.
  - Ovarian cystectomy may require conversion to oophorectomy with or without salpingectomy if there is uncontrollable bleeding, suspected malignancy, abscess, or necrosis.
  - About the possibility of malignancy and any plan for intraoperative or delayed evaluation by a gynecologic or surgical oncologist in the event of malignancy. Unless there is a surgical emergency, primary excision of suspected ovarian malignancy should be undertaken by a surgeon with specialized training in evaluation and management of gynecologic cancers.
  - There is a potential to decrease fertility after cystectomy especially for endometriomas due to excessive use of electrosurgery or inadvertent removal of normal tissue.
- Patients with significant comorbidities should undergo preoperative medical and anesthesia evaluation. For patients with significant comorbidities, surgery may need to be delayed to allow for proper preoperative optimization.
- Oophorectomy should be considered in perimenopausal and postmenopausal women undergoing surgery for ovarian cysts due to increased risk of malignancy with advancing age and as well as risk of recurrence of benign ovarian cysts.

SURGICAL MANAGEMENT

- Ovarian cystectomy is the treatment of choice for symptomatic benign-appearing cysts in women of reproductive age that do not resolve with conservative management.

Approach

- Laparoscopic approach is the gold-standard approach for suspected benign ovarian cystectomy.
- Laparotomy should be undertaken as clinically indicated due to large mass size, high suspicion for malignancy or known extensive adhesive disease, and other factors, such as combined cases for colorectal disease. Laparotomy should be the approach of choice if the surgical team has insufficient equipment, training, skill, and/or experience to safely attempt minimally invasive surgery.
- Ultrasound-guided transabdominal or transvaginal drainage of cysts may be considered for preoperative preparation in cases of large cysts with low suspicion for malignancy or for management of symptoms in patients with multiple functional cysts resulting from ovulation induction for infertility.

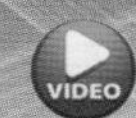

Procedures and Techniques (Video 11.1.1)

Operative huddle and patient positioning and surgical preparation (please see Chapter 5).

Laparoscopic ovarian cystectomy with or without robotic assistance

Vaginal field

- A Foley catheter should be placed sterilely in the bladder and secured to the drape to prevent traction on the urethra during the procedure. Position the urine collection bag so that the anesthesia team or circulating nurse can monitor the patient's urine output during the procedure.
- **For patients with a uterus, place a Hulka tenaculum into the uterus for uterine manipulation.**
- **A minimum of three trocars are used to perform ovarian cystectomy** and include a 12-mm trocar to accommodate a tissue extraction bag. Two additional 5-mm ports are used to decrease neuropathic injury and do not require fascial closure. In pregnant patients, patients with a large pelvic–abdominal mass or those with a previous midline incision, a left upper quadrant primary entry is recommended.

Pelvic field

Inspect the pelvis and collect pelvic cytology. Irrigate the pelvis with saline and collect pelvic washings for cytology. Inspect all pelvic structures and assess for adhesions, endometriosis, excrescences, or implants suspicious for malignancy. Lyse adhesions only as needed to achieve visualization. If malignancy is suspected, seek intraoperative consultation with gynecologic or surgical oncologist prior to proceeding with ovarian cystectomy or oophorectomy. If surgical oncology is not available, abort the procedure after collection of photographs, washings, and nondisruptive tissue biopsies, and refer the patient to a gynecologic oncologist for primary excision and staging.

Inspect the adnexa and identify the ovary containing the cyst

Using an atraumatic grasper, retract the utero-ovarian ligament.

Identify the ipsilateral ureter and vasculature

This ensures that these structures are safely away from the surgical field (Tech Fig. 11.1.1).

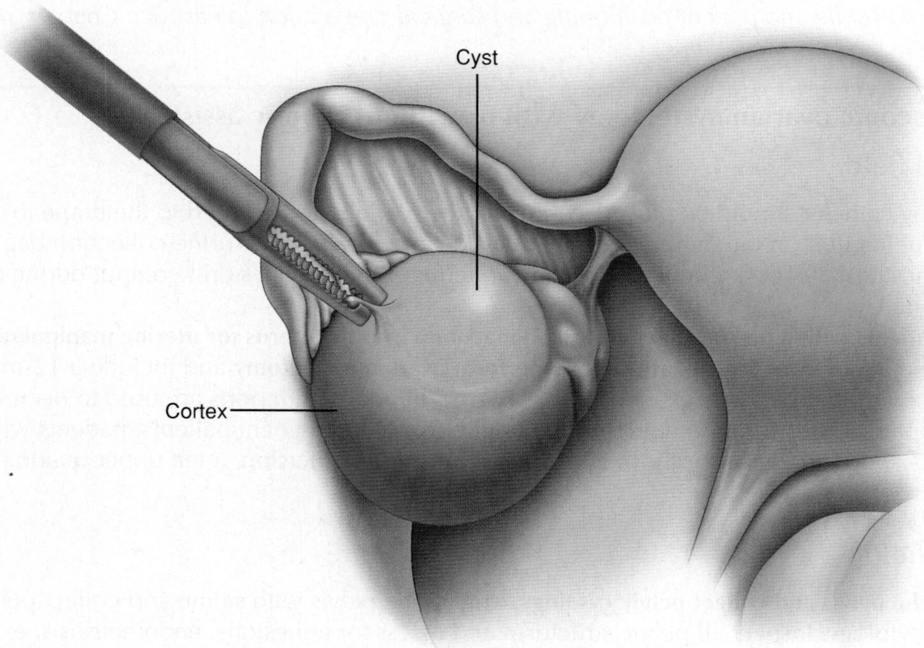

Tech Figure 11.1.1. Identify the ovarian cyst. Identify the ipsilateral ureter and vasculature to ensure that these structures are safely away from the surgical field.

Identify an optimal area for ovarian incision

Avoid the vascular hilum of the ovary (the meso-ovarium) and the ipsilateral fallopian tube (Tech Fig. 11.1.2).

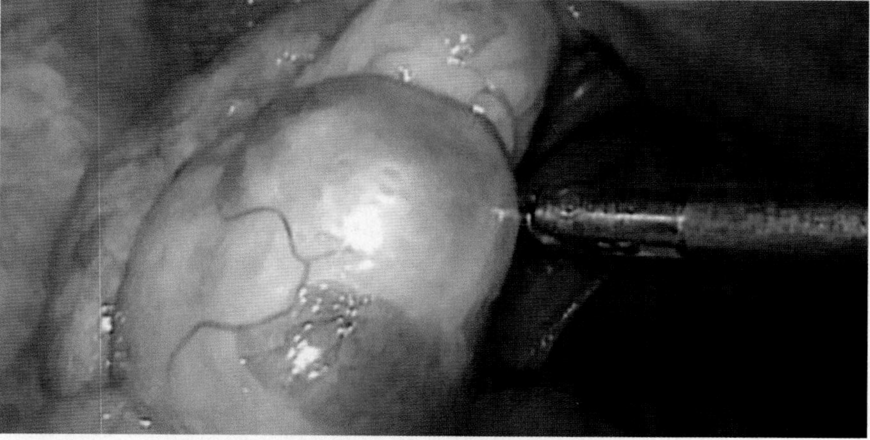

Tech Figure 11.1.2. Identify the optimal area for ovarian incision. Avoid the vascular hilum of the ovary (the meso-ovarium) and the ipsilateral fallopian tube.

Incise the ovarian cortex

Incise with the use of an electrosurgical instrument such as a monopolar needle set at low power (10 W) or bipolar instrument (Tech Fig. 11.1.3).

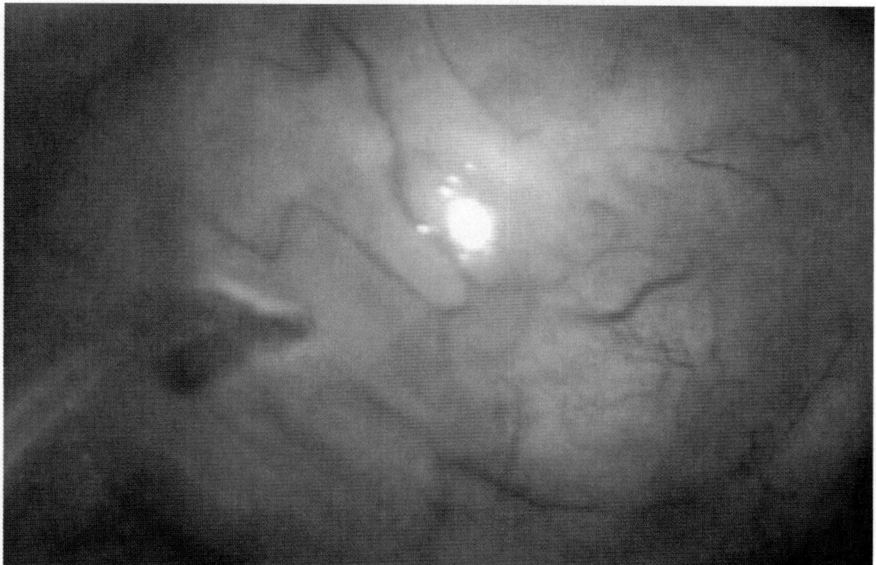

Tech Figure 11.1.3. Incise the ovarian cortex with the use of an electrocautery electrosurgical instrument such as a monopolar needle set at low power (10 W) or bipolar instrument. Choose an instrument with a small contact point, as tissue damage increases with increasing area contact with the electrode.

The size of the contact point of the instrument to the tissue is important, as tissue damage increases with the increasing size of the electrode.[5] The degree of tissue damage caused by electrical energy is also determined by the waveforms, the density of the current, and the duration of the energy application: longer application of current is associated with increased tissue damage.[5] Increasing levels of power also increase the degree of tissue damage.[5] Monopolar instruments such as monopolar needle, hook, or scissors should be used in pure cut or blended cut setting to dissect with minimal destruction of adjacent tissues. Pure cut setting has high-density, low-voltage current that minimizes thermal spread, while coagulation setting has low-density, high-voltage current with greater thermal spread and risk of destruction or injury to adjacent tissue. Blend 1 adds some coagulation effect to pure cut setting, while Blend 3 adds some cutting effect to a pure coagulation setting, while Blend 2 balances cutting and coagulation. In general, a lower power setting such as 45 W should be used, with increasing wattage only if a lower setting is ineffective. The harmonic scalpel, which cuts with high-frequency vibration, is also an option that minimizes damage to adjacent tissues.

Grasp the edge of the cortex with an allis, and extend the incision along the ovarian axis to expose the underlying cyst from pole to pole

In some cases, the suction–irrigation cannula can be introduced in between the cyst and cortex and fluid introduced to develop the plane (Tech Fig. 11.1.4).

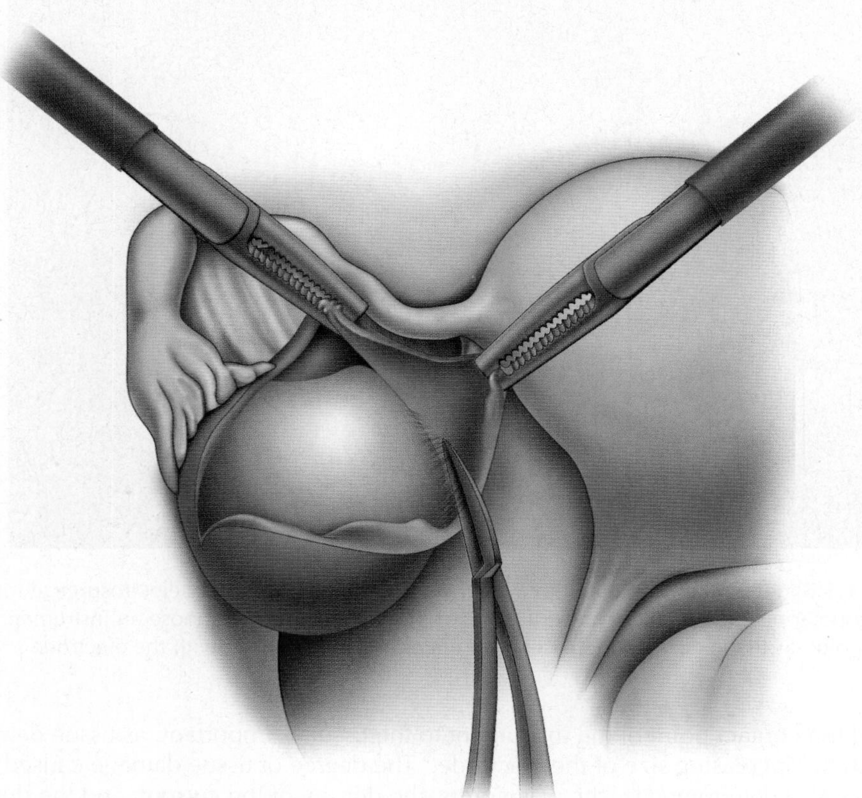

Tech Figure 11.1.4. Grasp the edge of the ovarian cortex and use a suction irrigator to irrigate and to develop a plane between the cortex and the cyst. Scissors or a monopolar needle may be used to extend the incision along the ovarian axis to expose the underlying cyst.

Lyse adhesion to the ovarian cortex with a blunt probe or suction irrigator tip

- **Lysis of adhesions should be done before the cystectomy.** The cyst wall easily yields to gentle pressure as there is little fibrosis compared to an endometrioma (Tech Fig. 11.1.5).
- Excessive use of electrosurgery causes destruction of the ovarian stroma and decreases fertility.
- Apply traction and countertraction (see Tech Fig. 11.1.6). Use blunt dissection and/or sharp dissection, applying electrocautery to bleeding vessels as needed while enucleating the intact cyst away from the normal ovarian stroma.

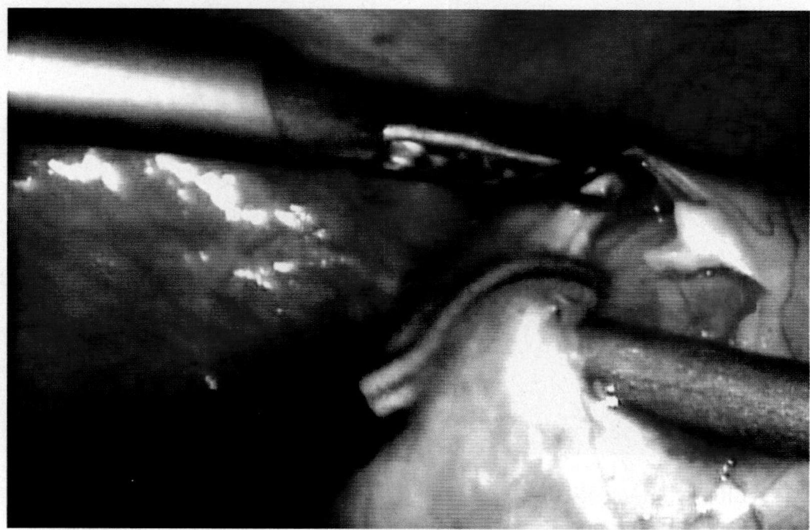

Tech Figure 11.1.5. Aqua dissection and adhesiolysis of the ovarian cortex with a blunt probe. Lysis of adhesions should be done before the cystectomy and easily yields to gentle pressure as there is little fibrosis.

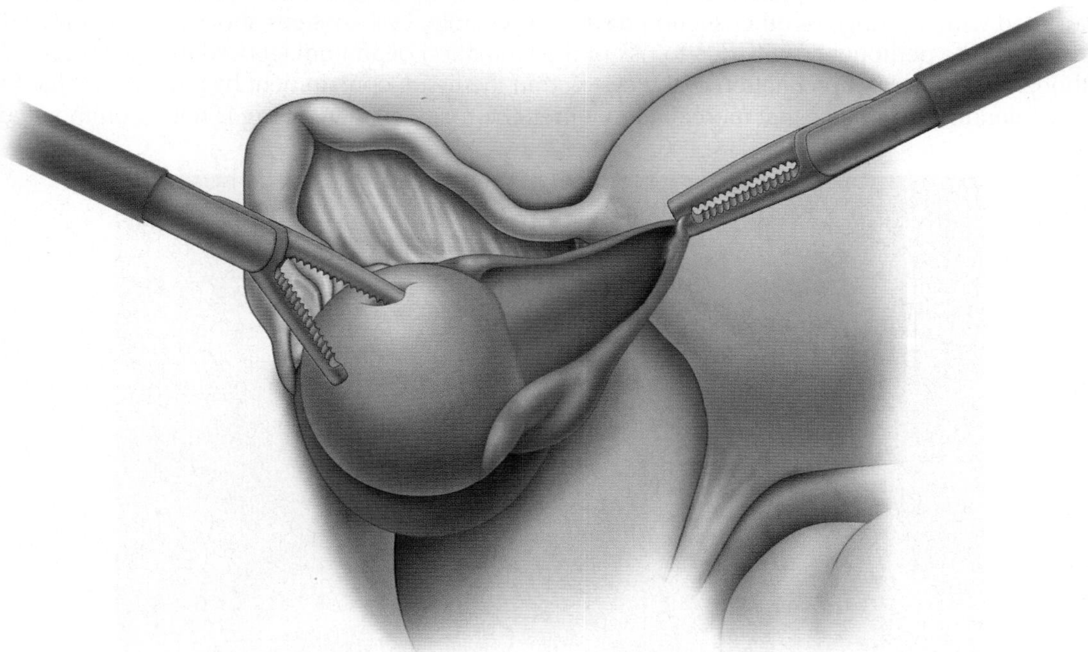

Tech Figure 11.1.6. Apply traction and countertraction. Use blunt dissection and/or sharp dissection, applying electrocautery to bleeding vessels as needed while enucleating the intact cyst away from the normal ovarian stroma.

Use traction and countertraction to enucleate the intact cyst away from the normal ovarian stroma (Tech Fig. 11.1.6)

Continue to bluntly enucleate the cyst until all ovarian attachments are lysed (Tech Fig. 11.1.7).

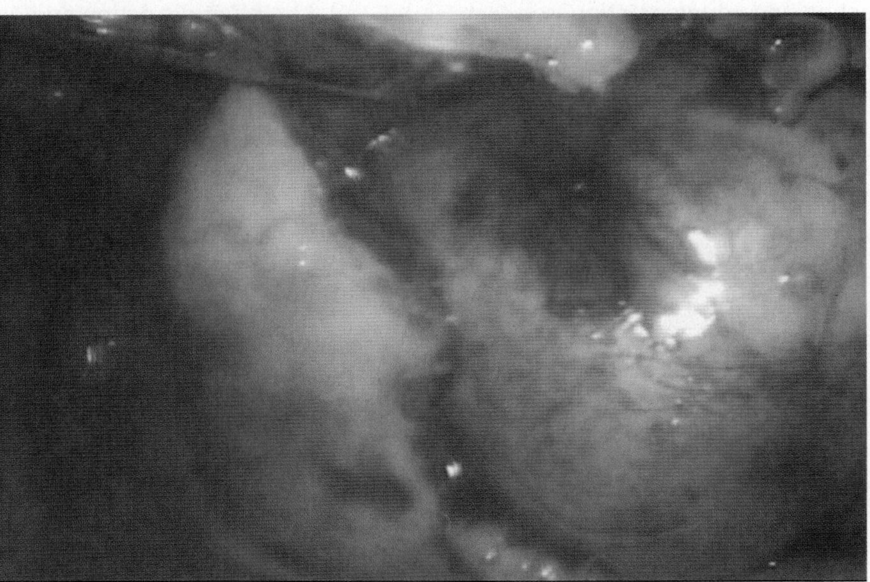

Tech Figure 11.1.7. Bluntly enucleate the cyst.

Place the cyst in a tissue extraction bag (Tech Fig. 11.1.8)

To facilitate removal from the abdominal cavity, the tissue extraction bag may be partially exteriorized at the skin, carefully opened to expose the surface of the cyst, and the cyst fluid may then be evacuated with a syringe or other suction device. If possible, cyst contents should not be allowed to spill into the peritoneal cavity due to risk of dissemination of an undiagnosed malignancy. Although we perform morcellation of the cyst within the tissue containment bag, be aware that the device manufacturer states that morcellation within the tissue extraction bag is not recommended.

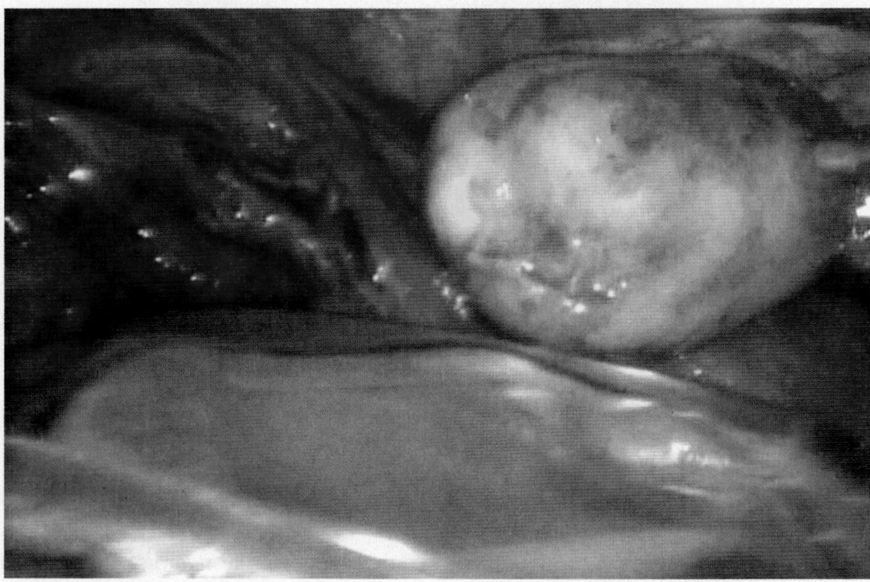

Tech Figure 11.1.8. Place the cyst within an endocatch bag for removal.

The manufacturer of the tissue extraction bag states that the surgeon should extend the abdominal wall incision to accommodate removal of the bag with the specimen intact.

For complex cysts with solid components, such as mature teratomas, extend the port site to ensure the bag does not rupture due to compression of solid material in the cyst. Rupture of the extraction bag will result in spillage of the cyst contents, leading to prolonged evacuation of extruded material from the peritoneal cavity, possible dissemination of undiagnosed malignancy, and the potential for retained material from a ruptured tissue extraction bag.

Irrigate the cyst bed and achieve hemostasis

- Use sparse radiofrequency electrical energy to achieve hemostasis. Sutures can be used within the cyst to achieve hemostasis. Do not place them through the cortex. Hemostatic agents such as FloSeal can also be used.
- Once the cyst bed is hemostatic, it is not necessary to re-approximate the ovarian edges. Although some areas of the remaining ovary will be very thin, stromal tissue should not be removed or trimmed as this may reduce oocyte reserve (see Tech Fig. 11.1.9).

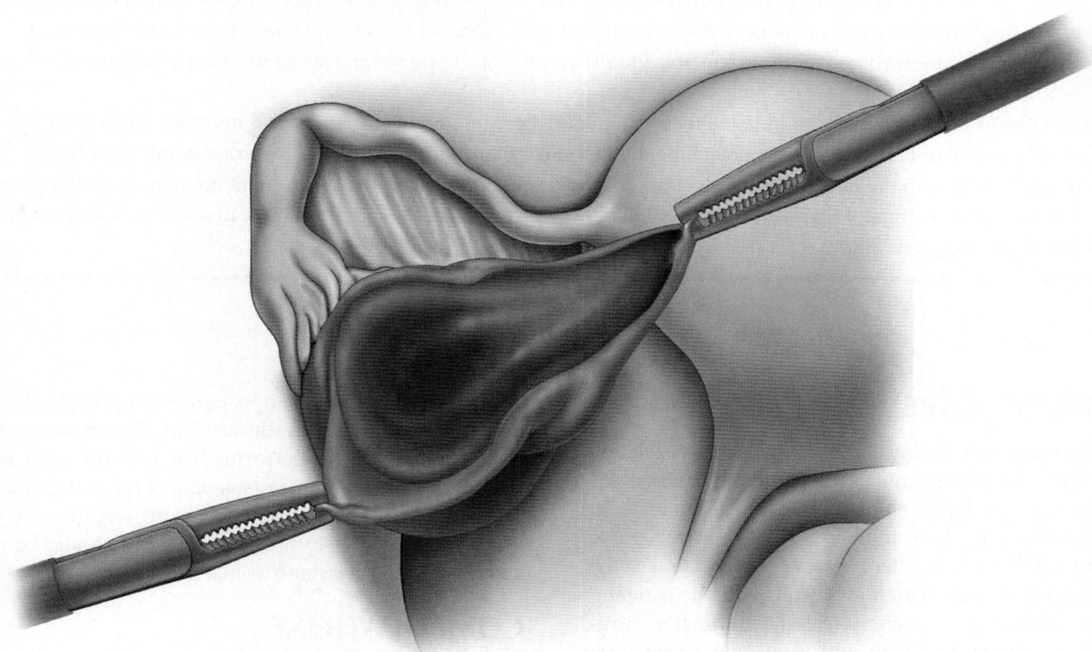

Tech Figure 11.1.9. Once the cyst bed is hemostatic, it is not necessary to re-approximate the ovarian edges. Although some areas of the remaining ovary will be very thin, stromal tissue should not be removed or trimmed as this may reduce oocyte reserve.

Irrigate and suction

- **Irrigate and suction the pelvis of any debris and perform a final survey to** ensure no extruded material or foreign bodies remain.
- Once hemostasis is confirmed, apply anti-adhesion barrier such as Interceed.
  - If you apply Interceed, the cyst bed must be perfectly hemostatic and irrigation fluid must be removed. The sheet of Interceed should be wrapped around the ovary alone. Do not wrap the tube with the ovary.
- Allow the pneumoperitoneum to escape and perform the first instrument and sponge count.
- Re-approximate fascial incisions greater than 10 mm and skin incisions.
- Remove instruments from the vaginal field and confirm hemostasis.

PEARLS AND PITFALLS

- ○ Correct plane identification is crucial to complete cystectomy. Identify and grasp the cyst wall and excise it from the surrounding ovarian stroma using traction–countertraction.
- ✕ Large dermoid cysts often rupture after extensive manipulation. Reduce content spillage by quickly grasping and elevating the leading edge of the cyst wall to avoid further extrusion and contamination. It the cyst is moderate in size, suction the contents directly from the cyst itself and avoid spillage into the pelvic cavity. If the cyst is very large and there is the potential for continual spillage, use an Endo-loop to secure the cyst wall closed and continue with the cystectomy.
- ○ Take the time to identify each plane. This improves surgical technique, reduces follicle damage, and decreases blood loss.
- ✕ About half of patients with ovarian torsion diagnosed at laparoscopy have had normal Doppler flow in an ovarian cyst demonstrated on a recent ultrasound study, so laparoscopy should be undertaken if there is a high suspicion for torsion based on clinical findings. Ovarian torsion typically presents with sudden onset severe pelvic pain and symptoms of peritoneal irritation such as nausea and/or vomiting. In some cases, patients will report similar episodes of pain for brief periods of time for days or weeks. Initial vascular findings in ovarian torsion include constriction in venous and lymphatic flow and may lead to ovarian edema, cyanosis, and tenderness to palpation. When encountering torsion in a patient at low risk for malignancy, detorsing the ovary should be undertaken followed by ovarian cystectomy to reduce risk of future torsion. Care should be taken to retain ovarian stroma even if tissue viability is questionable. Despite constricted blood flow, cyanotic ovarian tissue likely retains some viable stroma and should be salvaged to preserve ovarian function in women of reproductive age.
- ○ Unilocular cysts under 10 cm in diameter are generally benign, and in women with a normal CA125 level, it is permissible to drain the cyst laparoscopically to reduce morbidity from a large laparotomy incision. Make a small incision in the cyst surface with a laparoscopic scissor or monopolar instrument, then immediately insert a suction–irrigator tip in the cyst opening to quickly evacuate the cyst fluid. Cyst fluid is rarely helpful in histologic diagnosis and may be discarded.

POSTOPERATIVE CARE

- Initial postoperative care is dictated by surgical approach and by intraoperative or postoperative complications. Please see postoperative care for laparoscopic surgery in Chapter 5. In general, patients should be routinely evaluated in the office anywhere from 2 to 6 weeks after surgery for inspection of the incision sites and to review pathology results with the patient.
- For patients undergoing uncomplicated, minimally invasive surgery, discharge to home with oral pain medication is expected within 4 to 6 hours after surgery. Patients who experience increased perioperative bleeding, intractable nausea and/or vomiting, pain not controlled by oral analgesics, insufficient urine output, or other symptoms that preclude discharge to home, extended recovery is indicated. All patients should be given explicit instructions and contact information to seek urgent follow-up care in the event of severe pain, intractable vomiting, heavy bleeding, wound dehiscence, fever, or urinary retention.

OUTCOMES

Drainage alone or partial excision of ovarian cysts increases the likelihood that cyst fluid will re-accumulate and that the patient's symptoms will recur. Excision of an ovarian cyst with obliteration of any nonresectable cyst tissue reduces the likelihood of cyst recurrence. For patients with undiagnosed malignancy, spillage of cyst contents upstages the malignancy and worsens prognosis for survival. Therefore, ovarian cystectomy should not be performed in patients with multiple risk factors or signs/symptoms suspicious for malignancy. In young, reproductive-age women who desire fertility and suffer from symptomatic, large cysts, every attempt should be made to salvage remaining ovarian stroma.

COMPLICATIONS

- Known risks of ovarian cystectomy by any approach include anesthesia complications; hemorrhage and need for blood products; infection; intraoperative injury to gastrointestinal, genitourinary, vascular, and neural structures; and unplanned oophorectomy and/or salpingectomy with potential impact on fertility.
- In cases of excessive bleeding from the ovarian cyst bed, apply pressure to the area. If necessary, place a deep suture to re-approximate the tissue. If bleeding is localized and appears to be general oozing related to extensive dissection, consider applying a hemostatic agent like FloSeal.

The ureter is at particular risk of injury if there are adhesions of the ovary to the pelvic sidewall. Adhesiolysis and retroperitoneal dissection may be necessary to expose the ovary prior to ovarian cystectomy. For information about dissection of an ovary encased with extensive adhesions, refer to Chapter 11.3 Ovarian Remnant resection.

KEY REFERENCES

1. American College of Obstetricians and Gynecologists (ACOG). *Management of Adnexal Masses.* Washington, DC: American College of Obstetricians and Gynecologists (ACOG); 2013. (ACOG practice bulletin; no. 83.)
2. Levine D, Brown DL, Andreotti RF, et al. Management of asymptomatic ovarian and other adnexal cysts imaged at US: society of radiologists in ultrasound consensus conference statement. *Radiology.* 2010;256(3):943–954.
3. Grimes DA, Jones LB, Lopez LM, Schulz KF. Oral contraceptives for functional ovarian cysts. *Cochrane Database Syst Rev.* 2014;4:CD006134.
4. Hoo WL, Yazbek J, Holland T, Mavrelos D, Tong EN, Jurkovic D. Expectant management of ultrasonically diagnosed ovarian dermoid cysts: is it possible to predict outcome? *Ultrasound Obstet Gynecol.* 2010;36:235–240.
5. Davison JM, Zamah NM. *Electrosurgery: Principles, Biologic Effects and Results in Female Reproductive Surgery. Global Library of Women's Medicine, an educational platform for International Federation for Gynecology and Obstetrics.* 2008. 1756–22282008; 10.3843/GLOWM.10021

Chapter 11.2 Oophorectomy

Robert DeBernardo

GENERAL PRINCIPLES

Definition

Oophorectomy is the surgical removal of the adnexa or a portion of the adnexa. Typically this will involve removing the entire ovary and fallopian tube (adnexa) along with its vascular supply; however, in some conditions removing the fallopian tube alone, the ovary, or a portion of the ovary itself may be indicated. This chapter will focus upon removal of the entire adnexa recognizing that the techniques described can be applied to remove any portion of the adnexa.

Differential Diagnosis

- Prophylactic risk reducing surgery for breast, ovarian, or other genetic condition
- Benign adnexal tumors (serous or mucinous cystadenomas, teratomas, adenofibromas, among others)
- Endometriosis or endometriomas
- Tubo-ovarian abscess
- Borderline ovarian tumors
- Malignant ovarian tumors (epithelial, germ cell, or stromal tumors)

Anatomic Considerations

The steps of surgical removal of the ovary will be informed by the anatomy. Although it seems obvious, the anatomic relationships of the ovary to the uterus, ureter, iliac vessels, and bowel will to one degree or another become altered in pathologic situations. The degree of aberration will vary from case to case and across pathologic conditions; however, the basic surgical approach needs not vary. A detailed understanding of the normal anatomy of the adnexa and the surrounding structures is essential and will inform the surgeon on how to best approach the particular pathology at hand. The first step in any surgery is to restore the anatomy to normal. This can be especially important when preforming difficult surgery to remove the adnexa. Once adhesions are lysed and normal anatomic relationships reestablished, the level of complexity has been reduced allowing the surgeon to more easily remove the ovary.

The ovary is a retroperitoneal organ that resides in the pelvis. It is attached by a vascular pedicle to the uterine cornua (Fig. 11.2.1). Its arterial blood supply, however, originates off the aorta just distal to the renal vessels. The venous return runs adjacent to and inferior to the gonadal artery. These veins can become engorged in some pathologic conditions and often have multiple tributaries. The right gonadal vein empties into the vena cava directly; however, the left ovarian vein empties into the left renal vein (Fig. 11.2.2). The gonadal vessels travel toward the pelvis parallel to and adjacent to the ureter. Just like the ureter, the gonadal vessels cross the pelvic brim at the level of the bifurcation of the iliac vessels. The gonadal vessels are lateral and superior to the ureter at the pelvic brim. This relationship is difficult to appreciate unless the retroperitoneum overlying the gonadal vessels is opened (Fig. 11.2.3). The gonadal vessels insert into the ovary and, after passing by the ovary anastomose into the utero-ovarian pedicle at the cornua. The utero-ovarian pedicle contributes blood supply to the ovary and fallopian tube along its course. Again, while it may be difficult to appreciate, a layer of peritoneum covers the ovary and its blood supply, tube, and uterus.[1]

The concept of "restoring anatomy to normal" is predicated upon a complete understanding of these anatomic relationships. Expert pelvic surgeons understand and use the relationship between the gynecologic organs, the rectum, and the genital urinary system to inform their surgical decisions. The most important anatomic concept to recognize is that the bladder, ureters, and rectum, as well as the ovaries, tubes, and uterus are NOT located in the pelvis but in the retroperitoneum (Fig. 11.2.4). The

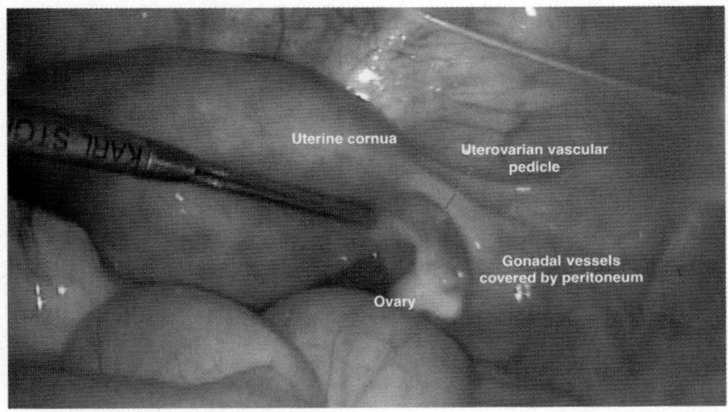

Figure 11.2.1. Utero-ovarian pedicle. The adnexa attach at the uterine cornua and share a rich vascular anastomosis with the uterine blood supply.

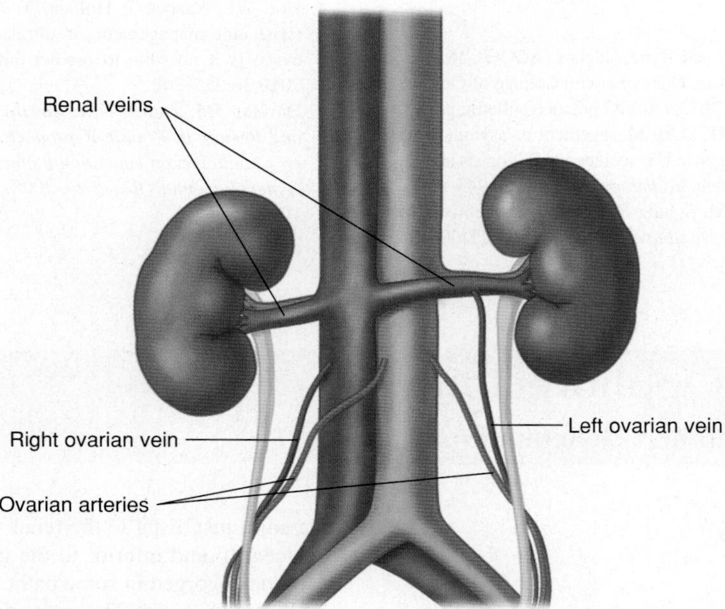

Figure 11.2.2. Ovarian vasculature. The ovarian arteries originate from the aorta beneath the renal vessels. Venous return on the right empties directly in the vena cava and on the left into the left renal vein.

rectosigmoid and ileum are the only true pelvic organs once we understand this anatomic relationship. In reality, for many operations this distinction is irrelevant. However, for complex ovarian surgery, it is critical to perform the operation quickly, safely, and with assurance that there has been no unintended injuries.

While this is a subtle distinction, it is an important one. When tackling a complex pelvic surgery with multiple adhesions and perhaps a pelvic mass adherent to the pelvic sidewall, recognizing this relationship will enable the surgeon to proceed judiciously. Lysing adhesions becomes easier when one recognizes that adhesions between loops of small bowel and to the rectosigmoid are inherently different than those to the adnexa or uterus. In fact, since there are no normal attachments of the ovaries to the true pelvic organs, these can be easily managed by following the course of bowel loops and sharply lysing adhesions free from the ovarian tumor or uterus. A systemic approach is often the best, beginning where the anatomy is normal and proceeding toward areas of complexity. With this approach, the surgeon continues until the anatomy becomes confusing, at which point

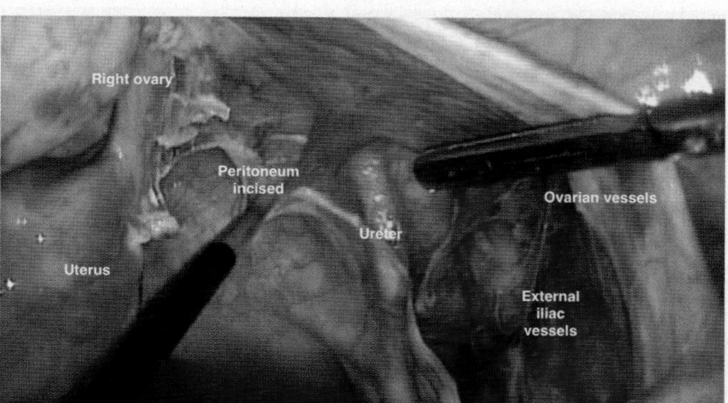

Figure 11.2.3. Pelvic sidewall. The peritoneum overlying the right pelvic sidewall is incised demonstrating the ureter, external iliac vessels, and the gonadal vessels (deviated laterally).

the focus changes to another area where the adhesions are less complex. With this approach, areas of adhesions that were initially difficult to lyse successfully, can more easily be managed (see **Video 11.2.1, Part A**). Careful dissection is important with attention to hemostasis as the planes between loops of bowel and the adnexa can be easily masked by blood. Sharp dissection offers some advantages over cautery because when the surgeon is in the correct anatomic plane there is little if any bleeding. In addition, there is no concern of thermal spread from cautery. Energy devices, such as harmonic or ligasure seal peritoneal edges together, are generally counterproductive when tackling adhesions.

Nonoperative Management

Nonoperative management of an adnexal mass is appropriate in certain situations and should be individualized based upon the patient. While conservative management of adnexal masses can occupy an entire chapter, a few guiding principles are worth discussing. In general, symptomatic or complex lesions should be managed surgically. In addition, an adnexal mass of 8 cm or larger is unlikely to resolve spontaneously and is at higher risk of torsion, making observation in these situations of questionable benefit. The risk of surgical intervention to manage the patient's symptoms and assess for malignancy must always be balanced by medical comorbidities, desire for future fertility, and to some extent loss of hormonal function. Repeat imaging at 6 weeks in premenopausal woman is reasonable when the adnexal mass is thought to be a hemorrhagic or functional cyst. If this lesion is still present at that point, it is less likely to resolve and surgical intervention is generally warranted.

IMAGING AND OTHER DIAGNOSTICS

- Imaging plays an increasingly important role of assessment of ovarian tumors. The most common preoperative imaging is ultrasound assessment. Not only is this noninvasive,

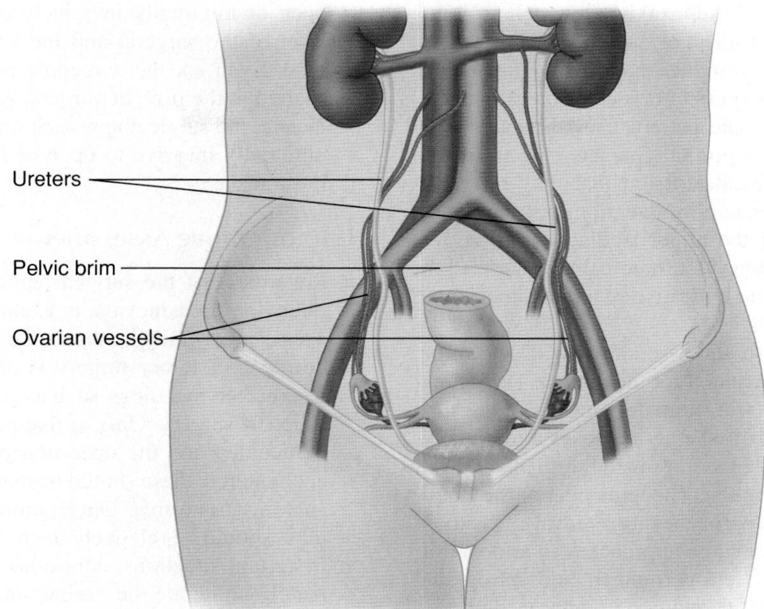

Figure 11.2.4. Course of ovarian vessels. The ovarian artery and veins run in the retroperitoneum adjacent to the ureter and cross the pelvic brim prior to supplying the ovary and anastomosing with the utero-ovarian pedicle.

inexpensive, and universally available, it does a reasonably good job of characterizing features of the ovarian mass. Simple cystic masses are almost always benign regardless of the size. The role of surgical intervention will vary based upon the patient; however, simple cystic masses that are 8 cm or greater or those with solid components are unlikely to resolve spontaneously. In most cases these should be removed. Based on ultrasound assessment, "complex" ovarian masses will encompass a broad range of tumors from a simple cystic lesion with septation(s) to a largely solid lesion with multiple small cysts. Many benign tumors can appear fairly complex on ultrasound such as endometriomas, adenofibromas, and mucinous cystadenomas. Additional imaging, such as MRI, rarely adds much to distinguish between these entities and cannot rule out malignancy. CT scans may be helpful in some situations. In reality, they do not offer any additional information about the adnexal mass; however, they can identify other high-risk features that the surgeon may need to be aware, such as hydronephrosis, ascites, adenopathy, omental implants, and other findings suggestive of ovarian malignancy.[2,3]

- Tumor markers are used frequently in the preoperative assessment of a pelvic mass. CA125, CEA, and CA19-9 are commonly ordered and may help appropriately triage patients to an oncologist. It is fairly common to see elevation of CA125 and to a lesser extent CEA and CA19-9 in patients with benign adnexal masses; however, these are rarely more than one or two standard deviations above the normal range. The use of a panel of tumor markers, such as ROMA, may increase specificity. A 40-year-old woman with a complex mass, history of worsening pain over several years, and a CA125 of 80 more likely has endometriosis than an ovarian malignancy. Nonetheless, care should be exercised in these situations. A management plan ought to be addressed preoperatively with the patient if malignancy is identified at the time of surgery. In certain situations, immediate assessment and management with gynecologic oncology is feasible. In situations where gynecologic oncology is not readily available and malignancy is identified at surgery, the best approach is often to make a diagnosis (remove the ovary or simply obtain a biopsy) and close the patient deferring definitive management to a later time. Studies have shown that the quality of surgery in women with ovarian cancer directly impacts survival. Patients managed by general surgeons, urologist, and gynecologist working in concert to stage or debulk ovarian tumors do not do as well as those managed by gynecologic oncology.[4]

PREOPERATIVE PLANNING

- Pathology that involves the adnexa will vary from relatively simple ovarian cystic lesions to complex masses that are densely adherent to the colon or pelvic sidewall. Obliteration of the cul-de-sac can present a difficult challenge to overcome when removing a pelvic mass. Often, while the surgeon may suspect they will be facing a complex case the question is how best to properly prepare. In some circumstances, it may be best to refer to patient to a specialist, especially if malignancy is a concern.
- Careful review of the patient's medical and surgical history is as important as preoperative imaging and tumor markers and the best place to start the preoperative assessment. While the differential diagnosis of an adnexal mass is broad, reviewing the patient's history can often time narrow down the possibilities. A reasonable approach is to first determine if the mass is likely benign or malignant. Age alone can be a useful piece of information, as epithelial ovarian cancer is quite rare in women younger than 40 without a personal or suspicious family history of malignancy regardless of tumor markers or complexity reported on sonography. Further, masses in prepubertal or adolescent patients carry a higher risk of malignancy and often should be approached cautiously. Menstrual

history is informative as well. Adnexal masses such as granulosa cell tumors, adenofibromas, or Sertoli–Leydig tumors among others may produce hormones that can alter menstrual function as well as produce symptoms such as breast tenderness, deepening voice, or male pattern hair distribution. A history of pain is another important characteristic to investigate. Acute pain may indicate torsion that may not only impact the urgency of operative intervention, but may alter sonographic appearance of the tumor leading one to be far more concerned of malignancy. Chronic pain in association with a complex mass may be indicative of an endometrioma and advanced endometriosis.

- The preoperative impression and assessment will determine the appropriate surgery best suited for the patient. This along with the surgeon's skill set will ultimately influence the surgical approach. Regardless of whether one uses a minimally invasive or an open approach, the steps in the surgical removal of the ovary should be the similar. The remainder of the chapter will focus on surgical approaches to removal of ovarian tumors. In general, there are three approaches to removal of the ovary: transperitoneal, retroperitoneal, and retrograde resection. Each has its benefits and certain approaches may be better suited to certain pathologic or anatomic conditions identified in the operating room. An expert pelvic surgeon should have all three approaches in their armamentarium.

SURGICAL MANAGEMENT

- The surgical removal of the adnexa will vary depending upon the nature of the pathology, patient characteristics, and the scope of other procedures that are being performed at the time of surgery. The indications for surgery will vary as will the complexity of the operation. When the adnexa are removed for prophylaxis such as in woman at high risk for ovarian cancer, the anatomy is generally normal and the operation is often straightforward. In women with benign adnexal masses, the surgery can be quite a bit more challenging depending upon the pathology found in the operating room. Some of the most complicated and difficult procedures are in women with advanced endometriosis or cancer. Prior surgery, diverticular disease or other conditions may lead to adhesive disease compounding the difficulty of oophorectomy. The surgeon's preoperative assessment is essential to plan the best surgical approach and to council the patient preoperatively regarding the extent of dissection and possible complications. After factoring all these variables, the surgeon then can select the best surgical approach.
- The surgical approach—open, laparoscopic, or robotic—is best decided upon after consideration of the aforementioned factors balanced by the surgeon's skill set. Minimally invasive surgery is generally associated with less postoperative pain, quicker recovery and return to baseline functional status, lower EBL, and lower infection rates. Unfortunately, in some instances, there may be higher complication rates such as unintended bowel or GU injury especially when tackling a challenging case. Resulting complications are as likely influenced by the surgeon's comfort and skill level with laparoscopy or robotics as they are with the pathology identified at the time of surgery. That being said, a good surgeon is aware of their limitations and should choose an approach that will best serve their patient. With this in mind, it may be equally reasonable to approach the same problem either open or minimally invasively depending upon the comfort level of the surgeon and the anticipated complexity of the case. Even so, the surgeon's preoperative assessment may change at the time of surgery. As the intraoperative findings dictate, the surgical approach may by necessity change from minimally invasive to open or from robotic to laparoscopic in some cases.[5]

Intraoperative Assessment

- Regardless of the surgical approach, the first step prior to removing the adnexa is to evaluate the abdomen and pelvis. This can generally be done quickly either laparoscopically or during exploratory surgery. A quick survey will identify any unexpected pathology such as adhesions that may impact the scope of surgery. Only at that point should the surgical plan be decided and the operation begins. Should adhesions be encountered, these should be managed first in order to restore anatomy to normal. Once completed, removing the adnexal mass should be relatively uncomplicated.
- In certain situations, adhesions may be dense or may completely obliterate the normal anatomic relationships such as with advanced endometriosis or a pelvic malignancy. Often, as in these two diseases, the peritoneum is involved with the disease process and restoring these planes is not possible. It is important to note that these processes generally do not invade through the peritoneum. In these circumstances, the knowledge that there is a layer of peritoneum between the ovaries and the rectosigmoid, for instance, can be used to the surgeon's advantage. Often the best approach is to enter the retroperitoneum laterally and cephalad to the pelvis. This offers several advantages. First, the surgery begins in an area without distorted anatomy. The blood supply to the ovary, which originates off the aorta just below the renal vessels, can be identified and isolated anywhere along its course. Many times, this is most easily accomplished at the pelvic brim or, if the pathology dictates, in the abdomen itself. The second advantage is the surgeon can now directly visualize the ureter and iliac vessels lessening the likelihood of injury (Fig. 11.2.5). The peritoneum can generally easily be separated from these retroperitoneal structures even in situations where dense inseparable adhesions are present in the pelvis proper. This approach, opening the peritoneum, entering the retroperitoneum, and isolating the IP, allows mobilization

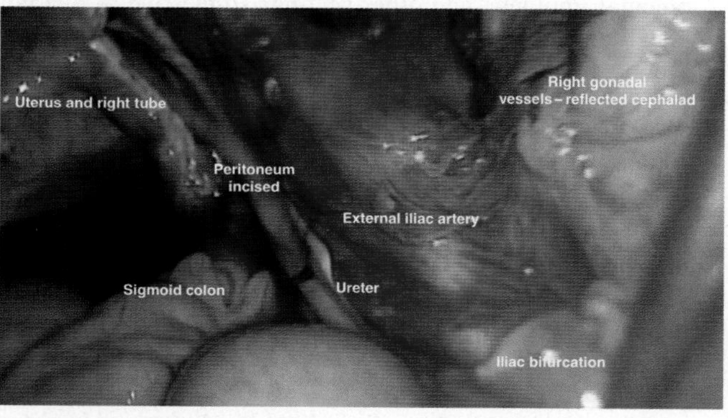

Figure 11.2.5. Retroperitoneum. The right pelvic sidewall was opened demonstrating the ureter crossing the common iliac artery. The utero-ovarian pedicle was divided and the ovary and gonadal vessels reflected cephalad.

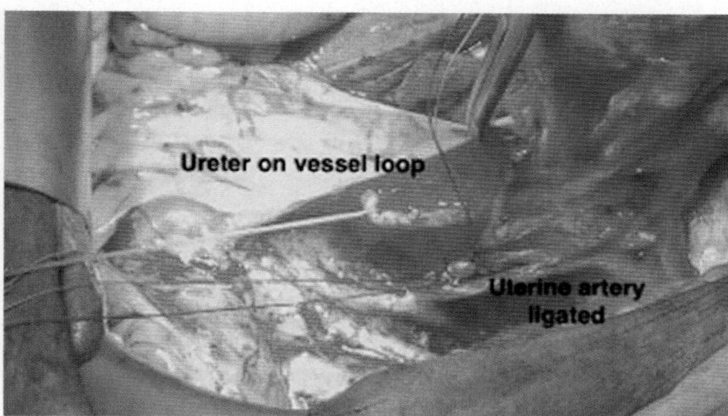

Figure 11.2.6. Ureterolysis. Once the retroperitoneum is developed, the ureter can be more easily dissected after placing a vessel loop and placing it on gentle traction.

of the ovarian mass from its lateral attachments. In certain cases, the ureter may be in harms way and at this point can be isolated with a vessel loop (Fig. 11.2.6). The ureter can be dissected free from the peritoneum completely to the insertion into the bladder separating it from the ovarian mass when necessary. Securing the vascular supply of the ovary early in the case also has the advantage of decreasing blood loss. Blood loss in addition to possibly compromising the patient's health will tend to obscure the surgical field complicating an already difficult dissection.

- Once the mass is mobilized medially, the surgeon can then focus upon ligating the remaining blood supply—the utero-ovarian pedicle, unless the uterus is being removed with the ovary itself. This pedicle has many venous channels and can be easily torn, leading to retroperitoneal hematomas. Securing this pedicle can be done in any variety of ways—suture ligation, energy such as bipolar or harmonic or with a vascular stapling device. Each method has its own advantages, cost, ease, speed, or vascular security. The manner in which this pedicle is secured is surgeon- and situation-dependent. After isolating this pedicle and ligating it, most complex adherent masses can be removed with gentle traction (see **Video 11.2.1**). Only in the situation of advanced endometriosis, ovarian malignancy, or diverticular abscess, resection of the rectosigmoid colon along with some or all of the pelvic peritoneum may be required. The major advantage to a radical resection with en bloc rectosigmoid resection is that all the peritoneum in the pelvis can be removed with the disease encapsulated (Fig. 11.2.7).

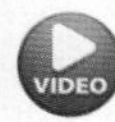

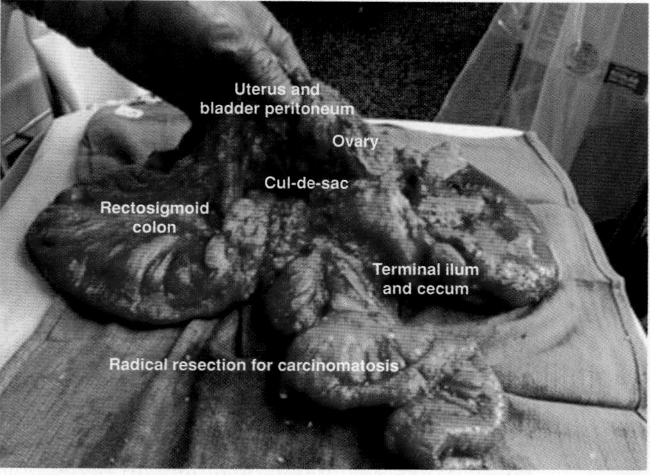

Figure 11.2.7. Radical en bloc resection. Radical resection is often the best approach to extirpate the pelvis of metastatic ovarian cancer.

Positioning

- Patient positioning for complex pelvic surgery should be done in low lithotomy if at all possible. Placing the patient in this manner will allow easy access to the bladder, vagina, and rectum without repositioning. We recommend prepping the perineum and vagina in all cases and placing the Foley and uterine manipulator (if applicable) after the patient has been prepped and draped.

Approach

- Transperitoneal approach: the most common approach to removing the adnexa, especially for simple benign lesions
- Retroperitoneal approach: an anatomic dissection that allows for safe resection of complex, adherent, and malignant tumors
- Retrograde resection: a relatively uncommon approach that is helpful in situations where the ureter cannot be identified at the pelvic brim or when taking the gonadal vessels.

Procedures and Techniques

Transperitoneal resection

The most straightforward approach is a transperitoneal resection. This is the most commonly preformed approach for removing a benign ovarian mass. This approach involves lifting the adnexa off the pelvic sidewall and placing its blood supply on tension. The ureter is identified through the peritoneum to assure it will not be injured. The ovarian vessels are ligated, most often, through the peritoneum. Typically an energy device, such as ligasure, is used to seal the gonadal vessels during MIS and a suture ligature is most often used when done during laparotomy.

The transperitoneal approach has several advantages, ease and speed among them. This technique works well when dealing with benign ovaries, simple cystic, or even solid masses that are not adherent to the ovarian fossa or pelvic sidewall. The major disadvantage to this technique is vascular sealing integrity. When elevating the ovarian vessels off the pelvic sidewall and using an energy device, the surgeon transects the vessels at an oblique angle resulting in a larger vessel to be sealed. In comparison, by opening the peritoneum and isolating the vessel, the vessels can be ligated perpendicular to their axis resulting in a smaller area and more secure vascular pedicle. This is an important distinction. A compromise in the vascular integrity of the gonadal vessels can lead to a retroperitoneal bleed requiring transfusion and occasionally reoperation (**Tech Fig. 11.2.1**).

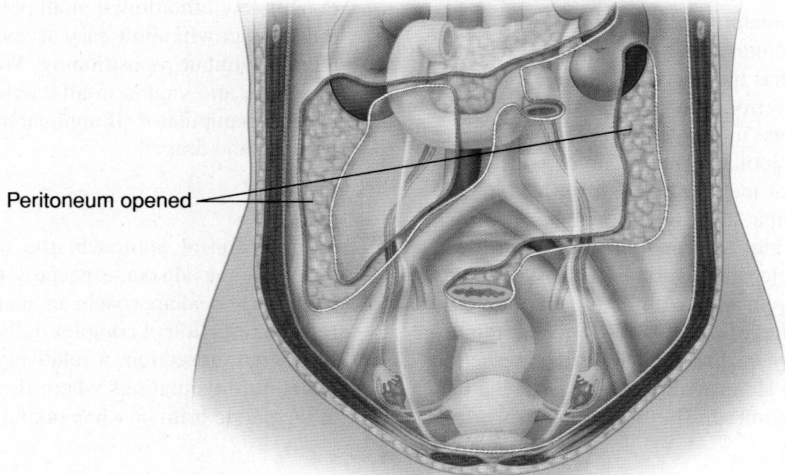

Tech Figure 11.2.1. The peritoneum. The peritoneum covers the aorta, IVC, as well as the ureters and gonadal vessels. It covers the pelvic viscera including the rectum, uterus, adnexa, and bladder.

Retroperitoneal resection

For more complex operations, a retroperitoneal approach is often the preferred surgical approach. While this is inherently more involved, it will often save time by identifying critical structures (ureter, iliac vessels) and avoiding unintended injury. By entering the peritoneum, this approach enables the surgeon to proceed with the anatomic dissection in the retroperitoneum on the opposite side of the ovarian pathology. Utilizing this technique, not only are the ureters and iliac vessels lateral to the dissection, but the adherent ovarian mass and peritoneum are now lifted off these critical structures as well. After securing the blood supply, the ovary can be removed, even if densely adherent to pelvic structure with relative ease and security in knowing a catastrophic vascular or ureteral injury has been avoided.

This technique relies upon the surgeon being comfortable operating in the retroperitoneum. To begin the operation, after lysing any adhesions and mobilizing the bowel out of harms way, the retroperitoneum is opened. This is best done lateral to the pelvic sidewall along the psoas muscle as there are no critical structures to inadvertently injure. On the left, it is most often necessary to mobilize the rectosigmoid from its peritoneal attachments to develop this space. While not always necessary, it is often helpful to mobilize both the left and right colon along Toldt's line. This facilitates identifying the gonadal blood supply and ureter as they cross the pelvic brim. By entering the retroperitoneum cephalad of any pelvic pathology, it is easier to identify these structures and dissect down toward the area of abnormality. Once the gonadal vessels are identified, they can be isolated and ligated. Again, this is typically done with suture in an open case and with an energy device when approached minimally invasively. Nonetheless, the principles are the same. The vessels should be isolated and transected perpendicular to their long axis yielding a secure vascular pedicle. Suture ligature is unnecessary and perhaps counterproductive as the IP can have extensive and tortuous venous channels that can be injured leading to retroperitoneal hematoma. After securing the vascular pedicle, the ovarian mass can then be mobilized from its pelvic attachments with less blood loss and the knowledge that the ureter has not been injured at that point (see **Video 11.2.1**).

In certain situations, the ureter is densely adherent to pelvic mass. In these circumstances, it is prudent to identify the ureter at the pelvic brim where it crosses the bifurcation of the external and internal iliac vessels (Tech Fig. 11.2.2). This is almost always the best place to identify the ureter because this anatomic relationship does not alter despite extensive pelvic and abdominal

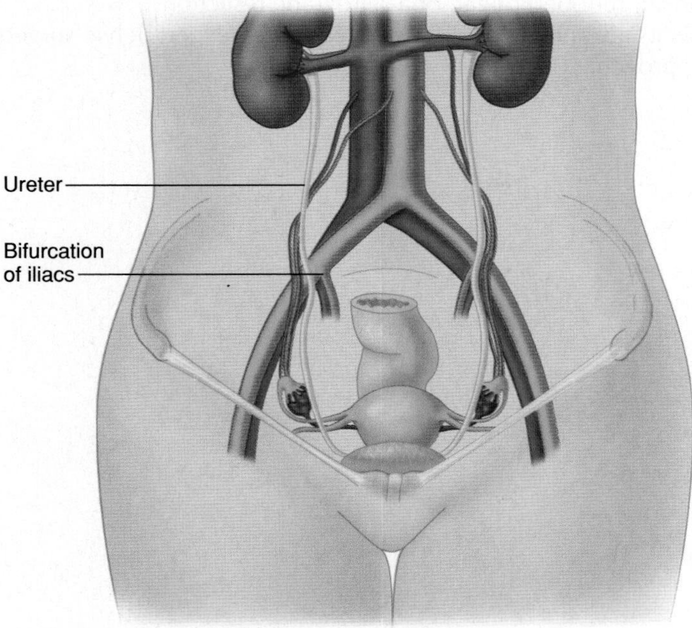

Tech Figure 11.2.2. The ureter. The ureter runs parallel to the ovarian vessels. It crosses the pelvic brim at the bifurcation of the common iliac artery. This is a convenient place to identify it and follow it into the pelvis.

diseases. Once the ureter is identified, it should be carefully dissected from the peritoneum leaving its adventitia intact and a vessel loop can be placed around it. With gentle traction, the ureter can be followed safely along its course and the ovarian mass dissected free.

This approach will generally then allows the surgeon to elevate the mass off the sidewall with the IP secure and ureter free of injury. The only remaining vascular pedicle is the attachment to the uterus. This can be ligated when leaving the uterus *in situ,* or can be left intact if the patient is undergoing hysterectomy. It is worth mentioning that this approach can be performed during MIS or laparotomy with slight variation in technique.

Retrograde resection

Perhaps the least common approach to removing an ovarian tumor is a retrograde dissection. This is similar to the retroperitoneal resection discussed above but essentially done in reverse. This may be helpful in situations where the surgeon cannot identify the ureter despite developing the retroperitoneal spaces. In such a case, inadvertent ligation of the ureter may occur when securing the gonadal vessels. This situation is not infrequently encountered in endometriosis or in patients with retroperitoneal fibrosis. Rather than proceeding with ligation of the IP, the surgeon can instead work from the uterine fundus in a retrograde fashion. The first step is to extend the retroperitoneal incision along the psoas muscle and external iliac vessel toward the round ligament. If the retroperitoneum is difficult to develop cephalad or the pathology is obscuring visualization of the ureter, the surgeon may have better luck moving inferiorly. Starting just cephalad to the round ligament and with traction on the uterine cornu medially, the retroperitoneum can often be entered. Dissection medially to develop the pararectal spaces is helpful to isolate the utero-ovarian pedicle and drop the ureter inferiorly. The utero-ovarian pedicle can be secured at this point allowing the ovarian mass to be mobilized cephalad in a retrograde fashion. With gentle traction and either cautery or sharp dissection, the mass can be lifted out of the pelvis, isolating the gonadal vessels. Once the ovarian pedicle can be seen at the pelvic brim, it can be safely ligated. With this technique, the ureter should remain free of harm despite the fact that it has not been previously identified. It is always good practice when using a retrograde approach once the mass has been removed to identify the ureter and follow it along the course of dissection to confirm that it has not been injured.

In summary, the approach to removing the adnexa is dependent upon a number of patient-related factors along with the pathology at hand. These will dictate the most judicious approach to utilize transperitoneal, retroperitoneal, or a retrograde resection.

Each approach has its advantages as discussed; however, expert pelvic surgeons should be familiar with each approach.

PEARLS AND PITFALLS

Restore anatomy to normal

- Prior to beginning the planned surgical procedure, restore anatomy to normal by lysing all adhesions and identifying normal anatomic landmarks.

Develop the retroperitoneal spaces

- Opening the retroperitoneum allows quick and accurate identification of the major blood vessels and ureter to assure they are out of harms way prior to surgical resection of the adnexa.

Mobilizing the rectosigmoid colon

- This can be a helpful maneuver when dealing with left-sided adnexal masses.

Use two hands when preforming complex laparoscopy

- The surgeon is better able to perform complex surgery using their two hands than trying to communicate with an assistant. Adding another trochar often can make a difficult case substantially easier.

POSTOPERATIVE CARE

- Postoperative care following oophorectomy depends more upon the surgical approach—open or MIS than on the operation itself. In general, when done robotically or laparoscopically removal of the adnexa is an outpatient procedure. In circumstances where laparotomy is required, we generally recommend rapid early feeding, ambulation, and minimization of IVFs.

COMPLICATIONS

- The most dreaded complication of oophorectomy is unintentional ureteral or bowel injury. The techniques described above will help minimize these complications; however, it should be recognized that in some cases these injuries are unavoidable given the pathology at hand. The key to avoiding morbidity is to recognize these injuries intraoperatively. Bowel or ureteral injury is relatively inconsequential when identified and properly repaired at the time of surgery. Delayed identification can be life threatening in addition to the need for emergent or repeat operations to address the complication. Proper surgical technique, a solid understanding of abdominal and pelvic anatomy, will allow a surgeon do perform complex cases with few injuries.

KEY REFERENCES

1. Conor D, et al. *Netter's Surgical Anatomy and Approaches.* Elsevier Saunders; 2014.
2. Valentin L, Ameye L, Franchi D, et al. Risk of malignancy in unilocular cysts: a study of 1148 adnexal masses classified as unilocular cysts at transvaginal ultrasound and review of the literature. *Ultrasound Obstet Gynecol.* 2013;41(1):80–89.
3. Goodrich ST, Bristow RE, Santoso JT, et al. The effect of ovarian imaging on the clinical interpretation of a multivariate index assay. *Am J Obstet Gynecol.* 2014;211(1):65.e1–65.e11.
4. Sölétormos G, Duffy MJ, Othman Abu Hassan S, et al. Clinical use of cancer biomarkers in epithelial ovarian cancer: updated guidelines from the European group on tumor markers. *Int J Gynecol Cancer.* 2016;26:43–51.
5. Chen I, Lisonkova S, Allaire C, Williams C, Yong P, Joseph KS. Routes of hysterectomy in women with benign uterine disease in the Vancouver Coastal Health and Providence Health Care regions: a retrospective cohort analysis. *CMAJ Open.* 2014;2(4):E273–280.

Chapter 11.3 Ovarian Remnant

Swapna Kollikonda

GENERAL PRINCIPLES

Definition

- Ovarian remnant syndrome (ORS) is the condition of persistent, histologically confirmed ovarian cortical tissue, in patients who have undergone oophorectomy. Kaufmann reported ORS in 1962 and it was described in 1970 by Shemwell and Weed.
- Follicular cyst, endometriosis, corpus luteum, serous cystadenoma, adenocarcinoma, clear cell carcinoma, and endometrioid carcinoma can exist in the ovarian remnant.
- Risk factors leading to ORS include poor surgical technique, altered pelvic anatomy secondary to adhesions from previous surgery, endometriosis, pelvic inflammatory disease, ruptured appendix, and inflammatory bowel disease. Increased incidence of ORS after laparoscopic oophorectomy may be because of improper use of looped suture ligatures or the linear stapler as per small study done by Nezhat et al.[7] Morcellation technique also contributed to increased risk by incomplete extraction of ovarian fragments resulting in implantation of ovarian tissue at different sites.
- Growing awareness and advanced imaging technology led to an increased detection of these cases.
- As there is a rise in laparoscopic ovarian surgeries, ovarian tissues can be implanted to port sites, anterior abdominal wall, and other abdominal organs leading to ORS.
- Usually, remnant ovarian tissue is encased in the scar tissue from prior surgeries, endometriosis, or PID. Expansion of this tissue can lead to chronic pain which is one of the

common presenting symptoms. Ovarian remnants can be found in 18% of patients with pelvic pain after oophorectomy.[1] Other less common presenting symptoms are pelvic mass, back pain, variable bowel symptoms, and ureteric compression symptoms. Symptoms usually start 1 to 3 years after oophorectomy.

Differential Diagnosis

- Residual ovary syndrome (secondary to retained ovary)
- Supernumerary ovaries (the development of extra ovaries during embryogenesis through the arrest of migrating gonocytes that contain ovarian follicle tissue)
- The most important concept in the differential diagnosis is to exclude other causes of chronic pelvic pain such as painful bladder syndrome, myofascial pelvic floor disorders, and irritable bowel syndrome.

Anatomic Considerations

- The ovarian remnant can also be found adherent to the lateral pelvic wall (most common), vaginal vault, bladder, bowel wall, ureter, or uterosacral ligament.

Nonoperative Management

- Suppression of ovarian tissue is the mainstay of treatment. This can be done by giving gonadotropin-releasing hormone analogues, danazol, birth control pills, depot medroxyprogesterone acetate injection, or etonogestrel implant. Levonorgestrel IUD can be considered if uterus is still present. None of these methods have been shown to be superior to other.
- Irradiation has also been used but is least favorable because of the risk of damage to surrounding tissue.

IMAGING AND OTHER DIAGNOSTICS

- Occasionally on pelvic examination we can palpate adnexal mass suggestive of ovarian remnant which needs to be confirmed by further imaging studies.
- Transvaginal ultrasound is the main stay and cost-effective modality of imaging.
- CT and MRI sometimes may help for preoperative preparation if the ovarian remnant is near to ureters, bladder, and bowel, or if ultrasound findings are inconclusive.
- FSH and estradiol levels can also supplement the diagnosis along with the imaging studies. The level of FSH and estradiol should be in premenopausal range (FSH <40 mIU/mL and estradiol >30 pg/mL). If patient is on hormone replacement therapy, stop estrogen at least 10 days prior to testing these hormone levels.
- Gonadotropin-releasing hormone analogue stimulation test is also helpful to diagnose the condition with an elevation of estradiol levels from day 1 to day 4 after receiving 3 days of leuprolide acetate (1 mg SC/d).

PREOPERATIVE PLANNING

- Intraoperative laparoscopic ultrasonography[8] may be helpful in detecting ovarian remnants especially in patients with distorted pelvic anatomy.
- Administration of clomiphene citrate (50 to 100 mg twice daily for 10 days) may help to make the ovarian tissue more prominent.
- Preoperative pyelography may also define status of ureter and can predict surgical obstacles.
- An informed consent should be obtained explaining all possible risks such as but not limited to infection, hemorrhage, injury to visceral organs, and major blood vessels. The consent should also include procedures such as resection of involved intra-abdominal organs with repair.
- Cystoscopy is indicated if ovarian remnant is near to bladder or requiring extensive ureterolysis and dissection of bladder. Administration of methylene blue or indigo carmine or sodium fluorescein will help visualization of ureteral jets during intraoperative cystoscopy.

SURGICAL MANAGEMENT

- Surgery is often mainstay of treatment because of side effects or inadequate response to medical therapy or if medical management is contraindicated or ovarian remnant is causing obstructive symptoms to urinary and gastrointestinal systems or any suspicion of ovarian cancer in the ovarian remnant.[6]
- Laparotomy, laparoscopy, or robotic-assisted laparoscopic routes have been used.
- Laparoscopy has been shown to be equally effective as laparotomy. There are advantages to laparoscopy as the magnification provided by the laparoscope through high-definition video technology, facilitates micro-dissection of tissue planes and easier identification of the remnant tissue. Increased intra-abdominal pressure helps decreasing the oozing of blood from the dissection and allows superior visualization of the retroperitoneal space.[3] In patients with multiple previous surgeries, laparoscopic approach may be less traumatic.
- Robotic-assisted surgery provides 3D view for adhesiolysis. Robotics also provides more magnification and flexibility of instruments but disadvantages include lack of tactile sensation and cost.

Positioning

- Lithotomy position in Allen stirrups is preferable for both laparotomy and laparoscopic approach. Proper positioning is important to avoid any nerve injuries.
- Arms should be tucked to patient's side in military position, semi-pronated, with adequate padding placement around bony prominences especially the elbows and wrists. It is important to avoid too much of abduction at shoulders to prevent brachial plexus injury.
- Adequate restraints should be placed around chest.
- Buttocks should be well supported at the edge of the table. Hips should be flexed to not more than 90 degrees at thigh and abducted to not more than 45 degrees to avoid obturator, sciatic, and femoral nerve injury. Appropriate padding is needed on lateral side of knee to avoid compression injury of common peroneal nerve. Knee should be flexed to 90 degrees with slight adduction. Feet also need good support with padding.
- Once the uterine manipulator is placed, the stirrups can be brought down to make thighs and abdomen at the same level, knees flexed to 90 degrees and thighs adducted in order to facilitate flexible movements of instrument.
- Assistants should avoid leaning on to the suspended inferior extremities during the surgery.
- Table should be kept flat for initial entry ports and then changed to Trendelenburg (less than 30 degrees) position for accessory ports.

- Use anti-skid methods such as vacuum beanbag, gel pad, etc. can be used to decrease movement during Trendelenburg position.

Approach

- Goal of surgical approach is high ligation of infundibulopelvic ligament after identifying and lateralizing the ureter by opening the retroperitoneal space and developing the para-rectal space.
- Entry into the retroperitoneal space can be achieved by the following two techniques:
  1. The peritoneum next to the round ligament is cut and the space entered.
  2. The second is to start at the pelvic brim under the ovarian vessels. The peritoneum is grasped, incised and the space entered.
- With either approach the ureter is identified and dissected from the pelvic brim to the level where the uterine artery crosses. Complete dissection of the ureter allows hemostasis to safely be achieved around the remnant dissection. The para-rectal space is identified with the ureter laterally, the rectum and mesorectum medially, and the pelvic floor at its base.
- The visible ovarian remnant should be removed along with surrounding healthy tissue to avoid any recurrence.
- In a study done by Fennimore et al.,[2] ovarian stroma extends up to 1.4 cm into infundibulopelvic ligament. So, isolating infundibulopelvic ligament at least 2 cm from ovarian tissue to clamp and cut plays a key role in prevention.

PROCEDURES AND TECHNIQUES

Ovarian Remnant Excision (Video 11.3) 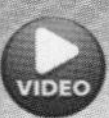

Time out

- Time out should be performed to ensure right procedure on right patient. Patient should be positioned as described above.

Preparation

- The operating area needs to be prepped and draped in a sterile fashion. The drapes should be laparoscopic favorable with slits to have access to perineum. Insert a 16-French Foley catheter for bladder drainage. In the presence of uterus, placement of uterine manipulator will help to identify vaginal fornices and vesicocervical space. If uterus is absent, a ring forceps with a sponge at the tip can be inserted. Placing EEA sizer in rectum can help to distinguish the margins of the rectum as vast majority of these patients have distorted pelvic anatomy from extensive adhesions as a result of prior predisposing conditions. The EEA sizer, uterine manipulator, and vaginal sponge stick need to be covered with sterile glove on the external part to allow grasping with sterile gloves. The role of ureteral stents is debatable given reports of possible ureteral injury due to its rigidity. Advantage of using fiber-optic ureteral stents which can illuminate ureters during surgery is also questionable because the camera lights need to be dimmed. When bowel adhesions are anticipated, preoperative bowel preparation can be beneficial, although this is still a challenged concept.

Port placement

- An orogastric tube should be inserted to decompress the stomach. The operating room table should be placed completely flat. Ensure that the electrosurgical pad has been placed on thigh. Local anesthetic such as 0.25% marcaine can be injected under the skin at port sites to give pain relief during and after surgery. For laparoscopic procedure, initial port is placed at the level of umbilicus, after insufflating with Veress needle, or directly with an optical trocar, or by an open (Hassan) technique. If the patient has a scar from prior midline abdominal incision, left upper quadrant entry at palmers point (3 cm below the rib cage at mid-clavicular line) is safe as the chance to encounter adhesions is minimal. Once intra-abdominal placement is confirmed by opening pressure less than 10 mm Hg, the peritoneal cavity is insufflated with CO_2 to a pressure of less than 15 mm Hg. Patient is then placed in Trendelenburg position. Three extra 5-mm ports are then inserted under direct vision, two on the right and one on the left side. The distance between these ports should be 8 to 10 cm to avoid collision and to get maximum mobility of instruments. Lateral ports are placed under direct vision by observing the inferior epigastric vessels (lateral umbilical ligament) about 8 cm from the midline and 5 cm upwards from the symphysis pubis to avoid injury to epigastric vessels. For the best visualization, insufflate through assistant port and evacuate smoke through the camera port.

Adhesiolysis

- Anticipate scar tissue and adhesions from prior surgeries. A survey of the peritoneal cavity is performed. Omental and bowel adhesions are taken down sharply and bipolar instruments are used for hemostasis. To clearly visualize ovarian remnants on the left side, the sigmoid colon needs to be mobilized medially from pelvic brim to cul-de-sac.

Locate ovarian remnant

- In many cases, the remnant ovary is adherent to the lateral pelvic side wall as shown in **Tech Figure 11.3.1**.

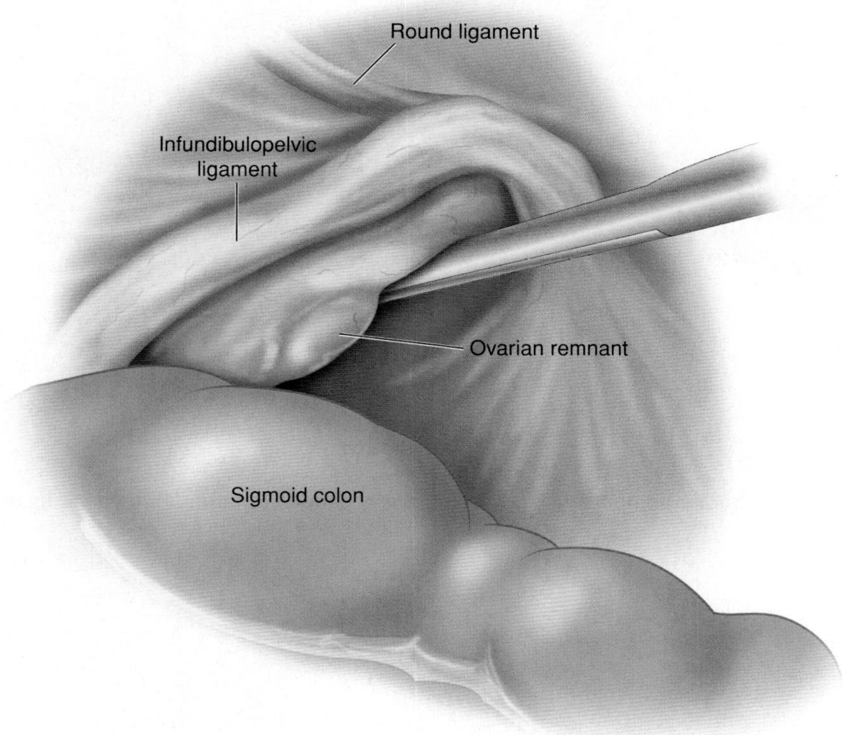

Tech Figure 11.3.1. Ovarian remnant adherent to lateral pelvic sidewall.

Identify landmarks, ureters, and excise ovarian remnant

- Identify the round ligament at its attachment to the deep inguinal ring and follow it medially. This is then coagulated, cut, and the retroperitoneal space entered (**Tech Fig. 11.3.2**). Extend the peritoneal incision cephalad parallel to infundibulopelvic ligament, along external iliac artery to open up the retroperitoneal space (**Tech Fig. 11.3.3**). The ureter is then identified in the retroperitoneal space on the medial leaf of the broad ligament below the infundibulopelvic ligament (**Tech Fig. 11.3.4A**). However, if there has been prior endometriosis surgery the ureter may not be as easily visualized. If the ureter is not visualized clearly, dissect peritoneum more cephalad and laterally toward pelvic brim. Once ureter is identified, dissect and trace ureter caudad all the way to area where the uterine artery crosses the ureter or to the trigone of bladder if the tissue is seen adherent to the bladder. During dissection of the para-rectal space, always keep the ureter and internal iliac branches on the lateral side wall. Avoid dissecting between the vessels. The infundibulopelvic ligament is skeletonized at least 2 cm from ovarian attachment, ideally cephalad to pelvic brim above the level of common iliac bifurcation. Create a window below infundibulopelvic ligament (**Tech Fig. 11.3.4B**) to coagulate and transect the ligament (**Tech Fig. 11.3.4C**). Try to remove adequate surrounding healthy peritoneal tissue margins to avoid any recurrence (**Tech Fig. 11.3.5**). Dissect ovarian remnant from ureter and surrounding vasculature before isolating from remaining surrounding tissue (**Tech Fig. 11.3.6**).

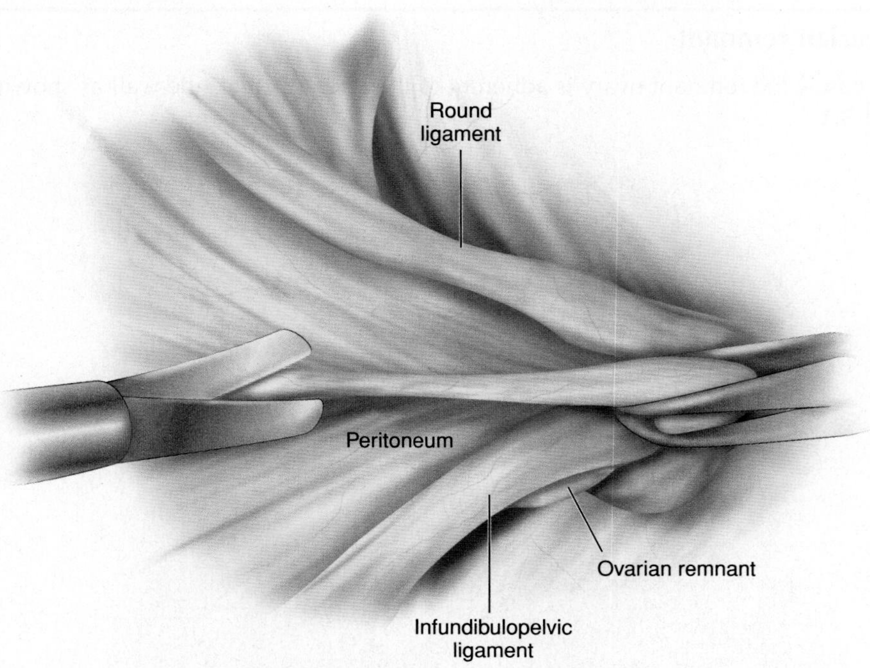

Tech Figure 11.3.2. Peritoneum next to round ligament and parallel to infundibulopelvic ligament.

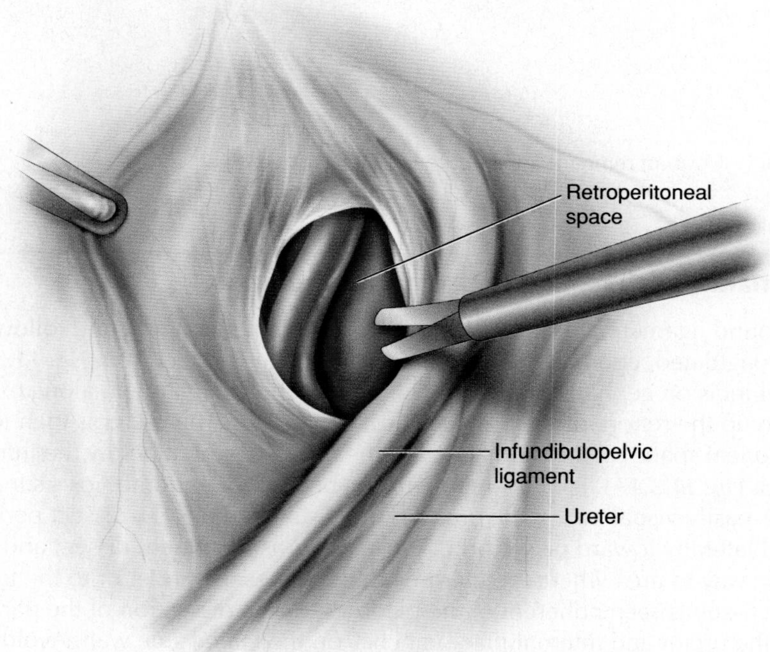

Tech Figure 11.3.3. Retroperitoneal space.

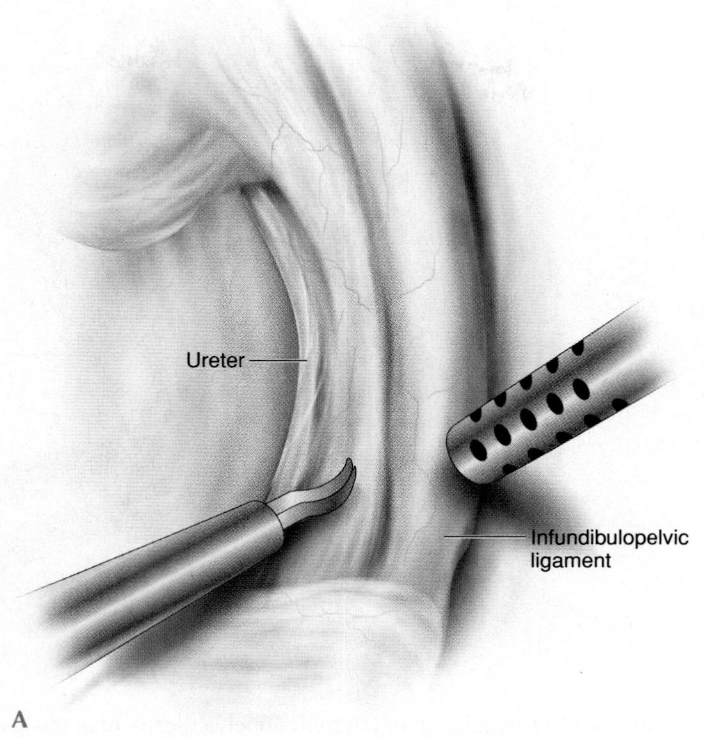

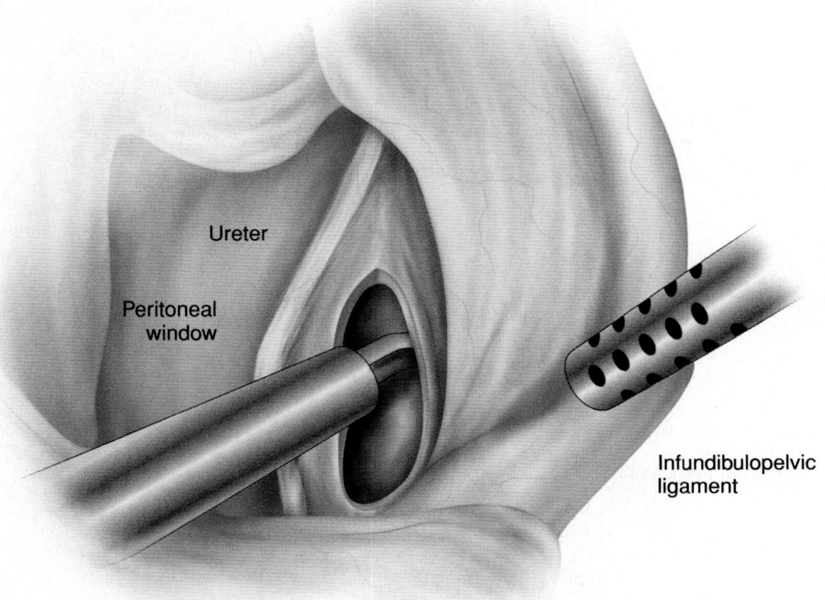

Tech Figure 11.3.4. **A:** Ureter below infundibulopelvic ligament on medial leaf of peritoneum. **B:** Isolation of infundibulopelvic ligament. (*continued*)

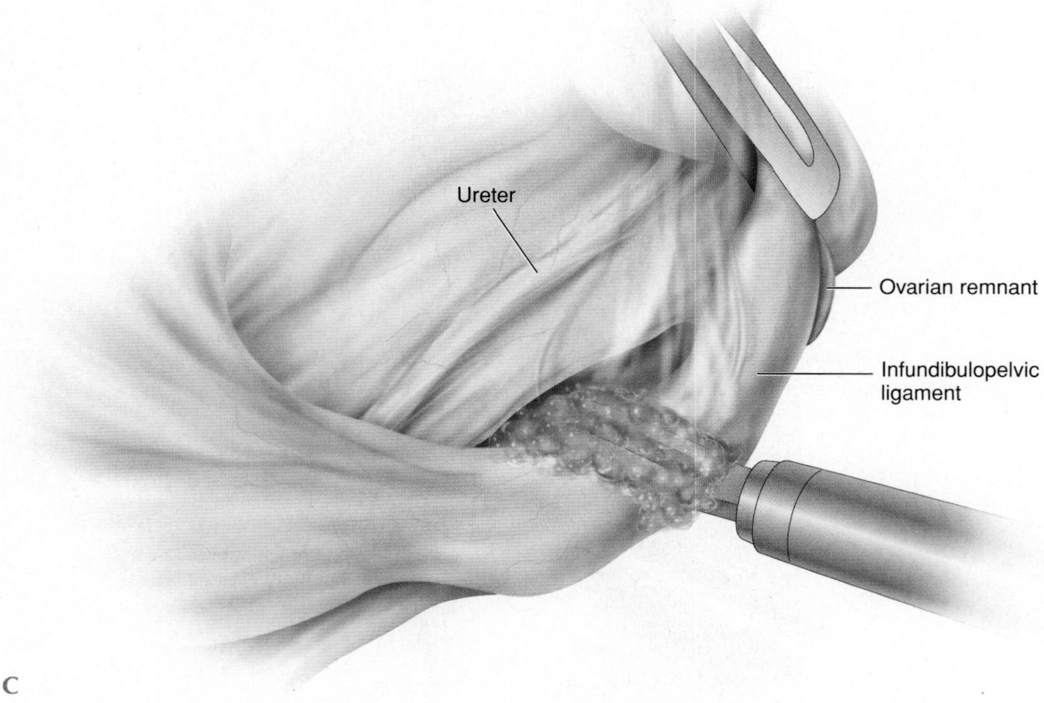

Tech Figure 11.3.4. *(continued)* **C:** Coagulation of infundibulopelvic ligament at the level of pelvic brim.

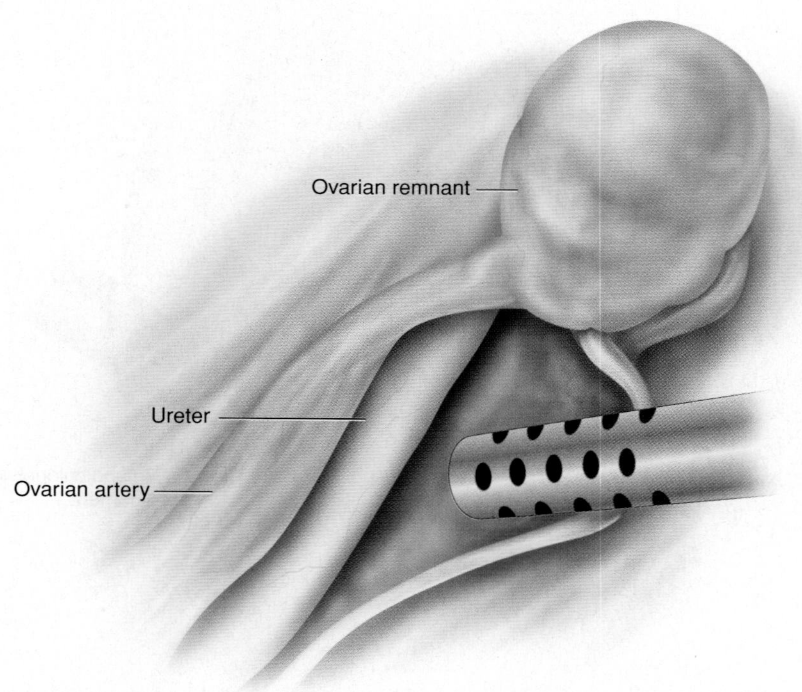

Tech Figure 11.3.5. Resection of ovarian remnant after separation from surrounding structures.

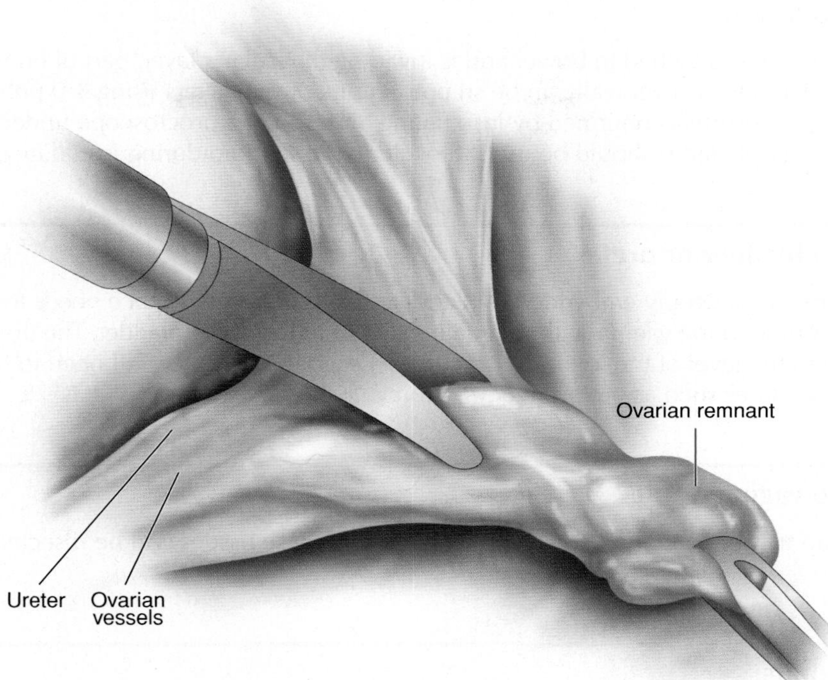

Tech Figure 11.3.6. Ovarian remnant in relation to ureter and ovarian vessels artery.

Removal of specimen

- It is also important to remove the tissue in one piece especially in case of endometriosis as it can implant and give rise to recurrence. Consider removing the specimen in a tissue containment bag if there is a possibility of malignancy. Ovarian remnant tissue should be sent for histopathology for confirmation.

Achieve hemostasis

- Attain adequate hemostasis either by bipolar energy for large vessels or monopolar energy for small bleeders. Irrigate and perform final check of the operating site for hemostasis after decreasing intra-abdominal pressure to 0 mm for 30 seconds.

Fascia and skin closure

- Close fascia of all the ports more than 8 mm with 0 polyglactin suture. Skin incisions are closed with 4-0 polyglactin 910 or poliglecaprone suture.

Distinct case scenarios

- Ovarian remnant can also be found adherent to vaginal vault, bladder, bowel wall, ureter, and uterosacral ligament. In this situation, pelvic spaces need to be opened up to clearly delineate structures and remove ovarian remnant without injury to surrounding organs.

If attached to bowel

- If ovarian remnant is attached to bowel and is invading muscularis layer, part of bowel wall has to be resected and the bowel wall can be sutured in one or two layers using 3-0 polyglactin suture. Air-tight closure is confirmed by insufflating air through a proctoscope under water. A laparoscopic bowel clamp should be used to occlude the sigmoid during insufflation.

If attached to bladder or ureter

- If ovarian remnant is deeply embedded in bladder, the vesicovaginal space needs to be dissected. A probe in the vagina will help delineate the limits of the bladder. The ureters should be dissected to the level of the trigone. Sometimes a segment of ureter will need to be removed requiring procedures such as ureteroneocystostomy.

If attached to vaginal vault

- When ovarian tissue is attached to vaginal vault, part of these tissues will be resected followed by repair.

Additional points

- Patients who had unilateral oophorectomy, FSH values are of no significance and many times we do not consider them to have ORS which can lead to continued distress and pain.
- Presence of large mass with elevated CA125 suggests malignant change, although normal CA125 cannot exclude the diagnosis. As the tumor is in retroperitoneal location, ascites seems to be a rare associated feature.[5]

PEARLS AND PITFALLS

- ○ Prevention of port site implantation of ovarian tissue.
- ✖ Use tissue containment bag to remove specimen without spillage of tissue and irrigation of port site with copious amount of normal saline.
- ○ Identifying ovarian remnant yet times can be challenging secondary to adhesions from prior surgeries and there is a higher possibility of ureteric injuries in the process of resection of ovarian remnant.
- ✖ Always first identify round ligament and try to open para-rectal space to visualize and dissect ureter away from ovarian remnant.
- ○ Left-side ovarian remnant is common as infundibulopelvic ligament on this side is short and lacks clear visualization due to sigmoid colon.
- ✖ Can be prevented by mobilizing sigmoid medially.
- ○ When severe periovarian adhesions are encountered blunt dissection can leave part of ovarian cortical tissue leading to recurrence.
- ✖ Always perform sharp meticulous dissection.

POSTOPERATIVE CARE

- Try to avoid parenteral pain medications. Consider oral NSAIDs and opioids. Resume regular diet. Remove the Foley as soon as possible unless you have created a cystotomy to excise the tissue. Discharge instructions for increase in abdominal pain, nausea, vomiting, and fever should be given. The patients should be followed up in 2 weeks.

OUTCOMES

- Surgical treatment for ovarian remnant or ovarian retention syndrome is effective but is most effective in patients with no other pain-related diagnoses.
- In a large study done at Mayo clinic by Magtibay et al.,[5] out of 186 only one had recurrence of ORS and 90% had resolution of symptoms when above surgical principles were followed which were originally described by Webb in 1989.[9]

COMPLICATIONS

- The incidence of injury to the bladder, ureter, and bowel at laparotomy for ovarian remnant is estimated to be 3% to 33%, with injuries to the ureter significantly greater by laparotomy than by laparoscopy.[3]
- A recent study of ovarian remnant managed by laparoscopy by Nezhat et al.[7] reported the rate of intraoperative complications at 5.8%, with four intraoperative complications in 69 laparoscopies. However, there were no ureteral injuries. This series and others[1,4] have demonstrated that the rate of complications with laparoscopic treatment of ovarian remnant is comparable to or lower than those reported in laparotomy.
- In a comparative study done by Zapardiel et al.,[10] between all surgical approaches laparoscopic route has less blood loss, lower postoperative complications, and shorter length of stay.

KEY REFERENCES

1. Abu-Rafeh B, Vilos GA, Misra M. Frequency and laparoscopic management of ovarian remnant syndrome. *J Am Assoc Gynecol Laparosc.* 2003;10(1):33–37.
2. Fennimore IA, Simon NL, Bills G, Dryfhout VL, Schniederjan AM. Extension of ovarian tissue into the infundibulopelvic ligament beyond visual margins. *Gynecol Oncol.* 2009;114(1):61–63.
3. Kamprath S, Possover M, Schneider A. Description of a laparoscopic technique for treating patients with ovarian remnant syndrome. *Fertil Steril.* 1997;68(4):663–667.
4. Kho RM, Magrina JF, Magtibay PM. Pathologic findings and outcomes of a minimally invasive approach to ovarian remnant syndrome. *Fertil Steril.* 2007;87:1005–1009.
5. Magtibay PM, Nyholm JL, Hernandez JL, Podratz KC. Ovarian remnant syndrome. *Am J Obstet Gynecol.* 2005;193:2062–2066.
6. Narayansingh G, Cumming G, Parkin D, Miller I. Ovarian cancer developing in the ovarian remnant syndrome: a case report and literature review. *Aust N Z J Obstet Gynecol.* 2000;40(2):221–223.
7. Nezhat C, Kearney S, Malik S, Nezhat C, Nezhat F. Laparoscopic management of ovarian remnant. *Fertil Steril.* 2005;83:973–978.
8. McIntyre RC Jr, Stiegmann GV, Pearlman NW: Update of laparoscopic ultrasonography. *Endosc Surg Allied Technol.* 1994;2:149.
9. Webb MJ. Ovarian remnant syndrome. *Aust N Z J Obstet Gynaecol.* 1989;29(4):433–435.
10. Zapardiel I, Zanagnolo V, Kho RM, Magrina JF, Magtibay PM. Ovarian remnant syndrome: comparison of laparotomy, laparoscopy and robotic surgery. *Acta Obstet Gynecol Scand.* 2012;91:965–969.

Chapter 11.4 Management of Adnexal Torsion

Marjan Attaran

GENERAL PRINCIPLES

Definition

- Adnexal torsion is defined as twisting of the ovary and/or tube around usually the utero-ovarian ligament and in case of the ovary the infundibulopelvic ligament (Fig. 11.4.1). It is responsible for 2.7% of all gynecologic emergencies. This number is likely an underestimate given that some patients fail to undergo surgery and thus a definitive diagnosis is not made. Patients typically present with sudden-onset lower abdominal pain that may be continuous or intermittent. The exact cause of adnexal torsion is not known. However, not uncommonly an adnexal mass such as an ovarian cyst, a hydrosalpinx, or a paraovarian cyst is present. In some instances, it is believed that an unusually long utero-ovarian ligament may lend itself to torsion. This diagnosis is usually made in reproductive-aged women, although it is not uncommon in premenarchal girls.
- As a result of the twisting about the gonadal vessels, venous flow is first compromised and thus the ovary becomes edematous. Once arterial flow is compromised, the ovary and tube will experience ischemia and possible necrosis.
- The classic signs of ovarian torsion are acute abdominal/pelvic pain accompanied by an adnexal mass and signs of peritoneal irritation. Other symptoms may include nausea and fever, although the latter may occur much later.
- The right side is most frequently affected by torsion possibly secondary to the fact that the sigmoid traverses to the left and reduces space for torsion to occur.

Differential Diagnosis

- The preoperative accuracy of adnexal torsion is at best 44% as noted in a study by Cohen,[1] where by only 29 out of 66 patients who underwent laparoscopy for presumed diagnosis of torsion in fact had adnexal torsion. Other causes of lower abdominal pain must be considered in the differential diagnosis. These include:
  - Ruptured ovarian cyst
  - Appendicitis
  - Pelvic inflammatory disease
  - Ectopic pregnancy
  - Colitis
  - Pyelonephritis
  - Nephrolithiasis
  - Degeneration of a fibroid

Anatomic Considerations

- In most cases of torsion an ovarian tumor is present. Cysts less than 5 cm are less likely to lead to torsion than larger cysts.
- In conditions where pelvic adhesions are likely, such as endometriosis and past pelvic inflammatory disease, there is less of a likelihood of torsion. However, hydrosalpingies may lead to an isolated twisting of the fallopian tube.
- Benign ovarian cysts are more likely to lead to ovarian torsion than malignant lesions, since malignant lesions can invade adjacent tissues thereby prohibiting movement and torsion.
- During early pregnancy as the uterus is growing the corpus luteum may twist upon itself.
- Ovarian torsion has also been described in patients with congenital anomalies such as elongated utero-ovarian ligament or abnormally located ovary due to müllerian agenesis.
- Patients undergoing ovarian stimulation are at increased risk for ovarian torsion secondary to the enlarged size of the ovaries. The diagnosis in this case is extremely difficult given the multicystic appearance of the ovaries bilaterally.

IMAGING AND OTHER DIAGNOSTICS

- Pelvic ultrasound is usually the first imaging tool utilized to assist with this diagnosis (Fig. 11.4.2).

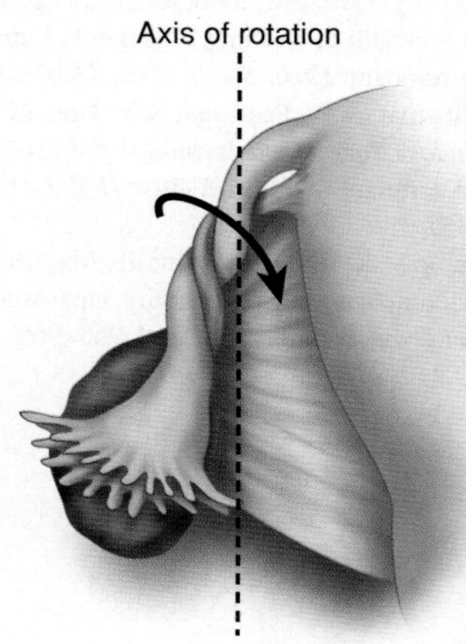

Figure 11.4.1. Ovary and tube twisted upon the utero-ovarian ligament.

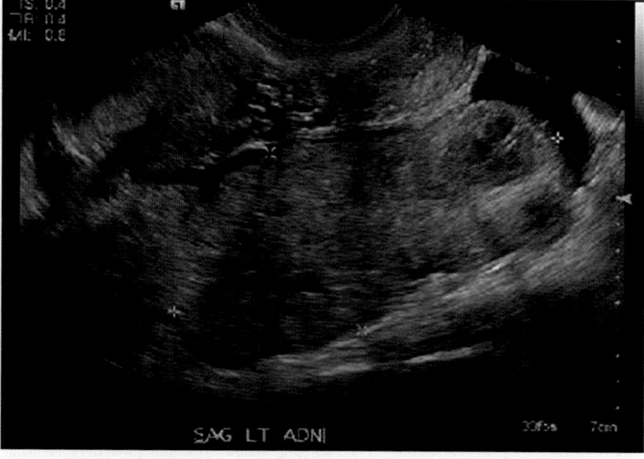

Figure 11.4.2. Transvaginal ultrasound image of torsed ovary.

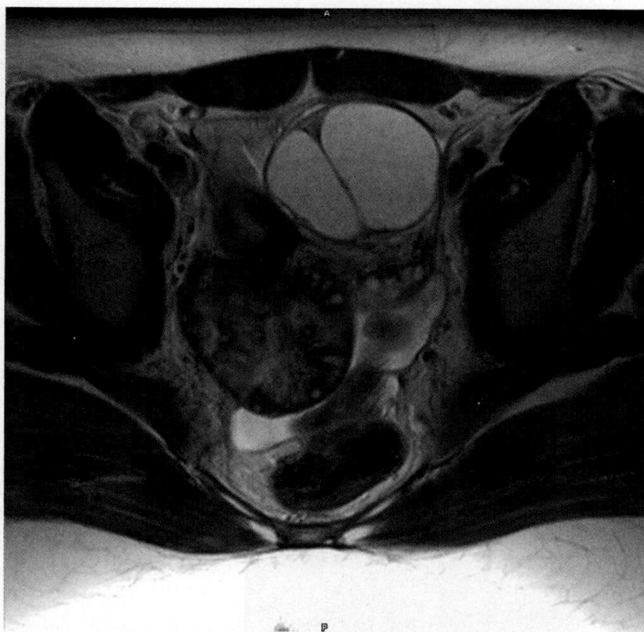

Figure 11.4.3. Swollen large right ovary.

- A transvaginal approach will provide better visualization of the ovarian vessels compared to the transabdominal approach.
- Indirect findings can include an enlarged ovarian/adnexal mass, multiple cystic structures in the periphery of the enlarged ovary, thickening of interfollicular tissue, and some fluid in the cul-de-sac or adjacent to the enlarged adnexa. The location of the ovary may also be abnormal. It may be located anterior to the uterus or on the contralateral side.
- The only direct ultrasound sign of torsion is the "whirlpool sign."[2]
- Doppler flow studies are routinely used to demonstrate flow in the ovaries. Doppler studies can miss torsion in 60% of cases but its positive predictive value is 100%. Thus while establishing the existence of flow to the ovaries may be reassuring; the clinical picture should direct the course of action. Lack of flow may be a late symptom of torsion, when not only venous but arterial flow is compromised.
- Given that the patient commonly presents to the emergency room with such symptoms the CT scan may be the first imaging study performed. Findings will include enlarged adnexa, fallopian tube thickening, ascites, and uterine deviation to the twisted side.
- MR findings on T2-weighted images include swollen ovarian stroma (the hyperintensity of the ovarian stroma is similar to that of water) (Fig. 11.4.3).

PREOPERATIVE PLANNING

- These cases are considered an emergency and should be performed as soon as possible.

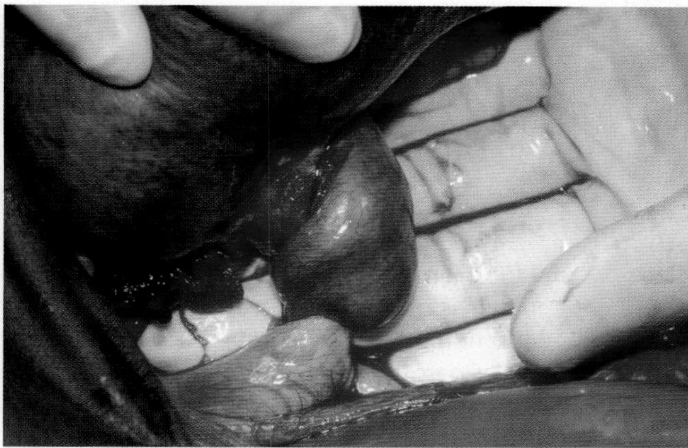

Figure 11.4.4. Twisted pedicle of large swollen ovary.

- The decision to proceed with surgery is based primarily on the clinical picture and suspicion of torsion.
- A discussion must occur with patient and family regarding their desire to preserve fertility. The younger the patient is the more important it is to address this issue.
- If a patient has had a prior history of torsion, there should be a discussion regarding possible need for oophoropexy.
- In a postmenopausal woman it is reasonable to discuss performing an oophorectomy. Only 2% of torsion cases are secondary to malignancy. However, this possibility does need to be addressed with the patient.

SURGICAL MANAGEMENT

- Once the diagnosis of ovarian torsion is entertained, surgery must be performed in an emergent manner. The purpose of surgery is to determine the exact cause of the symptoms and rule in or out the diagnosis of torsion. If torsion is identified, the goal is to untwist the adnexa. There is no evidence to suggest that the number of thromboembolic events increases in patients undergoing detorison of their adnexa.

Positioning

- In preparation for laparoscopy, the patient is placed in the dorsolithotomy position. The younger child and adolescent may be placed in the supine position.

APPROACH

- The typical approach to such patients is via laparoscopy. Once the diagnosis is confirmed, then one proceeds with detorsion and assessment of cause of torsion.
- However, laparotomy may be indicated if the mass is quite large or if there is concern for malignancy or spillage of cyst material (Fig. 11.4.4).

Procedures and Techniques (Video 11.4)

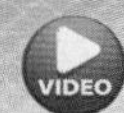

Detorsion

- Upon laparoscopic entry into the abdomen, the pelvis is assessed. The normal anatomy of the pelvis is noted as well as the area of concern. The direction in which the adnexa has twisted and number of times it has twisted is noted as is the size and color of the adnexa. In rare instances, the vessels supplying blood to the gonad have completely auto-amputated. But in the majority of cases the ovary can be easily untwisted (Tech Figs. 11.4.1 and 11.4.2).

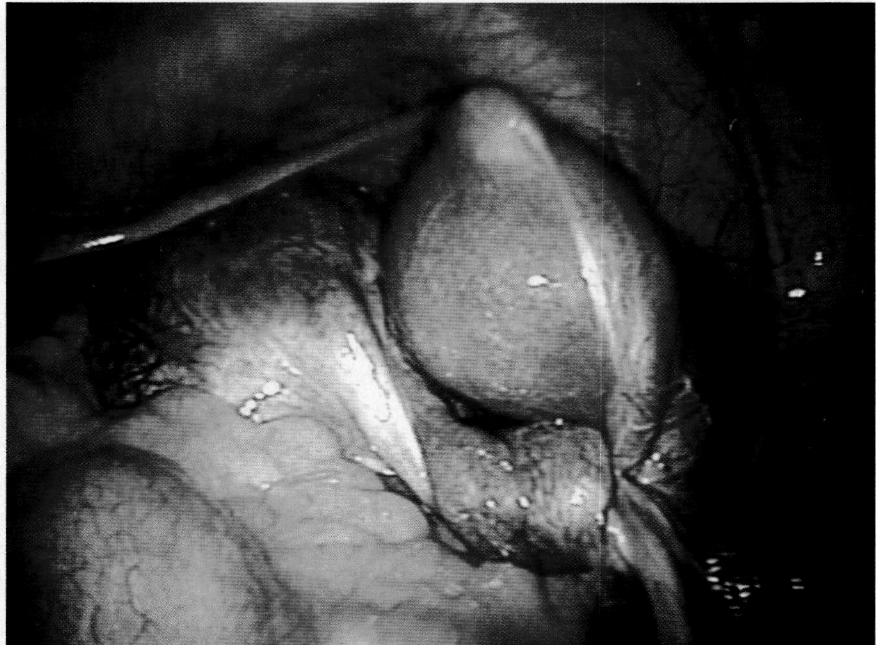

Tech Figure 11.4.1. Laparoscopic view of torsed right ovary.

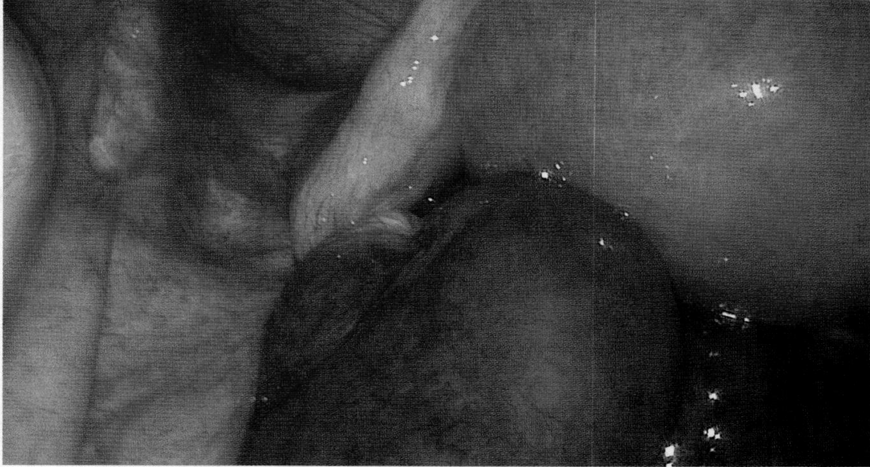

Tech Figure 11.4.2. Laparoscopic view of torsed left ovary after ovarian stimulation with gonadotropins.

- Using the two lower ports, blunt-tipped graspers are placed on either side of the mass and twisted in a reverse direction of the torsion. Usually the torsion is loose and gonad is easily placed back into normal position (Tech Fig. 11.4.3).

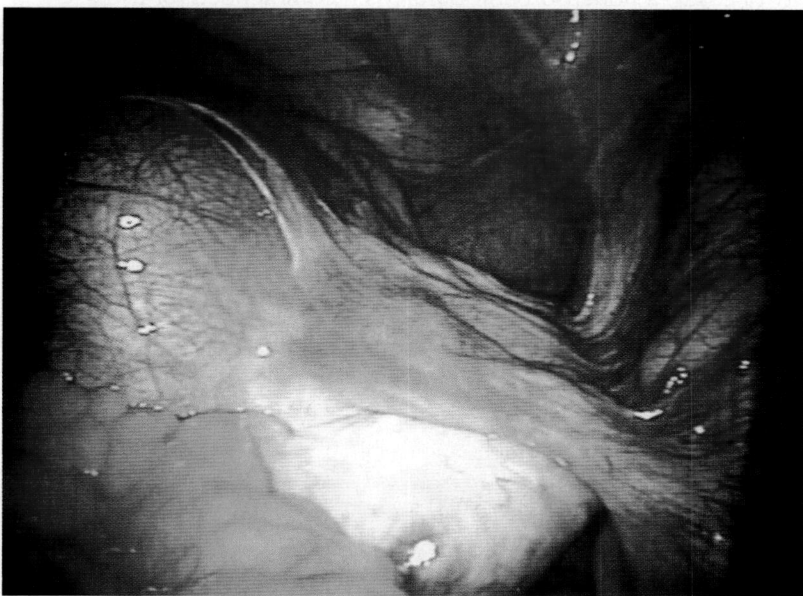

Tech Figure 11.4.3. Detorsed right ovary.

Assess for cause of torsion

- While waiting for the adnexa to reperfuse after detorsion, the affected adnexa are carefully examined for causes of torsion. Most commonly, an ovarian mass or cyst or paratubal cyst is noted that will need to be removed. Not uncommonly, the organ will appear so dark and swollen that it is difficult to clearly see a distinct mass or cyst. In such cases after untwisting the adnexa the procedure can be terminated and the patient followed carefully with follow-up ultrasound to assess the size and composition of the adnexa in the next couple of weeks. If a cyst is in fact seen, a planned operative laparoscopy and cystectomy can be performed.
- In the majority of cases, the adnexa will reperfuse dramatically and the color of the tissue will become pink.

Cystectomy/cyst aspiration

- If a distinct cyst is noted, the ovarian capsule on the cyst is cut using low-wattage current. The ovarian cortex is gently grasped and the cyst wall underneath is undermined and dissected away from the cortex. As the base of the cyst is approached, care must be taken regarding blood supply and small vessels coagulated. This can clearly be more difficult to assess the larger the size of the cyst. The goal is to remove the cyst wall intact and in its entirety without spill. An endocatch bag can be placed through one of the ports and the cyst is decompressed on the top of the bag and the cyst wall then removed from the abdomen. At times, a mini-laparotomy may be necessary to remove the cyst especially if bone fragments exist from a dermoid.
- In cases of large paratubal cysts, care must be taken to identify the course of the fallopian tube which in many instances is splayed very thin on the cyst and can easily be missed. Once again, an area away from the tube on the cyst is identified and the leaf of the broad ligament is grasped after incision is made, and the underlying cyst is dissected away. These cysts are typically clear and easily dissected and decompressed.
- In some instances, a larger looking ovary is noted secondary to polycystic ovarian syndrome or stimulation via gonadotropins. In these instances, only detorsion occurs and an assessment for possible oophoropexy.

Oophoropexy

- There is no consensus regarding the preferred technique or the timing of an oophoropexy.
- In the majority of cases, a nonabsorbable suture is recommended for use.
- In cases where the utero-ovarian ligament appears elongated, the proximal portion of the utero-ovarian ligament may be attached or plicated to its most distal portion via 2-0 nonabsorbable suture. This leads to shortening of this ligament thereby giving less mobility to the gonad. This is likely the preferred technique given that the anatomy of the pelvis is least distorted with this method. The relationship between the tube and ovary remains intact (Tech Fig. 11.4.4A,B).
- In some cases where the anatomy of the ligaments appears very normal but the size of the ovary is likely to remain large as in PCO-like ovaries, the meso-ovarium may be attached to the pelvic sidewall taking care to avoid the large pelvic vessels. This may again be performed with 2-0 nonabsorbable suture. There is some concern that the fallopian tube function may be compromised (Tech Fig. 11.4.5).
- In the pediatric literature, suturing the ovary to the posterior aspect of the uterine wall has been described.

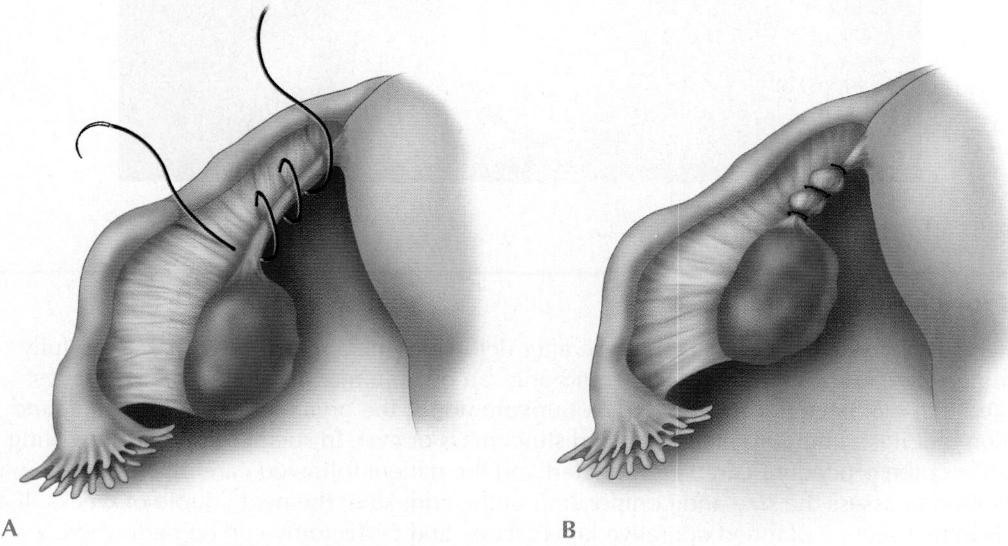

Tech Figure 11.4.4. A and B: Stich is applied to the proximal and distal portions of the utero-ovarian ligament and then inched down and tied. This results in shortening of the ligament.

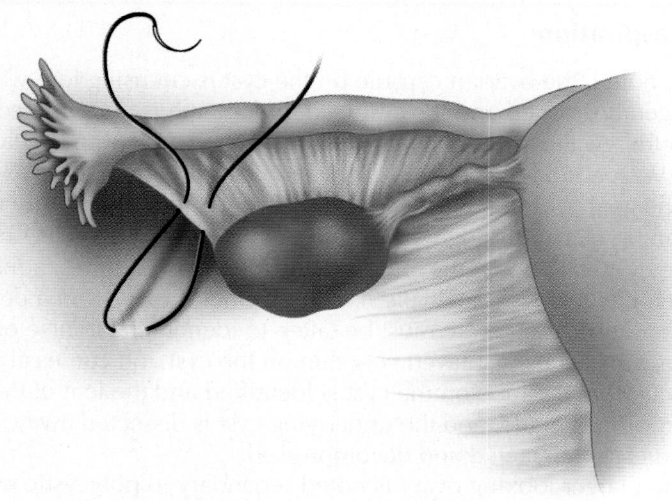

Tech Figure 11.4.5. Stich is placed in the meso-ovarium and then stitched to the peritoneum of the sidewall.

PEARLS AND PITFALLS

- Give time for the ovary to reperfuse.
- There is always some part of the ovary that can be salvaged.

POSTOPERATIVE CARE

- The immediate postoperative care is similar to a diagnostic laparoscopy. Typically when the patient awakens, the original pain from torsion is no longer present. They will need to be monitored for appropriate bowel and bladder function.
- Recurrence of pain and fever may indicate that the gonad has undergone necrosis. This is in fact a very rare occurrence.

OUTCOMES

- Ovarian function is preserved in 88% to 100% of patients that undergo detorsion of their adnexa.[3] Ovarian follicular development has been noted on ultrasound in such patients. In addition, ovaries have noted to look normal in a subsequent surgical procedure.[4]
- In cases where cystectomies were done successfully at the time of the detorsion, the pathology was consistent with functional cyst in 58% of cases.[4] In which case an argument can be made not to proceed with any intervention at the time of detorsion.
- Thus patients who have experienced torsion secondary to probable ovarian cyst may do well on combined oral contraceptive pills to prevent recurrence of a cyst.

COMPLICATIONS

- A very low probability of postoperative infection secondary to persistence of necrotic tissue has been reported.
- Loss of gonadal function may theoretically occur in cases of undiagnosed torsion.

KEY REFERENCES

1. Cohen SB, Weisz B, Seidman DS, Mashiach S, Lidor AL, Goldenberg M. Accuracy of the preoperative diagnosis in 100 emergency laparoscopies performed due to acute abdomen in nonpregnant women. *J Am Assoc Gynecol Laparosc.* 2001;8(1):92–94.
2. Valsky DV, Esh-Broder E, Cohen SM, Lipschuetz M, Yagel S. Added value of the gray-scale whirlpool sign in the diagnosis of adnexal torsion. *Ultrasound Obstet Gynecol.* 2010;36:630–634.
3. Oelsner G, Shashar D. Adnexal torsion. *Clin Obstet Gynecol.* 2006;49(3):459–463.
4. Oelsner G, Cohen SB, Soriano D, Admon D, Mashiach S, Carp H. Minimal surgery for the twisted ischemic adnexa can preserve ovarian function. *Hum Reprod.* 2003;18:2599–2602.
5. Sasaki KJ, Miller CE. Adnexal torsion: review of the literature. *J Minim Invasive Gynecol.* 2014;21:196–202.
6. Huchon C, Fauconnier A. Adnexal torsion: a literature review. *Eur J Obstet Gynecol Reprod Biol.* 2010;150:8–12.
7. Fuchs N, Smorgick N, Tovbin Y, et al. Oophoropexy to prevent adnexal torsion: how when and for whom? *J Minim Invasive Gynecol.* 2010;17:205–208.

Chapter 11.5 Ectopic Pregnancy and Salpingectomy

Lisa C. Hickman, Jeffrey M. Goldberg

GENERAL PRINCIPLES

Definition

- An ectopic pregnancy is one in which the embryo implants outside of the endometrial cavity. Ectopic pregnancies account for 1.5% to 2% of all pregnancies.

Differential Diagnosis

- The most common presenting symptoms of ectopic pregnancy include lower abdominal/pelvic pain (99%), delayed menses (74%), and vaginal bleeding (56%).[1] As such, the differential diagnosis is broad and should include both gynecologic and nongynecologic etiologies.
- For vaginal bleeding and/or pain in early pregnancy, the differential diagnosis includes:
  - Threatened, incomplete, complete and missed abortions
  - Subchorionic hematoma
  - Physiologic changes in early pregnancy
  - Gestational trophoblastic disease
- For lower abdominal/pelvic pain with or without vaginal bleeding, consider:
  - Adnexal torsion
  - Degenerating leiomyoma
  - Dysmenorrhea
  - Endometriosis
  - Hemorrhagic corpus luteum cyst
  - Pelvic inflammatory disease, tubo-ovarian abscess
  - Appendicitis
  - Cystitis
  - Diverticulitis
  - Inflammatory bowel disease
  - Irritable bowel syndrome
  - Nephrolithiasis

Anatomic Considerations

- The vast majority of ectopic pregnancies, 98%, are located in the fallopian tube, with 70% in the ampulla, 12% in the isthmus, 11% in the fimbriated end, and 2% in the interstitial (cornual) segment.[2] In these cases, the patient's clinical picture and diagnostic workup will largely direct the management plan. This will be further discussed in the sections below.

- Alternative locations of ectopic pregnancy, although rare, may require specialized treatment planning and can be associated with higher maternal morbidity. These include ovarian, cervical, abdominal, cesarean scar, rudimentary horn, and heterotopic pregnancies. Heterotopic pregnancies involve implantation of concurrent embryos in two separate locations, most commonly, an intrauterine and a tubal ectopic pregnancy.
- A pregnancy of unknown location refers to one in which the patient has an elevated serum hCG without evidence of a pregnancy on ultrasound. A pregnancy of unknown location can occur up to 20% of the time in women with first trimester pain and/or bleeding. Upon further workup, 21% will be ectopic, 53% will be spontaneous abortions, and 26% will be intrauterine pregnancies.[3] In a hemodynamically stable patient, one may trend hCG levels and perform repeat ultrasonography until the pregnancy location is determined; however, in a hemodynamically unstable patient or one with peritoneal signs, a diagnostic laparoscopy is warranted.

Nonoperative Management

- There are two primary nonoperative options for managing ectopic pregnancy: expectant management and medical treatment.
- Expectant management, which can be successful in nearly 20% of ectopic pregnancies, includes serial monitoring of hCG levels, follow up transvaginal ultrasonography if indicated, and cautious observation for changes in clinical status. Predicting the patients who will be best suited for expectant management can be difficult, so individuals who select this plan should be well counseled on the possibility for tubal rupture and the need for emergent surgery. Patients who can be considered for expectant management are asymptomatic and able to be compliant with the necessary follow-up. It has been suggested that expectant management outcomes are affected by the initial hCG level, with 90% of ectopic pregnancies spontaneously resolving when the baseline hCG is <1,000 IU/L and only 60% when the baseline hCG is <2,000 IU/L. Patients may continue to be followed expectantly as long as hCG levels are steadily decreasing and trending should continue until hCG becomes undetectable. If at any time hCG levels rise or plateau, medical or surgical management should be initiated.
- Medical management involves treatment with methotrexate, a folic acid antagonist that inactivates dihydrofolate reductase and thereby disrupts DNA and RNA synthesis. Similar to expectant management, patients best suited for medical management are lacking symptoms, hemodynamically stable and able to be compliant with follow-up. Absolute contraindications to methotrexate use include active pulmonary or peptic ulcer disease, alcoholism, breastfeeding, hematologic abnormalities, hepatic or renal dysfunction, immunodeficiency, and intolerance to the medication. In order to evaluate for eligibility, all patients should have a complete blood count, blood type, Rh antibody screen, serum creatinine, liver function panel, and transvaginal ultrasound prior to initiating methotrexate therapy. Use of methotrexate is thought to be most successful when the initial hCG level is less than 5,000 IU/L, the ectopic sac is less than 3 to 4 cm and there is no fetal cardiac activity.[4] There are several regimens of methotrexate dosing, including single, double, and multi-dose (**Table 11.5.1**). Numerous studies have compared efficacies of the different methotrexate regimens, and although both single and multi-dose regimens are effective in the treatment of ectopic pregnancy (88% vs. 93% success rate, respectively), a meta-analysis suggested that at least two doses are generally needed for successful ectopic management.[5] Regardless of the chosen regimen, all patients with properly decreasing serum hCG levels require measuring values weekly until hCG becomes undetectable. This on average takes 5 weeks, but may require up to 15 weeks of monitoring. A patient is considered to have failed methotrexate therapy if hCG levels rise or plateau any time after the initial measurements between days 4 and 7. Similar to expectant management, patients should understand warning signs and symptoms of tubal rupture, and the possible need for emergent surgery. Patients should be counseled to refrain from folic acid–containing supplements, NSAIDs, alcohol, excessive sunlight exposure, sexual intercourse, and strenuous physical activities while undergoing treatment with methotrexate. Lastly, patients should be provided with contraception for 3 to 6 months after successful treatment with methotrexate, as studies have shown that a single dose can take up to 8 months to be systemically cleared.
- In some circumstances, such as cervical, abdominal, cesarean scar, or interstitial ectopic pregnancies, one may chose to perform a more localized treatment by injecting an agent directly into the gestational sac under ultrasound or laparoscopic guidance. Methotrexate (50 mg/mL), potassium chloride (2 mEq/mL), and hyperosmolar (50%) glucose have all been successfully utilized, and function by delivering a high concentration of drug directly to the ectopic pregnancy. To

Table 11.5.1 Dosing Regimens for Methotrexate

Regimen	Methotrexate Dose	Administration Schedule	Monitoring Schedule	Additional Dosing
Single dose	50 mg/m^2 IM	Day 1	Day 1 (baseline), Days 4 and 7	Indicated if hCG levels do not decrease ≥15% from baseline
Two dose	50 mg/m^2 IM	Days 1 and 4		
Multi-dose	1 mg/kg IM 0.1 mg/kg (Leukovorin)	Up to 4 doses until hCG levels decrease ≥15% from baseline: Days 1, 3, 5, and 7 Leukovorin on Days 2, 4, 6, and 8	Day 1 (baseline), Days 3, 5, and 7	A maximum of 4 doses can be administered

perform localized injection, one must first aspirate the gestational sac contents and then inject ~10 mL of one of the aforementioned agents. In heterotopic pregnancies, direct injection with agents such as potassium chloride or hyperosmolar glucose provides a unique opportunity to manage the ectopic while decreasing the risk of interrupting the viable intrauterine pregnancy. Methotrexate injection should be avoided due to its known teratogenicity.

- Although limited data exists, uterine artery embolization, either alone or combined with medical or surgical management, has been safely and successfully used for the treatment of interstitial, cervical, and cesarean scar ectopic pregnancies.

IMAGING AND OTHER DIAGNOSTICS

- For the majority of ectopic pregnancies, the diagnosis can be quickly made with a quantitative hCG level and a transvaginal ultrasound. A serum progesterone level may provide additional information in cases where the viability of the pregnancy is uncertain.
- A quantitative hCG level can be assessed through a simple blood draw, and elevations in the maternal serum can be appreciated as early as 8 days after the LH surge. In normal pregnancies, hCG is produced by the syncytiotrophoblasts in a predictable manner, and levels increase in a linear fashion during the timeframe when an ectopic pregnancy may occur. A rise of at least 53% to 66% every 48 hours should be appreciated in normal pregnancies. Levels will continue to increase in this manner until they peak at approximately 100,000 IU/L, around 8 to 10 weeks of gestation. Pregnancies deviating from this trend on serial hCG monitoring are only indicative of an abnormal pregnancy and require further evaluation.
- Serum hCG assays are both highly sensitive and specific, with detection limits below 5 IU/L. Both false-negative and false-positive results are rare; however, in the case of a static and consistently elevated serum hCG level, one must evaluate for the presence of heterophilic antibodies. This diagnosis is made by obtaining a negative urine hCG. An additional consideration for cautious hCG interpretation is for individuals with an increased likelihood of a multifetal gestation, such as those who have conceived with the help of assisted reproductive technologies. In these cases, hCG levels will likely be elevated beyond that expected for the gestational age and may not be reliable for directing the expected findings on ultrasonography.
- Transvaginal ultrasonography can detect evidence of a pregnancy as early as 4.5 to 5 weeks gestational age, with the visualization of the gestational sac. At 5 to 6 weeks, a yolk sac can be seen, and between 5.5 to 6 weeks, a fetal heartbeat can be appreciated. Correlating the hCG level with ultrasonography helps to interpret the findings. Generally, sonographic evidence of an intrauterine pregnancy should be seen by day 24 if conception date is known, or with hCG levels between 1,500 and 2,000 IU/L, also known as the discriminatory zone.[6] A definitive diagnosis of an ectopic pregnancy is made when a gestational sac with yolk sac and/or fetal pole is appreciated outside of the endometrial cavity. Findings which are concerning for ectopic pregnancy include a complex adnexal mass, tubal ring, and free fluid in the posterior cul-de-sac; however, these alone are insufficient to diagnose an ectopic pregnancy. Color and pulsed Doppler ultrasonography can be helpful when a diagnosis is unclear. As arterial and venous blood flow is increased to a developing pregnancy, this technique may help differentiate an intrauterine pseudosac from an intrauterine pregnancy and an ectopic pregnancy from an ovarian or paratubal cyst.
- Serum progesterone levels should rise progressively throughout pregnancy. Assessment of this level can be helpful in distinguishing a normal from an abnormal pregnancy when the previous workup is inconclusive. Generally, a progesterone level of <5 ng/mL is suggestive of a nonviable pregnancy, whereas a level >20 ng/mL is consistent with a viable pregnancy. The limitation of this test, however, is that it cannot aid in elucidating the pregnancy location.
- Historically, culdocentesis was performed in the setting of an indeterminate ultrasound and a high clinical suspicion. A large bore spinal needle was inserted through the posterior vaginal fornix to aspirate the contents of the posterior cul-de-sac. An aspirate of blood is consistent with hemoperitoneum, a common sequela of tubal rupture. This test has largely fallen out of favor, not only because of its invasiveness, but also because it has an inferior sensitivity and specificity for hemoperitoneum as compared to transvaginal ultrasound.
- Special considerations for difficult diagnoses:
  - The diagnosis of extratubal ectopic pregnancies can be especially challenging given their rare incidence and sometimes unusual presentations. Specific criteria have been developed to assist with diagnosing interstitial, ovarian, cervical, and cesarean scar pregnancies (**Table 11.5.2**). The use of additional imaging modalities, such as MRI, may be helpful in establishing the pregnancy location.
  - Gracia and Barnhart[7] developed a helpful algorithm for the workup of a pregnancy of unknown location. If the hCG level is above the discriminatory zone and a pregnancy cannot be identified on ultrasound, a dilation and curettage can be performed. The absence of chorionic villi in the curettage and a continued rise in hCG confirms the presence of an ectopic pregnancy. If the hCG level is below the discriminatory zone, repeat hCG levels and a follow-up transvaginal ultrasound should be performed.

PREOPERATIVE PLANNING

- Since most patients have ready access to the above diagnostic testing, ectopic pregnancies are diagnosed early and fertility-preserving surgery can be performed in a controlled manner. It is very rare to see a hemodynamically unstable patient from massive hemoperitoneum due to a ruptured ectopic.
- If the patient is unstable, obtain a complete blood count and type and cross for the potential administration of blood products. Obtain venous access with two peripheral large-bore IVs for fluid resuscitation and place an indwelling Foley catheter to monitor urine output.
- For stable patients with an early unruptured ectopic pregnancy, a fertility-sparing salpingostomy may be planned. However, the patient should be consented for possible salpingectomy if the fallopian tube is significantly damaged or hemostasis cannot be achieved.

SURGICAL MANAGEMENT

- When deciding the best course for surgical management, one must consider the patient's clinical status, laboratory results, ultrasound findings, and fertility desire.

Table 11.5.2 Criteria for the Diagnosis of Interstitial, Ovarian, Cervical, and Cesarean Scar Ectopic Pregnancies

Ectopic Location	Prevalence	Diagnostic Criteria	Helpful Imaging Modalities	Management Options
Interstitial	2% of all ectopic pregnancies	• Eccentrically located GS >1 cm from the endometrial stripe • GS surrounded by a thin layer of myometrium measuring <5–8 mm	Ultrasound, MRI	• Laparoscopic cornuostomy • Systemic MTX • Direct injection
Ovarian	1–3% of all ectopic pregnancies	• A normal fallopian tube on the affected side • GS located in the ovary • Ovary and GS are connected by the utero-ovarian ligament to the uterus • Histologic confirmation of ovarian tissue in the GS wall	Ultrasound	• Laparoscopic excision of the ectopic • Case reports of systemic MTX
Cervical	<1% of all ectopics	• The GS is below the internal os • The uterine cavity is empty • The cervical canal is dilated and barrel shaped	Ultrasound, MRI	• Systemic MTX • Direct injection • Curettage with or without prior UAE
Cesarean scar	6% of all ectopics in women with a prior cesarean section	• Empty uterine cavity • GS in the anterior lower uterine segment • Absence or thinning of myometrium between the GS and bladder	Ultrasound, MRI	• Laparoscopy hysteroscopy or laparotomy • D&C • Systemic MTX • Direct injection • UAE
Abdominal	1.5% of all ectopics	• No specific criteria, common finding is absence of myometrium between the bladder and the pregnancy	Ultrasound	• Laparoscopy or laparotomy depending on the gestational age

GS, gestational sac; MTX, methotrexate; UAE, uterine artery embolization.

- In cases of tubal rupture, the fallopian tube is often damaged beyond repair and will require a complete salpingectomy. A salpingectomy should also be performed in the setting of recurrent ectopic pregnancy or prior surgery on the ipsilateral fallopian tube, uncontrollable intraoperative hemorrhage, or completed childbearing. In the latter case, the contralateral tube may be ligated for contraception.
- In patients who are clinically stable, but do not meet the criteria for medical management, a salpingostomy may be performed for individuals who desire future fertility, especially when the contralateral fallopian tube is surgically absent or appears functionally compromised.

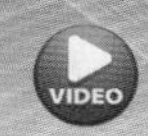

Procedures and Techniques (Videos 11.5.1 and 11.5.2)

Examination under anesthesia

- After general anesthesia is obtained, a gentle pelvic examination should be performed to ascertain the size, mobility, and positioning of the uterus, as well as to evaluate for fullness in the adnexa. Extreme care must be taken during adnexal palpation, as tubal rupture may occur if excessive pressure is exerted on the affected fallopian tube.

Patient positioning and creation of a sterile surgical field

- The patient should be placed in the low dorsal–lithotomy position using Allen-type stirrups with the legs in neutral position and the weight on the soles of the feet. The arms should be tucked at the patient's sides using a draw sheet. If the patient is obese, arm sleds may be indicated. The extremities are padded at pressure points to prevent neuropathy. Shoulder braces should be avoided, as these have the potential to cause a brachial plexus injury.
- Throughout the positioning process, one must communicate with the anesthesia provider to ensure that the patient's IV, pulse oximeter, and ventilation are not compromised.
- Intermittent pneumatic compression stockings should be placed on the lower extremities to help prevent deep vein thrombosis.
- The abdomen, upper thighs, and vagina are prepped and draped.
- Generally, prophylactic antibiotics are not indicated.

Insertion of a uterine manipulator

- A uterine manipulator may be inserted to facilitate exposure of the fallopian tubes. First, a bivalve speculum is inserted into the vagina. The anterior surface of the cervix is grasped with a single-toothed tenaculum to stabilize the cervix and straighten the uterine axis. A uterine sound may be used to assess the length and direction of the endometrial cavity. Gentle cervical dilation is performed if needed. A uterine manipulator is inserted, and the tenaculum and speculum are removed. No manipulator is placed in cases of heterotopic pregnancy so as not to disrupt the intrauterine pregnancy.
- An indwelling Foley catheter is placed to avoid bladder distention during surgery.
- A nasogastric or orogastric tube, placed by anesthesia, helps to ensure the stomach is decompressed during trocar insertion.

Abdominal entry

- The technique utilized for initial trocar placement is largely dependent on surgeon preference and expertise.
- Traditionally, initial entry through the umbilicus is chosen, as it is the thinnest portion of the abdominal wall. Mindfulness of the anatomical structures below is critical and vary based on the patient's habitus. This also determines the safest angle for trocar entry. Insert the trocar at a 45-degree angle in thin patients and 90 degrees in obese patients. There is no evidence that using a Veress needle or optical trocars reduces the incidence of complications with initial abdominal entry. Also, injecting local anesthesia at the trocar sites has not been shown to significantly reduce postoperative discomfort.

- Consider a left upper quadrant entry for patients at risk for having bowel adherent to the anterior abdominal wall beneath the umbilicus. These would include those with prior abdominopelvic surgery (especially with a midline laparotomy) or pelvic infection from pelvic inflammatory disease, Crohn's disease, or ruptured appendix. A 5-mm trocar is placed under the lowest rib in the mid-clavicular line. Again, an oro- or nasogastric tube must be inserted to decompress the stomach. An umbilical port may be safely placed under direct vision after assuring that it is free from adherent bowel. A 10-mm trocar is placed transumbilically to facilitate tissue extraction. After the initial trocar is inserted and intraperitoneal placement is confirmed, pneumoperitoneum is established with carbon dioxide gas and the patient placed in Trendelenburg positioning.
- A survey of the peritoneal cavity is important prior to inserting accessory ports. One should evaluate for any adhesive disease, inspect the anatomy, and identify the course of the inferior epigastric vessels. Also, transilluminate the abdominal wall with the laparoscope from within the pelvis to identify and avoid superficial vessels in the abdominal wall.
- Two accessory 5-mm ports should then be placed under direct laparoscopic visualization, one in each lower quadrant.

Salpingostomy versus salpingectomy

- For a salpingostomy, one can begin by grasping the affected fallopian tube with an atraumatic grasper and then injecting dilute vasopressin (20 units in 100 mL of injectable saline) into the mesosalpinx inferior to the pregnancy sac (Tech Fig. 11.5.1). A linear incision, 1 to 2 cm in length, can be made using monopolar needlepoint cautery on the antimesenteric side of the fallopian tube (Tech Figs. 11.5.2 and 11.5.3). Any instrument may be used to apply gentle pressure beneath the ectopic to help extrude the products of conception (POC) (Tech Figs. 11.5.4 and 11.5.5). This is preferred to manually removing the POC with graspers, which tends to cause

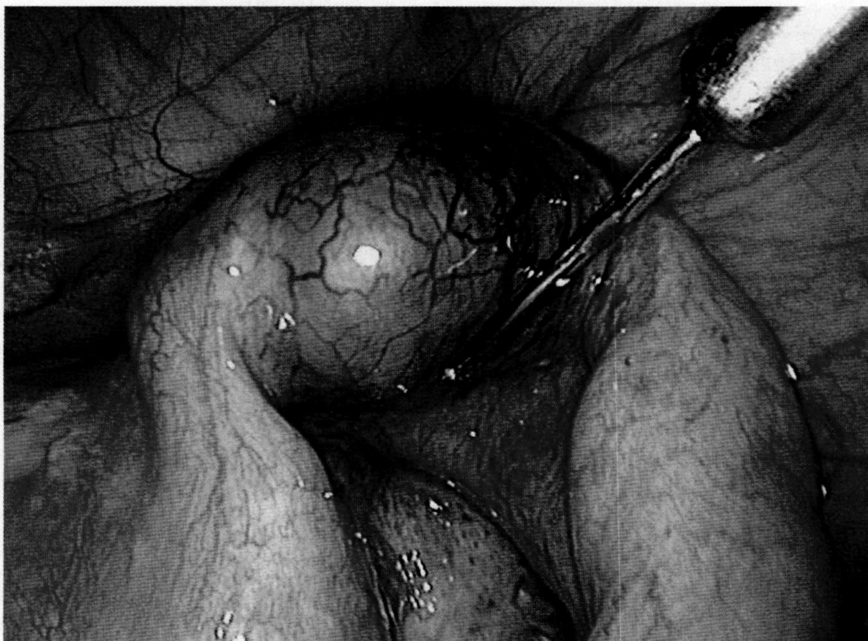

Tech Figure 11.5.1. Injecting vasopressin into the ectopic pregnancy.

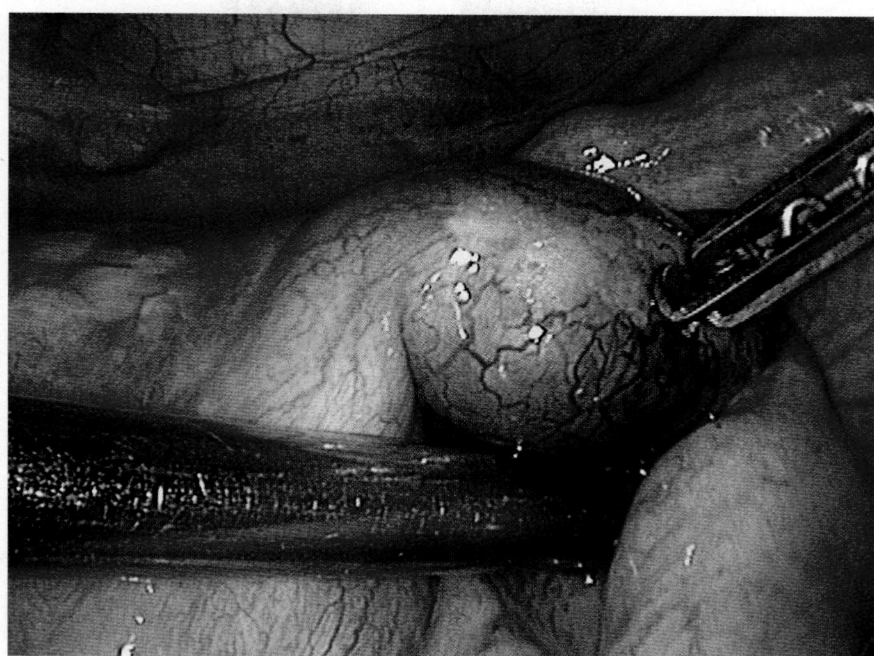

Tech Figure 11.5.2. Coagulating the superficial vessels.

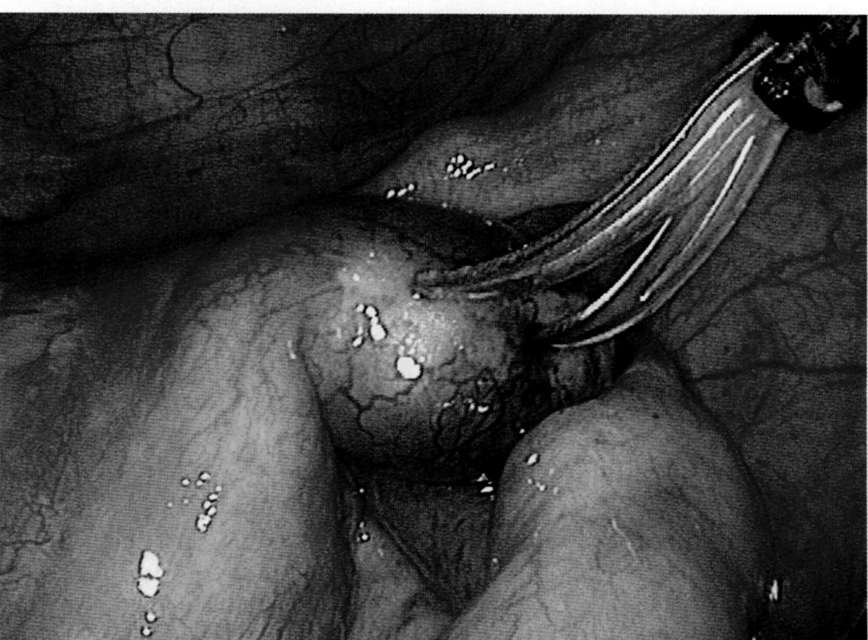

Tech Figure 11.5.3. Sharply incising the fallopian tube.

more bleeding. Once the POC is out, the tubal defect is irrigated and bipolar cautery is used sparingly to achieve hemostasis while limiting thermal damage (Tech Figs. 11.5.6 to 11.5.9). With the exception of the POC protruding though the fimbria, "tubal milking" should be avoided as it causes more damage to the fallopian tube than salpingostomy. Salpingectomy involves coagulating and dividing the proximal isthmic segment and serially coagulating and cutting the mesosalpinx. A bipolar grasper, such as a Kelppinger, may be used with scissors as well as any vessel-sealing device. The procedure can be performed from proximal to distal or distal to proximal depending on which is technically easier. It is of utmost importance to stay as close as

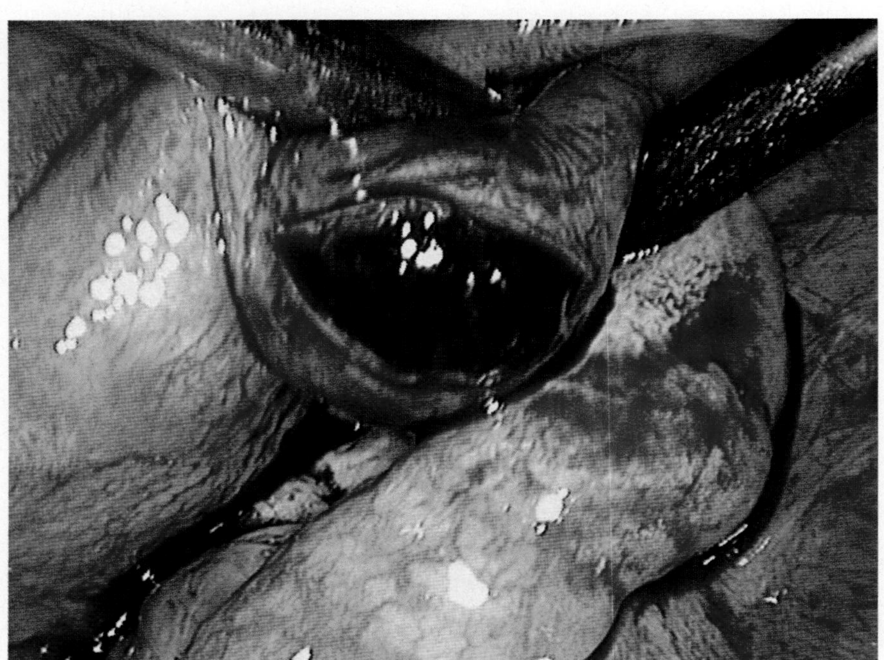

Tech Figure 11.5.4. Expressing the products of conception (POC).

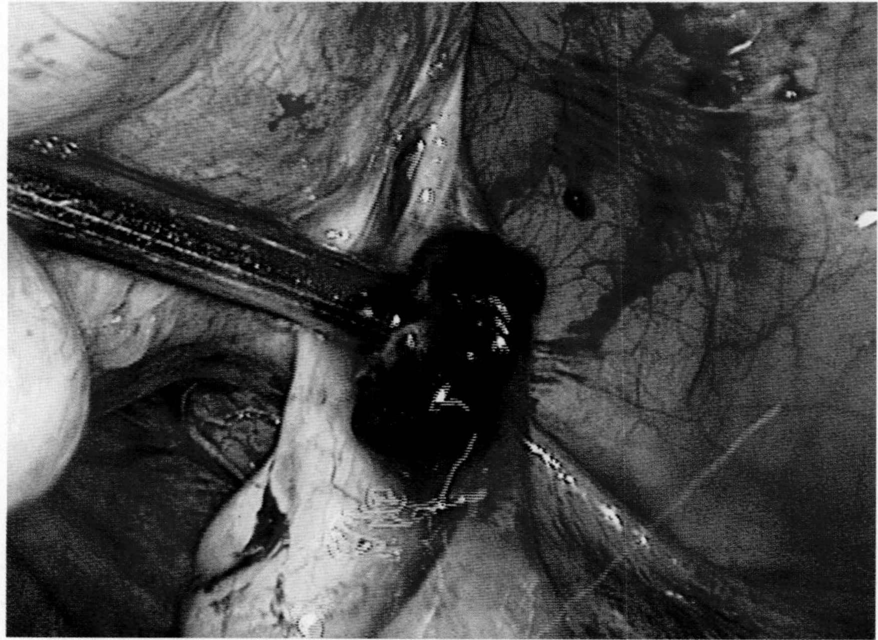

Tech Figure 11.5.5. POC ready for removal.

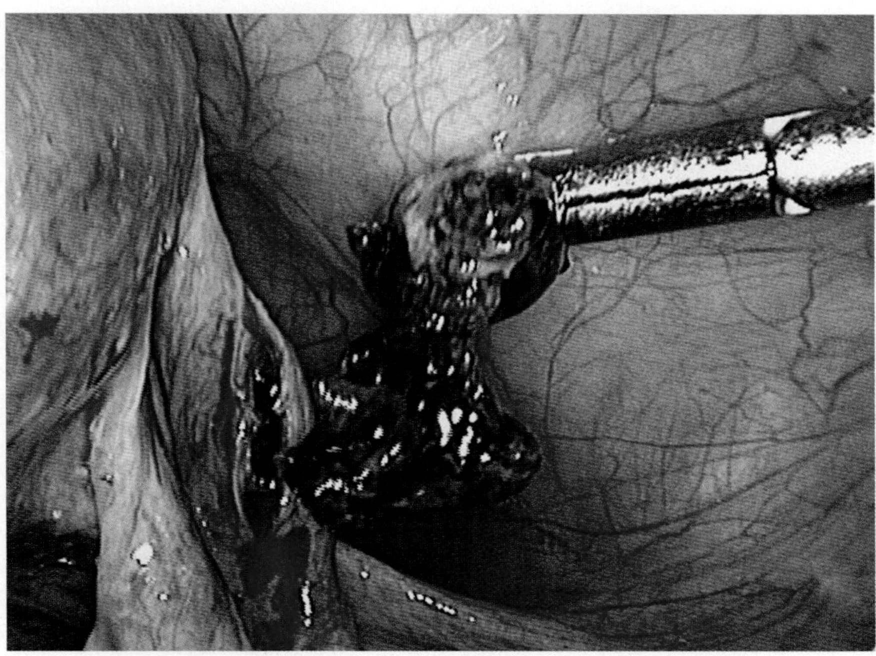

Tech Figure 11.5.6. Removing the POC from the fallopian tube.

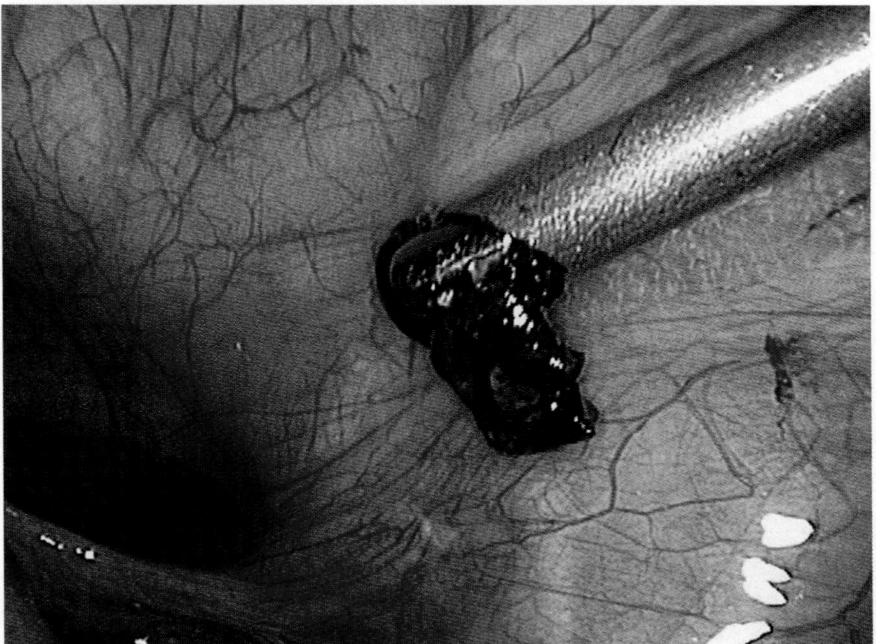

Tech Figure 11.5.7. Extracting the specimen.

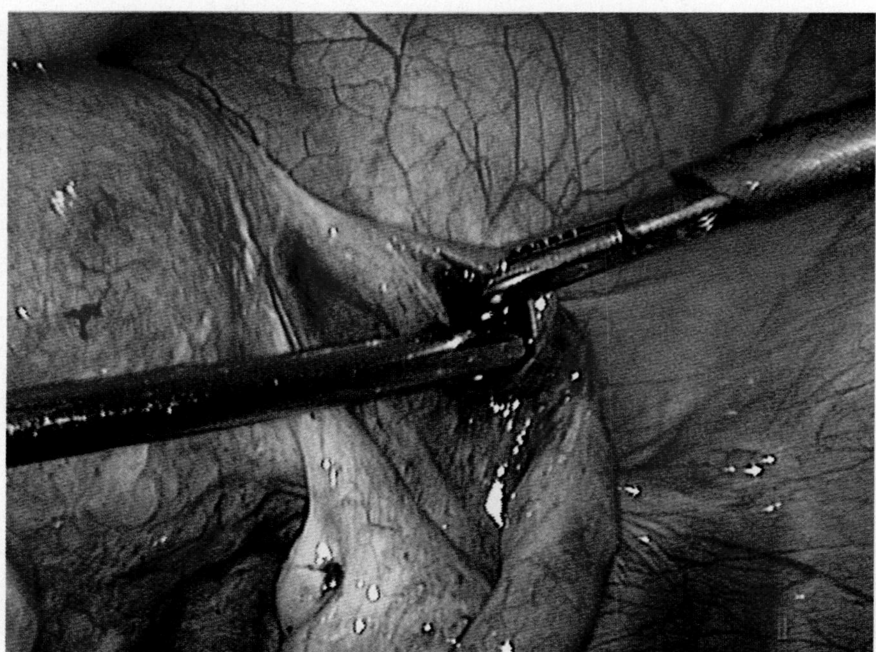

Tech Figure 11.5.8. Irrigating the fallopian tube.

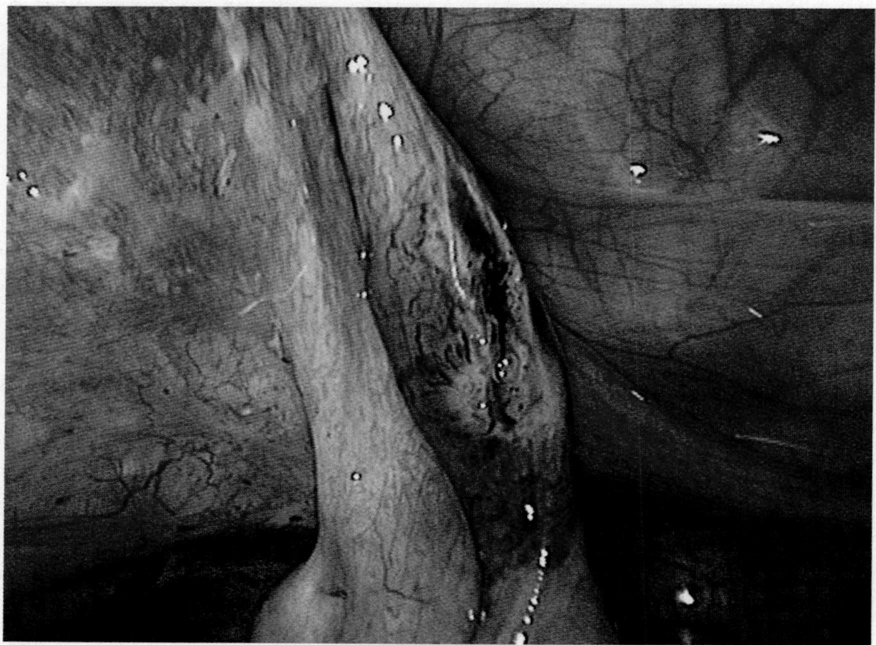

Tech Figure 11.5.9. Performing the final visual inspection of the fallopian tube at the end of the case.

possible to the fallopian tube to avoid compromising the ovarian vascular supply, which may lead to diminished ovarian reserve.

Retrieval of the specimen

- A 5-mm laparoscope is placed through one of the lower ports, or left upper quadrant port if used, and the specimen is extracted though the 10-mm umbilical port, with or without endoscopic bag. The key point is to avoid leaving any POC, which may develop a collateral blood supply and continue to grow.

Case completion

- The abdomen and pelvis should be copiously irrigated and the fluid aspirated. Bipolar cautery may be used if needed to assure complete hemostasis. Again, all POC should be removed, as failure to do so may result in persistent trophoblastic implants. The insufflation pressure can be decreased to ensure that no bleeding occurs under lower intra-abdominal pressures.
- The fascia of the 10-mm umbilical port must be closed with a delayed absorbable suture. This can be accomplished by placing the 5-mm laparoscope through one of the lower ports, removing the 10-mm port, and using an endoclose (Grice) needle or a Carter–Thomason device to suture the defect. Alternatively, it can be closed with a UR-6 needle on a conventional needle holder after all of the ports have been removed. The fascia should be closed with a delayed absorbable suture for any other port sites of 8 mm or greater to prevent a potential incisional hernia.
- The pneumoperitoneum is released, taking care to ensure that as much of the carbon dioxide gas is removed from the abdomen as possible for patient comfort postoperatively. All of the instruments are removed.
- The skin incisions can be closed with a delayed absorbable suture in a subcuticular fashion or with tissue adhesive.

POSTOPERATIVE CARE

- Same-day discharge to home may be appropriate if the surgical procedure was uncomplicated and the patient is doing well during the postoperative recovery. If a significant amount of blood loss occurred, observation overnight to follow vital signs and serial blood counts may be more appropriate.
- A patient may return to her preoperative diet and activities when she feels ready.
- Rh(D) immune globulin should be administered if indicated.
- Quantitative hCG levels should be followed weekly until negative if a salpingostomy is performed. Consider administering a dose of methotrexate (50 mg/m^2 BSA) to reduce the risk of persistent trophoblastic disease.
- Contraception should be provided if the pregnancy was unplanned. If pregnancy was planned, the patient should be instructed not to attempt to conceive until her hCG is negative and her menses resume.
- The patient should be informed that she is now at a higher risk for another ectopic and to call as soon as she conceives for close follow-up.

OUTCOMES

- A history of an ectopic pregnancy is a significant risk factor for recurrence, and approximately 15% of individuals will have a subsequent ectopic pregnancy. When stratified by treatment regimens, salpingostomy had a higher recurrence rate compared to salpingectomy and single-dose methotrexate (15%, 10%, and 8%, respectively).[8] It has been estimated that ~60% of individuals will have a successful pregnancy after an ectopic, regardless of the utilized surgical technique.[9]

COMPLICATIONS

- The primary complications in the management of ectopic pregnancies are related to the inherent risks associated with surgery. These include reaction to anesthesia, bleeding, infection, and unintentional injury to other organs, such as the bowel or bladder.
- The risk of incomplete removal of ectopic tissue is higher when surgery is performed at an early gestational age, the gestational sac diameter is small, tubal rupture occurred, salpingostomy is technically difficult, or insufficient irrigation is performed at the end of the procedure.[10] For salpingostomy, the risk of persistent ectopic pregnancy was estimated to be 3% to 20%. If a remnant of trophoblastic tissue remains in the abdomen, hCG levels may be persistently elevated. This can often be ameliorated with a dose of methotrexate postoperatively.

KEY REFERENCES

1. Alsuleiman SA, Grimes EM. Ectopic pregnancy: a review of 147 cases. *J Reprod Med.* 1982;27:101–106.
2. Bouyer J, Coste J, Fernandez H, Pouly JL, Job-Spira N. Sites of ectopic pregnancy: a 10 year population-based study of 1800 cases. *Hum Reprod.* 2002;17:3224–3230.
3. Barnhart KT, Gosman G, Ashby R, Sammel M. The medical management of ectopic pregnancy: a meta-anlysis comparing "single dose" to "multidose" regimens. *Obstet Gynecol.* 2003;101:778–784.
4. Menon S, Colins J, Barnhart KT. Establishing a human chorionic gonadotropin cutoff to guide methotrexate treatment of ectopic pregnancy: a systematic review. *Fertil Steril.* 2007;87:123–127.
5. Barnhart KT, Sammel MD, Takacs P, et al. Validation of a clinical risk scoring system, based solely on clinical presentation, for the management of pregnancy of unknown location. *Fertil Steril.* 2013;99(1):193–198.
6. Kadar N, Bohrer M, Kemmann E, Shelden R. The discriminatory human chorionic gonadotropin zone for endovaginal sonography: a prospective, randomized study. *Fertil Steril.* 1994;61(6):1016–1020.
7. Gracia CR, Barnhart KT. Diagnosing ectopic pregnancy: decision analysis comparing six strategies. *Obstet Gynecol.* 2001;97(3):464–470.
8. Yao M, Tulandi T. Current status of surgical and nonsurgical management of ectopic pregnancy. *Fertil Steril.* 1997;67(3):421–433.
9. Mol F, van Mello NM, Strandell A, et al. Salpingostomy versus salpingectomy in women with tubal pregnancy (ESEP study): an open-label, multicenter, randomized controlled trial. *Lancet.* 2014;383(9927):1483–1489.
10. Seifer DB, Gutmann JN, Grant WD, Kamps CA, DeCherney AH. Comparison of persistent ectopic pregnancy after laparoscopic salpingostomy versus salpingostomy at laparotomy for ectopic pregnancy. *Obstet Gynecol.* 1993;81:378–382.

Section VI

Surgical Management of Endometriosis

12 Surgery for Ovarian and Peritoneal Disease

M. Jean Uy-Kroh, Tommaso Falcone

GENERAL PRINCIPLES

Definition

- Endometriosis is a chronic, nonmalignant, condition characterized by pelvic pain and infertility that is hormonally mediated and responsive to hormone suppression and surgical excision. It is defined by the histologic identification of ectopic implants of endometrial glands and stroma. These implants are commonly found on the pelvic peritoneum, abdominal, and pelvic organs. Endometriosis can also be found within remote locations such as the thoracic cavity. The pathogenesis of endometriosis remains unclear.

Differential Diagnosis

- Adhesions, pelvic inflammatory disease, mittelschmerz, chronic pelvic pain, malignancy, hemorrhagic ovarian cyst.

Nonoperative Management

- Unfortunately, the only way to diagnose endometriosis is with tissue biopsies obtained during surgery. Once surgical pathology confirms ectopic endometriosis tissue, conservative nonoperative management with oral contraceptive pills and nonsteroidal anti-inflammatory drugs is recommended to inhibit ovulation and decrease pain. Other medications such as progestins, gonadotropin-releasing hormone agonists, and aromatase inhibitors may also be utilized to suppress the disease. Nonoperative medical management of this chronic disease is a cornerstone of treatment and should accompany surgical management.

IMAGING AND OTHER DIAGNOSTICS

Occasionally a speculum examination can reveal vaginal endometriosis implants that can be biopsied and confirm the diagnosis. More commonly, the pelvic examination yields suggestive but nonspecific findings of endometriosis such as decreased uterine mobility, a palpable adnexal mass, or rectovaginal and uterosacral nodules.

- Transvaginal ultrasound is the diagnostic imaging modality of choice for identifying ovarian endometriomas (Fig. 12.1). Rectal endometriosis can also be seen with transvaginal ultrasound, particularly with the addition of rectal contrast, and requires experienced sonographers and a high level of radiographic expertise.
- Small endometriomas are identified by abdominal or vaginal ultrasounds obtained at least 6 to 8 weeks apart to differentiate them from hemorrhagic corpus luteal cysts that usually involute during this time period. Larger endometriomas that are 4 to 5 cm or more in diameter are usually diagnosed by their characteristic homogeneous pattern (Fig. 12.2). The hypoechoic cyst may contain diffuse low-level echoes with septations and multiloculations and may not benefit from repeat imaging.
- Magnetic resonance imaging (MRI), with enterography, is reserved for equivocal ultrasound findings or for patients with a clinical history consistent with deep infiltrating endometriosis invading the bowel or bladder.
- Computed tomography (CT) is not a recommended imaging modality.
- For patients who desire fertility, have struggled with infertility, are 35 years of age or older, or have ovarian endometriomas, a serum anti-müllerian hormone level may be useful for fertility counseling.

Figure 12.1. 5.5-cm endometrioma identified by TVUS.

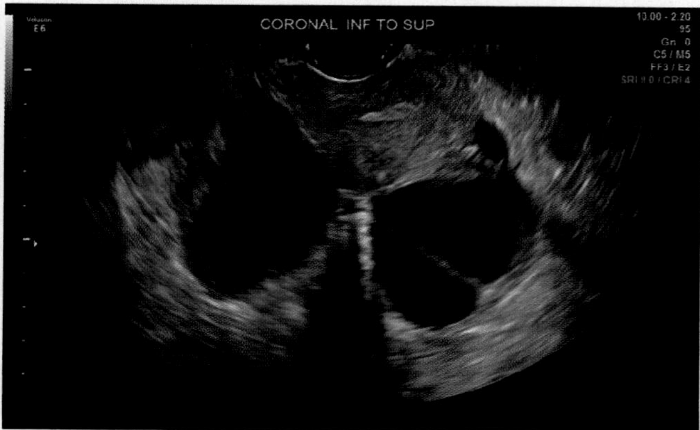

Figure 12.2. Bilateral 5-cm endometriomas identified by TVUS.

- Currently, there are no reliable serum markers for endometriosis. Ca-125 can be elevated in endometriosis and is not recommended unless there is a strong suspicion for malignancy.

PREOPERATIVE PLANNING

- An examination under anesthesia is performed to assess uterine position, sacral nodularity, and palpable adnexal masses that may affect incision length or laparoscopic trocar placement.
- Angled 30- or 45-degree laparoscopes can increase the range of surgical views, particularly for large adnexal masses.
- Cystoscopy is indicated when extensive sidewall adhesiolysis or ureterolysis is performed. Intraoperative intravenous indigo carmine or 10% sodium fluorescein, or presurgical administration of oral pyridium provides urine contrast for easy identification of the urine jets from the ureteral orifices.

SURGICAL MANAGEMENT

- Indications for surgical intervention may include the need to obtain tissue diagnosis, pain refractory to medical management, contraindications to medical therapy, to resect deep infiltrating endometriosis that is causing obstruction to the genitourinary or gastrointestinal tracts, to exclude malignancy in an adnexal mass, to improve pregnancy rates in infertile patients with suspected endometrioma, and to treat chronic pain in the infertile patient who desires pregnancy.
- Although endometriosis historically shares many characteristics that are similar to malignancy (tissue biopsy diagnosis, surgically staged condition, and it is colloquially referred to as recurrence of disease instead of persistence of disease) it is crucially important to remember that endometriosis is a *benign and chronic* condition. Application of malignant surgical principles such as debulking and cytoreduction tend to supersede the overall well-being of the patient. Surgical interventions for endometriosis must be thoughtful and tempered. Extreme surgical management that results in significant patient morbidity or decreased functionality is not encouraged.
- When endometriosis affects areas that are vulnerable to tissue damage and destruction, such as ovarian follicles, ablative techniques may be appropriate.
- Optimal endometrioma treatment in reproductive age women weighs inadvertent follicle destruction against endometrioma recurrence.
  - Current endometrioma surgical management is largely influenced by a Cochrane review that demonstrated endometriomas greater than 3 cm have a higher recurrence rate when ablated with bipolar energy versus cyst excision.
  - Recent investigations suggest that cyst fenestration and plasma vaporization may preserve antral follicles without compromising cyst recurrence or subsequent pregnancy rates.
  - While we await randomized, prospective investigation that confirms this claim, surgeons must reconsider their techniques to balance adequate treatment of symptomatic disease against unintentional reduction of the very fertility they wish to preserve.
- A key to both endometrioma and peritoneal endometriosis excision is identification and separation of endometriosis from healthy tissue.
- The goal of the surgery is paramount and should dictate the degree of surgical intervention.

For some patients, excision of a pelvic lesion to exclude malignancy is sufficient. For others, restoration of anatomy and resection of deep infiltrating disease are necessary.

Positioning

- Please see low lithotomy positioning described in Chapter 5.
- Laparoscopy: The patient's arms are gently tucked and extremities protected with padding. Her legs comfortably rest in neutral position in adjustable leg stirrups that allow for perineal access and manipulation of the uterus.

Approach

A minimally invasive, laparoscopic approach is the preferred surgical approach for this benign disease. Extensive adhesiolysis, excision, and ablation can be performed safely by an experienced laparoscopic surgeon.

Endometrioma Excision (Video 12.1)

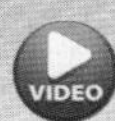

Identify anatomic landmarks

- First, perform an initial survey to identify landmarks—this is especially helpful in the case of distorted anatomy.
  - The bilateral medial and lateral umbilical ligaments are helpful to orient the anatomic space, to ensure safe dissection (Tech Fig. 12.1A–C). Perform adhesiolysis and expose the ureter.

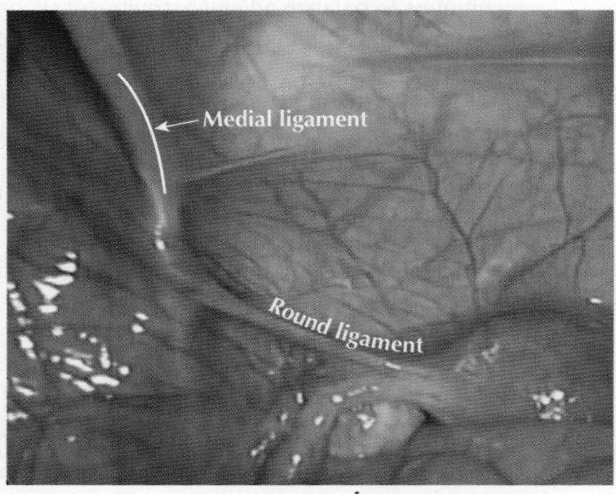

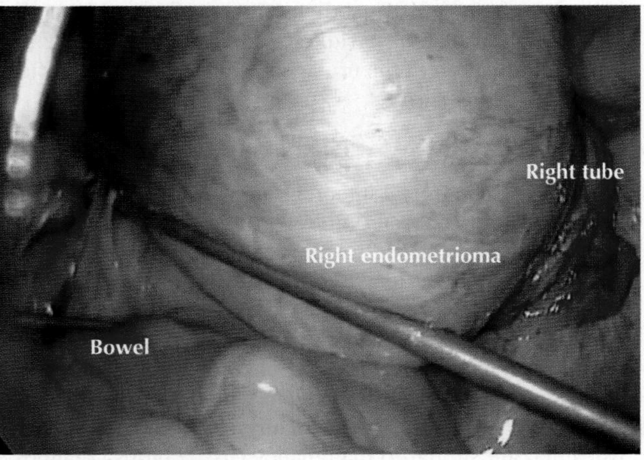

C

Tech Figure 12.1. **A:** The medial umbilical ligament contains the obliterated umbilical artery and points to the anterior division of the internal iliac artery. The lateral umbilical fold contains the inferior epigastric vessels. **B:** Distorted anatomy endometrioma right tube, and bowel. **C:** Endometrioma, myoma, left adnexa.

Incise the thinnest area of ovarian cortex overlying the endometrioma

- See Tech Figure 12.2.

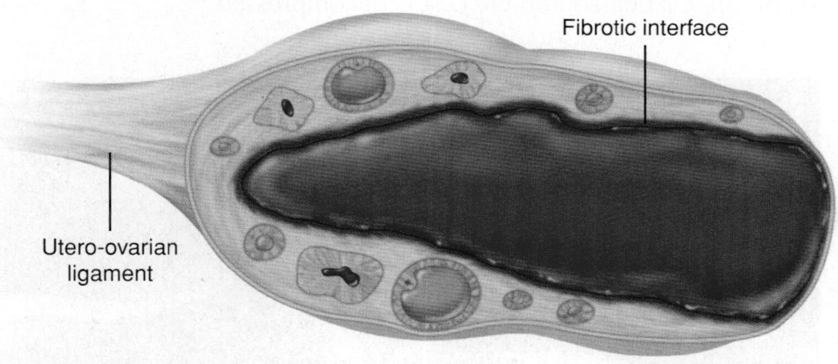

Tech Figure 12.2. Endometrioma with fibrotic interface.

Perform adhesiolysis of the fibrotic interface from the ovarian cortex and if necessary decompress the cyst

- The characteristic expulsion of old heme or "chocolate fluid" signals entry into the endometrioma and the contents are evacuated and the cyst is decompressed (Tech Fig. 12.3A,B).

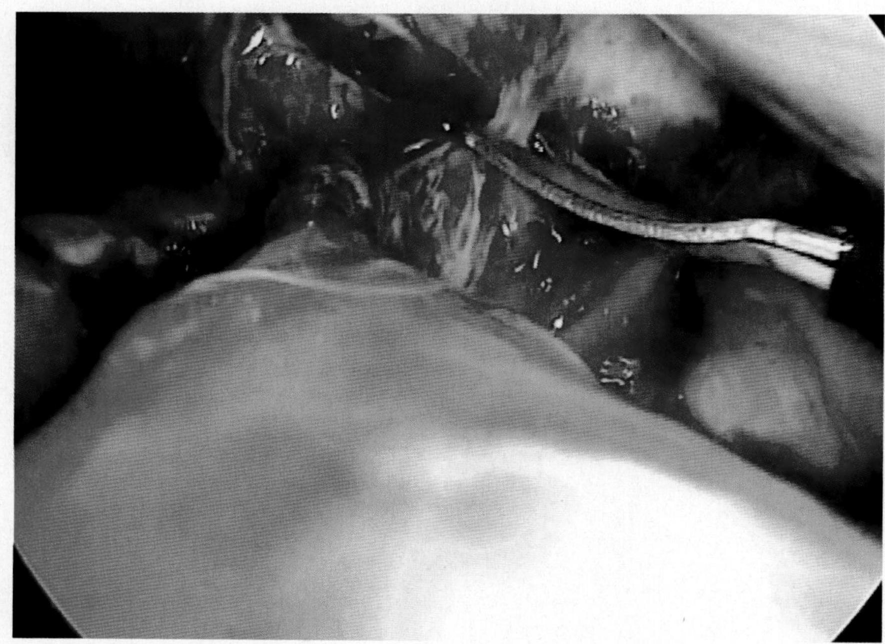

A

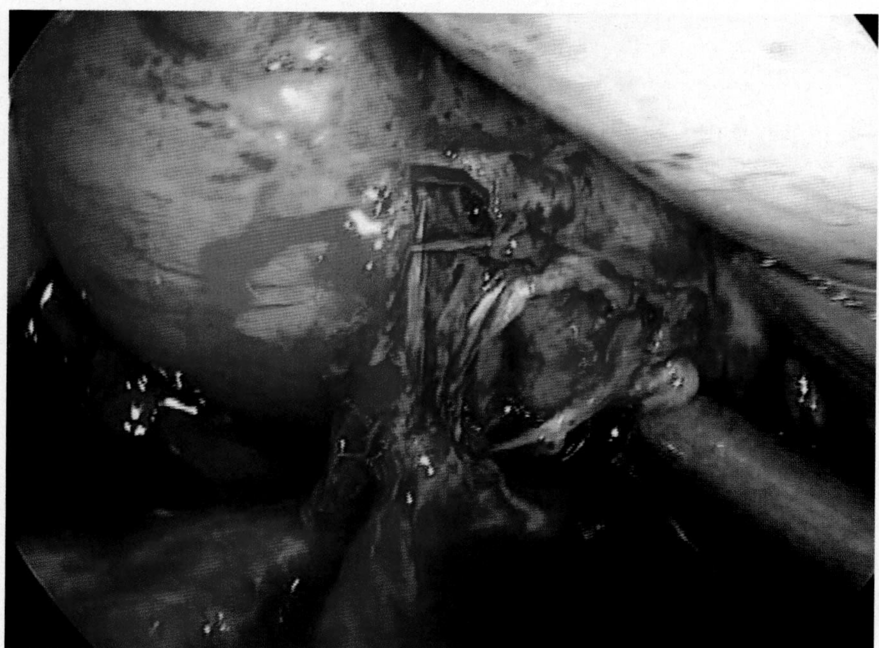

B

Tech Figure 12.3. A: Identify and incise the thin ovarian cortex, exposing the endometrioma. B: Evacuate and decompress the cyst.

Identify and bluntly separate the endometrioma from the ovarian parenchyma

- To reduce follicle destruction, meticulous, controlled, traction and countertraction are applied to the opposing tissue planes (Tech Fig. 12.4A). Large endometriomas will be turned inside out with progressive dissection.
- Forceful tissue separation causes "stripping" of ovarian follicles, therefore, this should be avoided.
- The endometrioma cyst wall will appear thick and white and adherent to ovarian tissue. Once in the correct cleavage plane, the cyst wall will easily yield and separate from ovarian parenchyma in bursts with blunt dissection (Tech Fig. 12.4B,C).

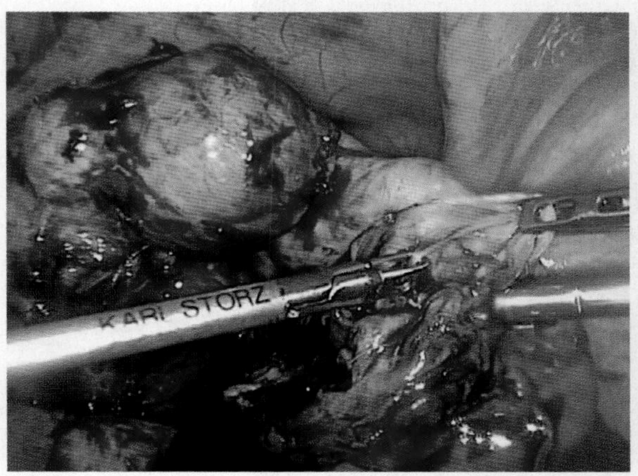

A

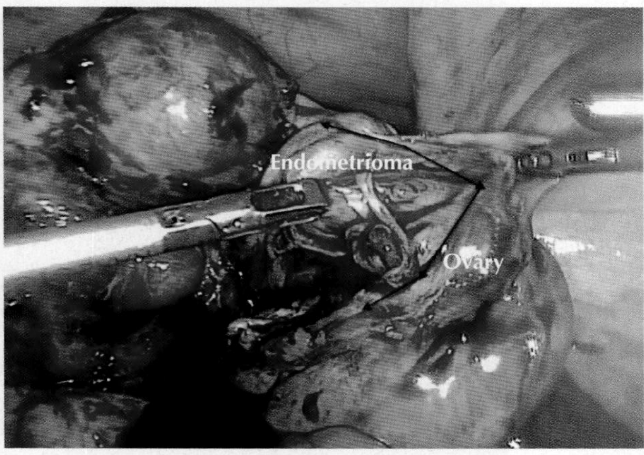

B

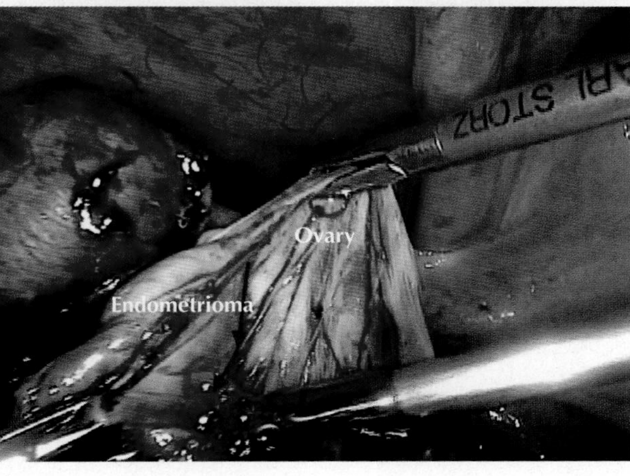

C

Tech Figure 12.4. A: Identify and bluntly separate the endometrioma from the ovarian parenchyma. B: Endometrioma cyst wall will be thick, white, and moderately adherent to ovary. C: Apply countertraction and gently sweep along the cleavage plane to separate the tissue.

Vaporize obstructing adhesions

- Once this technique no longer advances tissue separation, plasma energy can be employed to vaporize the obstructing adhesions (Tech Fig. 12.5).
  - Hold the handpiece 2 to 3 mm away and perpendicular to the adhesion.
- Continue to excise the cyst wall using these principles.
  - Apply sparse bipolar energy to fibrotic perihilar adhesions and incise with scissors.

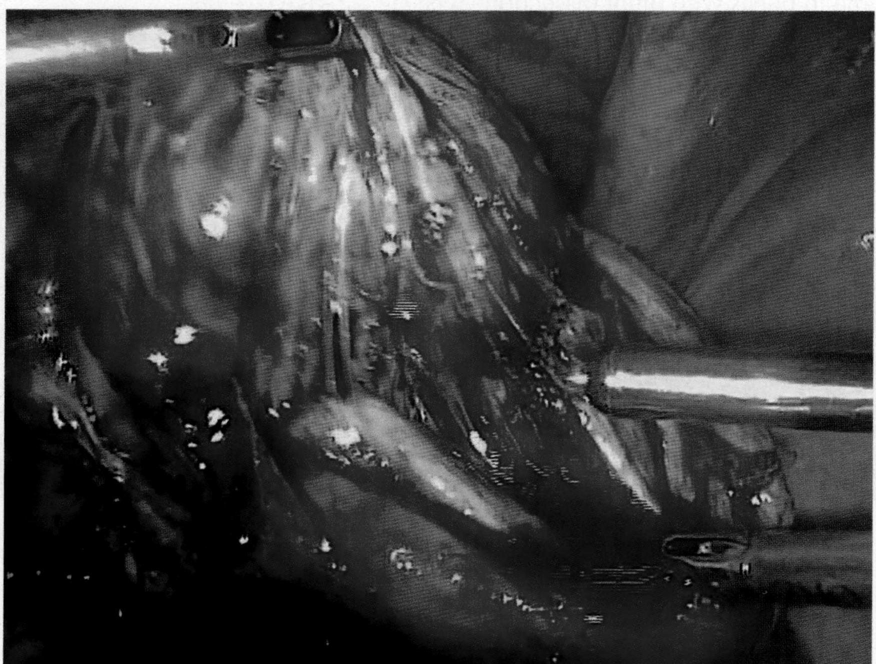

Tech Figure 12.5. Vaporize or ablate adhesions. Do not forcefully strip the tissue.

Achieve hemostasis

- Coagulate only active bleeding and resist the urge to "seal" the surface of the ovarian parenchyma (Tech Fig. 12.6).
  - Hold the handpiece approximately 8 to 10 mm away and perpendicular to the tissue.
- The area adjacent to the hilum contains numerous vessels.
  - Employ bipolar energy for vessels.

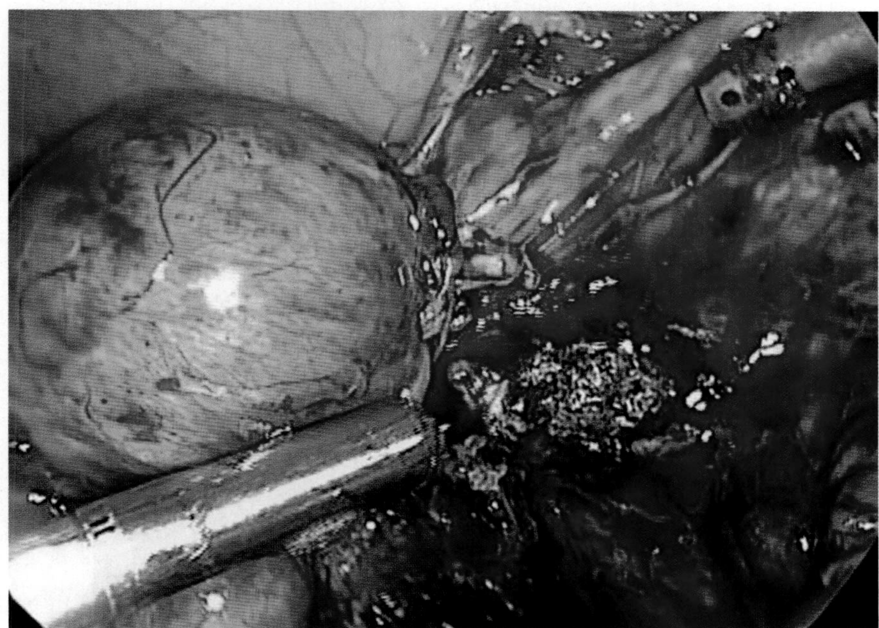

Tech Figure 12.6. Achieve hemostasis.

Remove the cyst wall, irrigate and perform final survey (Tech Fig. 12.7)

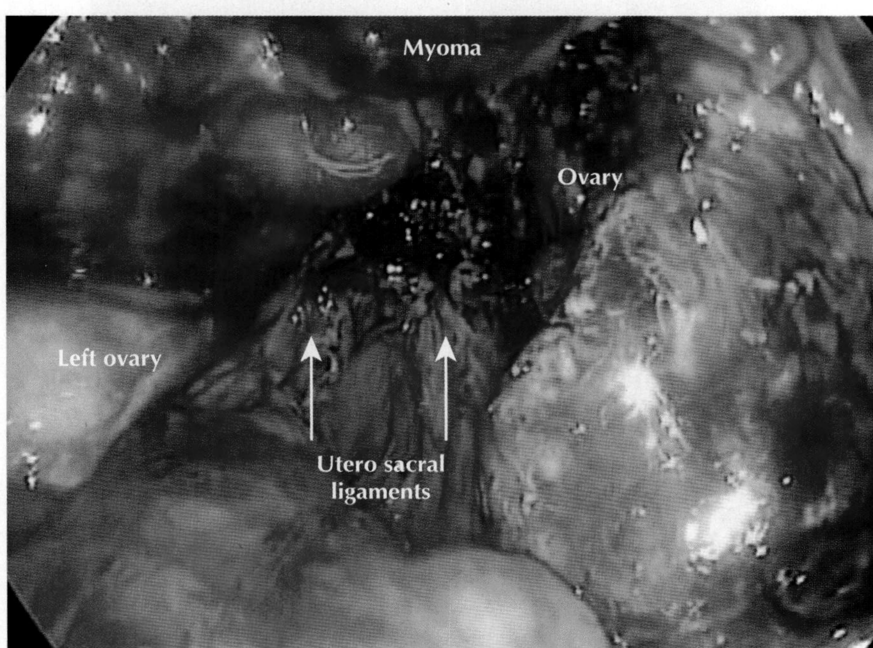

Tech Figure 12.7. Irrigate and perform final inspection.

Peritoneal Endometriosis Excision

Identify anatomic landmarks

- Locate vessels and ureters and note their distance from the target pathology. Perform adhesiolysis and ureterolysis. Evaluate the extent of endometriosis invasion.

Grasp the peritoneal endometriosis and apply traction

- Initially grasp only one thin cell layer of peritoneum.

Incise the peritoneum with either laparoscopic scissors, radiofrequency energy, or plasma energy

- Allow the pneumoperitoneum to dissect the tissue plane (Tech Fig. 12.8A,B).

A

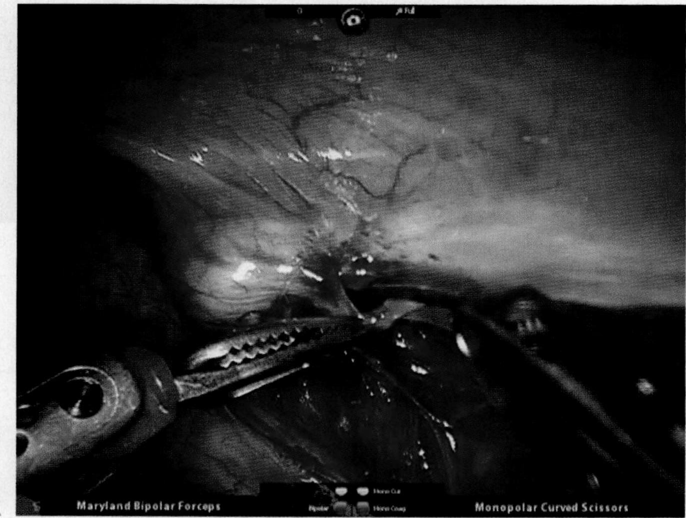

B

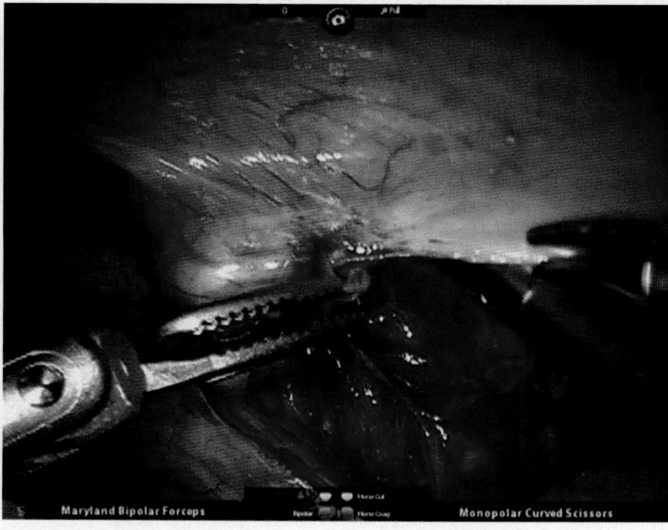

Tech Figure 12.8. A: Incise the peritoneum. B: Allow the pneumoperitoneum to separate the tissue.

Regrasp the tissue and apply traction away from the sidewall, leaving the area of deepest infiltration/nodule until the end

- To facilitate dissection, an assistant may apply countertraction with a laparoscopic grasper (Tech Fig. 12.9A,B).

A

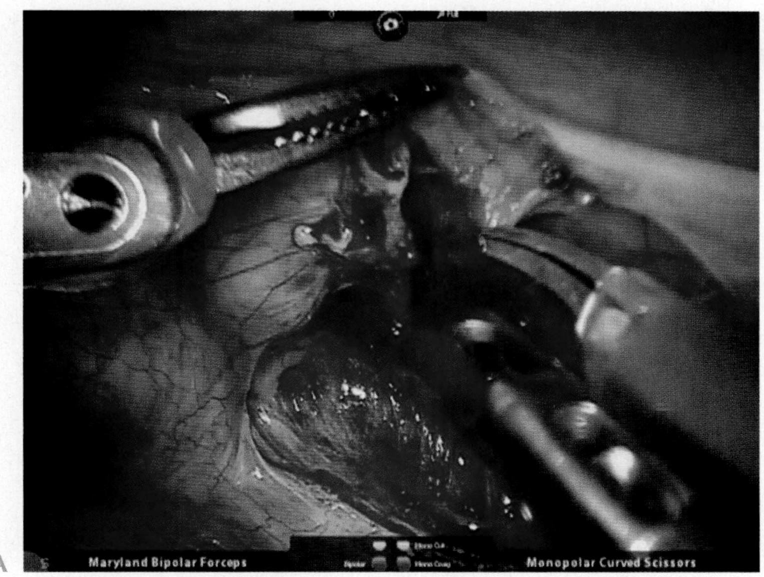

B

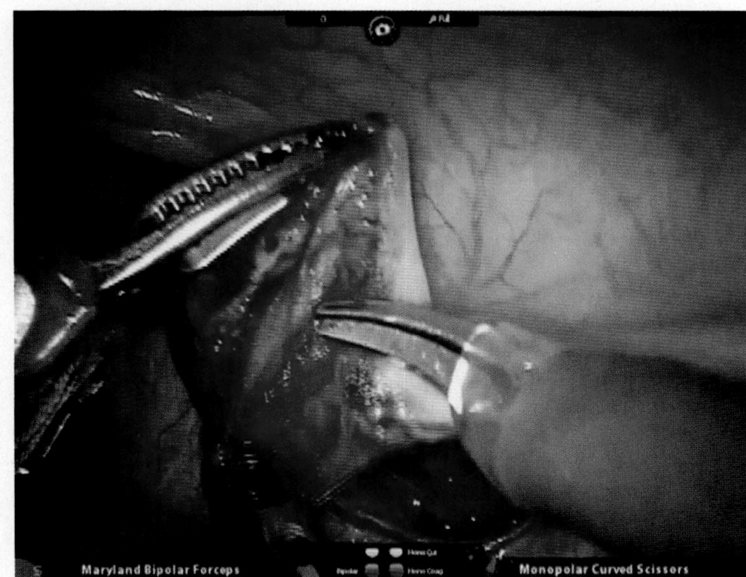

Tech Figure 12.9. A: Apply traction away from the pelvic sidewall. B: To facilitate dissection, apply countertraction with a laparoscopic grasper.

Once isolated, grasp the nodule to expose the deeper fibrotic attachments

- Excise the lesion from the surrounding healthy tissue.
- These attachments may range from cement-like concretions to sticky peritoneal whisps.

Obtain hemostasis using sparse radiofrequency energy, plasma energy, or a nonthermal hemostatic agent

PEARLS AND PITFALLS

- ○ Review pelvic anatomy vasculature in relation to ligaments and peritoneal folds. An understanding of vital structures and their usual relationships will aid in safe dissection when faced with severely distorted anatomy. For example:
  - Apply traction to the round ligament to identify the deep inguinal ring. Just medial and anterior to this insertion are the deep inferior epigastric vessels (contained within the lateral umbilical fold) that arise from the external iliac artery.
  - Follow the medial umbilical ligament past its intersection with the round ligament as it points toward the anterior division of the internal iliac artery.
- ✗ Do not rely solely on the uterus and adnexa as anatomic landmarks. Identify the median, medial, and umbilical ligaments to frame the pelvis. Then, identify the ureter and vasculature.
- ○ Identify and avoid incising the ovarium hilum. Premature entry into this vascular area will result in heavy and early blood loss that will complicate endometrioma excision.
- ✗ Abrupt brisk bleeding obscures the visual field, prolongs surgery, and compromises patient well-being. Therefore, immediately achieve hemostasis with plasma surface sealing or bipolar energy.
- ○ Grasp the peritoneal tissue to apply tissue traction. With an opposing blunt instrument, apply countertraction in a unidirectional, gentle sweeping motion to allow blunt dissection along natural cleavage planes which decreases blood loss.
- ✗ Avoid hydrodissection of the peritoneal tissue as it obscures tissue planes and hampers tissue excision.
- ○ After initial incision, allow the pneumoperitoneum to "poof up" the unscarred peritoneal tissue which creates an avascular space of areolar tissue.

POSTOPERATIVE CARE

- The majority of endometrioma and peritoneal endometriosis excision procedures may be performed as outpatient surgery. Postoperative care is similar to any other laparoscopic surgery. Immediate postoperative analgesia should include narcotic pain relief with concomitant stool softener and nonsteroidal anti-inflammatory drugs.
- All patients should receive secondary prevention, postoperative drug therapy to decrease disease persistence or recurrence. A myriad of oral contraceptive pills, progestins, GnRH agonists, aromatase inhibitors, Danazol, and hormone-secreting IUDS are available for this adjuvant medical therapy.

OUTCOME

- Incision and drainage of endometriomas has been abandoned due to endometrioma reformation. Endometrioma excision is currently the favored approach because of two randomized studies that revealed laparoscopic endometrioma excision was associated with a reduced recurrence rate of dysmenorrhea, dyspareunia, nonmenstrual pelvic pain, endometrioma recurrence and with a reduced requirement for further surgery compared to endometrioma ablation alone.
- Furthermore, for women attempting to conceive there was an increase in spontaneous pregnancy rate for those who had documented preoperative subfertility with endometrioma excision.
- Endometrioma ablation with novel plasma energy is promising but the results of a randomized study are still pending and further research is required.
- Endometrioma recurrence has been reported to be between 6% and 17%. Postoperatively, patients who took continuous oral contraceptive pills reduced endometrioma recurrence from 29% to 8% while those who used cyclic oral contraceptives reduced recurrence to only 15%.

COMPLICATIONS

- Inadvertent ovarian tissue destruction underscores the importance of surgical technique and expertise. Pathology specimens confirm that normal ovarian tissue is commonly removed with the endometrioma wall and the larger the cyst diameter, the more normal ovarian tissue is removed.
- Control brisk bleeding with direct pressure, suture ligation, vascular clips, and bipolar energy as needed. Large arterial bleeding cannot be controlled by topical hemostasis agents alone and heavy bleeding may necessitate oophorectomy if attempts to control bleeding are unsuccessful.
  - Nondiscrete bleeding of friable tissue can be achieved with topical hemostatic agents such as oxidized regenerated cellulose, thrombin, fibrin sealants, and microporous polysaccharide spheres. Caution and judicious use of these products is advised since some of these products have been implicated with causing widespread pelvic inflammation and bowel obstruction.
- Ureter injury may be recognized in the immediate postoperative period or may take up to 14 days to become apparent if due to thermal spread. Proficiency in ureterolysis is essential in order to safeguard the ureter and to avoid puncture and thermal injury. Intraoperative cystoscopy may provide some reassurance of ureteral integrity and allow for bladder evaluation.
- Thermal bowel injury is usually apparent by postoperative days 3 to 5. Route of repeat surgery depends on the patient's clinical condition but laparotomy may be required to optimally decrease contamination and to avoid further complications.

KEY REFERENCES

American College of Obstetricians and Gynecologists. Practice bulletin no. 114: management of endometriosis. *Obstet Gynecol.* 2010;116:223–236.

Falcone T, Lebovic DI. Clinical management of endometriosis. *Obstet Gynecol.* 2011;118(3):691–705.

Hart R, Hickey M, Maouris P, Buckett W, Garry R. Excisional surgery versus ablative surgery for ovarian endometriomata: a Cochrane Review. *Hum Reprod.* 2005;20(11):3000–3007.

Practice Committee of the American Society for Reproductive Medicine. Treatment of pelvic pain associated with endometriosis: a committee opinion. *Fertil Steril.* 2014;101:927–935.

Shakiba K, Bena JF, McGill KM, Minger J, Falcone T. Surgical treatment of endometriosis: a 7-year follow-up on the requirement for further surgery. *Obstet Gynecol.* 2008;111:1285–1292.

Endometriosis of Nongynecologic Organs and Extrapelvic Sites

13

M. Jean Uy-Kroh, Tommaso Falcone

GENERAL PRINCIPLES

Definition

Endometriosis is the presence of ectopic endometrial glands and stroma. Disease involvement is diverse and may be superficially limited or deeply infiltrative into organ systems such as the gastrointestinal and urinary tracts and the respiratory and musculoskeletal systems.

Differential Diagnosis

- Benign neoplasm
- Malignant neoplasm
- Overactive bladder
- Painful bladder syndrome
- Irritable bowel syndrome
- Inflammatory bowel disease
- Myofascial pain

Nonoperative Management

- Nonoperative management includes hormonal suppression with oral contraceptive pills, progestin therapy, or Levonorgestrol secreting IUD, gonadotropin-releasing hormone agonists, and off-label use of aromatase inhibitors. These treatments may provide symptomatic pain relief and reduce the size of lesions. However, even with optimal medical therapy many patients remain symptomatic due to fibrosis and infiltrating disease. Physical therapy and pain management procedures may also alleviate symptoms. Refractory pain and the uncertain neoplasm etiology lead many patients to undergo surgical resection and histologic confirmation of nonmalignant endometriosis.
- Bladder endometriosis warrants a trial of medical management. If there is a concern for obstructive uropathy, nephrostomy tubes and ureteral stents may also be used. Surgery is indicated for symptomatic patients who suffer from extrinsic obstruction, have contraindications to medical management, or who would benefit from ureteroneocystotomy.
- Bowel obstruction, ureteral stenosis, and pneumothorax caused by endometriosis implants typically require urgent surgical management in addition to palliative procedures (nasogastric tube, ureteral stent placement, and chest tube), concomitant medical management, and monitoring of electrolytes, kidney, and respiratory function.
- Postoperatively, we recommend continued hormonal suppression, no matter the disease location, and continue this therapy long term.
- One cautionary note: Asymptomatic patients with histologically confirmed endometriosis and extrapelvic or nongynecologic disease do not require surgical treatment and may be medically managed. Those with advanced disease may be followed with imaging if there is concern for advancing invasive disease.
- Conversely, a symptomatic patient without histologically confirmed endometriosis and imaging suggestive of endometriosis lesions must undergo a laparoscopic tissue biopsy at the very minimum to confirm the endometriosis diagnosis. The patient's quality of life, comorbid conditions, and lesion's mass effect should all be considered prior to surgical resection. It is crucial to confirm the endometriosis diagnosis by tissue pathology to avoid inappropriate medical management of a malignant neoplasm.

IMAGING AND OTHER DIAGNOSTICS

- Tumor markers such as CA125 are often elevated in patients with endometriomas. Therefore, we do not recommend this serum testing for a patient with known deep endometriosis extending more than 5 mm into the peritoneum and lesions with characteristic appearance of extraperitoneal endometriosis.
- Perform preoperative cystoscopy to assess bladder mucosal involvement if suspicious for this by the patient's history.
- Small-bowel endoscopy and colonoscopy rarely reveal transmural or mucosal endometriosis but may be useful to evaluate for differential bowel diseases, suspected malignancy, or bowel strictures secondary to endometriosis.
- Transvaginal and abdominal ultrasound can detect rectosigmoid and bladder endometriosis. This imaging requires experienced sonographers and a high level of radiographic expertise.
- Computed tomography (CT) is only useful for pelvic mass evaluation and ureteral obstruction but it is not useful for pelvic soft tissue evaluation. Instead, we prefer Magnetic Resonance Imaging (MRI), with enterography, for preoperative soft tissue evaluation (Figs. 13.1 to 13.4).

PREOPERATIVE PLANNING

- Patients with anterior abdominal wall disease can be examined easily in the office. Patient discomfort and habitus, however, may limit the utility of this examination.
- A rectovaginal examination should be performed to determine the presence of tissue thickening, masses, and nodularity. If the patient can tolerate a bimanual examination, this can also yield useful information such as a fixed, retroverted uterus, irregularity or tenderness of the posterior cul-de-sac and vaginal fornices.
- Occasionally, a speculum examination reveals pigmented endometriosis lesions that may be easily biopsied. Lesions that are deep to the vaginal mucosa should not be aggressively biopsied in the office as they may communicate with the rectum.

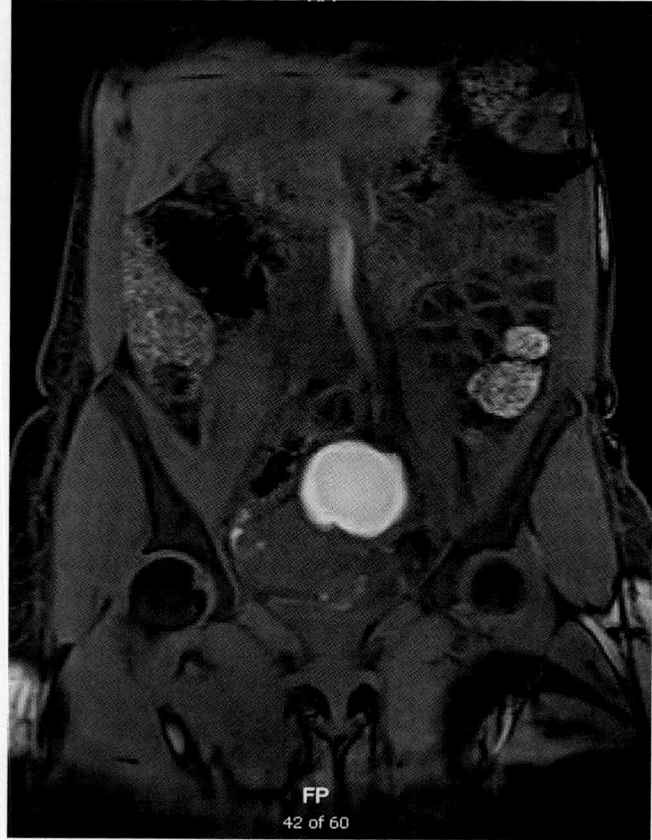

Figure 13.1. Endometriosis nodule of the bladder, MRI.

- We strongly advise referring these patients to a tertiary center with surgical experts experienced at managing nongynecologic endometriosis in an interdisciplinary fashion. Although endometriosis may present in anatomic locations that are surgically unfamiliar to gynecologists, it is important not to treat this benign, albeit tenacious, disease as an oncologic subset. Doing so places the patient at risk of decreased fertility, unnecessary

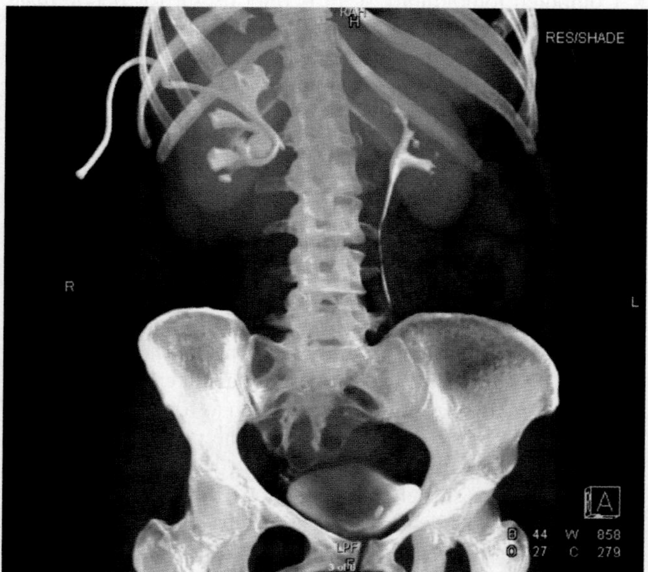

Figure 13.2. Right obstructive hydronephrosis, CT urogram.

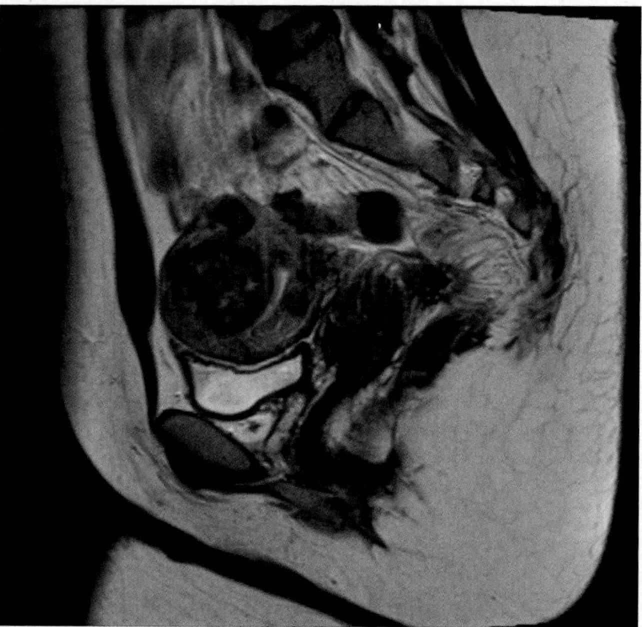

Figure 13.3. Obliterated cul-de-sac and spiculated endometriosis lesion, rectocervical disease, MRI.

intervention, and increased surgical risks. Surgical treatment is peppered with a myriad of known complications, many of which can be fatal if mismanaged. Even after successful surgical treatment, patients often require ongoing medical and ancillary treatments to abate the sequelae of their disease.

- The comprehensive medical and surgical management of patients suffering from extraperitoneal endometriosis should only be undertaken at large centers with the personnel and resources capable of providing complete care for the patient.
- Interdisciplinary treatment teams may include surgeons and physicians from urology, colorectal/general surgery, gastroenterology, plastic surgery, cardiothoracic surgery, physical therapy, and pain management.
- The goal of surgical extraperitoneal endometriosis management is to remove endometriosis and fibrosis and to restore the organ's function. Hysterectomy and salpingo-oophorectomy may also be considered depending on the age and desired future fertility of the patient.

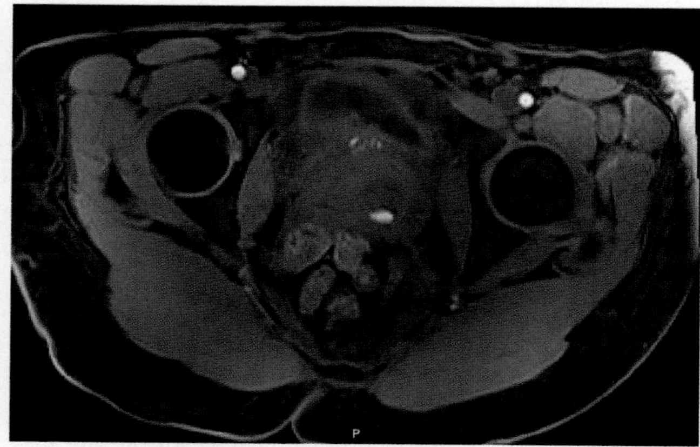

Figure 13.4. Rectrocervical endometriosis, MRI.

SURGICAL MANAGEMENT

Urinary System—Bladder and Ureter

- Approximately 0.3% to 6% of endometriosis cases have urinary tract involvement. Most commonly, endometriosis affects the bladder (84%), ureter (15%), kidney (4%), and urethra (4%).
- Symptoms include hematuria, vesical or suprapubic pain, dysuria, urinary frequency, and back pain that may be constant or cyclical especially at the time of menses.
- Imaging may reveal focal thickening of the bladder wall, edema, or a mass lesion. Cystoscopy confirms the absence or presence of mucosal involvement.
- Extrinsic ureteral compression is usually due to peritoneal fibrosis. Intrinsic ureteral compression is often caused by endometriotic implants on the muscularis of the ureter.
- Ureteral resection is often necessary if hydronephrosis exists.

Gastrointestinal System—Bowel and Rectum

- Rectocervical or bowel endometriosis is present in 5% to 12% of endometriosis cases and usually coexists with other endometriosis lesions. The most common bowel sites are the rectum and sigmoid colon, followed by the appendix and small bowel/ileum.
- Symptoms include dysmenorrhea, dyspareunia, bloating, constipation, diarrhea, dyschezia, and hematochezia.
- Based on anatomic location, bowel endometriosis can be divided into two subsets: rectocervical disease and disease affecting the bowel wall proximal to the rectosigmoid.
  - Rectocervical disease often requires uterosacral ligament excision and/or posterior cul-de-sac adhesiolysis.
  - Rectal nodule or local excision may confer equal pain relief compared to segmental rectal resection and with less postoperative gastrointestinal side effects.
- In general, bowel resection for endometriosis depends on the lesion size, depth of invasion, and the percentage of circumference involved. The smallest resection that eradicates the diseased area and maintains functional anatomy is preferred.
  - Perform a partial bowel excision (disc excision) if there is a:
    - unifocal lesion less than 3 cm.
    - lesion that involves less than 60% of the circumference of the rectum or sigmoid wall.
  - Perform a segmental bowel resection if there is:
    - deep invasion of the muscularis, or
    - a lesion larger than 3 cm or multiple nodules.
- The posterior vaginal fornix and pelvic sidewall require concomitant dissection and endometriosis resection.

Musculoskeletal System

- Iatrogenic endometriosis seeding occurs when the endometrium is breached during surgical procedures such as cesarean delivery. At that time, endometrial tissue can escape from the uterine cavity and implant along the fascia, muscle, subcutaneous fat, and other surfaces exposed during the surgery. The prevention, pathogenesis, and optimal treatment of musculoskeletal and abdominal wall endometriosis are unknown. Future areas for study include recurrence rates, optimal resection margins, and surgical techniques to decrease recurrence.

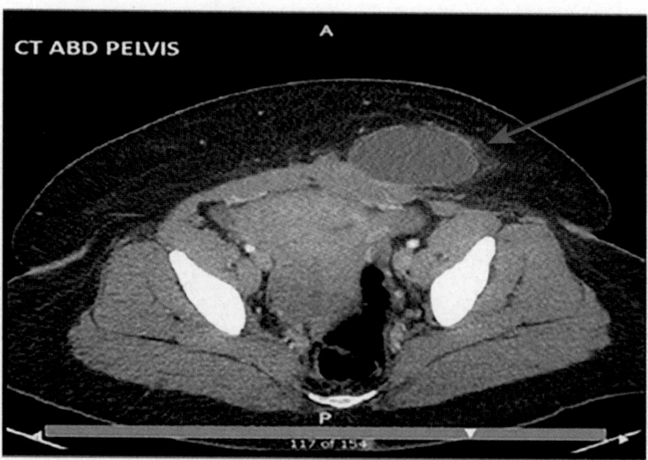

Figure 13.5. Abdominal wall endometriosis, CT abd pelvis.

- Symptoms: Cyclic or constant abdominal pain often with a palpable abdominal wall mass near a prior incision or trocar site.
- Seventy-five percent of patients report perimenstrual pain and have a history of cesarean delivery.
- Patients usually present in their mid-30s and their last surgery may be several months to years prior to clinical presentation. The mean mass size is 4 cm and is often misdiagnosed as an incisional hernia or granuloma.
- Perform CT to characterize the lesion (Figs. 13.5 and 13.6A,B).

Other Distant Sites

The enigmatic, and at times obstinate, nature of endometriosis can also affect distant sites and organs such as the diaphragm, lung, nervous and lymphatic systems. As with the pelvic counterparts, management of distant endometriosis should focus on minimizing the clinical sequelae of the disease and restoring/preserving organ function. The value of experienced, interdisciplinary surgical and medical management to yield optimal patient care is underscored.

- Symptoms of thoracic endometriosis include right-sided catamenial pneumothorax hemoptysis, chest pain, and dyspnea. Some patients are asymptomatic and do not require treatment. Co-management with an experienced interdisciplinary team that includes gynecologic, thoracic, vascular surgeons and neurosurgeons for disease resection in the respective distant organs is recommended (Figs. 13.7 and 13.8).

Positioning

- Patients should be placed in low lithotomy with leg stirrups (refer to Chapter 5 for laparoscopic patient positioning details). Alternatively, the patient may lie supine. Please refer to Chapter 8 for positioning details for an abdominal approach.

Approach

Preoperative Prophylaxis

- We recommend all patients receive venous thromboembolism (VTE) prophylaxis commensurate with their VTE risk. Administer antibiotics within 60 minutes before the

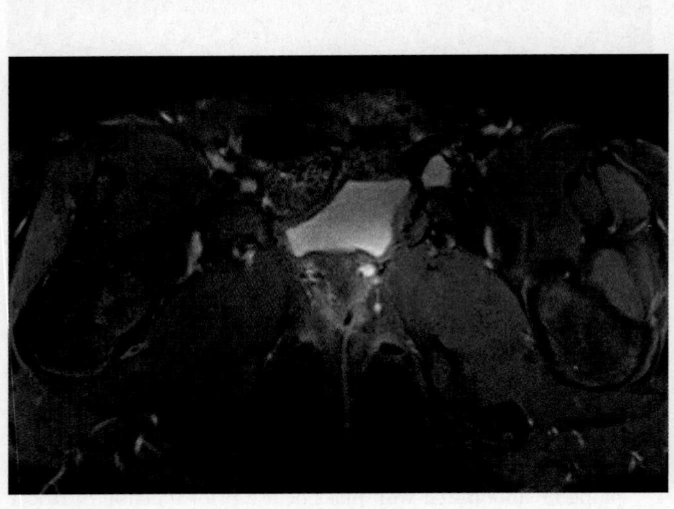

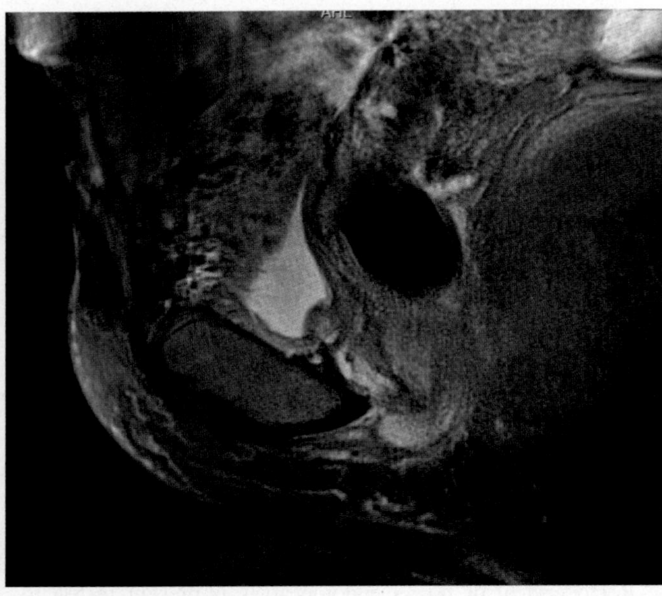

A B

Figure 13.6. A: Left rectus muscle seen anteriorly with spiculated endometriosis invasions into the bladder serosa, coronal, noncontrast MRI. (For intraoperative images, see Tech Fig. 13.38.) B: Left rectus muscle with poorly demarcated bladder interface, sagittal T2-weighted MRI. (For intraoperative images, see Tech Fig. 13.38.)

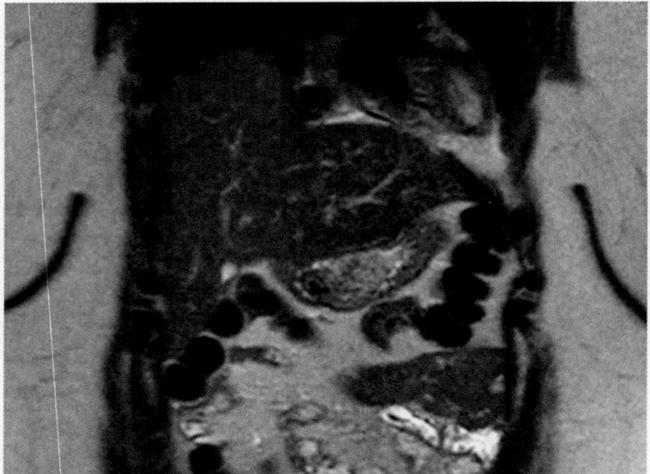

Figure 13.7. Right hydropneumothorax with liver herniation thru diaphragm due to endometriosis, coronal view MRI.

procedure and re-dose for major blood loss or prolonged procedures at intervals equal to 2.5 times the half-life of the antibiotic.

- Urinary tract and abdominal wall procedures:
  - Administer 2 g Cefazolin IV for patient less than 120 kg and 3 g for patients greater than 120 kg. Redose approximately every 4 hours during the procedure.
- Gastrointestinal tract:
  - Given variations in bowel preparation and antibiotic preferences, we recommend discussing this preoperatively with your colorectal surgeon.

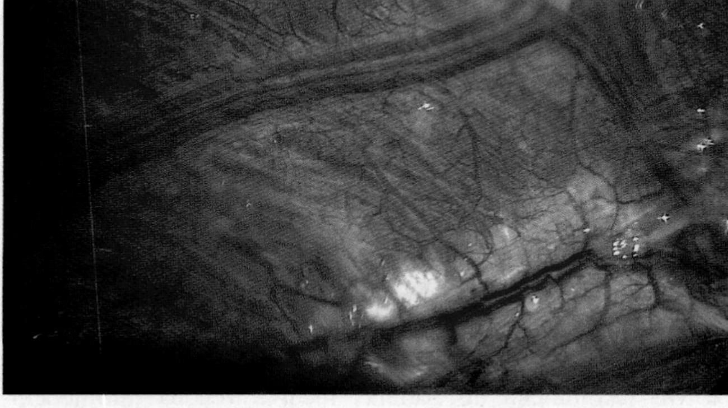

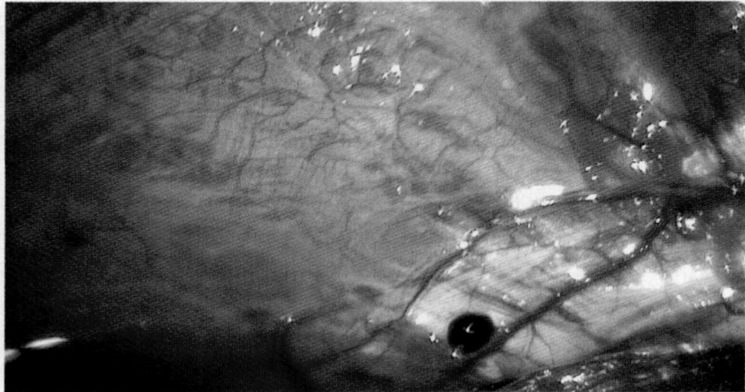

A B

Figure 13.8. A,B: Diaphragmatic endometriosis, note the diversity of lesions.

Procedures and Techniques: Urinary Tract Endometriosis Resection (Video 13.1)

Place a uterine manipulator of choice and a three-way Foley catheter into the bladder to allow for bladder instillation if needed throughout the surgery. See Chapter 5 for basic setup and entry for laparoscopy.

Superficial bladder peritoneum resection

- Grasp and sharply incise the normal bladder peritoneum (Tech Fig. 13.1).
- Dissect the loose areolar tissue and underlying structures off the peritoneum and around the endometriosis implant (Tech Fig. 13.2).
- Then excise the implant sharply or with radiofrequency or plasma energy.
- Perform cystoscopy to confirm ureteral patency and lack of mucosal involvement.

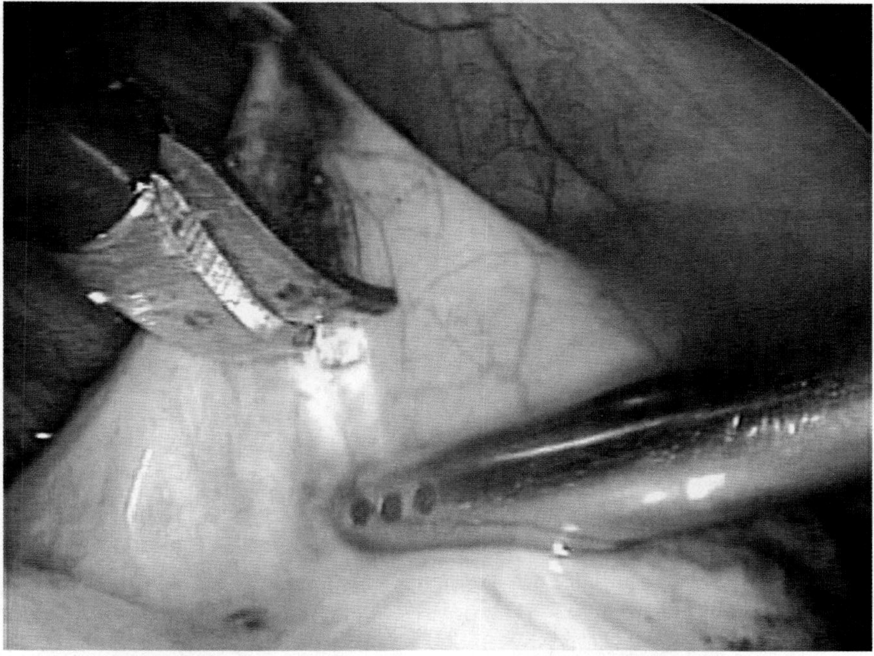

Tech Figure 13.1. Superficial peritoneal bladder lesion.

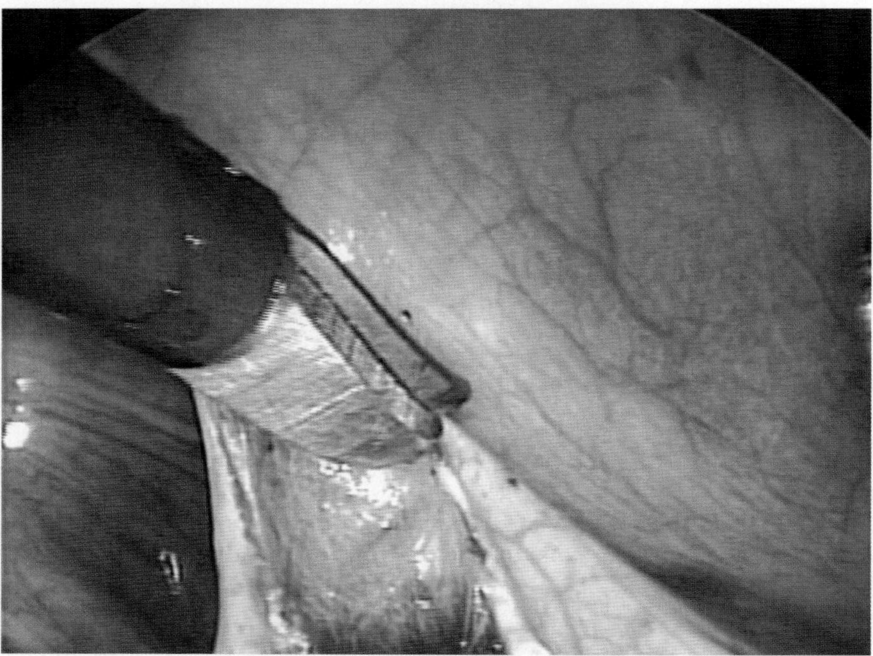

Tech Figure 13.2. Bluntly dissect loose areolar tissue.

Deep endometriosis resection involving the bladder muscularis

- An understanding of bladder anatomy is important for safe and efficient surgery (Tech Fig. 13.3).
- Begin laterally and sharply dissect the underlying nonfibrotic tissue away from the implant(s) (Tech Figs. 13.4 and 13.5).

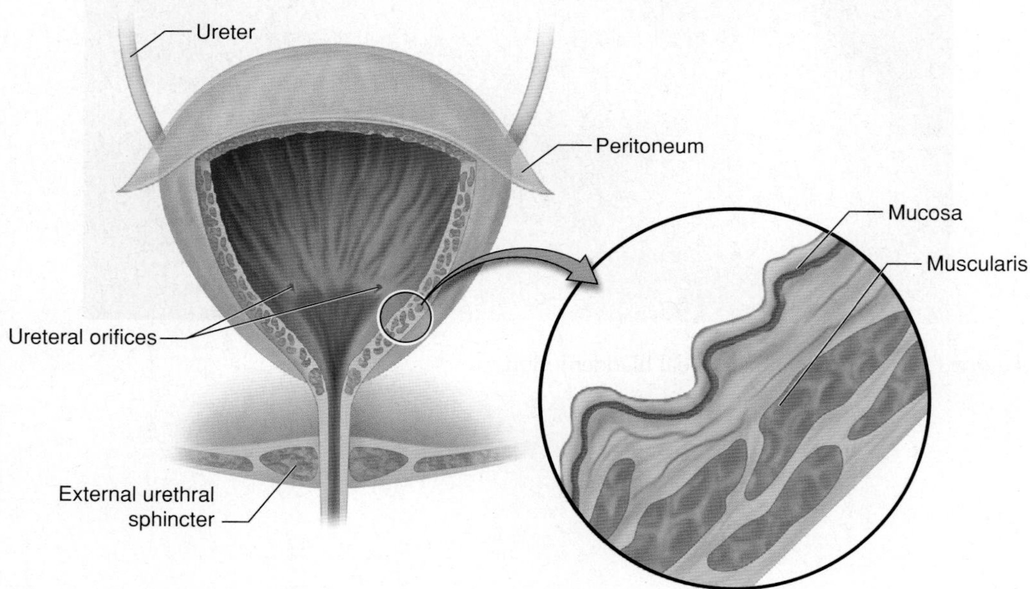

Tech Figure 13.3. Normal bladder anatomy and layers.

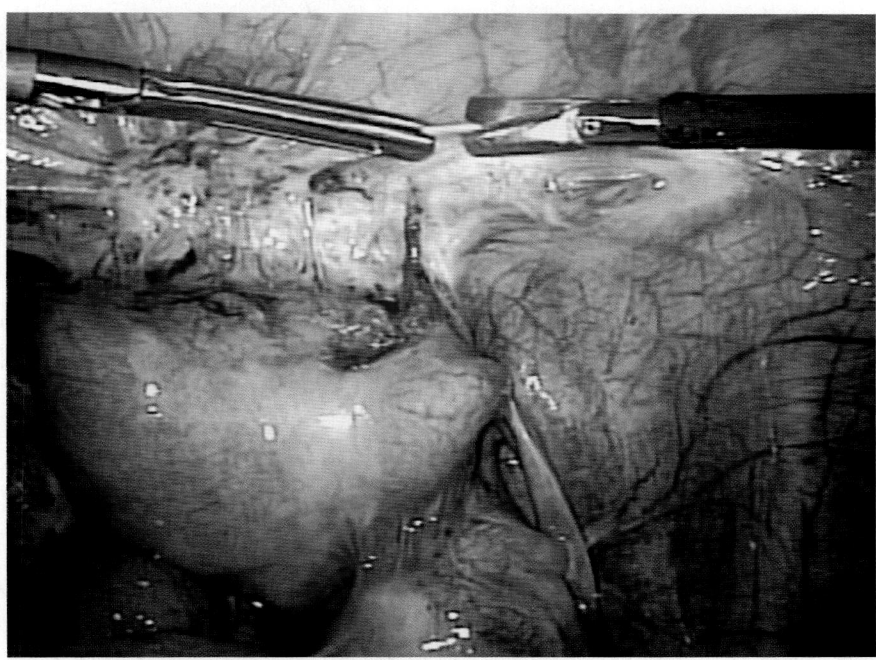

Tech Figure 13.4. Obliterated vesicouterine space with infiltrating endometriosis into the bladder muscularis.

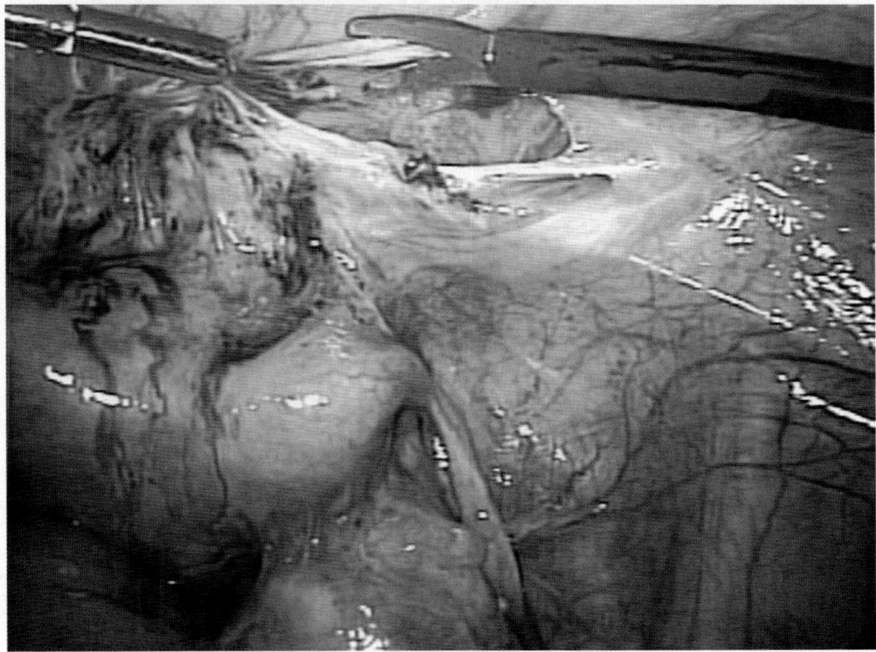

Tech Figure 13.5. Sharp excision of fibrotic adhesions.

- Grasp the abnormal tissue and press "toward the lesion" and not away (Tech Fig. 13.6).
- Identify the correct dissection plane: the nodule's interface to normal, healthy bladder tissue.
  - Push the uterus cephalad with a uterine manipulator to facilitate this plane dissection.
  - Once healthy tissue is encountered, bluntly dissect the tissue away from the fibrosis to minimize the loss of normal tissue and anatomy distortion (Tech Fig. 13.7).

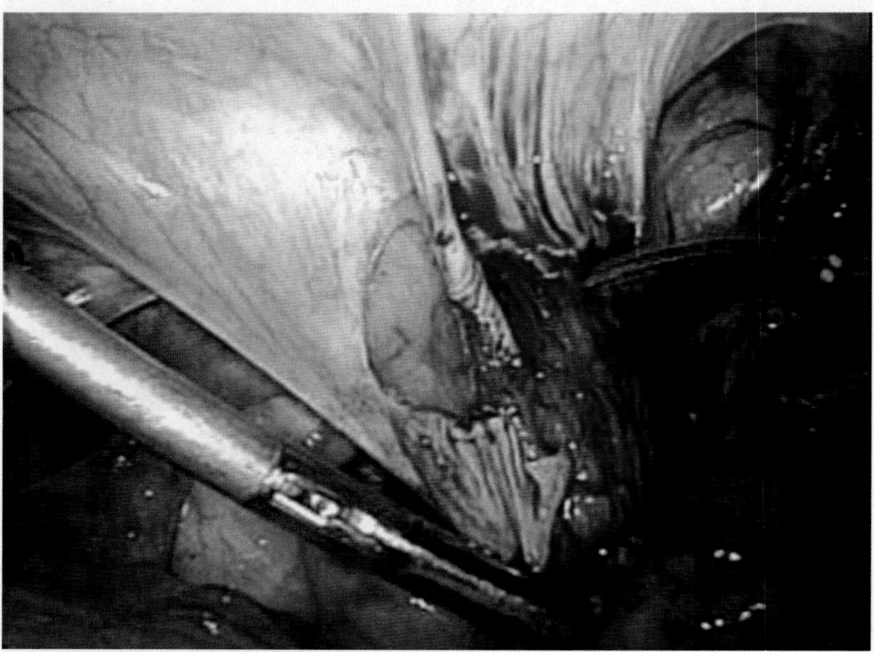

Tech Figure 13.6. Bladder resection technique and lesion isolation.

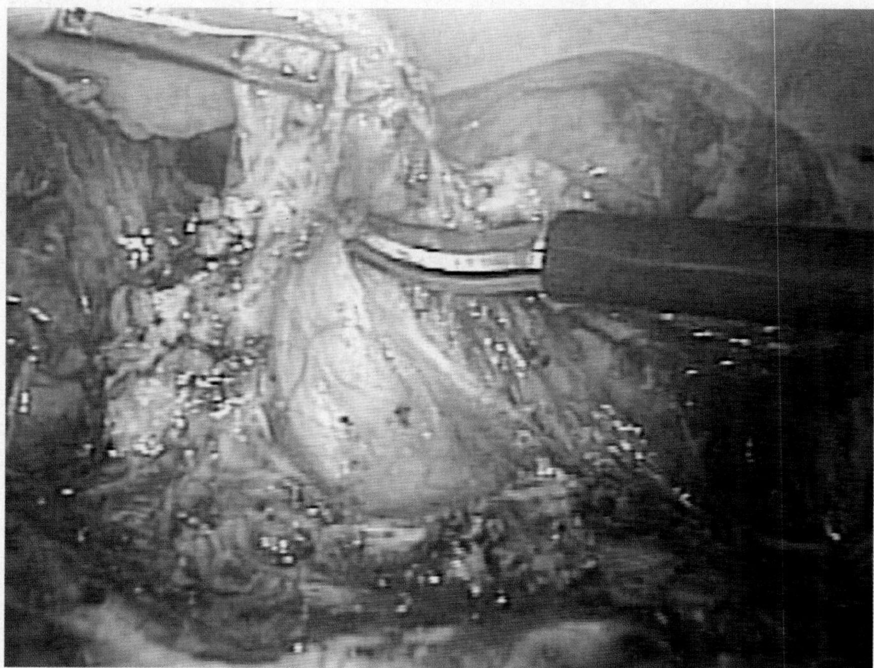

Tech Figure 13.7. Operative technique: proper plane dissection limits destruction to healthy tissue.

- Excise the nodule and the affected bladder peritoneum and bladder muscularis en bloc (Tech Fig. 13.8).
- The implant and the affected bladder muscularis may be excised without entering the bladder lumen (Tech Fig. 13.9A,B).

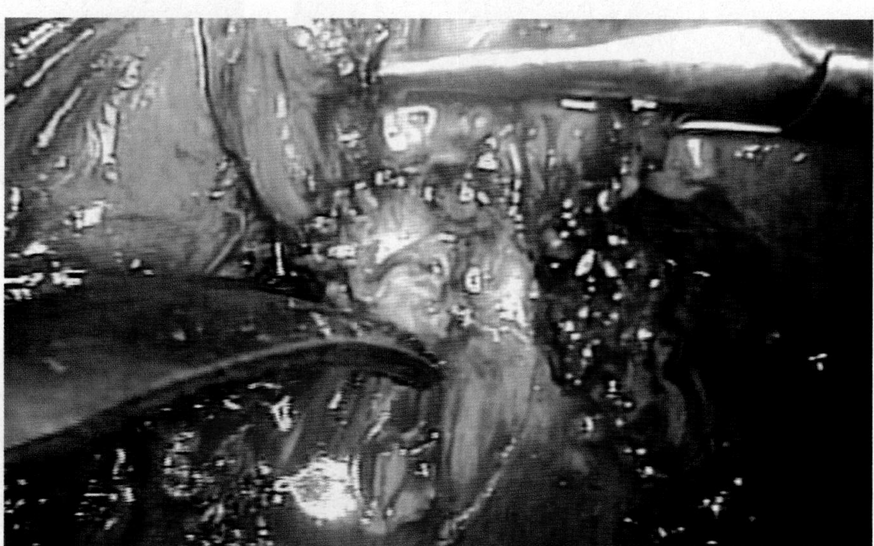

Tech Figure 13.8. Enbloc resection of endometriosis nodule, bladder peritoneum, and muscularis.

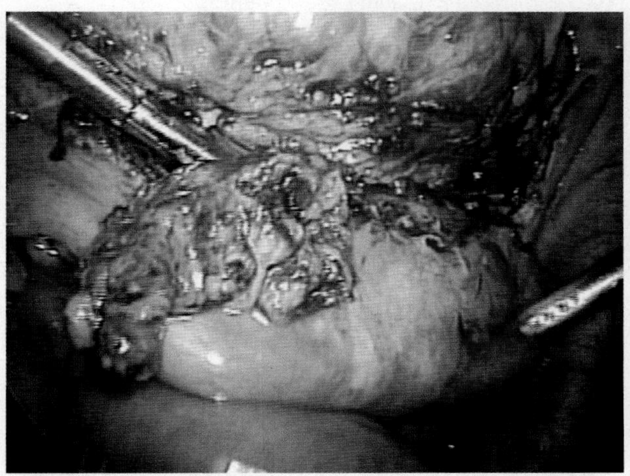

A

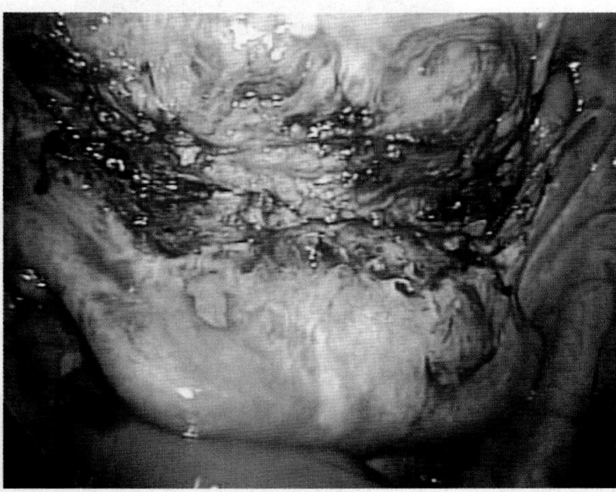

B

Tech Figure 13.9. A: Endometriosis implant and bladder muscularis (in Allis grasper). B: Final view of restored vesicouterine space not requiring cystotomy.

Deep endometriosis resection involving the bladder dome mucosa

- First, perform cystoscopy and place bilateral ureteral stents (Tech Fig. 13.10A,B).
- Create a cystotomy at the dome (Tech Fig. 13.11).
- Identify the intravesicular Foley catheter. Note the distance of the ureteral stents and ureteral orifices from the mucosal lesion (Tech Fig. 13.12A,B).
- Perform a partial cystectomy by circumscribing and then excising the transmural lesion sharply (Tech Fig. 13.13A,B).

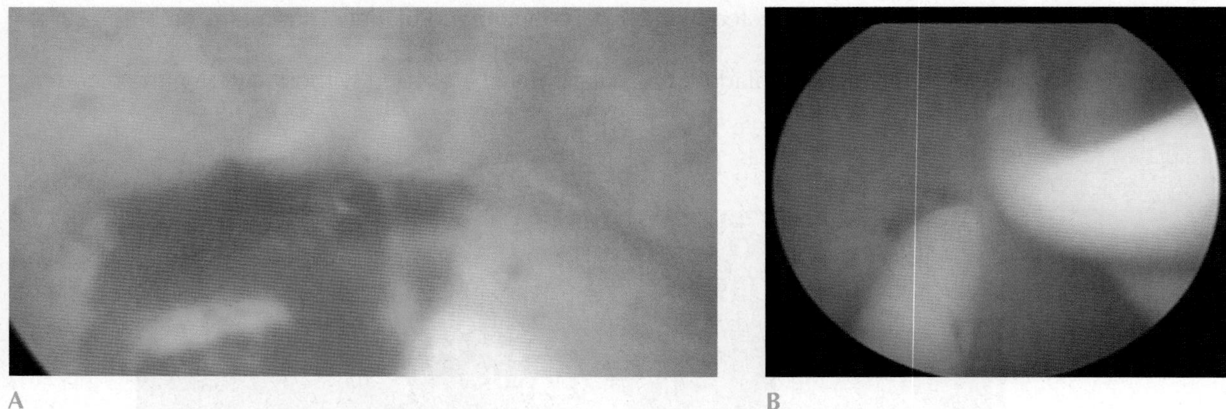

Tech Figure 13.10. **Cystoscopic views.** A: Bladder mucosa with posterior endometrial lesion. B: Double left ureter with separate stents.

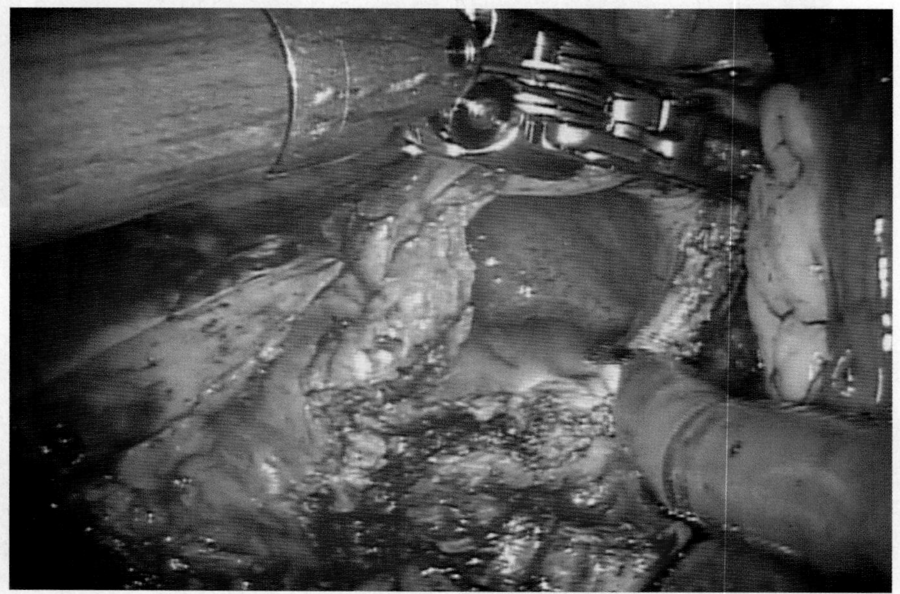

Tech Figure 13.11. Cystotomy at bladder dome.

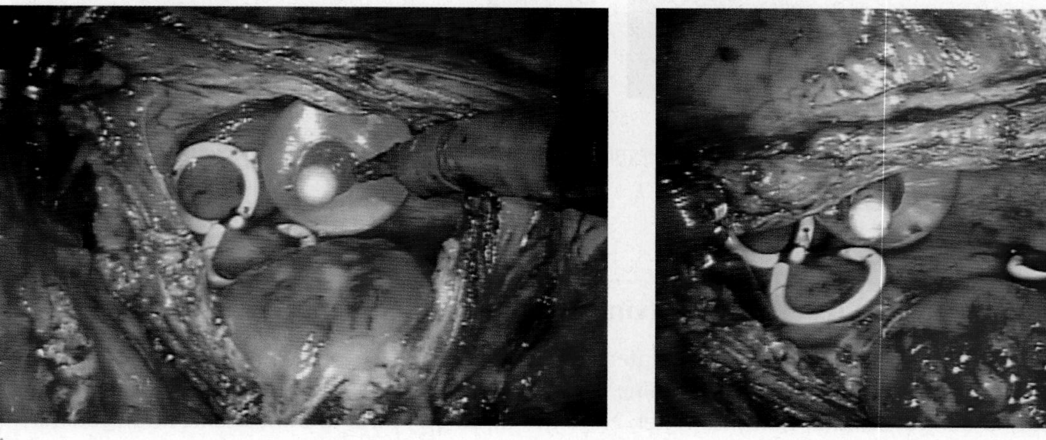

Tech Figure 13.12. A: Note the endometriosis nodule that extends from the dome to the posterior bladder wall, the two left ureteral stents, and the foley catheter. B: Complete intravesicular view. Note the distance between the orifices to the lesion.

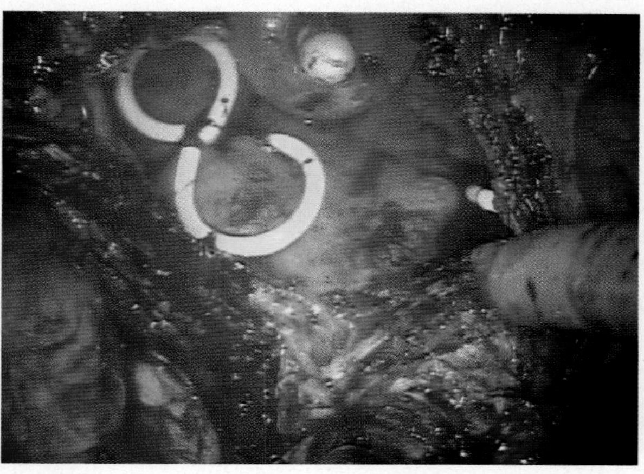

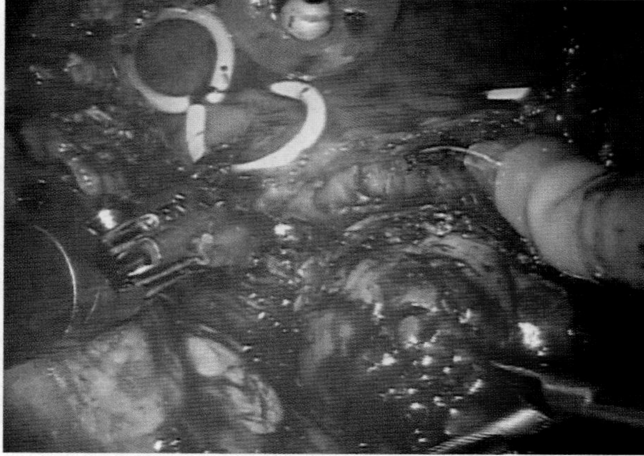

A B

Tech Figure 13.13. A: Circumscribe the transmural bladder lesion. B: Excise the nodule sharply and complete the partial cystectomy.

- Close the bladder defect in two layers.
  - Re-approximate the bladder mucosa with a 3-0 delayed absorbable running suture such as polyglactin 910 (Tech Fig. 13.14A).
  - Imbricate the bladder muscularis with 2-0 delayed absorbable suture.
- Retrograde fill the bladder with sterile solution and laparoscopically inspect the peritoneal cavity and bladder to ensure a watertight closure (Tech Fig. 13.14B).
- Place a Jackson–Pratt drain in the pelvis through a laparoscopic port site.
- Perform a cystogram 1 week postoperatively to confirm there is no extravasation from the bladder and remove the Foley catheter.

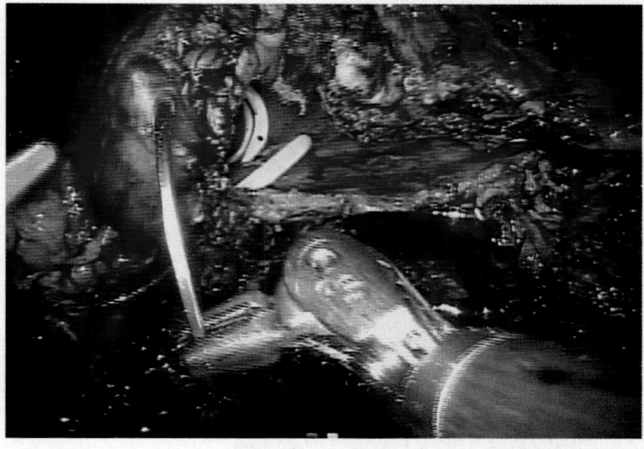

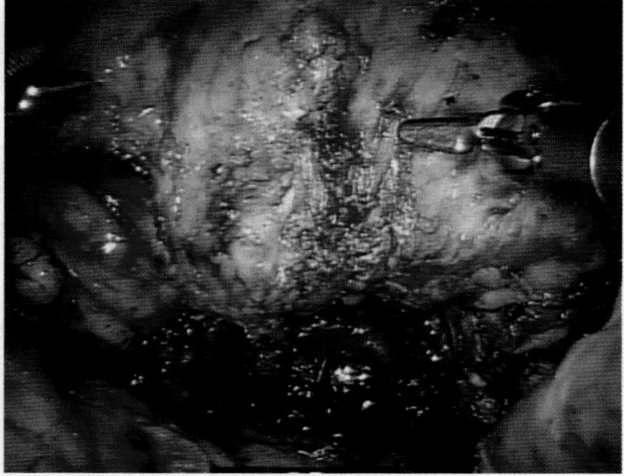

A B

Tech Figure 13.14. A: First layer of bladder closure. B: Imbricate and backfill the bladder.

Ureterolysis, ureter evaluation, and ureter procedures

- When endometriosis and fibrosis over lie the ureter, perform ureteral dissection and adhesiolysis (Tech Fig. 13.15A,B).
- Incise the peritoneum at the level of the pelvic brim (Tech Fig. 13.16).
  - Perform blunt dissection of the connective tissue.
- Identify and isolate the ureter on the medial leaf of the broad ligament.
  - Continue dissection to the level of the cardinal ligament.
- If endometriosis invades the adventitia, incise the adventitia while preserving the muscularis (Tech Fig. 13.17).
- Visually inspect the condition and functionality of the ureter (Tech Fig. 13.18).
- Identify any stricture, dilation, and note adequate perfusion and vermiculation.

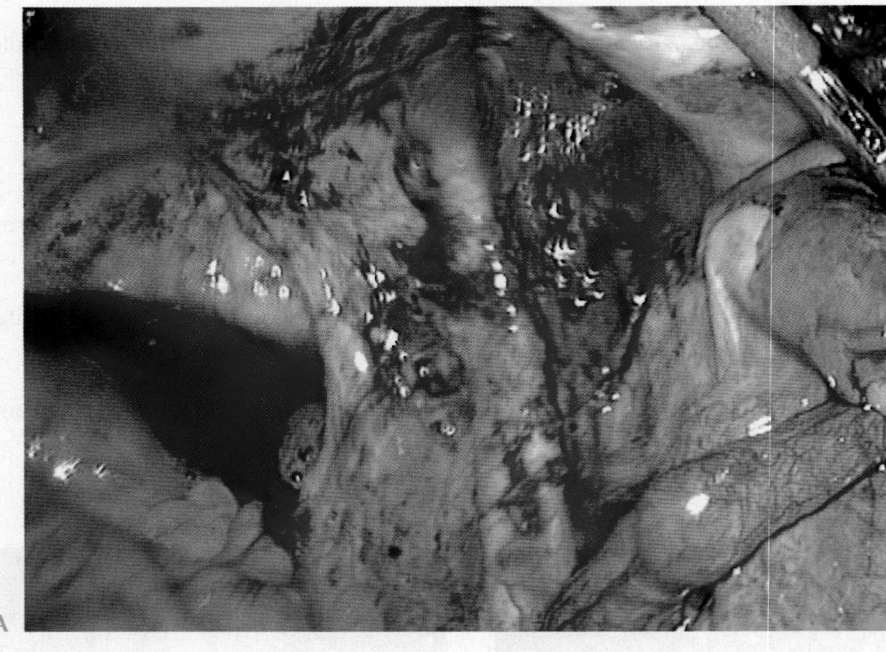
A

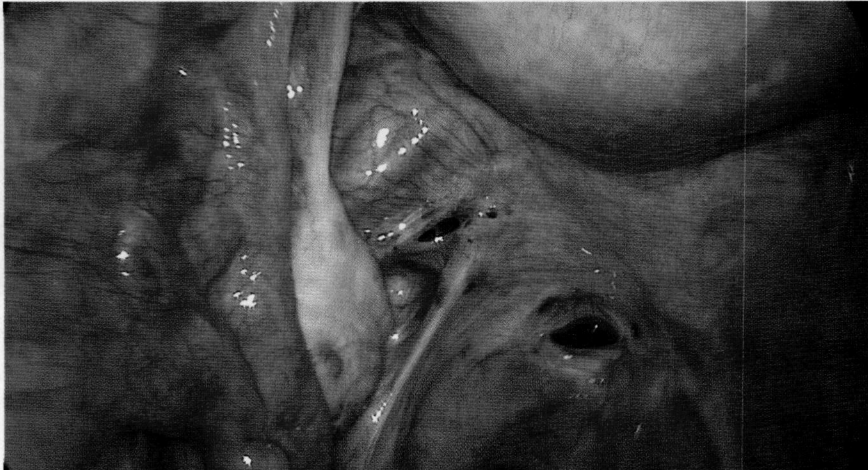
B

Tech Figure 13.15. Peritoneal endometriosis over (A) the right ureter and (B) the left ureter.

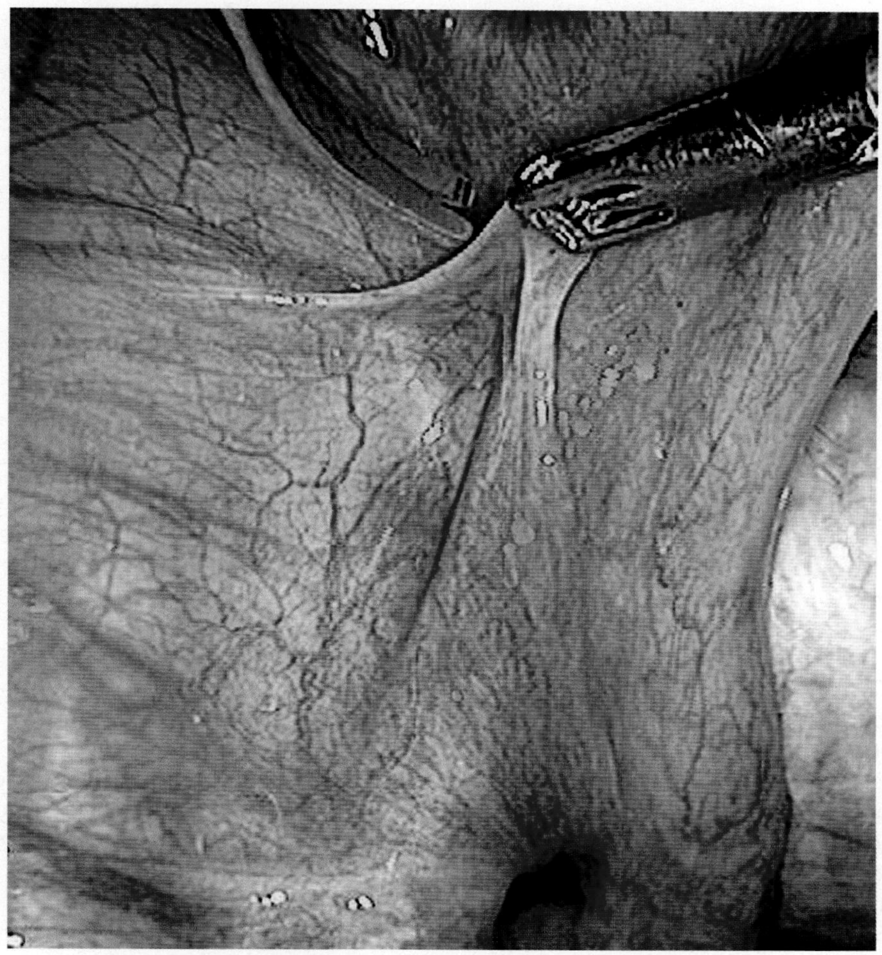

Tech Figure 13.16. Ureterolysis from the left pelvic brim.

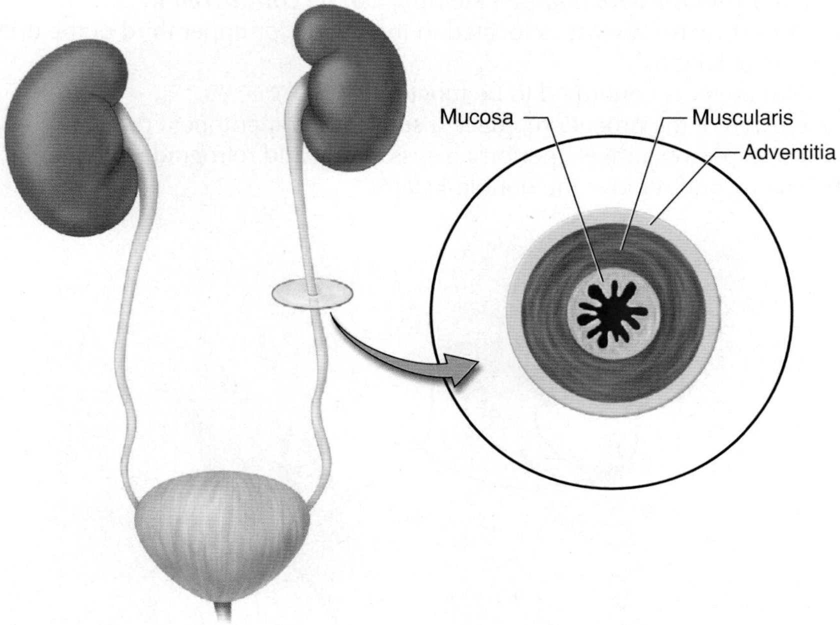

Tech Figure 13.17. Ureter layers.

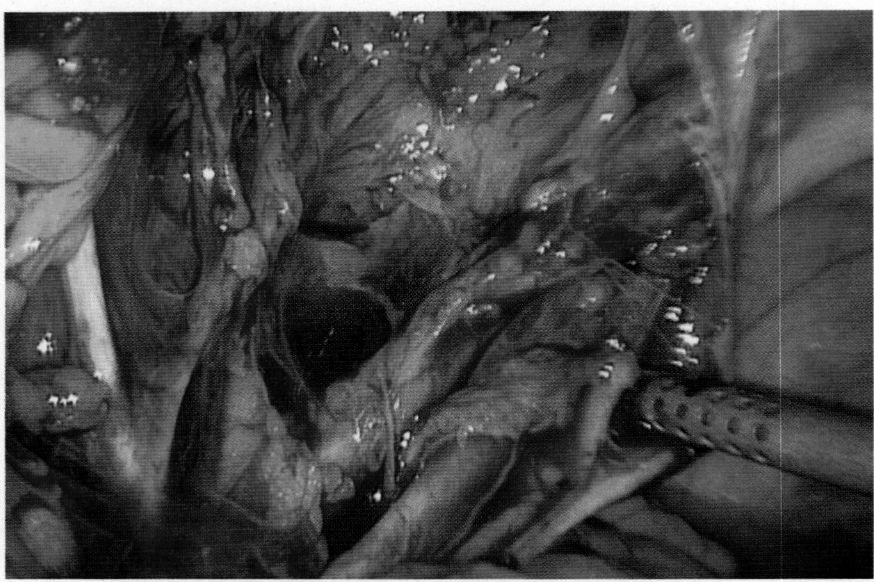

Tech Figure 13.18. Left pelvic sidewall dissection.

Ureteroneocystostomy allows for resection of the diseased distal ureter and reimplantation into the bladder

- The ureter is transected proximal to the stricture, spatulated, and directly anastomosed with the aid of a double-J stent. A psoas hitch or Boari flap may be needed to reduce tension on the anastomosis if proximal ureteral mobilization alone is inadequate. At the conclusion of the procedure, place a surgical intraperitoneal drain and maintain a Foley catheter.
- Approximately 1 week postoperatively remove the Foley catheter.
- Four to 6 weeks postoperatively perform a cystoscopy and retrograde pylogram to confirm adequate healing and to remove the double-J stents. Alternatively, the stents may be removed and a CT urogram obtained to confirm ureteral patency.

Ureteroureteral anastomosis with double-J stenting can be considered if:

- The stenosis or obstructive disease is located in the middle or upper third of the ureter and there is sufficient ureteral length.
- The contralateral ureter is confirmed to be functional (Tech Fig. 13.19).
  - At the conclusion of the procedure, place a surgical intraperitoneal drain.
  - Four to 6 weeks postoperatively perform a cystoscopy and retrograde pylogram to confirm adequate healing and remove the double-J stents.

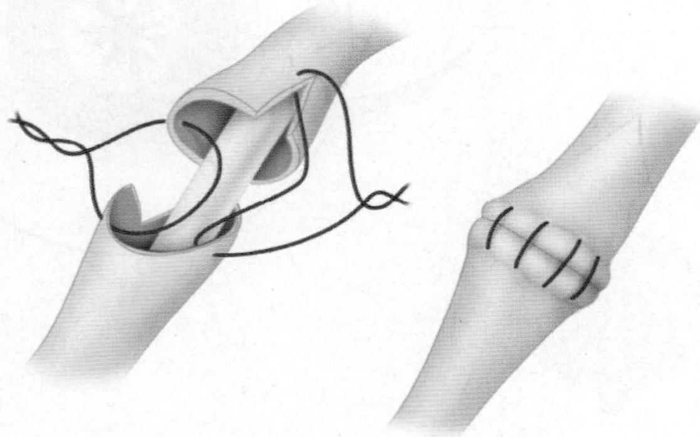

Tech Figure 13.19. Simplified ureteroureteral anastomosis: spatulate and suture the segments over a stent.

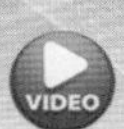

Procedures and Techniques: Gastrointestinal Tract Endometriosis Resection (Video 13.2)

Rectocervical endometriosis resection

- Identify anatomic landmarks such as the ureters and uterosacral ligaments bilaterally. Assess the extent of organ involvement (Tech Figs. 13.20 and 13.21).
- Develop the pararectal spaces with blunt dissection and then sharp dissection once fibrosis and endometriosis are encountered.
  - The pararectal space is defined laterally by the internal iliac vessels, medially by the rectum and ureter, posteriorly by the sacrum, and anteriorly by the cardinal ligaments and uterine arteries (Tech Fig. 13.22).

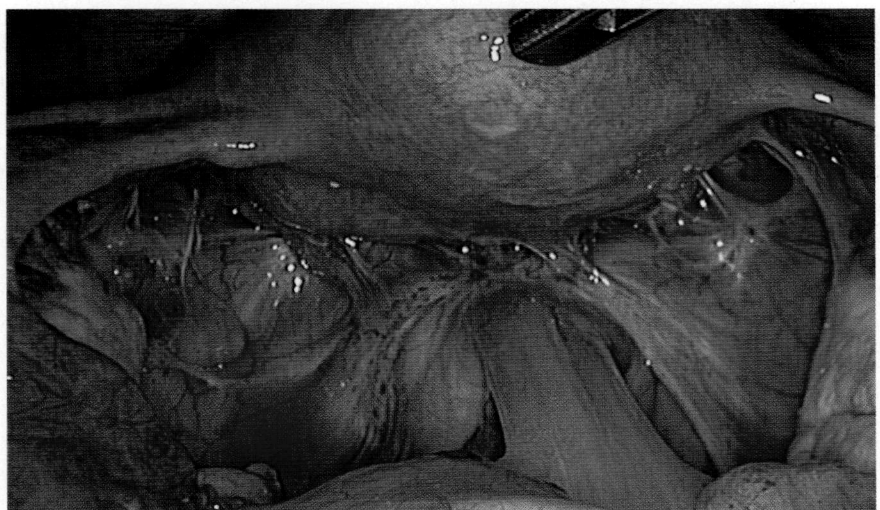

Tech Figure 13.20. Obliterated cul-de-sac.

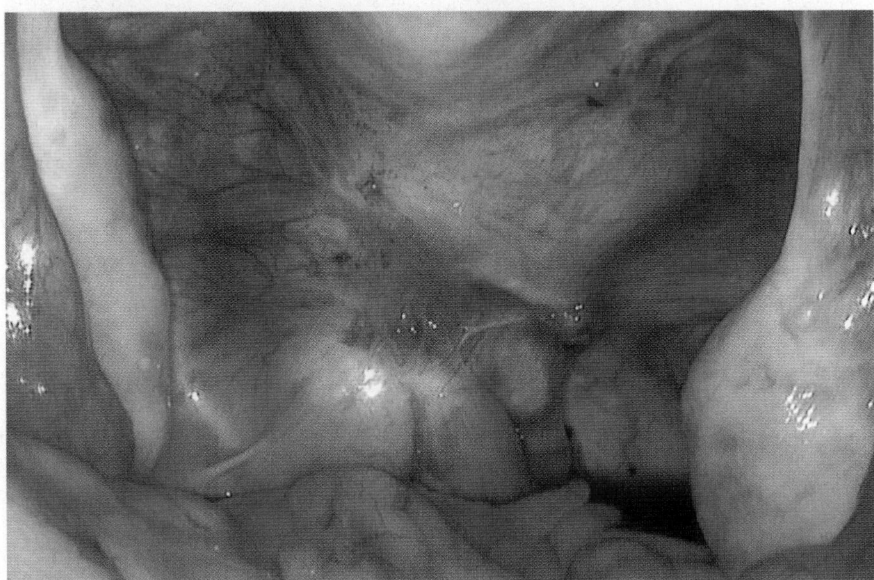

Tech Figure 13.21. Obliterated cul-de-sac with endometriosis rectal nodule.

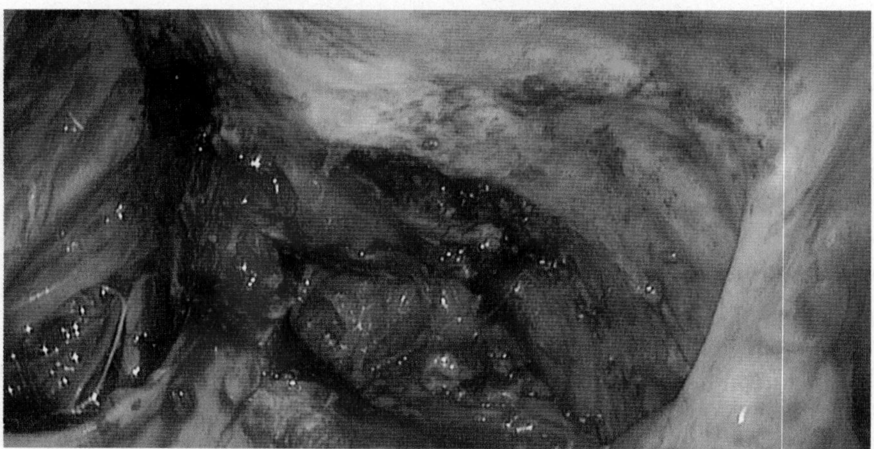

Tech Figure 13.22. On the left, pararectal space dissection. In the midline, cul-de-sac dissection.

- Dissect the rectum from the posterior uterus and vagina.
  - This is facilitated by applying caudad pressure on the posterior vaginal fornix with a vaginal sponge stick. To push the rectum toward the sacrum place a reusable end-to-end anastomotic (EEA) sizer into the rectum (Tech Figs. 13.23 and 13.24).
- Excise the endometriotic plaque and adjacent fibrosis.
  - While viewing the lesion laparoscopically, we recommend manual palpation of the vaginal fornices, and posterior vaginal wall to verify complete excision of diseased tissue.
  - If vaginectomy is inherent to the procedure take care to suture the vaginal tissue in a transverse fashion to avoid vaginal stenosis or foreshortening of the vagina.
- Assess the anterior rectal wall and rectum and colon to determine if further discoid or segmental resection is necessary.
- Restore normal anatomy (Tech Fig. 13.25).

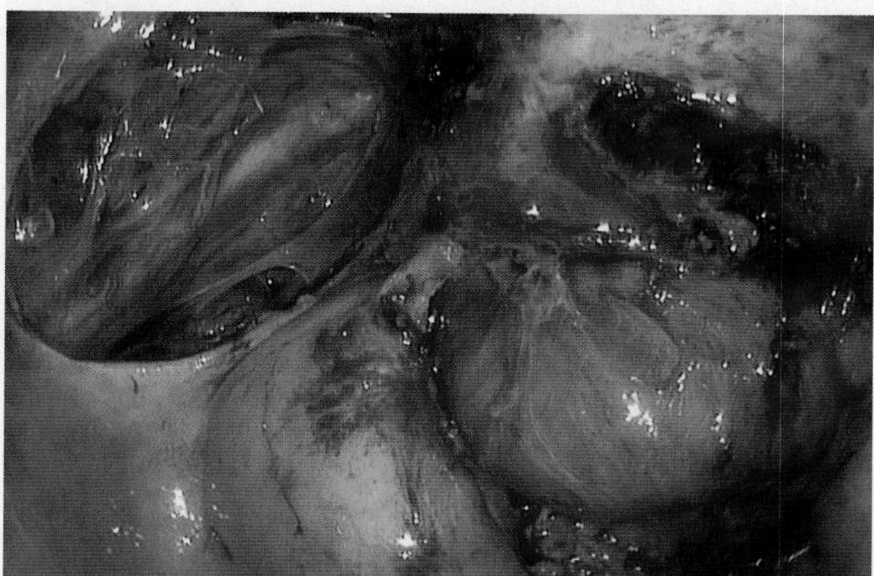

Tech Figure 13.23. Sponge stick in vagina to identify the posterior fornix area (compare to Tech Fig. 13.22).

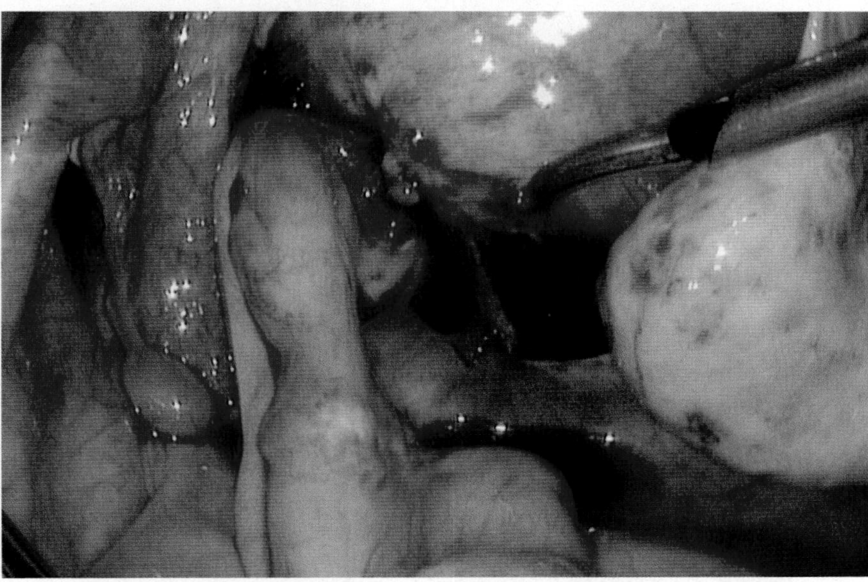

Tech Figure 13.24. Rectal probe during dissection directed to the patient's left to identify the right pararectal space.

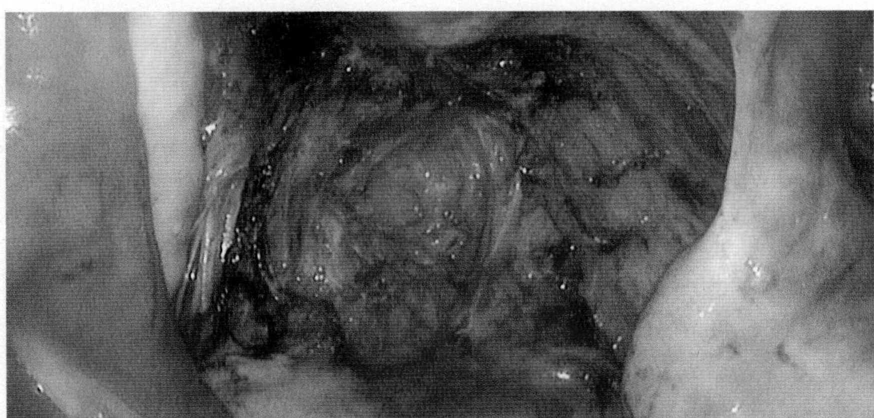

Tech Figure 13.25. Final appearance: restored cul-de-sac anatomy.

Bowel endometriosis focal resection

- An understanding of colon and rectum anatomy is important for safe and efficient surgery (Tech Fig. 13.26).
- Evaluate the lesion size, penetration depth, and circumferential involvement.
- Lesions limited to the serosa can be shaved by sharply excising the lesion with scissors or electrosurgery.
  - Grasp the lesion and excise only the fibrotic and endometriotic tissue.
- Inspect the integrity of the bowel for muscularis invasion.
- Imbricate the serosa as needed taking care not to stenose the underlying layers and bowel lumen.
- Then assess bowel integrity.
  - Perform intraoperative endoscopy or air insufflation with intraperitoneal water instillation to inspect anastomotic integrity and to confirm a watertight closure.

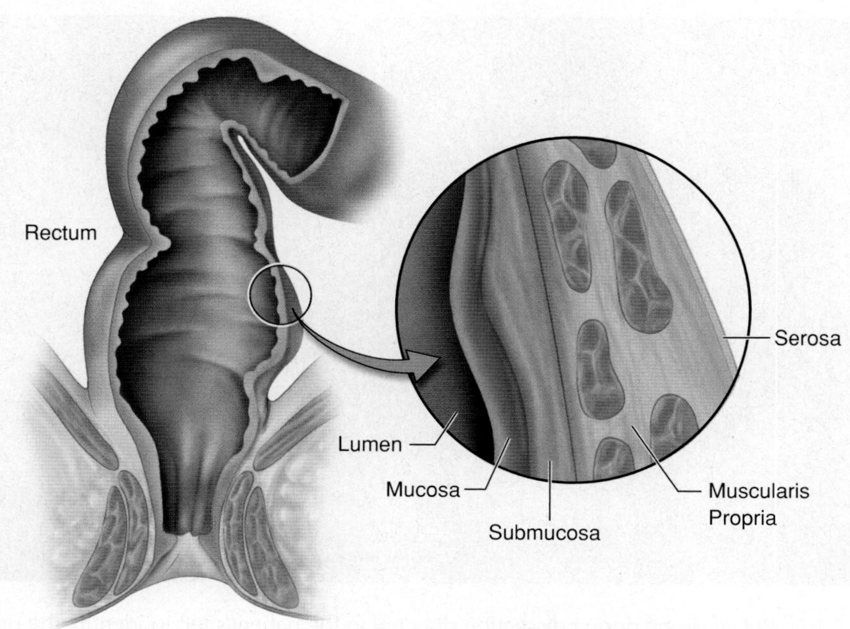

Tech Figure 13.26. Layers of the rectum.

- Full-thickness discoid resection can be performed if:
  - The lesion penetrates deeper than the superficial serosa and involves less than 60% of the bowel circumference.
- Place a rectal probe or sizer in the rectum to aid in bowel dissection. The sizer also acts as a backstop when sharply excising the full-thickness lesion. Grasp the lesion and excise only the fibrotic and endometriotic tissue (Tech Fig. 13.27).

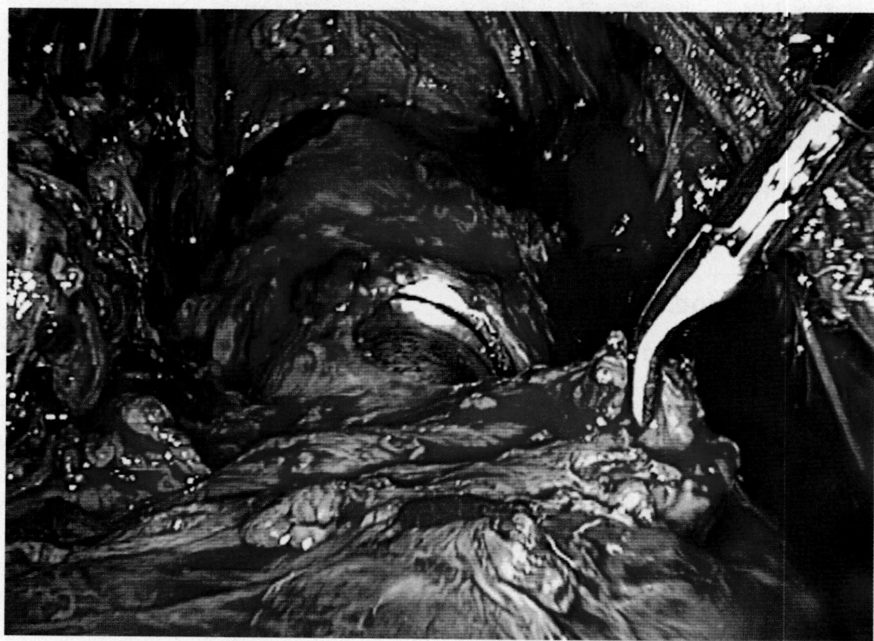

Tech Figure 13.27. Full-thickness (discoid) resection with visible EEA sizer.

Repair the enterotomy with a two-layer closure

- The suture line should be placed perpendicular to the lumen of the bowel (Tech Fig. 13.28).
- Use 3-0 delayed absorbable, interrupted sutures to close the defect with full thickness, incorporating all bowel wall layers.
- Imbricate the second layer with 2-0 or 3-0 delayed absorbable or permanent interrupted sutures, also known as a Lembert stitch (Tech Fig. 13.29).
- Assess bowel integrity (Tech Fig. 13.30).

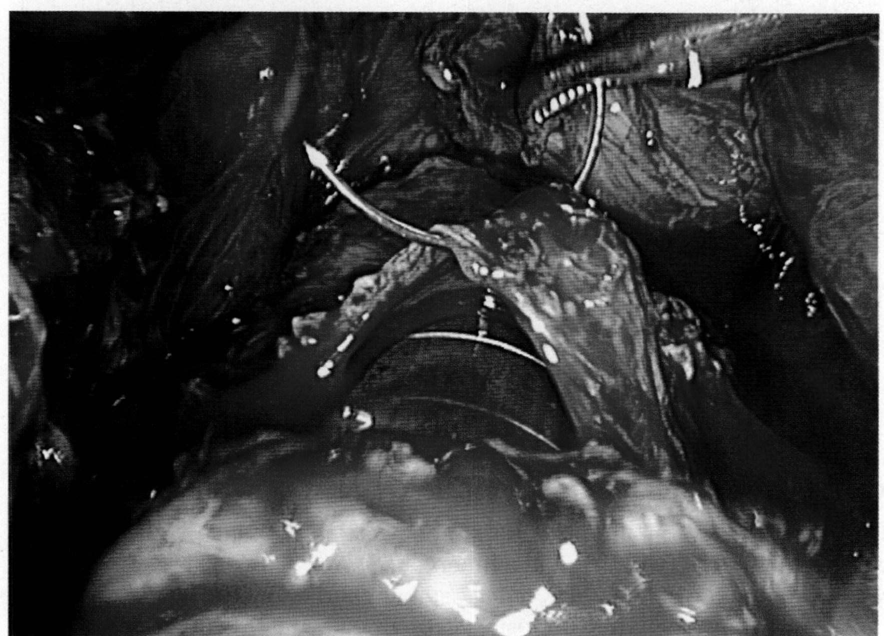

Tech Figure 13.28. The first of two-layer enterotomy closure with suture line perpendicular to the bowel lumen.

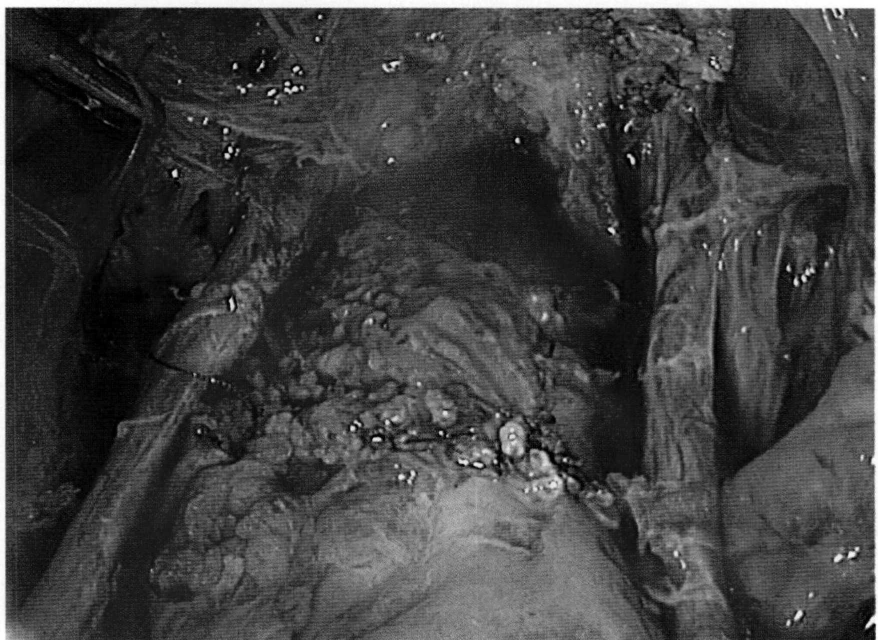

Tech Figure 13.29. Lembert stitch.

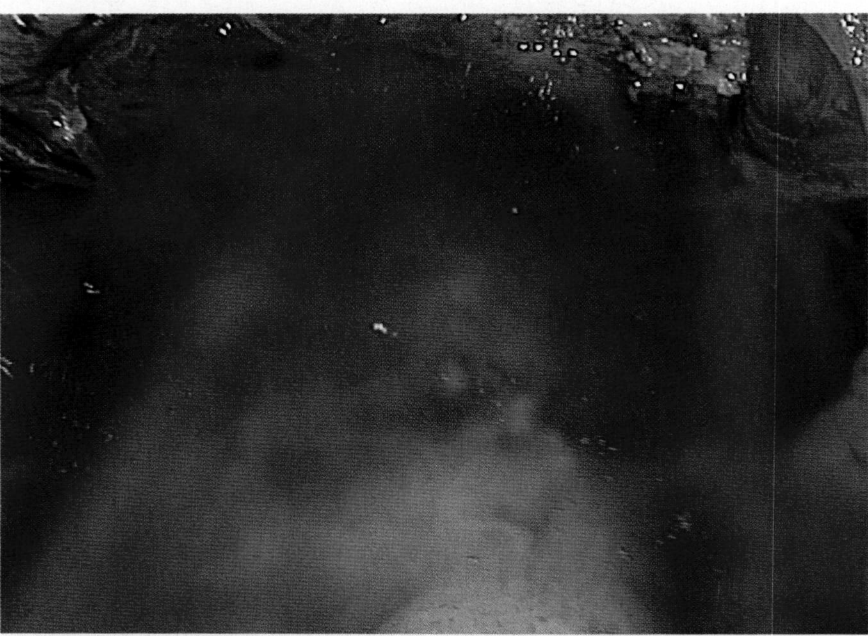

Tech Figure 13.30. Watertight enterotomy closure.

Bowel endometriosis segmental resection

- Identify the segment of colon and/or rectum to be resected with involved disease.
- Mobilize its pertinent retroperitoneal attachments.
- Select the proximal and distal margins of the segment and divided with a linear stapler taking into account tissue thickness when choosing stapler height (Tech Fig. 13.31).
- Achieve hemostasis of major vascular structures with suture ligation and divide the remaining mesentery with an advanced energy source.

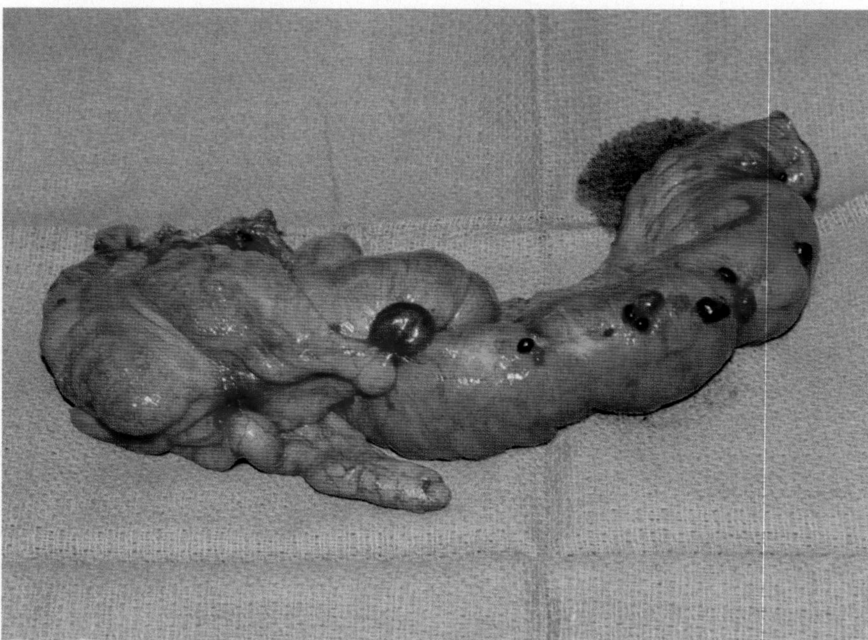

Tech Figure 13.31. Resected bowel segment.

- Complete the reconstruction by means of hand-sewn, linear-stapled, or circular-stapled techniques.
  - For an EEA technique, insert the anvil into the proximal limb (Tech Fig. 13.32).
  - Place a monofilament suture in a purse-string configuration and tie it to secure the anvil in place (Tech Fig. 13.33).

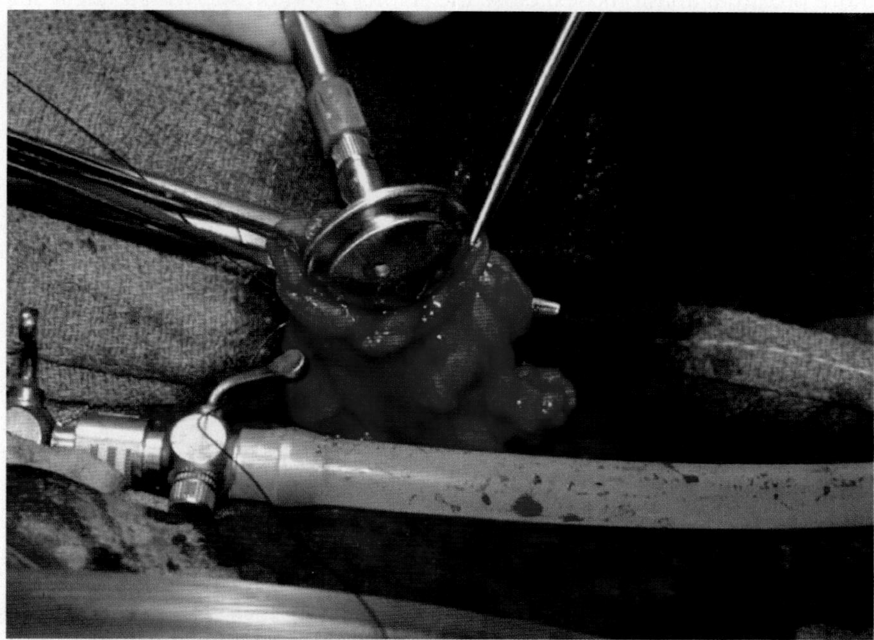

Tech Figure 13.32. EEA technique: Anvil in the proximal segment.

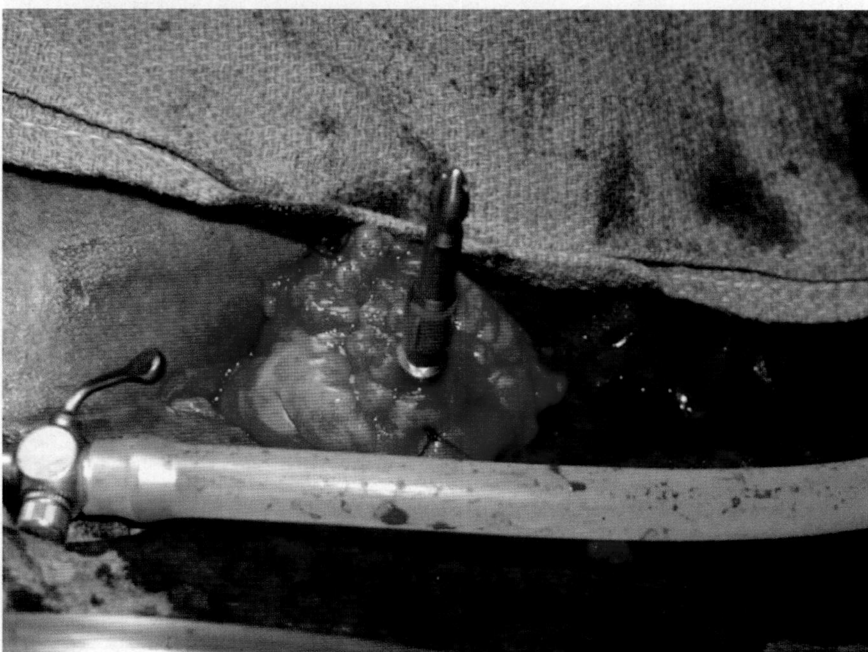

Tech Figure 13.33. EEA technique: Anvil secured with purse-string suture.

- Insert the stapler handle into the distal limb.
  - This is accomplished transanally for lower anastomoses, including colorectal or coloanal, or through the cut end of bowel for a more proximal anastomosis, such as an ileocolic anastomosis.
- Mate the stapler and anvil (Tech Fig. 13.34).
- Engage the device to create the circular stapled anastomosis.
  - For more proximal anastomoses, close the stapler insertion site with a linear stapler in the standard fashion. Some surgeons prefer to oversew the staple lines.

- Assess bowel integrity as described above.

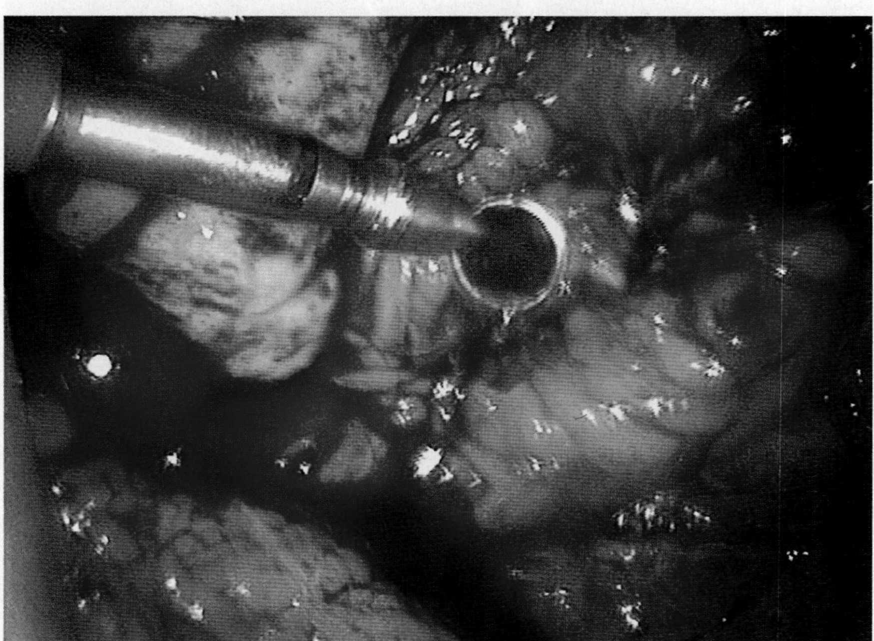

Tech Figure 13.34. EEA technique: Mate stapler and anvil.

Procedures and Techniques: Musculoskeletal/ Anterior Abdominal Wall

Abdominal wall endometriosis resection

- While the patient is awake and lying supine, mark the site of pain and palpable mass with the patient's assistance in the operating room.
- Induce anesthesia and perform routine sterile surgical preparations.
- Inject local anesthetic and, if possible, use the prior surgical incision.
- Once the scar is visually identified, palpate the lesion to identify its borders.
- Grasp the mass and perform adhesiolysis of the surrounding fibrotic tissue with a monopolar instrument (Tech Fig. 13.35).
  - Frequently palpate the mass and surrounding tissue to ensure no residual endometriosis remains *in situ*.
  - If the fascia is entered, mark the location with a delayed absorbable suture for easy re-approximation and identification.
- Continue with meticulous dissection until the lesion is completely excised (Tech Fig. 13.36).
- The nodule contains a variety of glandular, fatty, and fibrotic tissues (Tech Fig. 13.37).
  - Re-approximate the fascia with delayed absorbable suture.
  - Place interrupted sutures to re-approximate the dead space if the subcutaneous tissue measures greater than 3 cm.
  - The dermis may be re-approximated with either staples or suture.

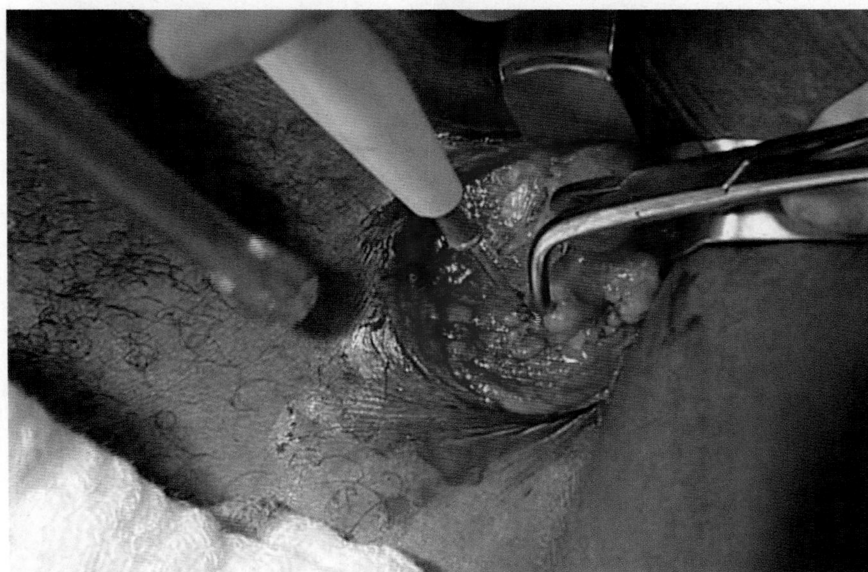

Tech Figure 13.35. Grasp and excise the endometriosis.

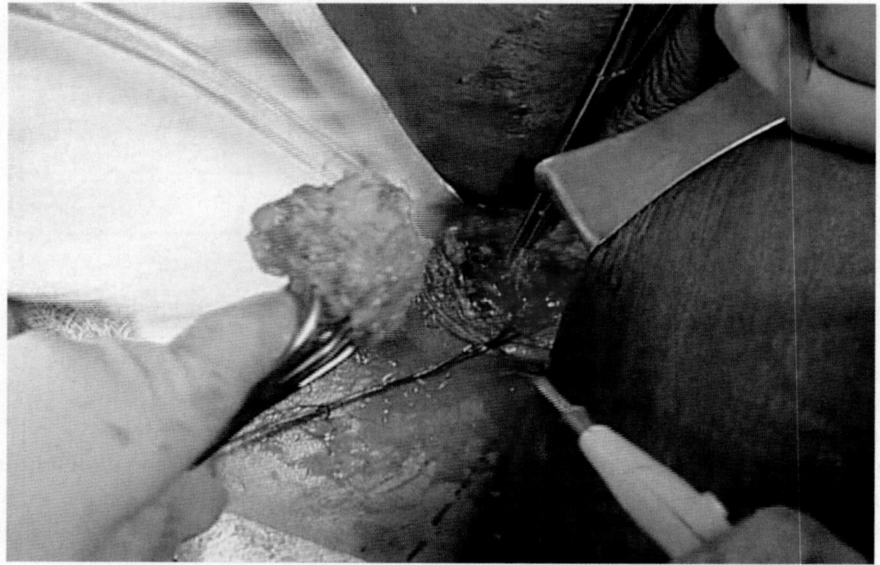

Tech Figure 13.36. Endometriosis nodule in towel clamp (left) and suture marking the fascia entry.

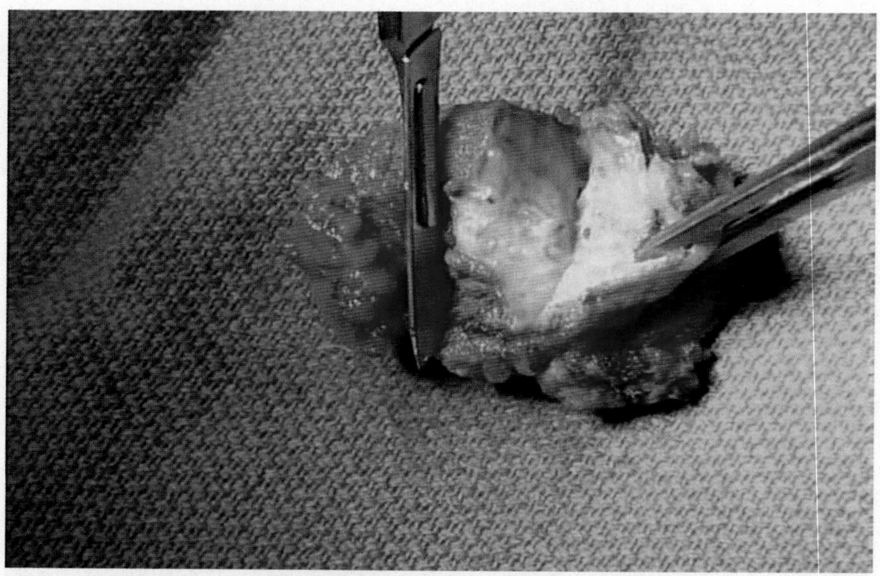

Tech Figure 13.37. Abdominal wall endometriosis nodule, bivalve.

Advanced abdominal wall techniques

- When the endometrioma encompasses a large surface area or invades multiple layers through the muscle, fascia, and into underlying viscous (Tech Fig. 13.38), advanced techniques to close the abdominal wall may be required.
  - A component separation allows for medialization of the rectus fascia, which results in tension-free re-approximation of the fascia.
    - Dissect and identify the insertion of the external oblique muscle fascia into the rectus. Incise the aponeurosis of the external oblique fascia. This can be performed from the costal margin down to the pubic symphysis.
    - Re-approximate the anterior rectus sheath at midline with interrupted delayed absorbable suture.
  - If mesh is needed, select the appropriate type and size and secure it with interrupted sutures taking care not to injure the underlying bowel and organs. The mesh may be placed in an intraperitoneal location, with closure of the fascia above it. Alternatively, the mesh may be placed in a retro-rectus position. This requires opening of the posterior rectus sheath and dissection of this plane laterally. Once developed, the posterior rectus sheath is closed with absorbable suture. The mesh is inserted and secured with suture. Then, close the anterior fascia (Tech Figs. 13.39 and 13.40).
  - Place drains if needed.
  - Re-approximate the skin with suture or staples.

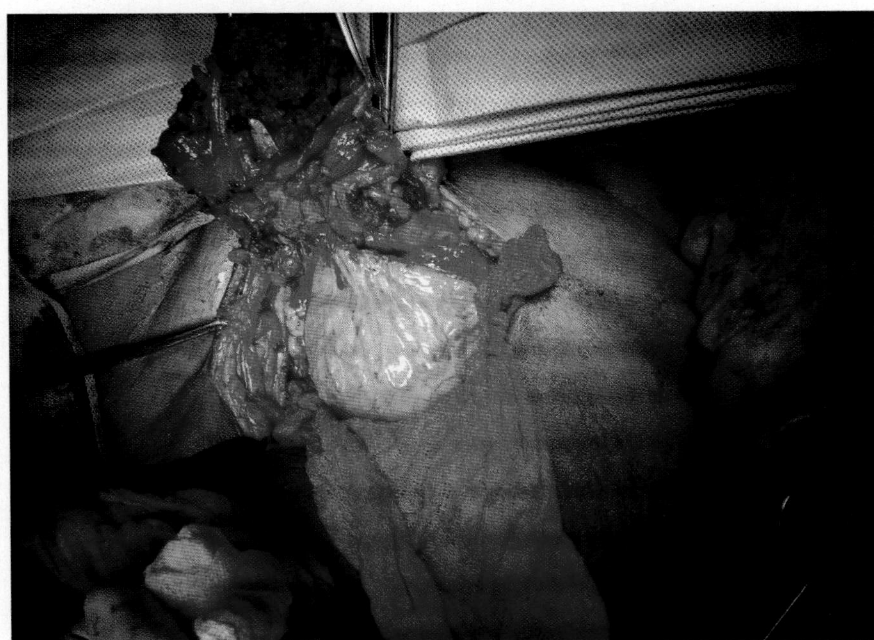

Tech Figure 13.38. Rectus muscle, fascia, subcutaneous tissue, and abdominal endometrioma adherent to bladder. A 31-year-old G5P4 presented with 10 months of severe cyclic pain. Her history was significant for a cesarean delivery 5 years prior. MRI revealed an infiltrative mass that measured 10 cm × 6 cm × 4 cm in the distal rectus abdominis muscles. The mass had notable spiculated margins and a halo of edema with increased T2 signaling that crossed midline and was just below her previous Pfannenstiel incision (Fig. 13.6A,B). The mass encompassed 60% of the left rectus muscle and stretched from just above the pubic symphysis to above her umbilicus.

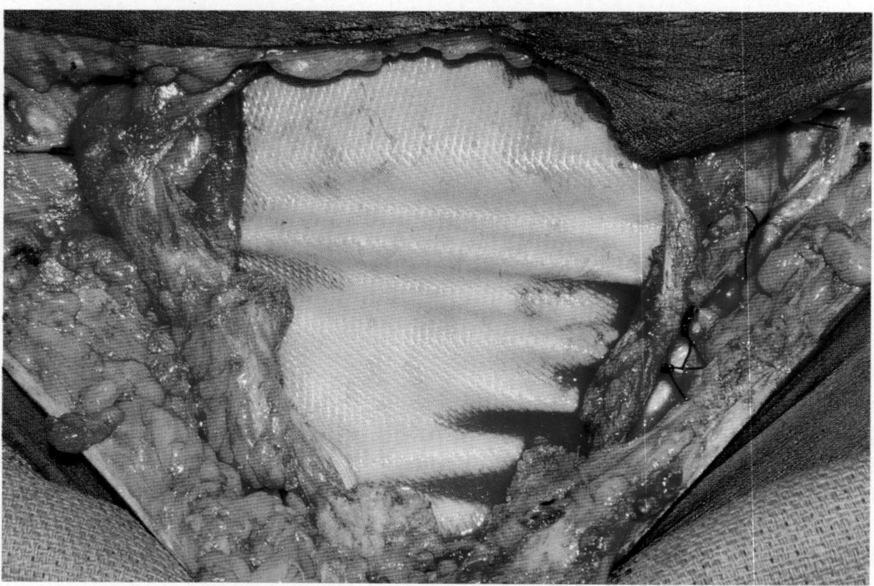

Tech Figure 13.39. Mesh for large anterior abdominal wall defect, retracted caudad.

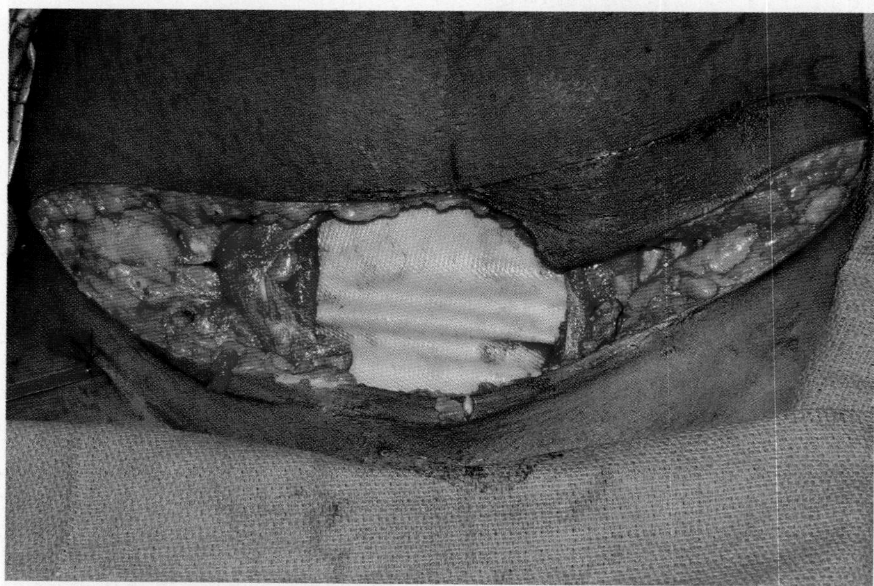

Tech Figure 13.40. Large abdominal endometrioma resection required advanced closure techniques and mesh.

PEARLS AND PITFALLS

- Consider a preoperative biopsy to confirm the diagnosis of benign extraperitoneal endometriosis prior to a respective surgery.
- Clearly outline the goals of the extirpative surgery (relieve obstruction, mass excision, pain reduction), complications, possibility of recurrence, and postoperative chronic treatments. Even in emergent cases, poor preoperative counseling and collaborative patient goal setting may undermine long-term outcomes despite excellent surgical technique.
- Always dissect and identify the ureters before initiating adhesiolysis or excisional procedures.
- Bladder and rectocervical endometriosis is complicated by dense scarring and aberrant anatomy. Begin dissections lateral to the lesions in the perivesical and perirectal spaces, respectively.
- Repair ureterostomy with interrupted 4-0 polydioxanone sutures and place a ureteral stent.
- Extensive debridement of the ureteral adventitia may result in devascularization of the ureter.
- Visual and frequent tactile evaluation of the musculoskeletal mass will aid in adhesiolysis and dissection
- Large fascial defects may require mesh, component separation, and abdominal wall reconstruction. Preoperative imaging and surgical team planning are important.

POSTOPERATIVE CARE

Urinary Tract Endometriosis Resection

- Remove the surgical drain once its output is minimal. If there is any concern for urinary collection from the pelvic drain send the fluid for creatinine evaluation before the drain is removed.

Gastrointestinal Tract Endometriosis Resection

- Clear diet is started on postoperative day 1 and is advanced ad lib. IV patient-controlled analgesia is typically used until the patient is transitioned to oral medications.

Musculoskeletal/Anterior Abdominal Wall

- As with all extraperitoneal endometriosis, regardless of their location, we recommend continued, hormonal suppression in the immediate postoperative state and continue this therapy for long term. If the resection site is large, the patient may require overnight admission for several days and may benefit from postoperative rehabilitation and physical therapy. Postoperative care should be individualized and focus on early ambulation and improved functionality.

OUTCOMES

Urinary Tract Endometriosis Resection

- A large comparison of ureterolysis, ureteroureteral anastomosis, ureteroneocystotomy, and bladder resection outcomes has yet to be performed. This could be due to several reasons including the belief that ureteral endometriosis is a separate entity from bladder endometriosis. In general, urinary tract endometriosis surgery is well tolerated with few complications.

Gastrointestinal Tract Endometriosis Resection

- Most excisional rectovaginal endometriosis case series report excellent short-term pain relief in 70% to 80% of patients. At 1 year postoperatively, however, approximately 50% of the patients required hormonal or analgesic treatment. A quarter of the patients undergo a subsequent operation.

Musculoskeletal/Anterior Abdominal Wall

- There are several case reports and reviews of abdominal wall endometriomas in cesarean section scars and laparoscopic trocar sites. As mentioned earlier, the recurrence rates, optimal resection margins, and surgical techniques to decrease recurrence are unknown and warrant further investigation.

COMPLICATIONS

Urinary Tract Endometriosis Resection

- Urinary tract complications include ureteral injury, fistula, and leakage.

Gastrointestinal Tract Endometriosis Resection

- Gastrointestinal tract complications include bladder denervation, rectovaginal fistula, anastomotic leak, and pelvic abscess. In general, the larger the resection, the higher the complication rate. The major complications from radical endometriosis resection are listed in **Table 13.1**.

Table 13.1 Major Complications from Radical Rectocervical Endometriosis Surgery

Complication	Rate
Neurogenic bladder dysfunction due to parasympathetic nerve disruption	4–10%
Rectovaginal fistula formation	2–10%
Inadvertent rectal perforation	1–3%
Anastomotic leakage	1–2%
Pelvic abscess	1–2%
Postanastomotic rectal stenosis	0.5–1%
Postanastomotic ureteral stenosis	0.5–1%

Adapted from: Vercellini P, Somigliana E, Viganò P, Abbiati A, Barbara G, Crosignani PG. Surgery for endometriosis-associated infertility: a pragmatic approach. *Hum Reprod*. 2009;24:254–269.

Musculoskeletal/Anterior Abdominal Wall

- Case reports of malignant transformation are rare and the frequency is unknown. The major postoperative complications from abdominal wall resection include hematoma, seroma, hernia, and surgical site infection.

KEY REFERENCES

1. Abrao MS, Petraglia F, Falcone T, Keckstein J, Osuga Y, Chapron C. Deep endometriosis infiltrating the recto-sigmoid: critical factors to consider before management. *Hum Reprod Update.* 2015;21(3):329–339.
2. Chapron C, Dubuisso JB. Laparoscopic management of bladder endometriosis. *Acta Obstt Gynecol Scand.* 1999;78:887–890.
3. Duepree HJ, Senagore AJ, Delaney CP, Marcello PW, Brady KM, Falcone T. Laparoscopic resection of deep pelvic endometriosis with rectosigmoid involvement. *J Am Coll Surg.* 2002;195(6):754–758.
4. Fedele L, Bianchi S, Zanconato G, Bergamini V, Berlanda N, Carmignani L. Long-term follow-up after conservative surgery for bladder endometriosis. *Fertil Steril.* 2005;83:1729–1733.
5. Falcone T, Lebovic DI. Clinical management of endometriosis. *Obstet Gynecol.* 2011;118:691–705.
6. Horton JD, Dezee KJ, Ahnfeldt EP, Wagner M. Abdominal wall endometriosis; a surgeon's perspective and review of 445 cases. *Am J Surg.* 2008;196:207–212.
7. Jerby BL, Kessler H, Falcone T, Milsom JW. Laparoscopic management of colorectal endometriosis. *Surg Endosc.* 1999;13(11):1125–1128.
8. Vercellini P, Crosignani PG, Abbiati A, Somigliana E, Viganò P, Fedele L. The effect of surgery for symptomatic endometriosis: the other side of the story. *Hum Reprod Update.* 2009;15:177–188.
9. Vercellini P, Somigliana E, Viganò P, Abbiati A, Barbara G, Crosignani PG. Surgery for endometriosis-associated infertility: a pragmatic approach. *Hum Reprod.* 2009;24:254–269.

Section VII

Vulvar and Perineal Surgery

14 Vulvar Biopsy and Excision of Vulvar Lesions

Oluwatosin Goje

GENERAL PRINCIPLES

Definition

- Vulvar lesions represent a wide spectrum of disorders found in the vulvar and perianal regions.[1,2] The correct diagnosis is based on clinical history, physical examination, and sometimes laboratory tests. The greatest challenge is to differentiate what is normal, or a normal variant, from the abnormal and also to identify potentially serious disease or infection.[3] The most concerning vulvar lesions are intraepithelial neoplasia (VIN) and cancer. The most bothersome are the lichen diseases that are characterized by intense pain and pruritus.

Differential Diagnosis

- Vulvar dermatoses: These are inflamed, scaling skin diseases of the vulvar and fall into two morphologic groups: papulosquamous disease and eczematous disease. Papulosquamous diseases are well demarcated and usually show little evidence of rubbing and scratching while eczematous disease has poorly demarcated borders, and characterized by excoriations or thickening of skin from rubbing.
- Infectious vulvar lesions may result from candida or herpes simplex virus (HSV) infection. Acquisition of human papilloma virus (HPV) and syphilis may manifest as condyloma accuminata and condyloma lata, respectively. In turn, these lesions are treated with antifungal, antiviral, and antibiotics.
- Other benign vulvar lesions include lichen planus, lichen sclerosus, lichen simplex chronicus. Lesions may also develop from chronic irritation secondary to contact/allergic irritants.
- Vulvar ulcers: Ulcers are deep with the defect extending into the dermis. They could be infectious or noninfectious. Examples of noninfectious ulcers include Behcet's disease, apthous ulcers, complex aphthosis, and Crohn's disease. Vulvar ulcers are often treated with steroids and immunotherapy such as tacrolimus.
- Premalignant or malignant vulvar lesions include vulvar intraepithelial neoplasia (VIN), melanoma, basal cell carcinoma, and squamous cell carcinoma. At the very minimum, these lesions require biopsy and excision.

Nonoperative Management

- There are no special considerations prior to performing a vulvar biopsy, but patients undergoing excisional biopsy may need to be optimized. Controlling blood sugar in diabetics improves wound healing, anti-coagulated and chronically immunosuppressed patient needs a multidisciplinary approach for optimization prior to surgery. If a patient is anti-coagulated and the international normalized ratio is within the therapeutic window, the procedure can be performed, but physician must have electrical or chemical cautery available for hemostasis.

IMAGING AND OTHER DIAGNOSTICS

- Diagnosis should be made prior to initiating treatment. It is imperative for the clinician to ascertain if the etiology is infectious in nature. This may lead to ancillary blood tests, vulvar and vaginal swabs for culture, polymerase chain reaction (PCR), and biopsies. For example, a patient with vulvar ulcer should be screened for syphilis and HSV using serology. The ulcer should be swabbed and sent for HSV culture or PCR, and dark-field microscopy. Ulcer should be biopsied and sent to pathology.
- Vulvar colposcopy: High-grade intraepithelial lesions of the vulvar (HSIL) or VIN are usually multifocal and located on the nonhairy part of the vulvar. Lesions may be raised and variegated with hues of white, red, pink, brown, or grey. Thorough vulvar colposcopy identifies additional lesions and assists in biopsy planning.
- Perform colposcopy by covering the area with gauze soaked in 3% to 5% acetic acid for 3 to 5 minutes. Abnormal areas may appear white (acetowhite) and should be biopsied.[4] Other areas may present with irregular borders and uneven pigmentation. VIN usually presents as sharply marginated flat-topped papules and plaques (see Pearls and Pitfalls section).
- Vulvar biopsy should also be performed on lesions with the following: asymmetry, color variation, irregular borders, rapid change in size or appearance, and bleeding or nonhealing ulcers.
- Recalcitrant, nonimproving lesions must be biopsied. A common scenario is an elderly woman who was adequately treated for candida infection but continues to experience persistent itching. On examination, her vulva remains erythematous, with or without fissures and excoriations. Such a patient may have contact or allergic dermatitis, lichen sclerosus, or a premalignant lesion.
- Diagnostic vulvar biopsies are office procedures, whereas wide local excisions are performed in the operating room to ensure all affected tissues are excised down to the subcutaneous tissue level.
- Prior to procedure, discuss the indication and steps of the procedure with the patient. Counsel her on the risk of pain, bleeding, infection, scarring, and the possibility of a nondiagnostic sample. Finally, obtain the patient's written consent.
- Ensure all equipment and supplies are arranged and available (**Table 14.1**).

Table 14.1 Biopsy Box Supplies

Biopsy Box Supplies
Baby shampoo/povidone–iodine, or chlorhexidine solutions
Lidocaine injection (1–2%) with or without epinephrine
Surgical gloves
Lidocaine gel 2%
Disposable drape
Syringe—30-gauge tuberculin syringe (1 mL) or 1- or 3-mL syringe
Needles—22–25 gauge (draw up solutions), 25–30 gauge (for injection)
Sterile gauze 2 × 2 or 3 × 3 or 4 × 4
Disposable surgical Scalpel #15
Disposable Keyes punch biopsies, 3–6 mm
Small tissue forceps and Metzenbaum or Iris scissors or disposable kit with forceps and scissors
Needle drivers
3-0 and 4-0 Vicryl suture
Alcohol swabs
Bandages and band-aids
Formalin specimen bottle
Patient instructions
Surgical marking pen
Silver nitrate sticks/Monsel's solution
Hyfrecator/electrosurgical unit

- Depending on the biopsy area, we recommend applying topical anesthetic to increase patient comfort.
- If the site involves keratinized skin, apply topical anesthesia (lidocaine cream) for at least 30 to 60 minutes. If the site is confined to the mucous membrane, 20 minutes of topical anesthesia is sufficient. Application of 2% lidocaine gel or 2.5% prilocaine cream desensitizes the skin and allows painless injection of 1% to 2% lidocaine into the site. Lidocaine with or without epinephrine can be used, lidocaine solution with epinephrine may reduce bleeding, but do not use epinephrine around the clitoral area.
- Position the patient on an examination table with lower extremity stirrups and prep the area of interest with chlorhexidine, povidone–iodine, or baby soap solution (depending on patient's allergy profile) (Fig. 14.1).
- Inject 1 to 3 mL of 1% to 2% lidocaine (local anesthetic) using a small needle (27- to 30-gauge needle) into the dermis to form a bleb or wheal under the lesion and beyond its edges (Fig. 14.2). Wheal formed should be wider in diameter than the biopsy instrument used. Test for appropriate anesthesia using a forceps prior to biopsy; in general, adequate anesthesia is achieved about 2 minutes post lidocaine injection.

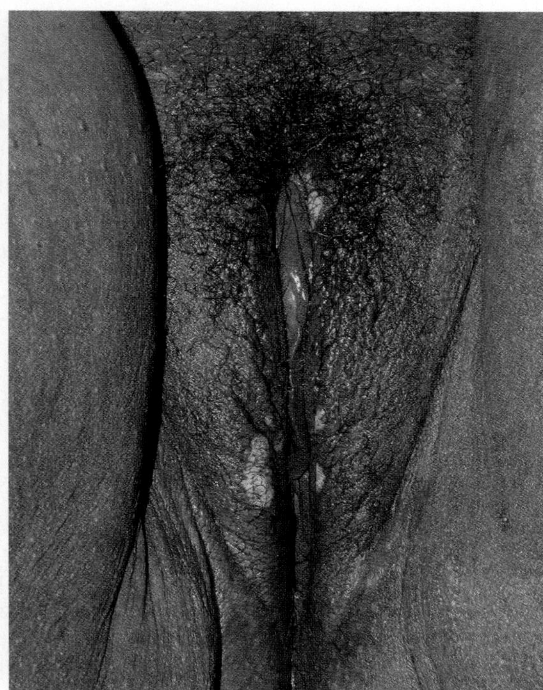

Figure 14.1. Positioning of patient and preparation of biopsy site.

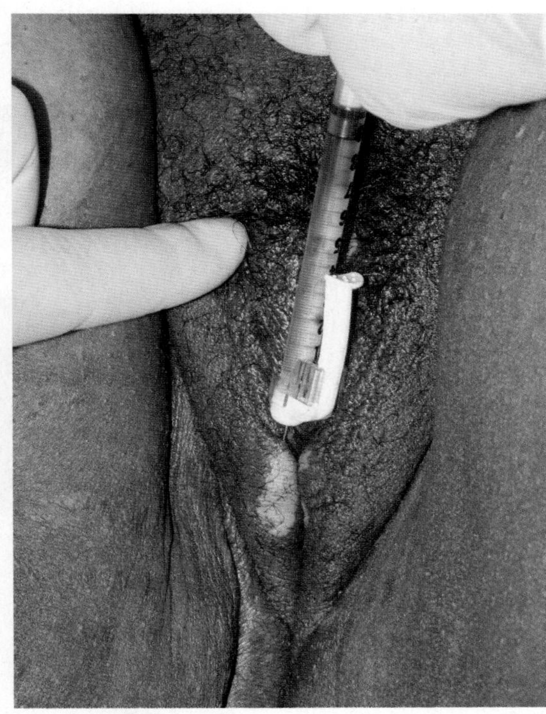

Figure 14.2. Injecting anesthetic solution under the lesion to create a wheal or bleb.

Procedures and Techniques

Vulvar sampling can be performed using these different instruments and techniques: punch biopsy (Keyes punch biopsy), cervical biopsy forceps, suture and scissors technique, or wide local excision. Table 14.1 highlights the basic supplies needed.

A punch biopsy

This is a disposable instrument which removes a core-shaped piece of tissue.[5] Use this instrument when all skin layers are needed to make a diagnosis. It is available in different sizes and most commonly used diameters are 3 to 6 mm. Select the appropriate size of punch biopsy based on the lesion.

Using sterile gloves and technique test the patient's analgesia. Once it is confirmed to be adequate, position your nondominant hand to stretch the skin perpendicular to the lines of least skin tension. Then place the biopsy instrument perpendicular to the skin and firmly press down on it while simultaneously twisting the instrument 360 degrees until the tissue yields, indicating it has reached the subcutaneous fat and a full-thickness biopsy has been obtained. Stabilize the tissue with forceps and excise the tissue from its base with Metzenbaum or Iris scissors (Tech Fig. 14.1).

Apply moderate pressure and possibly a hemostatic agent (silver nitrate or Monsel's solution) to achieve hemostasis. Electrocautery may be used to stop bleeding if needed. Re-approximate larger biopsies (>4 mm) with suture to prevent scarring (Tech Fig. 14.2A,B).

If decision is made to re-approximate the defect, most patients will need a single stitch to close the defect; make sure to evert the skin edges, the underlying dermis from both edges should touch. This compensates for future contracture of the wound and produces a flat scar.

For large defects, start suturing in the middle of the wound and work toward the edges to prevent "dog ears" of the wound. If tension is noticed during the repair, undermine the edges of the wound by 2 to 3 mm to prevent tension.

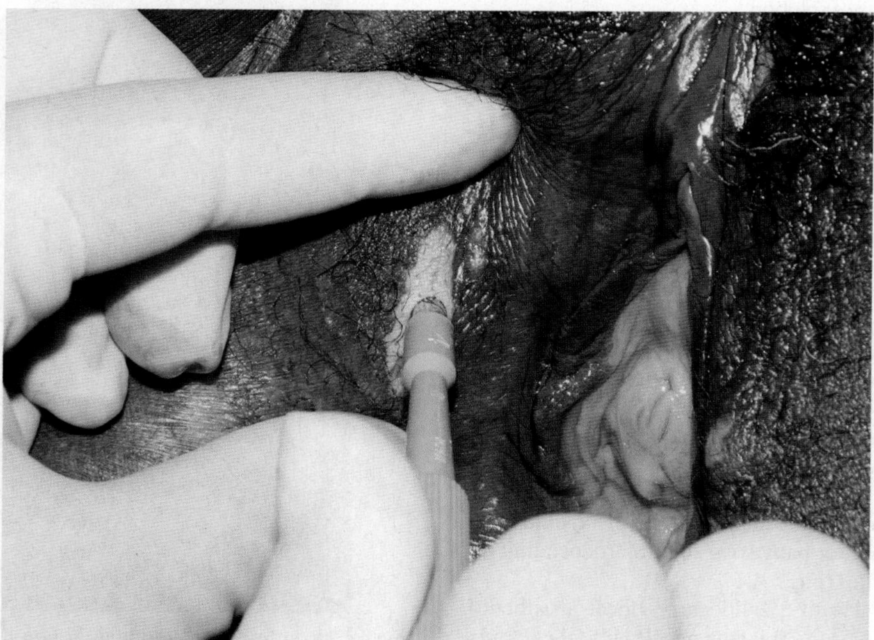

Tech Figure 14.1. 4-mm Keyes punch biopsy technique.

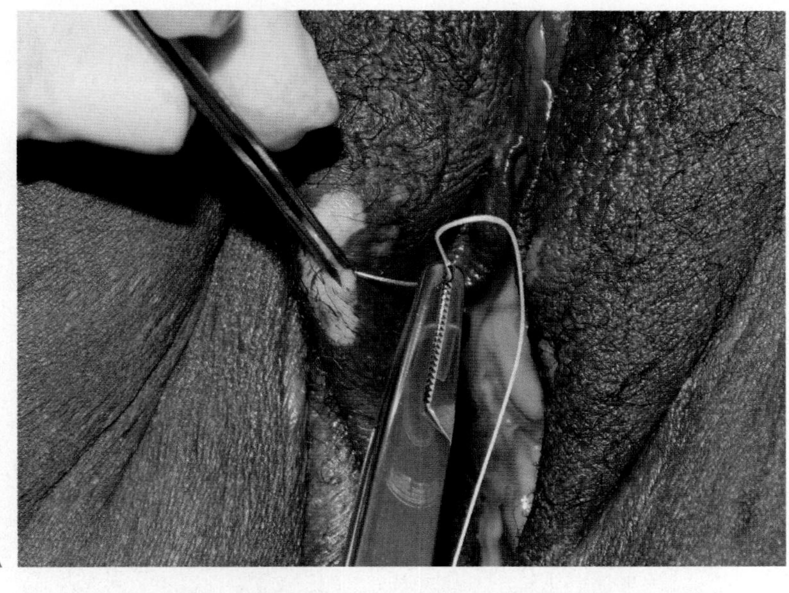

A

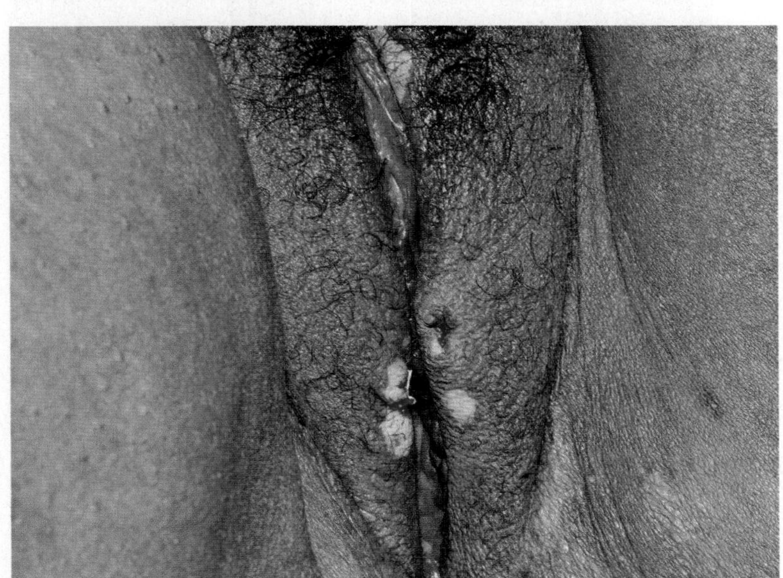

B

Tech Figure 14.2. A and B: Suturing of a defect >4 mm.

A Tischler biopsy forceps

- The same used for cervical biopsy may also be used for vulvar lesion biopsies.
- Simply grasp the lesion within the open jaws of the biopsy forceps and squeeze the handles together to excise the specimen.

The suture and scissors technique

- For fragile tissue, place a 3-0 or 4-0 absorbable suture in the lesion and apply gentle traction to elevate the tissue. Then excise the lesion from its base using a small scissors (Tech Fig. 14.3A,B). Take care to excise under the suture to avoid cutting the suture itself.
- Regardless of the biopsy method, achieve hemostasis with any combination of firm pressure, suture, and a chemical hemostatic agent such as Monsel's solution or silver nitrate or electrical coagulation.

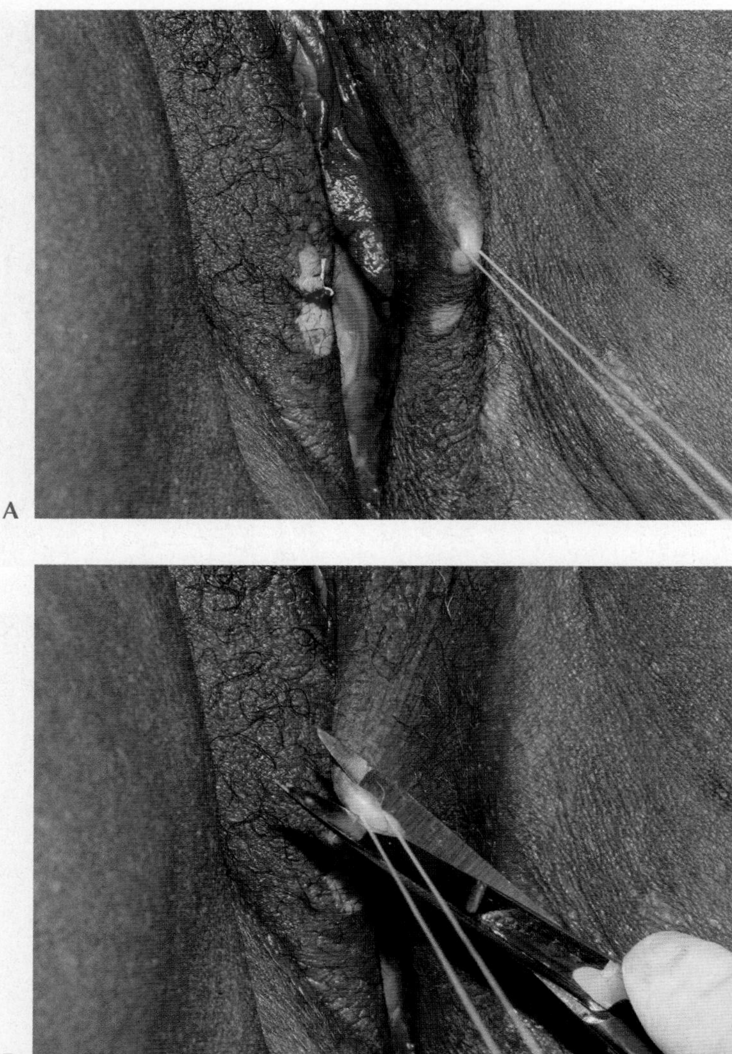

Tech Figure 14.3. A and B: The suture and scissors method of vulvar biopsy.

Excisional biopsy

This technique is ideal for lesions that need complete removal for diagnostic or therapeutic purposes. It requires the greatest amount of time and expertise.

It is usually performed under general or regional anesthesia. Position the patient with lower-extremity stirrups. Prep the patient in a standard surgical fashion. Using a marking pen, draw an ellipse around the lesion and include a 2 to 5 mm circumferential margin of normal/healthy skin.[4] Apply a sharp stimulus to test the patient's level of analgesia. Using a no. 15 scalpel, begin at one

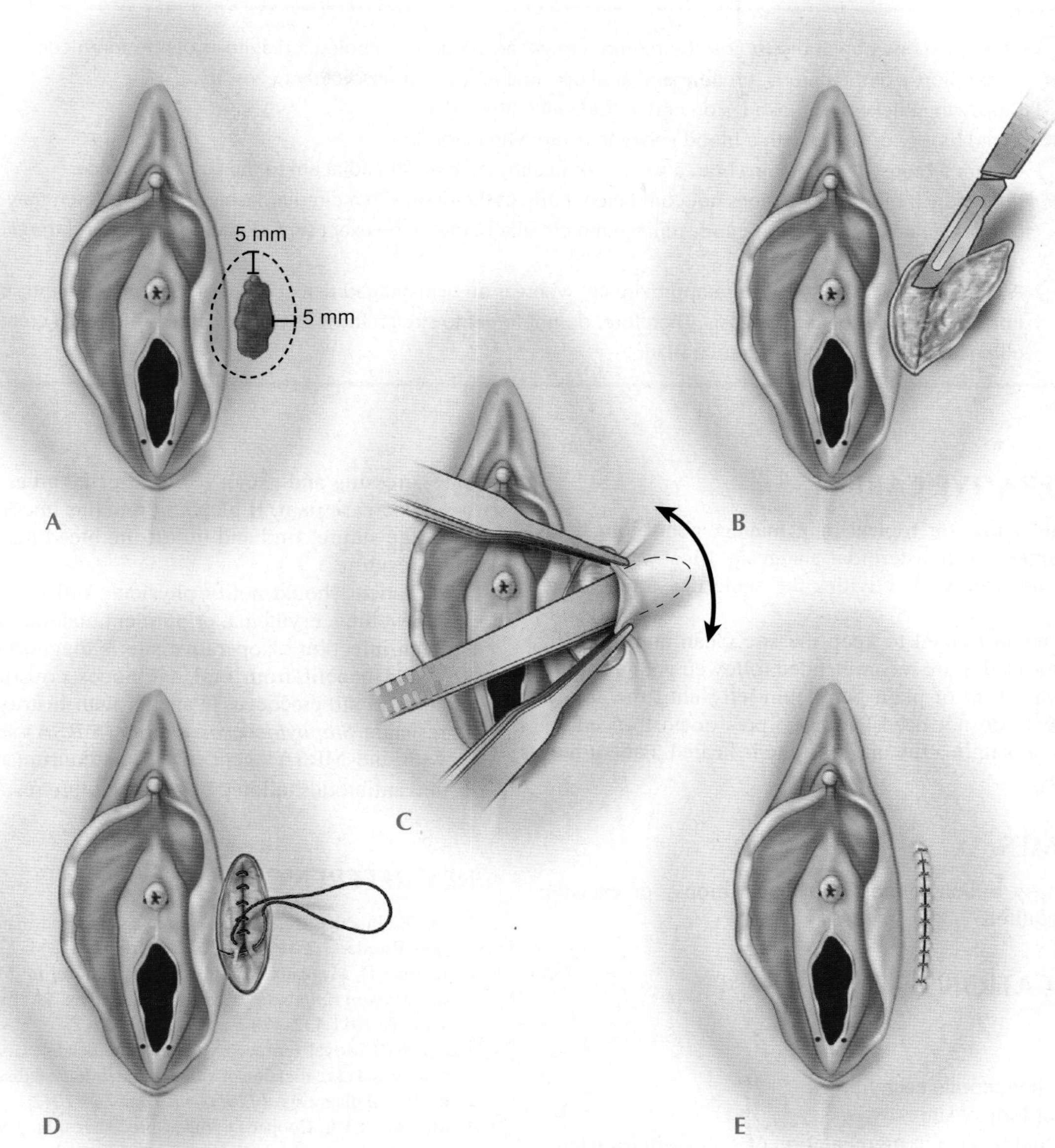

Tech Figure 14.4. Illustration of excisional biopsy.

apex and place firm, consistent, downward pressure on the scalpel perpendicular to the skin. Take the incision down to the subcutaneous adipose tissue and continue along the ellipse. Once the excisional biopsy is removed, this adipose tissue will be exposed. Take care to excise a uniform depth from apex to apex and avoid decreasing excisional depth at the apices. Lift the edge of the excised tissue with forceps and undermine the sample at the level of subcutaneous fat with a scalpel or scissors. Use a microfine needle tip to apply electrical coagulation sparingly to obtain hemostasis and to minimize thermal destruction of the tissue (**Tech Fig. 14.4**). Using a 4-0 absorbable suture, close from the middle of the defect to the edges to prevent "dog ear." Depending on the depth of the wound, defect may need to be closed in two layers with the subcutaneous space closed first with interrupted stitches before the skin is everted and closed.

PEARLS AND PITFALLS

- ○ More than one punch biopsy may be required to get an accurate pathologic diagnosis of a lesion/ulcer.
- ✗ Avoid biopsy of the clitoris, urethra, and anal opening unless it is absolutely necessary.
- ○ Biopsy the thickest area of a lesion and include ulcerated edge.
- ✗ Avoid biopsy of areas with a blood vessel to avoid a hematoma.
- ○ Obtain a biopsy that contains both a section of healthy normal skin adjacent to the suspicious ulcer.
- ✗ If the punch biopsy blade does not completely transect the dermis in a circular fashion, the specimen may be of inadequate depth. If this occurs, replace the circular blade in the exact same location and extend the biopsy depth.
- ○ A circular defect is difficult to re-approximate, whereas an oval-shaped defect has less tension along the suture line and provides better cosmesis. Therefore, do not forget to stretch the skin prior to punch biopsy to create an elliptical incision from the circular blade.

POSTOPERATIVE CARE

Apply 2% lidocaine for topical pain management along with over-the-counter oral nonsteroidal analgesia. Most patients are able to resume work and activities the same day after vulvar biopsy.

Patients are instructed to keep the site clean and dry. Sitz baths two times a day are recommended followed with an application of a thin film of plain petroleum jelly until the area is healed. Patients do not need antibiotic pre- or postprocedure. Avoid taking a bath in a tub until the site is healed. Patient may take showers.

OUTCOMES

- If the biopsy is nondiagnostic, a repeat biopsy or excision may be required.

COMPLICATIONS

- Infection
- Pain
- Bleeding, hematoma, ecchymosis
- Scarring of biopsy site
- Irritation and change in pigmentation of skin from Monsel.
- Controlling complications:
  - Bleeding can be controlled by applying pressure for 5 minutes and or suture ligation of bleeding vessels. The risk of hematoma can be reduced with pressure dressing and use of ice to affected area, which may also decrease pain. If bleeding remains uncontrolled, remove the suture, find and tie off the bleeding vessel, and then resuture.
  - Patient should notify physician office if severe pain and swelling, erythema, or purulent malodorous discharge.
- If an infection of operative site is diagnosed, most patients would benefit from oral antibiotics covering staphylococcus and streptococcus. Patients with history of methicillin-resistant *Staphylococcus aureus* (MRSA) should be treated with anti-MRSA agent like trimethoprim/sulfamethoxazole and antibiotics tailored based on culture results if applicable.

KEY REFERENCES

1. ACOG Practice Bulletin No. 93. Diagnosis and management of vulvar skin disorders. *Obstet Gynecol.* 2008;111(5):1243–1253.
2. Haefner H, Mayeaux EJ. Vulvar abnormalities. In: Mayeaux EJ, Cox T, eds. *Modern Colposcopy.* 3rd ed. Philadelphia, PA: Lippincott, Williams, Wilkins; 2011:432–470.
3. Lynch PJ, Moyal-Barracco M, Scurry J, Stockdale C. 2011 ISSVD terminology and classification of vulvar dermatological disorders: an approach to clinical diagnosis. *J Low Genit Tract Dis.* 2012;16(4):339–344.
4. Mayeaux EJ Jr, Cooper D. Vulvar procedures: biopsy, bartholin abscess treatment, and condyloma treatment. *Obstet Gynecol Clin N Am.* 2013; 40(4):759–772.
5. Mayeaux EJ. Punch biopsy of the skin. In: Mayeaux EJ, ed. *The Essential Guide to Primary Care Procedures.* Philadelphia, PA: Wolters Kluwer: Lippincott, Williams, Wilkins; 2009:187–194.

Bartholin Duct and Gland Surgery

Megan Lutz

15

GENERAL PRINCIPLES

Definition

The physiologic Bartholin gland is a nonpalpable structure 12 mm deep to the vaginal mucosal surface. Two bilateral glands drain into orifices located at 5 and 7 o'clock positions between the hymenal ring and labia minora. The misnomer, Bartholin cyst, is often used to describe the obstructed and dilated, but sterile and nonpainful, Bartholin gland and duct. An encapsulated Bartholin abscess may elicit vulvar pain with sitting or walking. Less frequently, a Bartholin abscess may be associated with fevers or chills. Progression is not always the necessary path to abscess formation.

Differential Diagnosis

- Bartholin adenocarcinoma or squamous cell carcinoma
- Folliculitis
- Leiomyoma
- Lipoma
- Vulvar dysplasia/cancer
- Vaginal dysplasia/cancer
- Skene's and Gartner duct cysts
- Necrotizing fasciitis
- Perirectal abscess
- Canal of Nuck cyst
- Fibroma
- Epidermal inclusion cyst

Anatomic Considerations

The Bartholin gland, also known as the greater vestibular gland, is located in the superficial compartment of the vulva, near the introitus. The gland comprised of mucinous acini, and the duct is a combination of transitional epithelium, mucinous cells, and squamous epithelium. The orifices are lined with squamous epithelium. Supplying the gland are numerous branches of the inferior pudendal artery. Deep to the gland is a thick network of anastomosing venous channels, known as the vestibular bulb. It is this erectile tissue of the vestibular bulb that contributes to the bloody nature of the Bartholin gland excision. Occasionally, during large gland excisions, other surrounding structures can be appreciated. The ischiorectal fossa is a relatively avascular area that has notorious potential for infection to manifest and spread to surrounding pelvic compartments.

Nonoperative Management

Management may entail observation, sitz baths, antibiotics, silver nitrate ablation, CO_2 laser vaporization, epithelialization with Word or Jacobi ring, marsupialization, and excision. None has proven to be superior, but ideal treatment would be fast, safe, performed with local anesthesia in outpatient setting, and with low recurrence and fast healing. Observation is sufficient for the painless Bartholin duct cyst that may even reach several centimeters in size in the otherwise-healthy individual under the age of 40. If the patient has no signs of systemic infection, advise sitz baths alone for the spontaneously draining abscess or pointed abscess that is almost ready to drain. Antibiotic therapy is the first-line treatment for an abscess that is not yet matured for drainage and is the second-line therapy for an abscess that has not clinically improved after drainage. Evaluate the need for antibiotics as adjunctive treatment at the time of drainage. Patients with the following comorbidities and/or sign and symptoms should be treated with antibiotics at the time of drainage: diabetes, immunosuppression, pregnancy, high MRSA risk, recurrent infection, or signs of cellulitis or systemic infection. A broad-spectrum antibiotic that covers Gram-negative and Gram-positive organisms over anaerobes such as amoxicillin clavulanate 875 mg PO q12h for 7 days, or trimethoprim sulfamethoxazole 800/160 PO q12h for 7 days is sufficient. For augmented MRSA and Bacteroides coverage, consider adding clindamycin 300 mg PO four times a day for 7 days. An Israeli study by Kessous et al. confirmed *Escherichia coli* as the most common organism cultured from 43.7% of Bartholin gland infections. Empiric treatment with amoxicillin clavulanate was associated with recurrence averages between 32 and 50 months. Historically, Bartholin abscesses were attributed to sexually transmitted infections, but recently, this notion has been disproven by Hoosen, Tanaka, and Kessous. STD testing may be offered at the time of Bartholin abscess presentation but antibiotic choice should not empirically encompass *Neisseria gonorrhea* or *Chlamydia trachomatis*.

Characteristics of an abscess, that require prompt operative, rather than nonoperative management, include abscess recurrence, pain and erythema, fever, and fluctuance. Of note, although incision and drainage (I&D) may offer symptomatic relief of an acutely painful abscess, I&D alone, although described in some studies, is generally not recommended because it confers no long-term benefit and increases the risk of recurrence up to 38%. Instead, drainage with the goal of epithelializing an egress tract from the gland is preferred. This may be accomplished with silver nitrate ablation, CO_2 laser, Word catheter or Jacobi ring placement, or marsupialization. The following patients and conditions require biopsy in addition to drainage: women over 40, immune-compromised patients, history of Paget's disease, history of any gynecologic malignancy, and those with recurrent abscess formation. Complete surgical excision should be performed instead of biopsy in postmenopausal women and when the Bartholin mass is firm and irregular.

Silver Nitrate Ablation

Various silver nitrate techniques have been described, all with the goal of gland destruction. A silver nitrate technique from Turkey was compared to marsupialization and found to have similar recurrence rates (26% and 24%) and time to recurrence (2 and 1.5 months); however, the side effects of the treatments differed. Chemical burn and hematoma formation occurred, compared to discharge from marsupialization.

CO_2 Laser

CO_2 laser treatment is an outpatient procedure performed under local anesthesia. The laser is used to vaporize, fenestrate, or excise Bartholin lesions with a recurrence rate of 10%. It is less optimal for lesions which are hyperechogenic, multiloculated, and with wall thickness 0.5 to 1.5 mm. Ultrasound, CO_2 laser accreditation, and pre- and postprocedure antibiotics are necessary for this technique. Specific social factors significantly associated with likelihood of recurrence were elevated stress, use of synthetic clothing, and use of condoms.

Indwelling Devices: Word Catheter or Jacobi Ring

Drainage of the obstruction coupled with placement of a Word catheter or Jacobi ring, both of which are placed in the outpatient setting under local anesthesia, have recurrence rates of 4% to 17%.

Biopsy

Any Bartholin gland enlargement in the woman over 40 is considered malignant until proven otherwise by biopsy. In any of these procedures, a biopsy of the superficial gland wall can be excised with sharp scissors and submitted to pathology; however, biopsies must be amply large to be of use.

Marsupialization

Although its role is largely replaced by outpatient Word catheter placement; marsupialization offers guaranteed epithelialization of the Bartholin gland in the setting of recurrent abscess formation and is an option with less morbidity than Bartholin gland excision. Perform marsupialization after the patient has failed one to two Word catheters or Jacobi ring placements, and when the gland is not acutely inflamed, to avoid risk of infection.

Excision

Bartholin gland excision is quintessentially one of the bloodiest of the small gynecologic procedures. Excision is rarely required for the young patient, as the sequelae often can include dyspareunia from either lack of lubrication due to removal of the mucin-producing cells, or more commonly, from obstruction of any residual duct. In women over 40, where malignancy is of greater concern, gland excision permits a definitive evaluation and is chosen when other methods have failed; however, biopsy is still preferred over excision. Adenocarcinoma of the Bartholin gland is exceedingly rare, comprising 1% of all vulvar cancers. Nearly 50% of suspected adenocarcinomas of the Bartholin gland are in fact squamous cell carcinomas. If the deeper gland surface is palpated to have a mass, consider excision due to proximity to underlying vestibular bulb. If a mass persists after a normal biopsy result, perform excision. Ulceration and persistent dyspareunia, a solid mass, or a mass in a slightly different location than the usual Bartholin duct could be other indications of Bartholin malignancy that require excision of the entire gland for definitive diagnosis.

IMAGING AND OTHER DIAGNOSTICS

- Imaging is not routinely utilized for Bartholin pathology. History and physical examination dictate management decisions.

PREOPERATIVE PLANNING

- Perform a pelvic examination under anesthesia with careful attention to the size, shape, and direction of the Bartholin gland prior to surgical management. Include a rectal examination to evaluate the proximity of the gland to the rectum in cases of excision.

SURGICAL MANAGEMENT

Epithelialization

Creating an intentional fistula, or epithelialization of a Bartholin gland abscess, is superior to simple I&D as the fistula prevents future abscess formation.

Silver Nitrate Ablation

- This outpatient technique is performed with local anesthesia.
- The gland is incised, two stay sutures are placed to retract the gland margins and a 0.5 × 0.5 cm piece of silver nitrate is placed in the cavity. The sutures are then tied to re-approximate the gland.
- At day 3, the sutures and silver nitrate are removed. Antibiotics are only prescribed in the case of abscess.

CO_2 Laser

- The laser is used to create a 10 to 15 mm circular lesion on the overlying mucosal surface, and after drainage, the gland surface, including all loculations, is vaporized with a depth of 2 mm, excised, or left fenestrated.

Word Catheter

- The Word catheter is a latex-free silicone-based indwelling device.

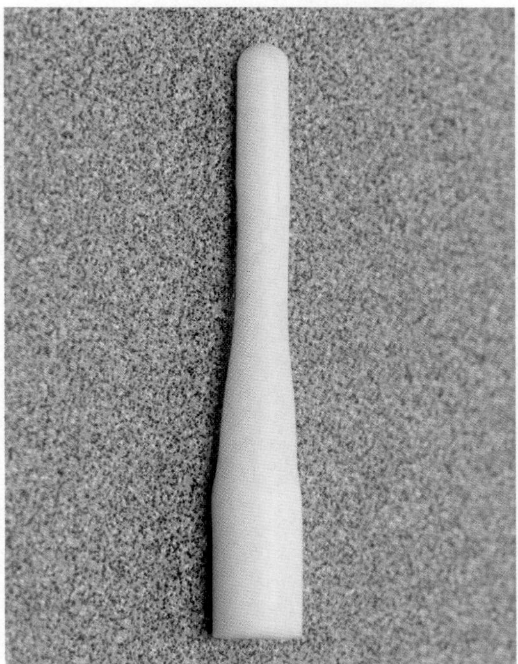
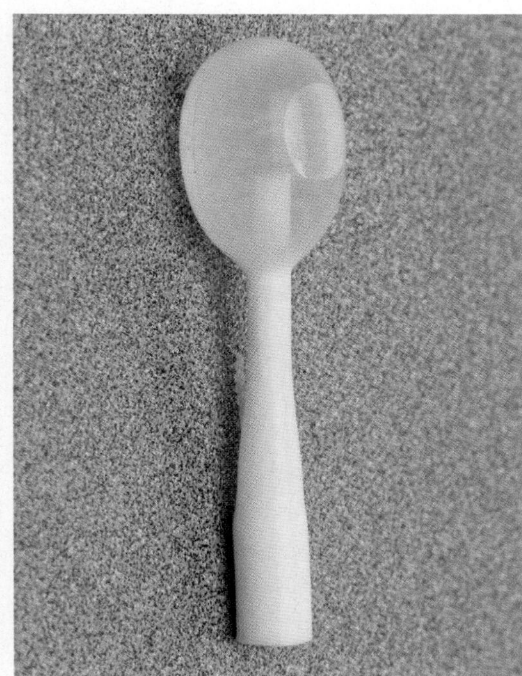

Figure 15.1. A and B: Inflate the Word catheter with 3 mL of sterile liquid.

- Cleanse the mucosa overlying the Bartholin gland and vaginal mucosa with antiseptic solution and then retract open.
- Inject the mucosa near the hymenal ring that is overlying the Bartholin gland with 1 to 2 cc of 1% lidocaine without epinephrine. Depending on the size of the gland, exposure to the mucosa may best be accomplished by applying pressure to reflect the gland out of the vagina.
- Make a 2 to 3 mm incision with the 11 blade scalpel over the most gravity-dependent mucosa ideally inside, but if necessary on or just outside the hymenal ring.
- Probing inside the gland is not recommended, as this can overly stretch the length of this incision, and then the Word catheter will fall out.
- Allow the contents of the abscess to drain, then insert the deflated catheter. Inflate the balloon with up to a maximum of 3 mL of sterile liquid, not air. Use caution so as not to puncture this tiny balloon with either the syringe upon inflation or by over-distention.
- Remove the syringe and tuck the catheter inside the vagina. The Word catheter should remain in place for 3 to 4 weeks, to ensure the tract becomes epithelialized and ideally prevent future obstruction (Fig. 15.1).
- If the gland size is too small to accommodate the Word catheter, other indwelling drainage options are available. If office supplies are at hand, the gland can be marsupialized. Otherwise, I&D will have to suffice until further management can be planned.

Jacobi Ring

The Jacobi ring is an alternative to the Word catheter. It is a tubular structure with a threaded suture that is passed into and out of the gland through two separate incisions and then tied into a 360-degree ring. The ring establishes an egress and promotes prolonged fenestration.

- Construct the ring catheter from 7 cm of an 8-French rubber T tube threaded with a 20 cm length of 2-0 silk suture.
- Cleanse the area and inject local anesthetic, then make a 3-mm incision with the 11 blade scalpel on the mucosal surface.
- Pass a hemostat through the abscess to tunnel and make the indentation for the second incision.
- Pull one end of the Jacobi ring through the abscess incisions. Tie the two ends together. Use caution not to tie too tightly, as ischemia can occur (Fig. 15.2).

Positioning

- The patient is placed in the dorsal–lithotomy position with careful attention not to hyperflex or hyperextend the legs and hips. The patient is then prepped and draped in the usual fashion for a vaginal procedure.

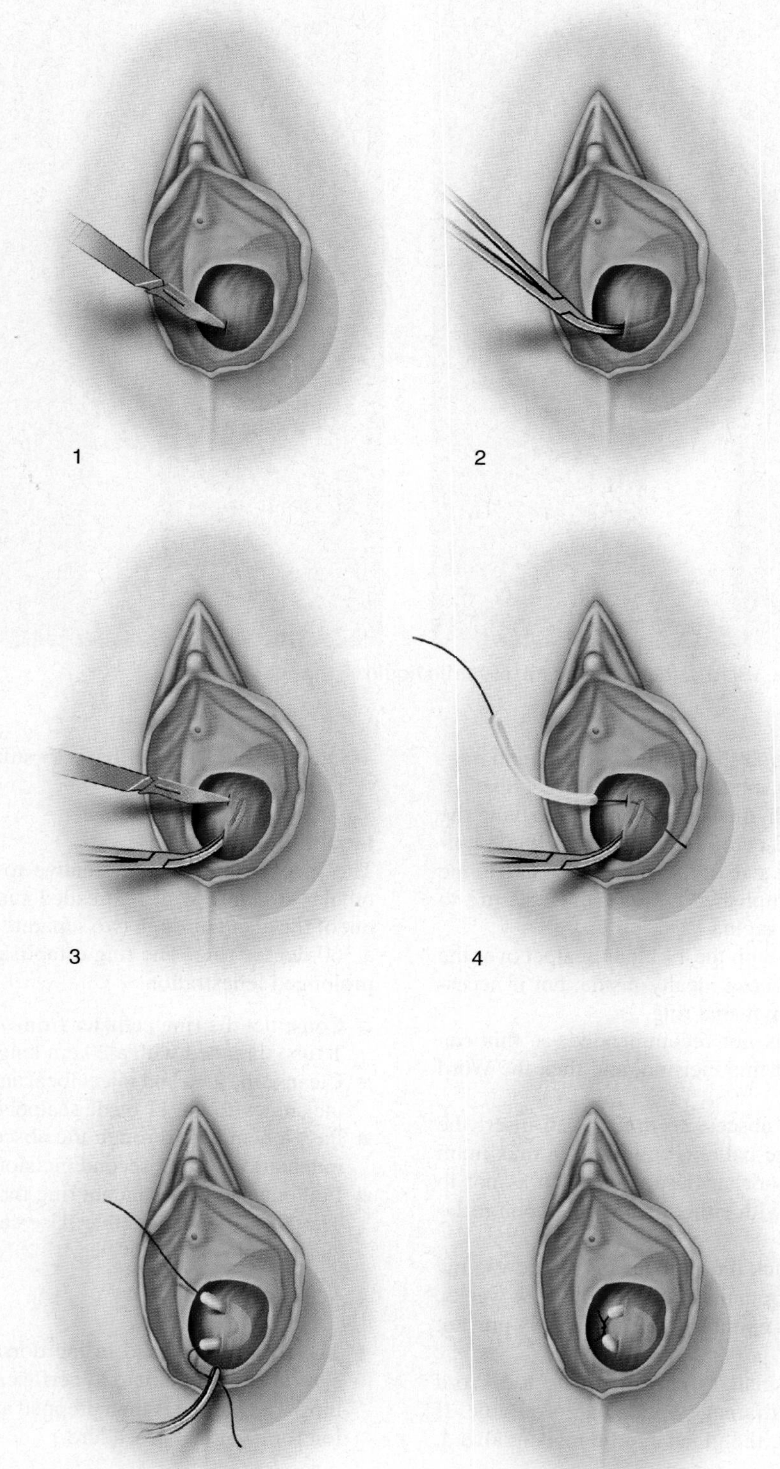

Figure 15.2. Steps for Jacobi ring insertion for epithelialization of the Bartholin gland.

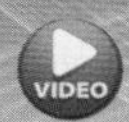

Procedures and Techniques (Video 15.1)

Biopsy

- Biopsy is performed by excision of cyst wall at the time of drainage when a small sample of gland wall can be excised with the scalpel. During marsupialization, send the elliptical portion of gland wall to pathology.

Marsupialization

- Marsupialization is performed under local or general anesthesia. Perform a digital vaginal examination to delineate the borders of the gland.
- With a 15 blade scalpel, make a generous vertical incision the length of the cyst along the hymenal ring.
- To incise and drain the gland, make an elliptical incision through the wall of the gland.
- Evert gland edges and mucosal edges with atraumatic grasping forceps, then suture the wall of the gland to squamous epithelium of the introitus laterally and to vaginal mucosa medially with interrupted horizontal mattress stitches with 3-0 polysorb. Place sutures at least 5 mm from everted glandular wall to epithelial tissue to increase success of marsupialization procedure (Tech Fig. 15.1).
- Potential consequences are infection and recurrence of cyst if the opening scars shut.

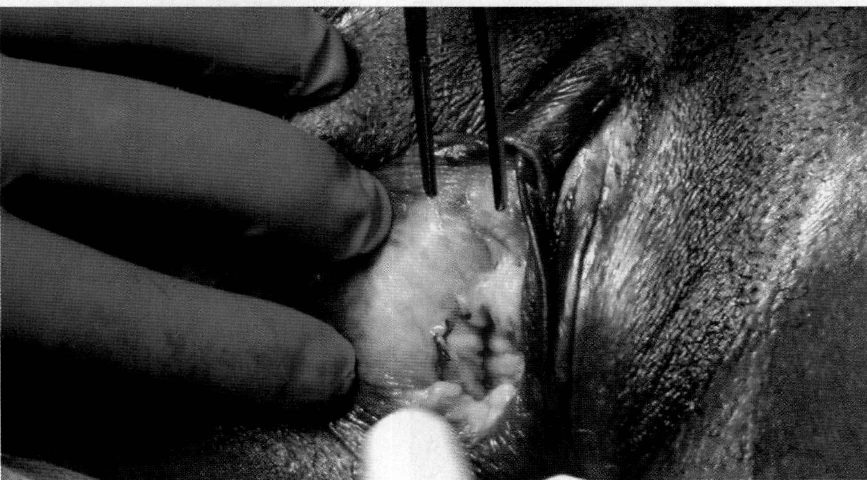

Tech Figure 15.1. The hymenal ring is the preferred location for epithelialization, marsupialization, and the initial incision of gland excision due to optimal tissue healing and cosmesis. Photo courtesy of M. Walters, MD.

Bartholin gland excision

- Begin the procedure with a digital rectovaginal examination to appreciate the borders of the gland and proximity to the vaginal wall and rectum. The deep base of the gland is supplied by branches of the inferior pudendal artery, a branch of the internal iliac artery. The vestibular bulb drains the gland and is a network of venous channels.
- Empty the bladder with straight catheterization.
- Retract the labia laterally with Allis clamps.
- Inject 1% lidocaine with epinephrine into the mucosa along the hymenal ring, but notably, not into the gland.
- Over the vaginal mucosal side of the gland, just on or inside the hymenal ring, use a 15 blade scalpel to create a superficial long vaginal mucosa incision, with careful attention to avoid simultaneously incising the gland (Tech Fig. 15.2). The mucosa is the preferred site because it heals faster and is less painful than the epidermal vulvar skin. Retract the mucosa and expose the gland. Infection may fuse the borders between the gland and mucosa.

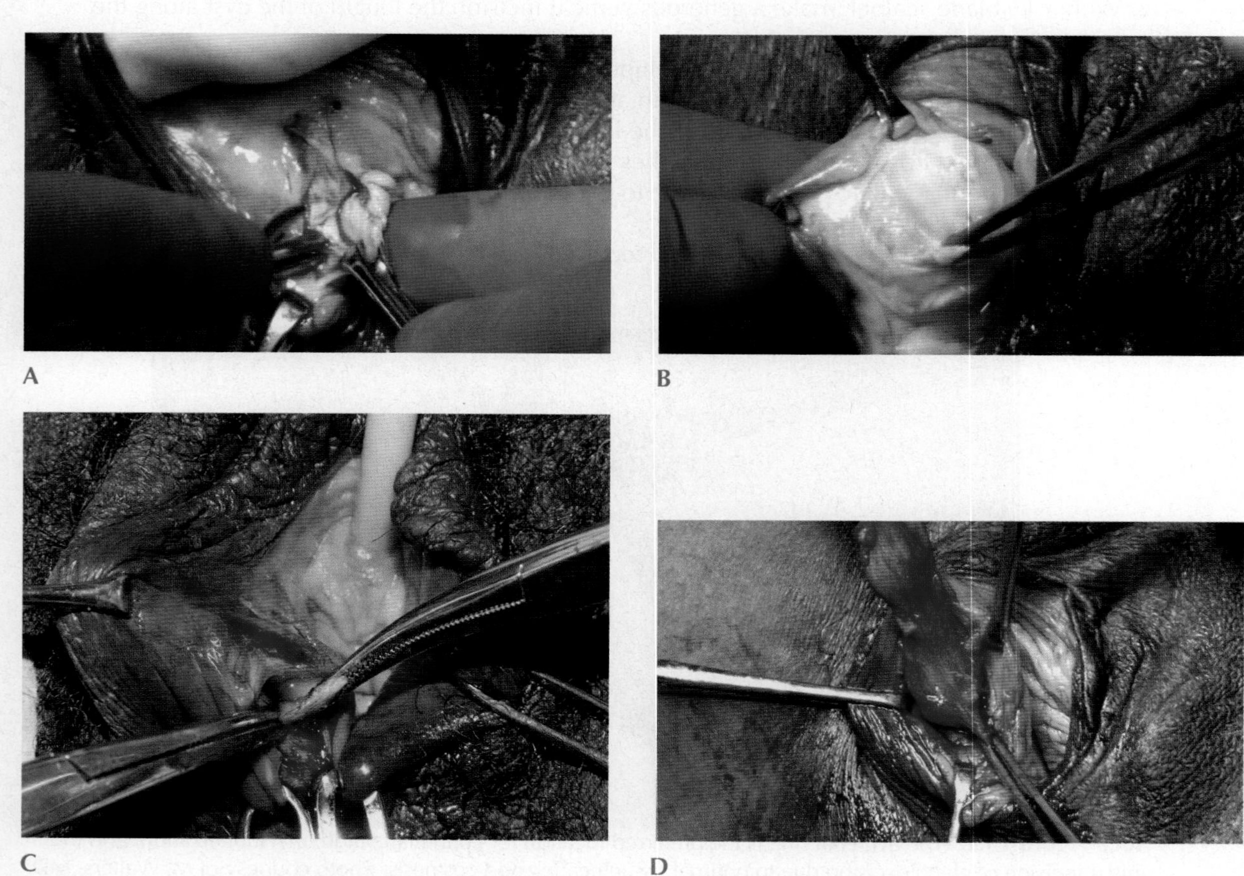

Tech Figure 15.2. A–D: Bartholin gland excision. The initial incision should extend the entire length of the gland. Whereas the gland is well delineated in (B), the other surgical circumstances may be complicated by gland fusion with surrounding tissue (C), in which case, methylene blue can be helpful in defining gland borders. Isolate, clamp, and tie all pedicles at the base of the gland, as branches of the inferior pudendal artery are sure to exist here (D). Photo courtesy of M. Paraiso, MD and M. Walters, MD.

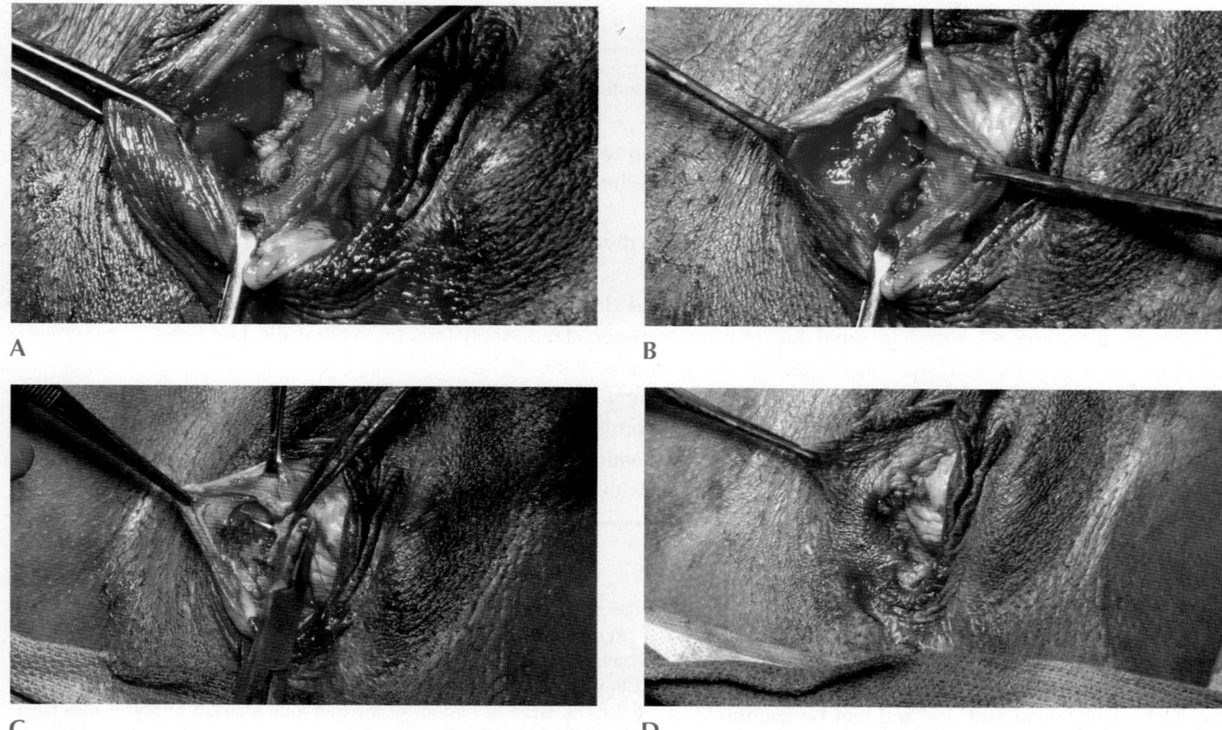

Tech Figure 15.3. A–D: Closure after gland excision occurs in multiple layers. Re-approximating the dead space is an initial measure to prevent bleeding from the venous network comprising the vestibular bulb. Photo courtesy of M. Walters, MD.

- Delineate the plane between mucosa and gland with traction and countertraction and Metzenbaum scissors. Dilute methylene blue can be injected for purposes of demarcating the gland during excision (Tech Fig. 15.2). Grasp and retract the gland wall with the Allis clamp to facilitate dissection and visualization of blood supply.
- Bleeding must be anticipated and hemostasis must be achieved with each step. Clamp any vascular pedicles with a fine-tipped clamp, cut, and suture ligate with 3-0 absorbable suture (Tech Fig. 15.2).
- Entire removal of the gland is crucial, as residual glandular tissue may cause recurrence of cyst or abscess and may be responsible for chronic pain. Evaluate for multiloculated remaining abscess. If the margins of the gland are fused to surrounding tissue because of infection, open the gland, place a finger in the gland, and proceed with dissection from this angle. A lacrimal duct probe can be inserted into the gland to mark the gland.
- Once the entire gland is removed, hemostasis must be achieved, namely with suture ligation, but also with electrosurgery, hemostatic agents, and, ultimately, obliteration of the dead space with a multilayered closure. Electrocautery alone is insufficient. Once a bleeding vessel retracts and bleeding continues, dissect further and tie the vessel. The entire cavity must be closed with interrupted 3-0 absorbable suture, in multiple layers (**Tech Fig. 15.3**). Use caution to avoid placing a stitch through the labia. Interrupted stitches are preferred over running stitches as running stitches may cause abnormal scarring and pain.
- If necessary, in the circumstance of infected gland with purulent drainage, a drain may be stitched into the wound closure with 5-0 interrupted absorbable suture to ensure drainage.
- Close the vaginal mucosa with interrupted 3-0 delayed absorbable suture around the drain. Perform a rectal examination at the conclusion of the case to ensure the rectum and vaginal wall are free of suture. Remove the drain on postoperative day 3 or 4.

PEARLS AND PITFALLS

✗ The Word catheter is likely to fall out if the balloon is perforated by overfilling, if the incision is made too wide, or if the depth of the deflated gland is too shallow.

○ Cook medical manufacturing instructions indicate the maximum volume of the bulb is 3 mL.

○ The preferred location of Bartholin surgeries is on or inside the hymenal ring for the purposes of tissue healing, cosmesis, and pain.

✗ Surgeries performed outside the hymenal ring can result in distorted anatomy, which can contribute to chronic pain.

○ Keeping the abscess intact during excision allows for easy delineation of borders and gland removal.

○ If the abscess is entered, keep a lacrimal duct probe in the open gland. Apply traction to the walls. Use fine clamps and fine scissors to delineate borders for the remainder of the excision.

○ Achieve hemostasis with each step of excision with the clamp, cut, and tie suture ligation technique.

✗ Unidentified sources of bleeding can result in hematoma formation and postoperative complications.

○ Evaluate carefully for multi-loculated abscess and remove entire abscess upon excision.

✗ Residual gland after excision will have incomplete results with abscess reformation and chronic pain.

POSTOPERATIVE CARE

- Postoperative perineal lavage bottles are recommended and wound packing is not necessary. Drainage is to be expected. The area should be kept clean and dry and can be accomplished with the cool setting of the hair dryer. Pelvic rest is recommended for 4 weeks.

COMPLICATIONS

- Vulvar hematoma from the vestibular bulb at the base of the gland can spread to even the mons pubis. Postoperative hematoma is most commonly managed with bed rest, ice packs, and pressure dressings.
- Chronic pain from gland excision may result from obstructed residual gland or from suture placement. Reoperation may be required at a later point if the introitus is considerably narrowed, wherein vestibulectomy or scar revision may be necessary.

KEY READINGS

Baggish MS, Karram MM. *Atlas of Pelvic Anatomy and Gynecologic Surgery.* St. Louis, MO: Elsevier/Saunders; 2011.

Benedetti Panici P, Manci N, Bellati F, et al. CO_2 laser therapy of the Bartholin's gland cyst: surgical data and functional short- and long-term results. *J Minim Invasive Gynecol.* 2007;14:348–351.

Cobellis PL, Stradella L, De Lucia E, et al. Alcohol sclerotherapy: a new method for Bartholin gland cyst treatment. *Minerva Gynecol.* 2006;58:245–248.

Di Donato V, Bellati F, Casorelli A, et al. CO_2 laser treatment for Bartholin gland abscess: ultrasound evaluation of risk recurrence. *J Min Invas Gynecol.* 2013;20(3):346–352.

Ergeneli MH. Silver nitrate for Bartholin gland cysts. *Eur J Obstet Gynecol Reprod Biol.* 1999;82:231–232.

Gennis P, Li SF, Provataris J, et al. Jacobi ring catheter treatment of Bartholin's abscesses. *Am J Emerg Med.* 2005;23(3):414–415.

Heller DS, Bean S. Lesions of the Bartholin gland: a review. *J Low Genit Tract Dis.* 2014;18(4):351–357.

Kessous R, Aricha-Tamir B, Sheizaf B, Steiner N, Moran-Gilad J, Weintraub AY. Clinical and microbiological characteristics of Bartholin gland abscesses. *Obstet Gynecol.* 2013;122(4):794–799.

Kushnir VA, Mosquera C. Novel technique for management of Bartholin gland cysts and abscesses. *J Emerg Med.* 2009;36(4):388–390.

Mayeux EJ Jr, Cooper D. Vulvar Procedures biopsy, bartholin abscess treatment, and condyloma treatment. *Obstet Gynecol Clin North Am.* 2013;40:759–772.

Omole F, Simmons BJ, Hacker Y. Management of Bartholin's duct cyst and gland abscess. *Am Fam Physician.* 2003;68:135–140.

Ozdegirmenci O, Kayikcioglu F, Haberal A. Prospective randomized study of marsupialization versus silver nitrate application in the management of Bartholin cysts and abscesses. *J Min Invas Gynecol.* 2009;16(2):149–152.

Penna C, Fambrini M, Fallani MG. CO(2) laser treatement for Bartholin's gland cyst. *Int J Gynaecol Obstet.* 2002;76:79–80.

Stevens DL, Bisno AL, Chambers HF, et al., Infectious Diseases Society of America. Practice guidelines for the diagnosis and management of skin and soft-tissue infections. *Clin Infect Dis.* 2005;41:1373–1406.

Tanaka K, Mikamo H, Ninomiya M, et al. Microbiology of Bartholin's gland abscess in Japan. *J Clin Microbiol.* 2005;43:4258–4261.

Wechter ME, Wu JM, Marzano D, Haefner H. Management of Bartholin duct cysts and abscesses: a systematic review. *Obstet Gynecol Surv.* 2009;64(6):395–404.

Yuce K, Zeyenloglu HB, Bükülmez O, Kisnisci HA. Outpatient management of Bartholin gland abscesses and cysts with silver nitrate. *Aust N Z J Obstet Gynaecol.* 1994;34(1):93–96.

Word Catheter Silicone Bartholin Gland Balloon. Medical Devices for Minimally Invasive Procedures. Cook Medical, 2012. Web. Nov. 8, 2016.

Vestibulectomy and Hymenectomy Surgery

Natalia C. Llarena, Mark D. Walters, M. Jean Uy-Kroh

16

GENERAL PRINCIPLES: VESTIBULECTOMY FOR VULVODYNIA

Definition

- Vulvodynia refers to "vulvar pain of at least 3 months duration without clear identifiable cause, which may have potential associated factors."[1] *Vulvodynia* is further characterized by distribution as *generalized, localized* (i.e., vestibulodynia or clitorodynia), or *mixed,* and by stimulus as *provoked, spontaneous,* or *mixed. Vestibulodynia* is a subset of localized vulvodynia, and refers to discomfort in the vestibule region. Patients often describe the pain as "burning or cutting" in nature. Provoked pain may be elicited by sexual contact, clothing pressure, fingertip pressure, or tampon use. The onset of vulvodynia is either *primary* or *secondary* and the temporal pattern is specified as *intermittent, persistent, constant, immediate,* or *delayed* (**Table 16.1**).
- The misnomer vestibulitis is no longer used since inflammatory changes are not associated with the condition.
- The etiology of vulvodynia remains unclear, but it is likely multifactorial and may include central and peripheral neurologic mechanisms, neuroproliferation, and musculoskeletal and hormonal disorders.[2] In addition, patients with vulvodynia have an increased rate of comorbid chronic pain disorders, including fibromyalgia, irritable bowel syndrome, temporomandibular joint disorder, and interstitial cystitis.[3,4]

Table 16.1 Characteristics of Vulvodynia

Distribution	Localized (vestibulodynia, clitorodynia, hemivulvodynia) Generalized (whole vulva) Mixed
Stimulus	Provoked (physical contact—sexual contact, tampon insertion) Spontaneous (no specific trigger) Mixed
Onset	Primary Secondary
Temporal Pattern	Intermittent Persistent Constant Immediate Delayed

Adapted from Bornstein J, Goldstein A, Coady D. *Consensus Terminology and Classification of Persistent Vulvar Pain.* International Society for the Study of Vulvovaginal Disease; 2015;1–4.

Differential Diagnosis

- Vulvar infection (e.g., candidiasis, herpes)
- Inflammatory vulvar disorders (e.g., desquamative inflammatory vaginitis (DIV), lichen planus, lichen sclerosis, immunobullous disorders, severe atrophy)
- Neoplastic vulvar disorders (e.g., Paget's disease, squamous cell carcinoma)
- Neurologic disorders (e.g., herpes neuralgia, spinal nerve compression)

Nonoperative Management

- Vestibulectomy is the most effective available treatment for localized, provoked vestibulodynia, but is reserved for patients who have failed less invasive modes of management. We do not offer surgical treatment for generalized, unprovoked vulvodynia. A number of nonoperative treatments exist, but few data are available from randomized controlled trials comparing the effectiveness of these strategies.[2,5] Medical approaches to vulvodynia and vestibulodynia include localized, topical application of lidocaine (5% ointment at bedtime for 7 weeks) and use of estrogen cream.[5] In addition, off-label topical compounded gabapentin ointment may be used. Although topical corticosteroids are not useful, injections of bupivacaine (0.25%) provide relief for some patients.[4] Oral therapies including amitriptyline and gabapentin are commonly used. Additionally, biofeedback and pelvic floor physical therapy often benefit these patients.[2]

IMAGING AND OTHER DIAGNOSTICS: VESTIBULECTOMY FOR VULVODYNIA

- *Vulvodynia* often occurs in the absence of visible findings; therefore, it is critical to perform a detailed history and physical examination to exclude other etiologies of vulvar pain.
  - A detailed history often reveals the most significant clues that guide successful treatment. Questionnaires help collate a comprehensive history that includes the location, onset, duration, quality, temporality, and severity of the pain, aggravating and relieving factors, and prior therapies (see Table 16.1).
  - Inquire about the functional impact her pain has had on her sexuality, quality of life, and her relationships as well as her treatment goals.
  - Symptoms that suggest an alternative diagnosis include abnormal vaginal bleeding or discharge, vulvar itch, pain with bowel movements, or neurologic symptoms suggestive of pudendal neuralgia.[6]

    - A history of atopic or inflammatory skin conditions may suggest a dermatologic cause of vulvar symptoms. Any history of vulvovaginal trauma (including birth trauma) or recurrent vulvar candidiasis should also be elicited.
    - Sexual history, including dyspareunia and history of abuse or trauma.
    - Vulvar hygiene regimen, including use of soaps and feminine products that may contribute to discomfort, and type of undergarment fabric worn.
- Physical examination.
- Even a visual inspection of the perineum can evoke trepidation and fear for patients who suffer from vestibulodynia; therefore, patience and patient partnership are essential to performing a successful examination. Patients can aid in the examination by holding magnifiers, mirrors, retracting their own anatomy, and identifying the exact location of the most tender sites. This method also alleviates patient anxiety and provides her a measure of control during the examination.
    - Perform a magnified, visual inspection, without any tactile stimulus, from the mons to the anus to evaluate for infectious, inflammatory, or neoplastic etiologies of vulvar discomfort. Note any skin erosions, plaques, erythema, fissures, nodules, ulcers, and architectural changes such as loss of labia minora, burying of the glans clitoris, and agglutination.[6] Of note, bilateral erythema surrounding the Bartholin ducts and minor vestibular ducts is typically a normal finding and may not be relevant to the diagnosis of vulvodynia.[7]
    - Colposcopic investigation of the vulva with biopsies should be considered when symptoms are refractory to therapy, the diagnosis is unclear, or there is a suspicion for malignancy. Furthermore, the traditional, routine use of dilute acetic acid should be reconsidered as it rarely improves tissue examination and more often causes pain exacerbation and significant patient discomfort.
    - Although a patient may have concomitant disease such as genital warts or cysts in addition to vulvodynia, the findings must not account for vulvar pain.
    - Cotton swab testing is used to identify and diagram painful areas. Introduce the soft q-tip swab to the patient's nongenital skin such as the inner thigh. Confirm that this q-tip palpation is perceived as soft and nonpainful. Explain to the patient the series of palpations that will ensue and indicate her answer choices for each palpation. Then, use the moistened q-tip to first palpate lateral to Hart's line and then medial to Hart's line. Palpate the vestibule at 1 and 11 o'clock positions near the Skene's ostia and then at 4 and 8 o'clock positions at the Bartholin's ostia. Finally, palpate the vestibule at 6 o'clock. Locations of the pain should be diagrammed and documented in the patient's medical record to assist with monitoring the pain over time.[2]
    - Gently palpate the levator muscles with one finger in the vagina to examine for muscle tightness, tension, or tenderness.
- Vulvodynia cannot be diagnosed by laboratory or imaging studies. However, a saline wet prep, vaginal pH testing, and cultures for aerobic bacteria, yeast, and herpes can help rule out atrophic, inflammatory, or infectious vaginitis.

PREOPERATIVE PLANNING: VESTIBULECTOMY FOR VULVODYNIA

- *Vaginismus* is a spasm of the levator ani that contributes to dyspareunia and difficulty with vaginal penetration. Vaginismus frequently occurs in association with vulvodynia; however, data suggest that surgery is less effective in this patient population.[2,8] Pelvic floor physical therapy, dilators, and trigger point injections may benefit these patients.
- Sexual counseling may be considered preoperatively, as it may reduce vaginismus, and has been shown to improve outcomes after vestibulectomy.[8]
- Prior to anesthetizing the patient in the operating room, painful areas of the vestibular mucosa should be identified with a cotton swab and marked to target excision.

SURGICAL MANAGEMENT: VESTIBULECTOMY FOR VULVODYNIA

- Vestibulectomy (Fig. 16.1) is typically performed for localized, provoked vulvodynia that has failed medical management. In general, it is more effective for secondary than primary localized vulvodynia. However, there are no evidence-based guidelines regarding a treatment algorithm, in large part because the etiology of vulvodynia is unknown and both medical and surgical treatments are understudied.[5] Among the studied interventions, surgical management has the most robust evidence and has been shown to be significantly more effective than medical management. Future randomized studies comparing operative techniques and outcomes may further our understanding of how best to surgically manage these patients and their pain.
- Patient selection is critical for ensuring the success of vestibulectomy. Careful consideration must be given to operating on patients with mixed vulvodynia or concurrent vaginismus, in whom the procedure has lower success rates.[2,8]

Approach

- Several approaches to surgery for vestibulodynia have been described, including local excision, total vestibulectomy, partial vestibulectomy with vaginal flap, and perineoplasty.[2,5,8] Local excision involves identification and removal of painful vestibular tissue, including tissue at the base of the hymen, without vaginal advancement. A total or partial vestibulectomy identifies and excises painful vestibular mucosa, then mobilizes the distal vagina to cover the excised area. In a total vestibulectomy, the incision typically extends from the periurethral region to the fourchette, although in some cases a limited incision from the fourchette partially up the labia minora may be sufficient. Finally, the perineoplasty includes a vestibulectomy with extension of the tissue excision to the perineum. Vestibuloplasty, in which the vestibule is denervated but painful tissue is not excised, is not an effective procedure. Partial vestibulectomy with vaginal flap is the procedure best described in the literature and most commonly performed. It will be the focus of the technical discussion that follows.

Positioning

- The patient should be placed in the dorsal lithotomy position using adjustable stirrups to allow access to the vestibule and perineum. Care should be taken to avoid hyperextension or hyperflexion of the lower extremities.

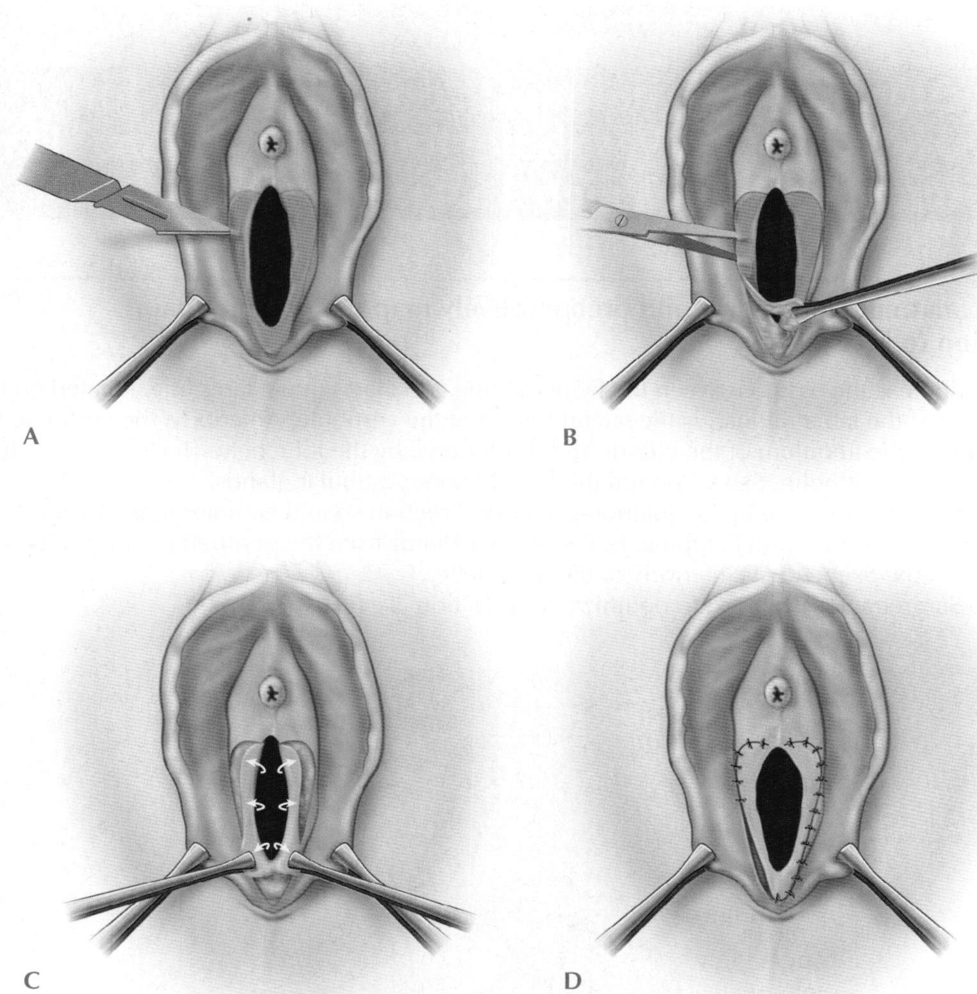

Figure 16.1. Total Vestibulectomy in four steps. **A:** Incise the vestibule and create a vaginal flap. **B:** Excise vestibular tissue. **C:** Advance the vaginal flap. **D:** Place interrupted sutures to secure the vaginal flap.

Procedures and Techniques: Vestibulectomy for Vulvodynia/Partial Vestibulectomy with Vaginal Flap (see Tech Fig. 16.2, Video 16.1)

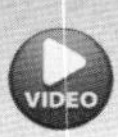

Identify anatomic landmarks and preoperatively map the patient's pain and region to be excised

- The vestibule is the tissue between the hymenal ring and Hart's line. Hart's line, located on the inner fold of the labia minora, is the lateral border of the vestibule. Anteriorly, the vestibule is bordered by the frenulum of the clitoris and, posteriorly, by the fourchette (Tech Fig. 16.1). It comprises the Bartholin, Skene, periurethral, and minor vestibular glands.
- The extent of the incision in the anterior–posterior direction should be determined by the patient's preoperative pain mapping, but typically extends from the periurethral area at the opening of the Skene ducts inferiorly to the fourchette.
- A Lone Star retractor is placed to optimize visualization (Tech Fig. 16.2).

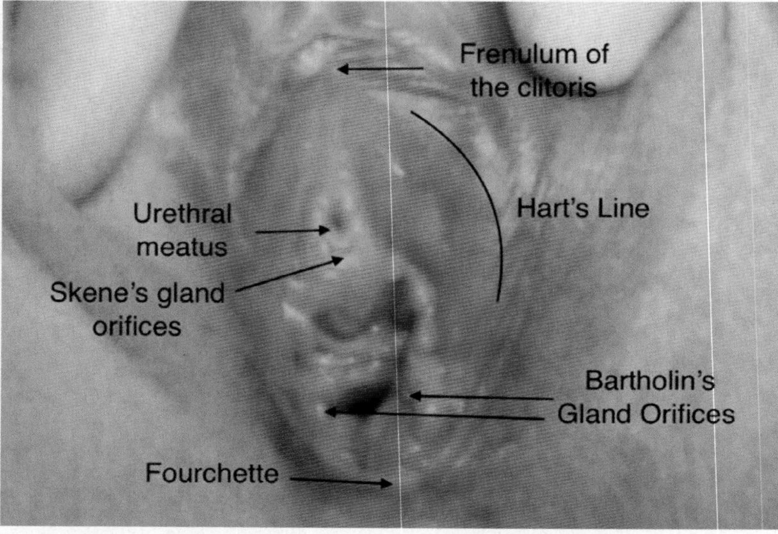

Tech Figure 16.1. Vestibular anatomy.

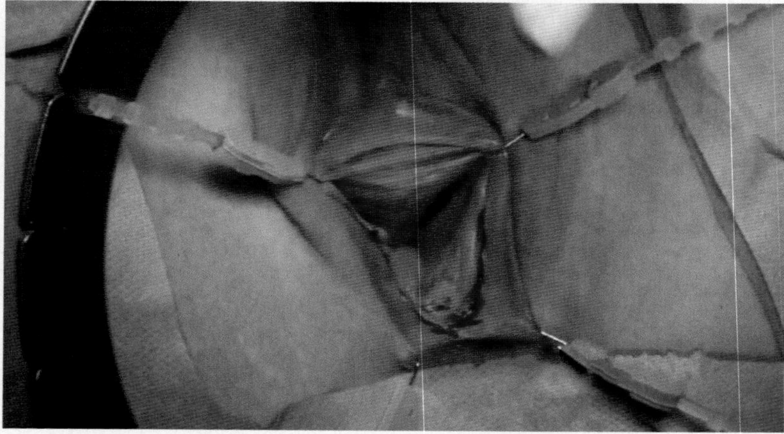

Tech Figure 16.2. The Lone Star retractor assists with visualization.

Incise the vestibule

- Prior to making the initial incision, a solution of lidocaine 0.5% with 1:200,000 of epinephrine is injected into the vestibule subcutaneously and subdermally to assist with hydrodissection and hemostasis (Tech Fig. 16.2).
- A U-shaped vestibular incision is made (Tech Fig. 16.3) over the marked tissue with a no. 10 scalpel. The lateral border of the incision is made along Hart's line, the lateral border of the vestibule, and the medial border of the incision is made proximal to the hymeneal ring. Care must be taken when incising the periurethral area to avoid damaging the urethra.
- The Bartholin glands should be palpated for any nodular or cystic component. If cysts or nodules are present, the gland should be removed.

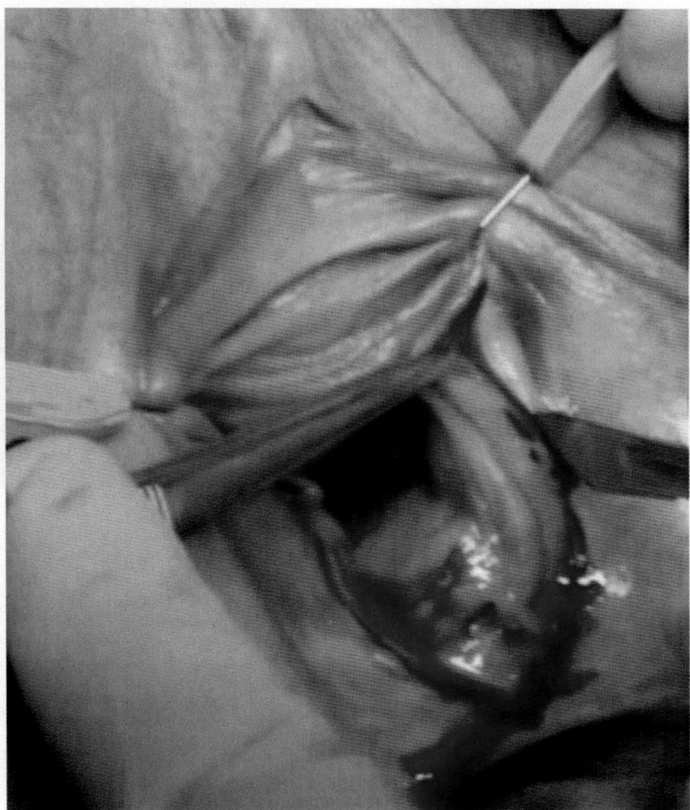

Tech Figure 16.3. Vestibular incision.

Create the vaginal flap

- Dissect the posterior vaginal wall epithelium from the underlying tissue to create a vaginal flap. This may be accomplished using Allis clamps and Mayo scissors taking special care to avoid damaging the rectum.

Excise the vestibule

- Excise the U-shaped region of the vestibule including the skin, hymen, and the minor vestibular glands (Tech Fig. 16.4).

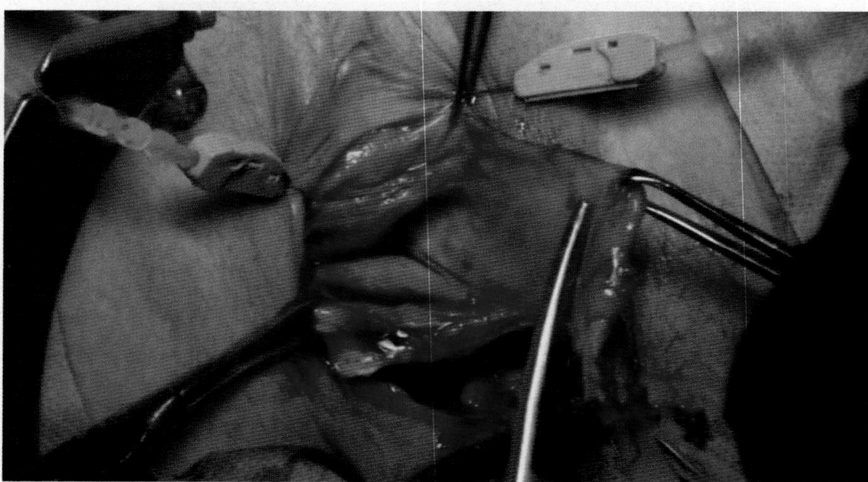

Tech Figure 16.4. Vestibular excision.

Mobilize the vaginal flap

Mobilize the flap distally to cover the defect; it must be advanced adequately to avoid placing excessive tension on the incision line (Tech Fig. 16.5A,B).

- Excellent hemostasis must be achieved to prevent hematoma and wound dehiscence.

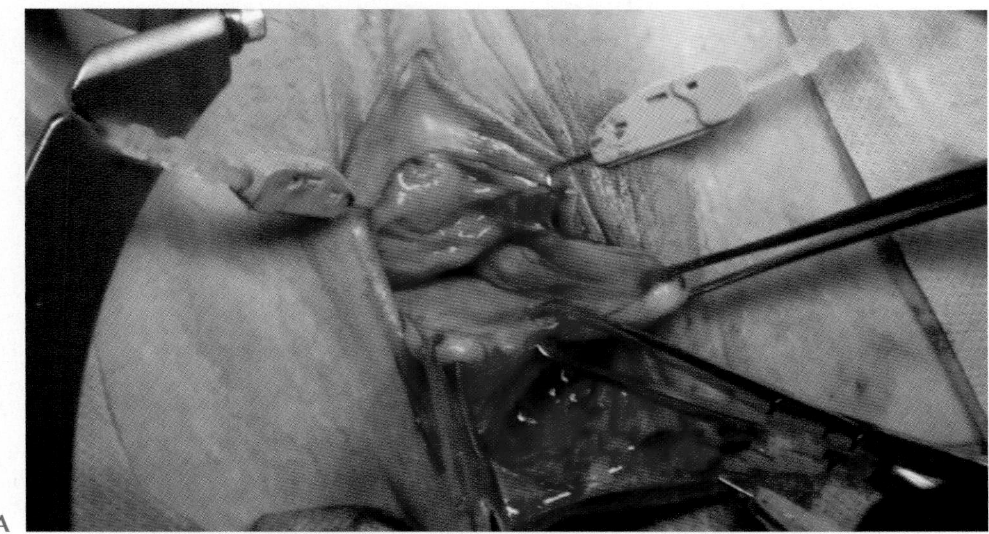

A

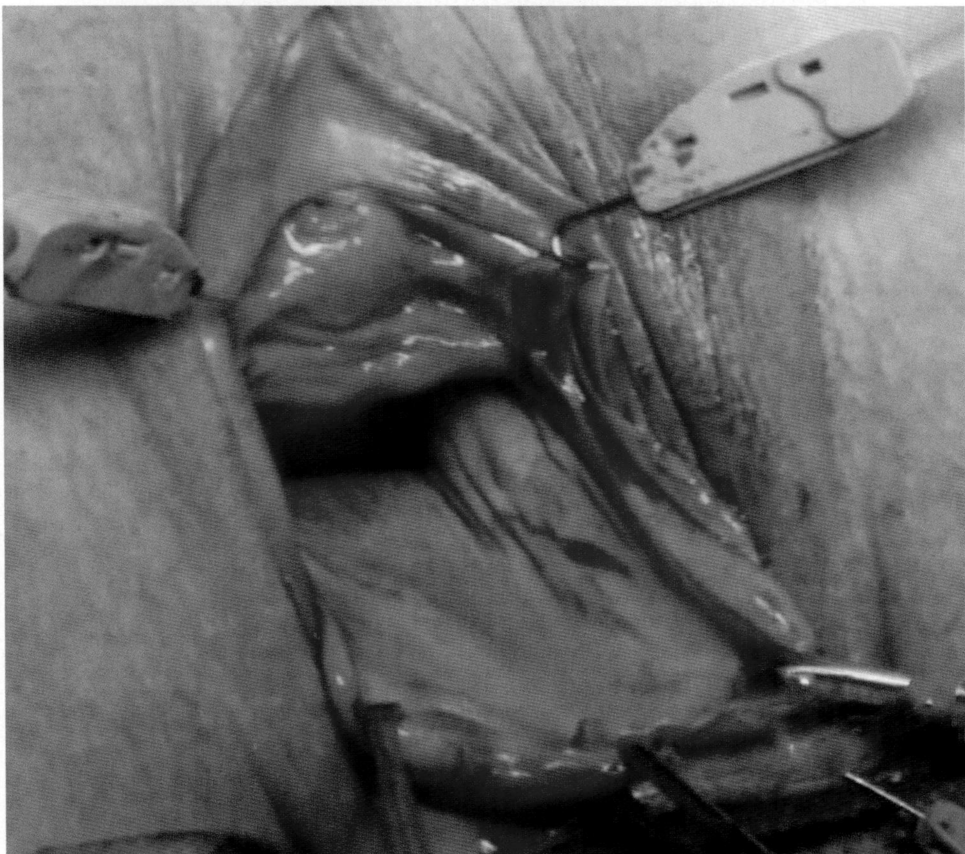

B

Tech Figure 16.5. **A** and **B:** Advancement of the vaginal flap.

Wound closure

- The closure is accomplished in two layers (Tech Fig. 16.6). First, place a deep layer of interrupted 3-0 absorbable sutures (Vicryl or Polysorb) in a U-shaped fashion to facilitate approximation of the vaginal wall to the edge of the vestibular defect. Second, re-approximate the vaginal epithelium to the perineal skin using interrupted 4-0 absorbable sutures.

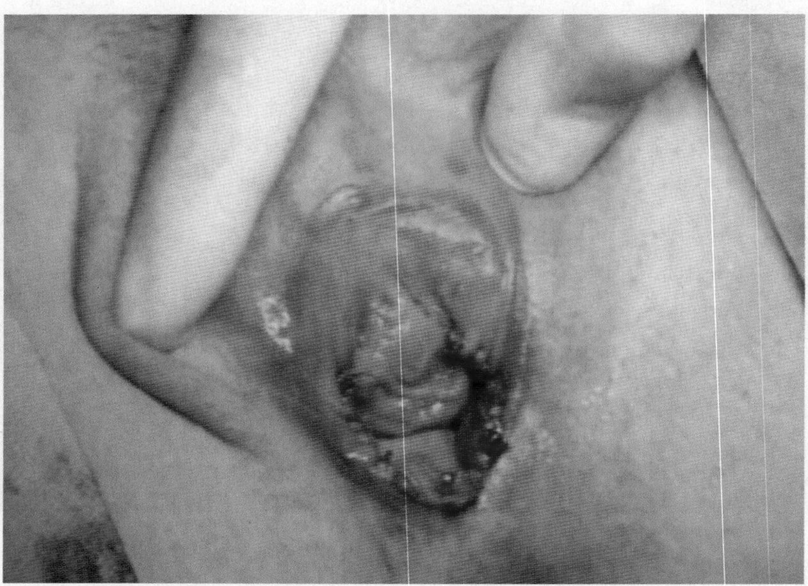

Tech Figure 16.6. Wound closure.

PEARLS AND PITFALLS: VESTIBULECTOMY FOR VULVODYNIA

○ Outlining the area of excision may be done either in the operating room or in the clinic. Prior to anesthetizing the patient in the operating room, map out and mark painful regions of vestibular mucosa to appropriately target areas for tissue excision. The anterior–posterior extent of the incision should be based on pain mapping. Alternatively, if done in the clinic, be sure to descriptively document the excision margins.

✖ If the incision is extended to the opening of the Skene ducts, take care to avoid urethral injury. Similarly, the incision should never be extended too far toward the anus since chronic fissuring and anal sphincter weakness may result.

○ Prior to incising the vestibule, lidocaine with epinephrine may be injected subcutaneously and subdermally to assist with hydrodissection and hemostasis.

✖ Take care to ensure that the vaginal flap is not under excessive tension when it is approximated to the edge of the excised vestibule. If it is under excessive tension, it may result in postoperative vestibular contraction and dyspareunia.

○ Ensure that excellent hemostasis is achieved prior to wound closure. This may be done using coagulation or suture. Inadequate hemostasis may result in hematoma or wound dehiscence.

POSTOPERATIVE CARE: VESTIBULECTOMY FOR VULVODYNIA

- Vestibulectomy is performed as an outpatient procedure.
- Patients should receive immediate postoperative analgesia with nonsteroidal anti-inflammatory medications and narcotics, if necessary. Local injection of bupivacaine and epinephrine intraoperatively into the labia and peri-incisional regions can help minimize pain as well as intraoperative bleeding. Sitz baths and ice packs also assist with pain control.
- Patients should receive a stool softener and be advised to eat high-fiber foods to avoid constipation.
- Use of a vaginal dilator may help reduce vestibular contraction and pain. This can be instituted a few weeks after surgery in the office when the pain has subsided and after an examination and instructions.
- Patients should be advised to abstain from intercourse for 6 to 8 weeks, or until a postoperative visit when the incision is evaluated for appropriate healing.

OUTCOMES: VESTIBULECTOMY FOR VULVODYNIA

- Prospective studies evaluating the resolution of vulvar pain after vestibulectomy report success rates ranging from 61% to 83%.[5] These studies vary in terms of how they define success, some reporting a positive outcome only after complete resolution of symptoms, and others equating success with a "significant improvement" in symptoms.[8]
- One prospective study comparing vestibulectomy to no treatment and to nonsurgical treatments found that 79% of patients who had surgery experienced a significant improvement in pain, whereas only 48% of patients who received nonoperative treatment and 12% of patients who received no treatment, experienced an equivalent improvement in pain.[9] Similarly, a randomized controlled trial comparing vestibulectomy to cognitive behavioral therapy (CBT) and to biofeedback found a 68% rate of complete relief or great improvement of pain with vestibulectomy versus a 39% improvement for the CBT group and a 36% improvement for the biofeedback group.[10]
- Some data suggest that up to 15% of women experience a minor postsurgical complication, such as pruritis, hematoma, local infection, or Bartholin duct stenosis, and as many as 17% of patients require a follow-up surgery.[11]

COMPLICATIONS: VESTIBULECTOMY FOR VULVODYNIA

- Complications are typically minor, and may include the following:
  - Blood loss
  - Wound infection or dehiscence
  - Bartholin gland cyst formation
  - Failure to reduce vulvar pain
  - Vaginal stenosis
  - Vaginismus

GENERAL PRINCIPLES: IMPERFORATE HYMEN

Definition

- The hymen is a remnant of the connection between the sinovaginal bulbs and the urogenital sinus. During normal fetal development, the inferior aspect of the vaginal endplate canalizes to allow for an opening between the vaginal canal and the perineum.[12] An imperforate hymen is the result of perforation failure during the fetal period. Other hymeneal abnormalities include microperforate, cribriform, and septate hymens.
- In the neonatal period, infants with imperforate hymen may have mucocolpos due to secretion of mucus in response to maternal estradiol. This may manifest as a bulging mass at the vaginal introitus. Often the mass is asymptomatic and regresses spontaneously.
- During adolescence, patients may accumulate menstrual blood behind the imperforate hymen resulting in hematometra

and hematocolpos. They may present with a blue bulge at the vaginal introitus, cyclic abdominal pain, an abdominal mass, constipation, or urinary obstruction.

Differential Diagnosis

- Transverse vaginal septum
- Distal vaginal atresia
- Vaginal agenesis
- Hymeneal cyst
- Labial adhesions

IMAGING AND OTHER DIAGNOSTICS: IMPERFORATE HYMEN

- Imperforate hymen is evident on physical examination. The condition is occasionally diagnosed during the neonatal period or childhood, but diagnosis is often delayed until adolescence, when patients present with amenorrhea, abdominal pain, or an abdominal mass associated with hematometra. Examination of the genitalia during childhood by pediatricians is advised to allow for appropriate management of imperforate hymen and avoidance of symptoms with the onset of menarche. We recommend referral to a pediatric gynecologist or gynecologist with surgical experience when this diagnosis is made.
- Rarely, the diagnosis of imperforate hymen is made on prenatal ultrasound, when bladder outlet obstruction is noted due to mucocolpos.[13]
- When an imperforate hymen is noted on physical examination, obtain a transabdominal or transvaginal pelvic ultrasound to evaluate for hematocolpos, and to exclude more complex anomalies such as a vaginal septum or Müllerian agenesis. If a Müllerian anomaly is detected, we recommend pelvic MRI and renal ultrasound.
- We recommend surgical and medical referral to a pediatric gynecologist or gynecologist experienced with imperforate hymen and Müllerian anomaly management.

SURGICAL MANAGEMENT: IMPERFORATE HYMEN

Positioning

- The patient should be placed in the dorsal lithotomy position using adjustable stirrups. Care should be taken to avoid hyperextension or hyperflexion of the lower extremities.
- The labia must be retracted to allow for adequate visualization of the hymen.

Approach

- The goal of the hymenectomy, or hymenotomy, is to open an imperforate hymen sufficiently to allow for the passage of blood and mucus, and sexual intercourse, without causing excessive scarring or narrowing of the vaginal introitus. The technical aspects of this procedure are discussed below.
- Surgical treatment should not be undertaken without preoperative imaging to exclude Müllerian disorders (i.e., vaginal atresia or transverse vaginal septum) that would require other appropriate treatments.
- Treatment of hematocolpos with needle aspiration is not recommended due to the risk of infection and inadequate drainage.
- Imperforate hymen may be surgically corrected at the time of diagnosis, including during infancy and childhood. However, if a child is asymptomatic, it is reasonable to delay surgery until after the onset of puberty but before menarche. Timing the surgery before menarche is critical to avoid the symptoms associated with hematometra and hematocolpos.

Procedures and Techniques: Imperforate Hymen/Hymenectomy

Incise the hymen

- Make a cruciate incision from 10 to 4 o'clock and from 2 to 8 o'clock in the anterior to posterior direction. A cruciate rather than a vertical incision reduces the risk of injury to the urethra and the rectum.

Excise the hymenal tissue

- Sharply excise the four triangular hymenal leaflets created. When excising the entire hymen, slightly undermine the vaginal epithelium to facilitate a tension-free closure and to reduce scar formation.

Irrigate the vagina

- Irrigate the vagina with sterile saline.

Wound closure

- Over-sew the edges of the excised hymenal leaflets to achieve hemostasis by placing interrupted, 3-0 delayed absorbable sutures. Do not perform a running, interlocking closure as it may cause scarring and narrowing of the introitus.
- Two percent lidocaine jelly may be applied to the vaginal introitus for pain relief postoperatively.

POSTOPERATIVE CARE: IMPERFORATE HYMEN

- Hymenectomy is performed as an outpatient procedure.
- Patients should receive postoperative analgesia with nonsteroidal anti-inflammatory medications. Lidocaine jelly may be applied to the vaginal orifice. Sitz baths may also assist with pain control.
- If hematocolpos or mucocolpos existed, patients should be counseled that drainage from the vagina for several days after the procedure is normal.
- Vaginal dilation may be useful postoperatively before initiation of sexual intercourse.

KEY REFERENCES

1. Bornstein J, Goldstein A, Coady D. ISSVD, ISSWSH and IPPS Consensus Terminology and Classification of Persistent Vulvar Pain and Vulvodynia. *J Sec Med.* 2016;13(4):607–612.
2. Haefner HK, Collins ME, Davis GD, et al. The vulvodynia guideline. *J Low Genit Tract Dis.* 2005;9(1):40–51.
3. Lamvu G, Nguyen RH, Burrows LJ, et al. The evidence-based vulvodynia assessment project. A national registry for the study of vulvodynia. *J Reprod Med.* 2015;60(5–6):223–235.
4. Reed BD, Harlow SD, Sen A, Edwards RM, Chen D, Haefner HK. Relationship between vulvodynia and chronic comorbid pain conditions. *Obst Gynecol.* 2012;120(1):145–151.
5. Landry T, Bergeron S, Dupuis MJ, Desrochers G. The treatment of provoked vestibulodynia: a critical review. *Clin J Pain.* 2008;24(2): 155–171.
6. Sadownik LA. Etiology, diagnosis, and clinical management of vulvodynia. *Int J Womens Health.* 2014;6:437–449.
7. Haefner HK. Report of the international society for the study of vulvovaginal disease terminology and classification of vulvodynia. *J Low Genit Tract Dis.* 2007;11(1):48–49.
8. Haefner HK. Critique of new gynecologic surgical procedures: surgery for vulvar vestibulitis. *Clin Obstet Gynecol.* 2000;43(3):689–700.
9. Granot M, Zimmer EZ, Friedman M, Lowenstein L, Yarnitsky D. Association between quantitative sensory testing, treatment choice, and subsequent pain reduction in vulvar vestibulitis syndrome. *J Pain.* 2004;5(4):226–232.
10. Bergeron S, Binik YM, Khalife S, et al. A randomized comparison of group cognitive–behavioral therapy, surface electromyographic biofeedback, and vestibulectomy in the treatment of dyspareunia resulting from vulvar vestibulitis. *Pain.* 2001;91(3):297–306.
11. Schneider D, Yaron M, Bukovsky I, Soffer Y, Halperin R. Outcome of surgical treatment for superficial dyspareunia from vulvar vestibulitis. *J Reprod Med.* 2001;46(3):227–231.
12. Miller RJ, Breech LL. Surgical correciton of vaginal anomalies. *Clin Obstet Gynecol.* 2008;51(2):223–236.
13. Bajaj M, Becker M, Jakka SR, Rajalingam UP. Imperforate hymen: a not so benign condition. *J Paediatr Child Health.* 2006;42(2006): 745–747.

Section VIII

Hysteroscopy, Uterine Sterilization, and Ablation Procedures

17 Diagnostic Hysteroscopy

Linda D. Bradley

GENERAL PRINCIPLES

Definition

- Hysteroscopy is a minimally invasive transcervical procedure to provide panoramic visualization of the vagina, endocervix, endometrial cavity, and tubal ostia.
- Hysteroscopy can be performed for diagnostic or therapeutic indications.
- Diagnostic hysteroscopy with small-caliber hysteroscopes ideally can be performed in the office. However, diagnostic hysteroscopy can also be performed in an ambulatory surgical center or operating theatre.

Anatomic Considerations

- Hysteroscopy is generally well tolerated in an office setting.
- Anatomic findings that may impact the ability to perform diagnostic office hysteroscopy include:
  - Overweight and obese patient may have difficulty in keeping their legs comfortable in stirrups.
  - Knee braces may be better suited for obese patients or those with limited lower extremity mobility.
  - Limited lower extremity mobility may impair comfortable positioning for the patient.
  - Vaginal length may be greater in obese women. A rigid hysteroscope may not be long enough to reach the cervix. A flexible hysteroscope may be a more suitable option for obese patients due to its longer working length.
  - Cervical stenosis may limit the ability to insert the hysteroscope comfortably in an office setting.
  - Increased risk of cervical stenosis noted in:
    - Menopausal women (medically induced or natural)
    - Patients with a prior LEEP or cone biopsy
    - Nulliparous patients
    - Prior C/section
  - Excessive menstrual bleeding may obscure visualization during hysteroscopy:
    - A fluid management distention system is not required for brief diagnostic procedures. Therefore, visualization may be hampered without the ability to vary the intrauterine pressure.
    - The inability to vary the intrauterine pressure significantly debris, clots, and heavy bleeding can obscure findings.
  - Uterine distention is more difficult in patients with an enlarged uterus greater than 14 to 18 gestational weeks on bimanual examination.

IMAGING AND OTHER DIAGNOSTICS

- Diagnostic hysteroscopy is often performed to evaluate:
  - Abnormal uterine bleeding
  - Postmenopausal bleeding
  - To clarify equivocal ultrasound or MRI results
  - Postoperative evaluation
  - Müllerian anomalies
- Several diagnostic studies including endometrial biopsy and medical therapy for abnormal bleeding may precede hysteroscopy.
  - When medical therapy for abnormal bleeding fails, it is possible that the patient has a focal lesion including an endometrial polyp, intracavitary fibroid, endometrial hyperplasia, or endometrial malignancy.
  - If multiple medical or hormonal treatments do not resolve bleeding abnormalities, then hysteroscopy should be considered.
- Diagnostic hysteroscopy should be considered in patients who have had a levonorgestrel intrauterine device placed for heavy menses (without an endometrial evaluation) and whose IUD expels. It is possible that an intracavitary lesion is the culprit for the expulsion. Before replacing another IUD, a quick hysteroscopy can confirm intracavitary anatomy.
- Transvaginal ultrasound imaging is helpful in evaluating the endometrium in reproductive-aged patients and menopausal patients.
  - TVUS imaging may miss one-sixth of intracavitary lesions in reproductive-aged patients with abnormal uterine bleeding.
  - If hysteroscopy is not routinely available, ideally SIS would be recommended because it has greater sensitivity in evaluating the endometrial cavity compared to TVUS.
  - If SIS is not available, then patients with a normal endometrial echo on TVUS and who continue to have abnormal bleeding would benefit from hysteroscopy.
  - Menopausal patients with persistent bleeding despite a negative endometrial biopsy and thin endometrium echo (4 mm or less) should be scheduled for office hysteroscopy if SIS is not available.
    - A thin endometrial echo of less than 4 mm in a menopausal patient is unlikely to be associated with an endometrial malignancy. However, endometrial polyps conform to the endometrial cavity, creating a false negative result.
  - Patients presenting with a hematometria also benefit from diagnostic hysteroscopy after drainage of the hematometria.

- If SIS findings are equivocal, hysteroscopy can be helpful in evaluating the endometrium.
- MRI of the pelvis with and without contrast is sensitive in detecting intracavitary fibroids. However, endometrial and endocervical polyps are not detected as well with MRI. Therefore, patients who have abnormal bleeding which cannot be explained with MRI would benefit from hysteroscopy.

PREOPERATIVE PLANNING

- A urine pregnancy test is required on the day of the procedure for all reproductive-aged patients.
- Diagnostic hysteroscopy ideally should be scheduled in the proliferative phase in ovulatory patients. The endometrium is thin during the early proliferative phase and leads to a decrease in false positive results.
- Reproductive-aged patients who bleed incessantly with a pattern of bleeding consistent with an anovulatory cycle may benefit from an endometrial biopsy and short course of progesterone therapy to halt the bleeding. Once progesterone therapy is stopped, the patient will have a withdrawal bleed. At the conclusion of the withdrawal bleeding diagnostic hysteroscopy can be scheduled. Improved visualization occurs with this strategy.
- Menopausal patients can be scheduled for diagnostic hysteroscopy at any time.
- Cervical cultures for sexually transmitted disease are not routinely required. However, patients queried on a case-by-case basis to determine if needed.
- There are no specific laboratory tests necessary for an office hysteroscopy (except pregnancy testing). It is likely that routine labs including a CBC with platelets and TSH would be ordered as a part of the evaluation of abnormal uterine bleeding. However, it is not needed for scheduling hysteroscopy.
- Follow required surgical laboratory protocols if the diagnostic procedure is performed in the ambulatory care center or operating room.

SURGICAL MANAGEMENT

- Indications for office hysteroscopy:
  - Abnormal perimenopausal and postmenopausal bleeding
  - Evaluation of thickened endometrium on TVUS
  - Equivocal endometrial findings noted with MRI, SIS, or TVUS
  - Failure to respond to medical therapy
  - Infertility evaluation
  - Postoperative evaluation of the endometrial cavity following surgical procedures such as myomectomy, dilation and curettage, or an intrauterine procedure
  - Retained products of conception
  - Location of foreign bodies (IUD, suture, migration of cerclage)
  - Leukorrhea
  - Evaluation of the endometrium following uterine fibroid embolization
  - Sterilization
  - Endocervical lesions
  - Endometrial polyps
  - Evaluation of the endometrium in women on Tamoxifen therapy
  - Submucosal fibroids
  - Müllerian anomalies (e.g., uterine septum)
  - Evaluation of C/section scars
  - Following uterine perforation to determine if the perforation has healed
  - Location of hysteroscopic inserts to determine if migration or expulsion into the uterine cavity has occurred.
- Contraindications
  - Viable pregnancy
  - Cervical cancer
  - Known uterine cancer
  - Active pelvic inflammatory disease
  - Acute endometritis
  - Untreated sexually transmitted disease
  - Patient apprehension for office-based procedure
  - Excessive vaginal bleeding and clotting that would likely preclude an adequate view of endometrium

Positioning

- The patient is supine with legs placed in stirrups
- The arms can rest at her side or across the abdomen
- Her buttock should be placed at the end of the table

Approach

- Hysteroscopy can be performed in the office without anesthesia.
- Hysteroscopy can be performed in an ambulatory surgical center when an office procedure is not available or patient preference.
- Hysteroscopy can be performed in a standard operating theatre for:
  - High-risk patients who cannot tolerate an office setting
  - Excessive bleeding
  - Hemodynamically unstable patients
  - Unable to tolerate a vaginal procedure in the office

Procedures and Techniques (Video 17.1)

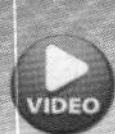

Time out

- Identify patient and proposed procedure.
- Confirm negative pregnancy test in reproductive-aged patients.
- Confirm that the patient has no history of an active herpes infection.
- Determine the last menstrual period.
  - Ideally, in reproductive-aged patients diagnostic hysteroscopy should be performed in the early proliferative phase.
- Describe the procedure to the patient and answer questions if needed.

Perform a bimanual examination and inspect cervix

- The patient is prone on the examination table with legs in stirrups.
- The buttock should be at the end of the table.
- Place an absorbable pad under the patient to absorb fluids. It is helpful to have a small tray attached to the table to collect any overflow of fluid.
- Provide a heating pad and place on the abdomen.
- An electrical table is helpful to vary the height and to be able to place the patient in Trendelenburg position if a vasovagal reaction occurs.
- Determine uterine size, position, exclude cervical motion tenderness.
- Visualize cervix and exclude mucopurulent discharge.

Vaginoscopy

- Vaginoscopy is an emerging technique to introduce the hysteroscope into the cervix without use of a speculum. This may decrease pain and discomfort for some select patients.
- A vaginal speculum and cervical tenaculum are not used.
- The hysteroscope is placed in the lower vagina and the distention medium fills the vagina. Vaginal distension does not provoke pain. The hysteroscope is advanced to the posterior fornix, then retracted a little, to direct the hysteroscope to the external uterine orifice.
- Once the cervix is visualized, the hysteroscope is advanced into the endocervical canal and then the uterine cavity.

Traditional introduction of the hysteroscope

- The open-sided speculum is placed in the vagina and the cervix cleansed with an antiseptic solution.
- If the ectocervix appears patulous, the hysteroscope can be inserted under direct visualization without dilation or placement of a single-tooth tenaculum.
- If the cervix is stenotic:
  - Grasp the cervix with an atraumatic single-tooth tenaculum.
  - An os dilator can gently probe the endocervix.
- Attached the light cord, camera, distention media, hysteroscopic tubing to the hysteroscope.
- White balance the camera.
- Flush the IV tubing with the sterile saline solution or CO_2.

Distention media options for diagnostic hysteroscopy

- Saline or lactated ringers can be used for diagnostic hysteroscope.
  - With small-caliber hysteroscopes, a fluid pump system is not needed because the procedures are very brief lasting usually less than 5 minutes.
  - Sterile IV tubing can be attached to the hysteroscope and the fluid administered manually with sterile 60-mL syringes.
- Hysteroscopic CO_2 administered via a hysteroscopic insufflator.
  - The flow rate with a hysteroscopic insufflator is less than 100 mL/min.
  - Never use a laparoscopic insufflator.

Insert the hysteroscope under direct visualization

- Introduce the hysteroscope into the endocervix and slowly advance the hysteroscope (**Tech Fig. 17.1**).

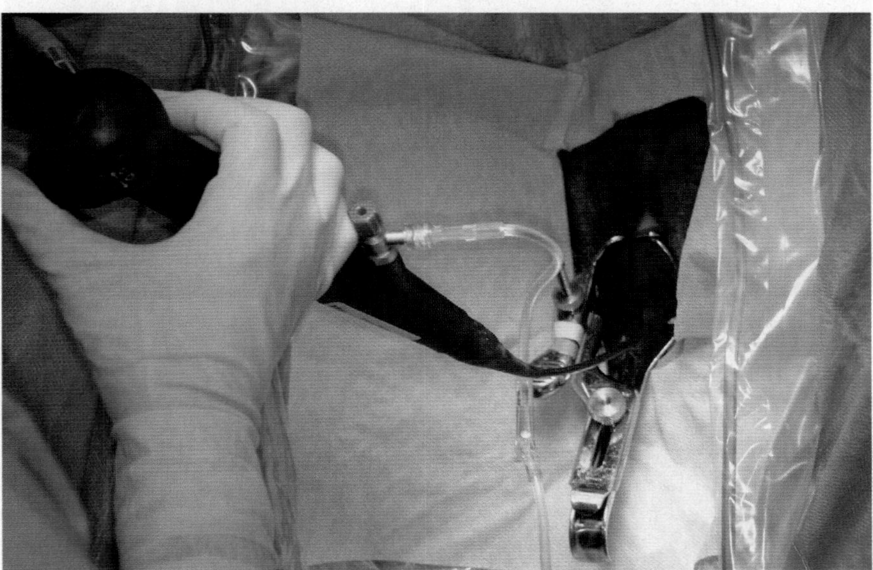

Tech Figure 17.1. Introduce the hysteroscope.

Inspect the endocervix and endometrial cavity

- Take a circumferential inspection of the endocervix.
- Identify all endometrial landmarks including panoramic view from lower uterine segment, tubal ostia, fundus, endometrial cavity, and endocervix (**Tech Figs. 17.2** to **17.4**).
- Describe all lesions noted, size, and location (**Tech Figs. 17.5** to **17.13**).
- Deflate the uterine cavity intermittently during the procedure.
- If there is active bleeding, then saline can be infused and bloody fluid aspirated.
- Discard the bloody fluid in the tubing and reinfuse with fresh saline.
- Take a final inspection of the endometrial cavity and endocervical cavity as the hysteroscope is removed.
- Document all findings in the electronic medical record.

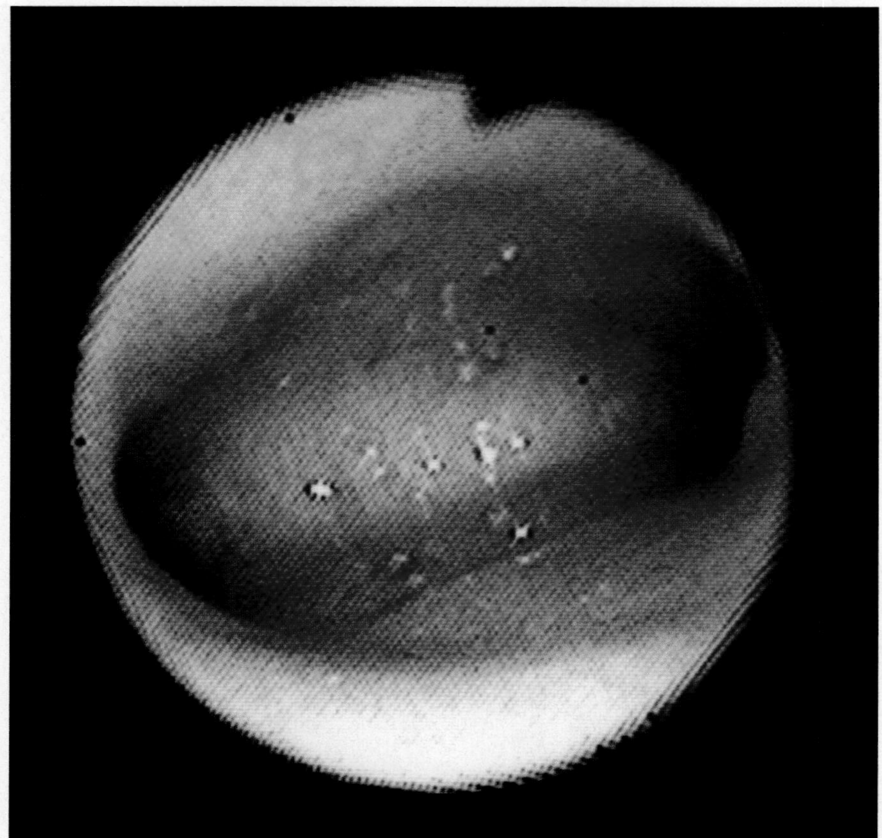

Tech Figure 17.2. Endometrial landmarks: panoramic view.

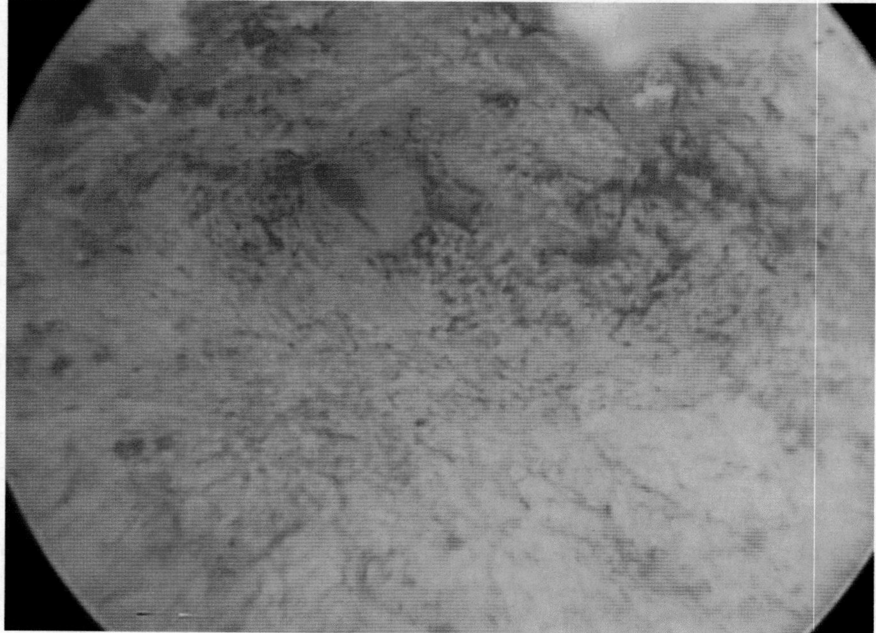

Tech Figure 17.3. Endometrial landmarks: tubal ostia.

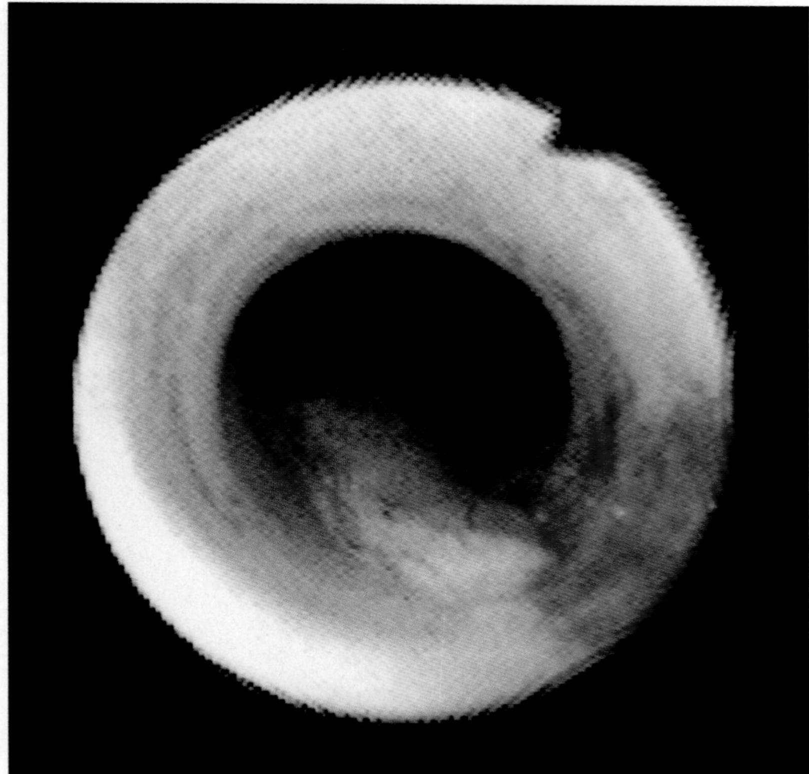

Tech Figure 17.4. Endometrial landmarks: endocervix.

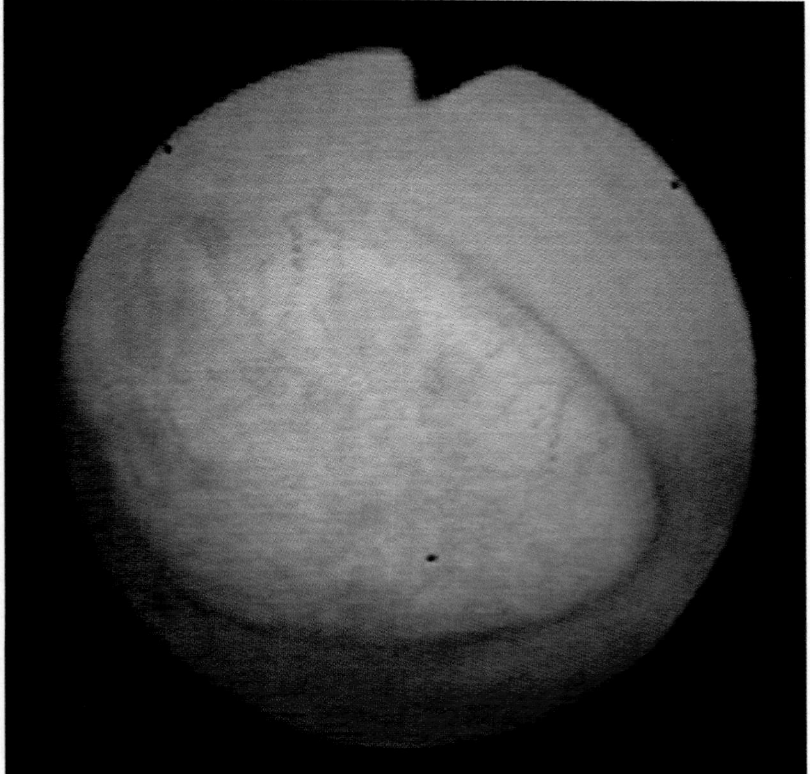

Tech Figure 17.5. Intracavitary fibroid.

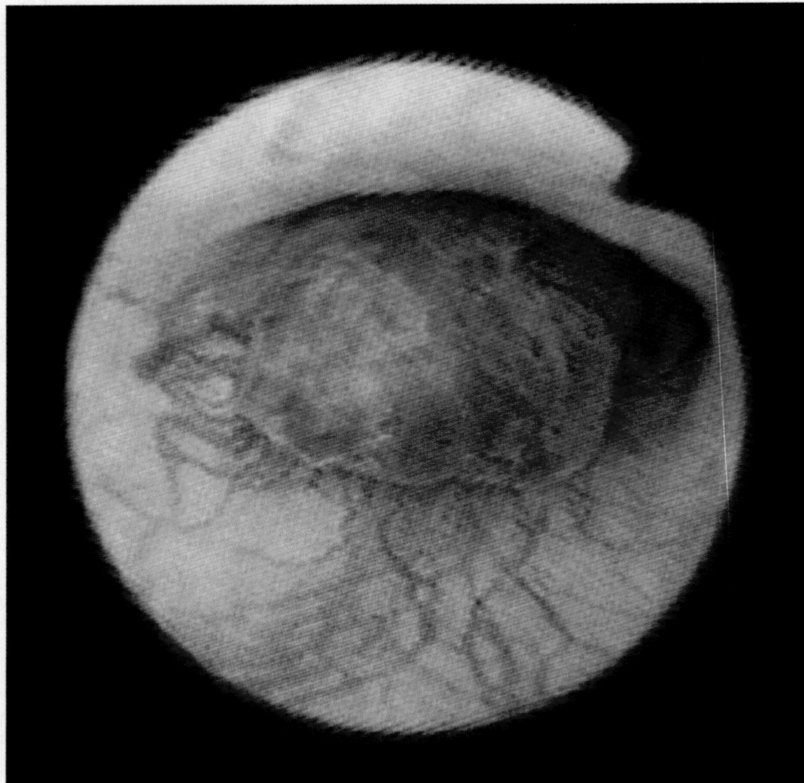

Tech Figure 17.6. Hemorrhagic polyp through endocervix.

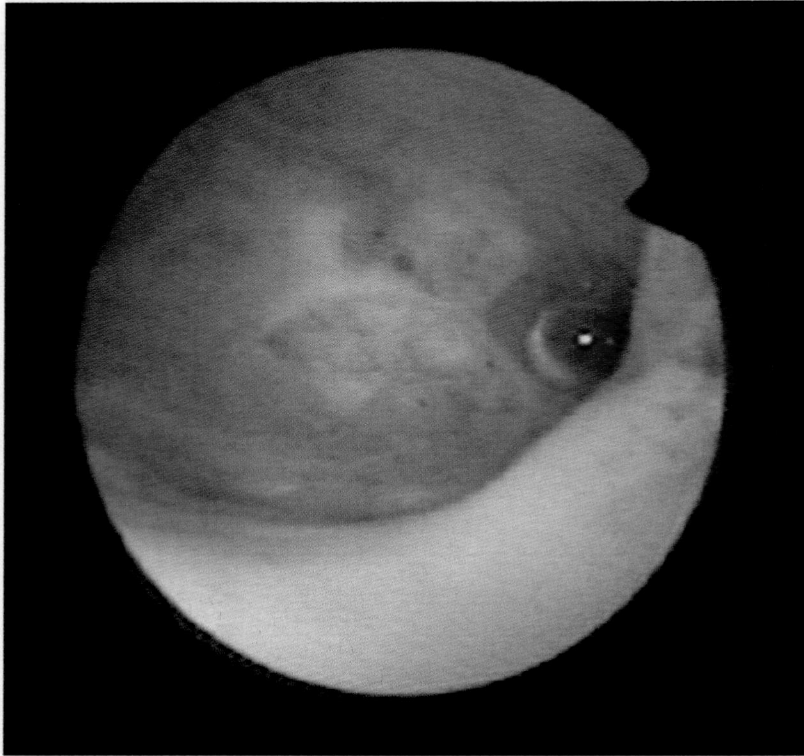

Tech Figure 17.7. Healing endometrium status postfibroid resection.

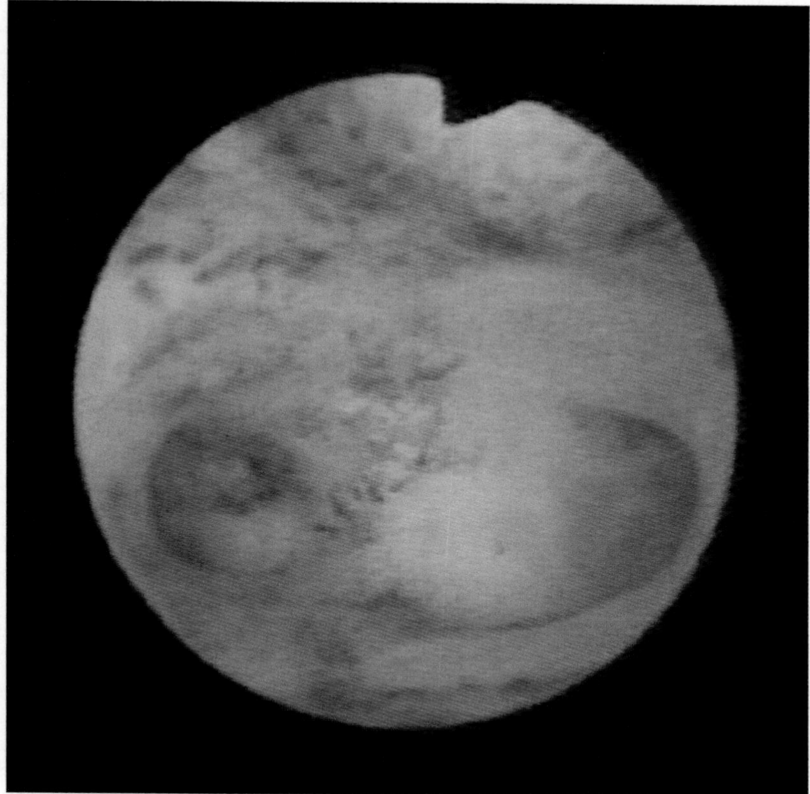

Tech Figure 17.8. Fundal adhesions.

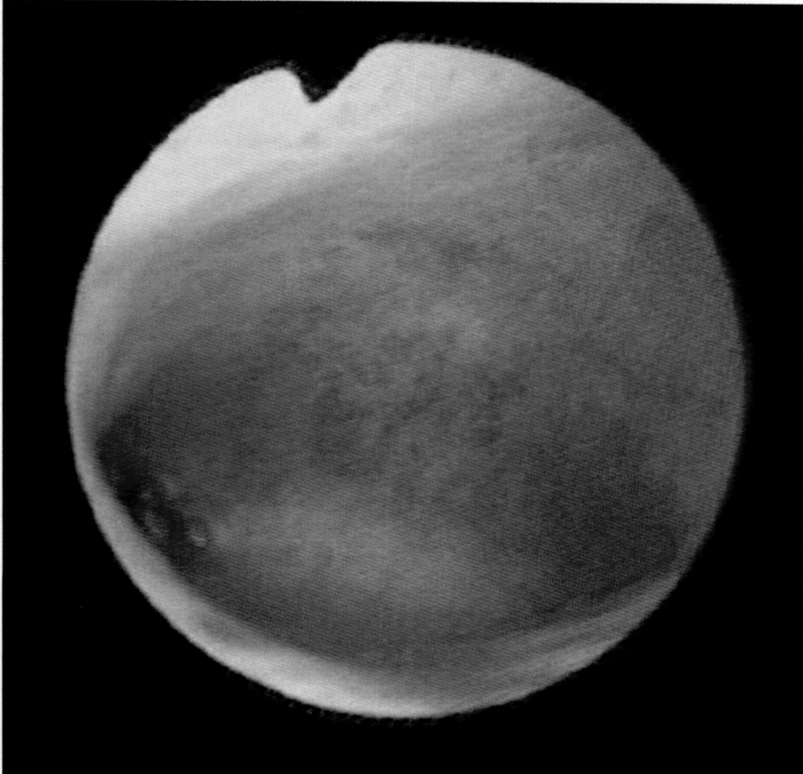

Tech Figure 17.9. Panoramic view from lower uterine segment of normal anatomy.

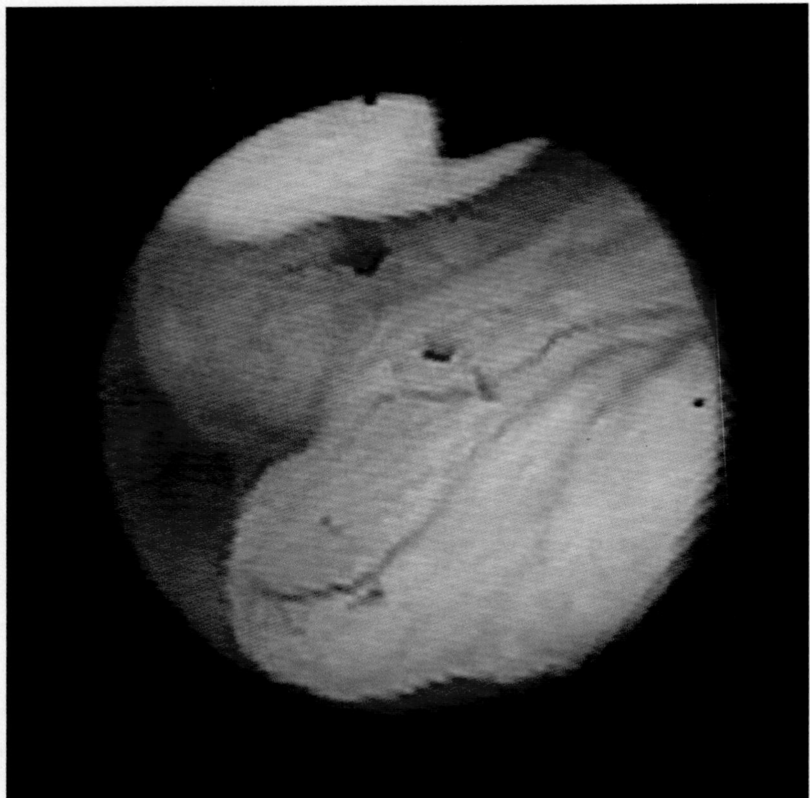

Tech Figure 17.10. Polyp close-up demonstrating vessels.

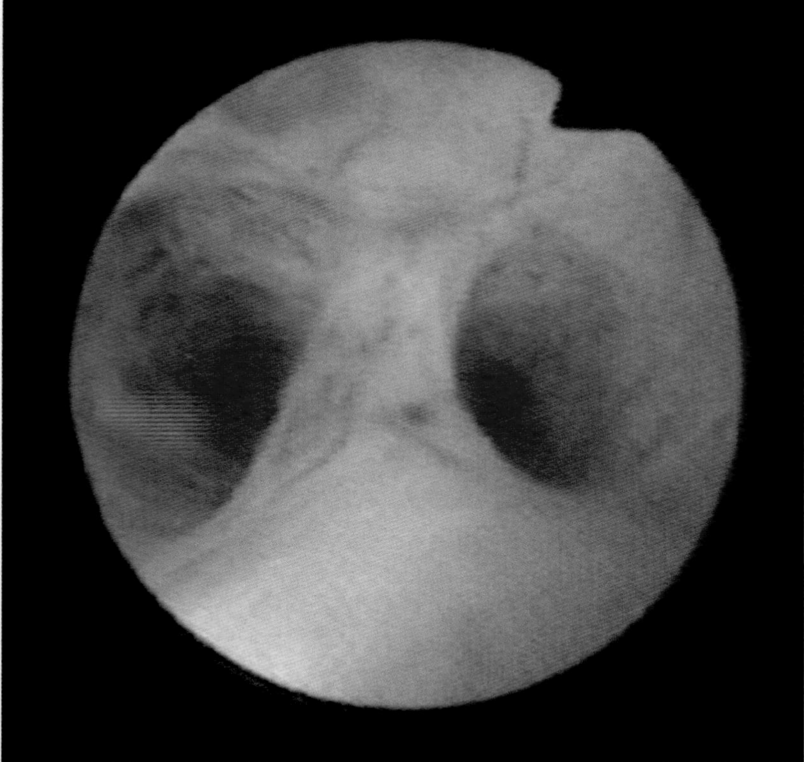

Tech Figure 17.11. Endocervical adhesion.

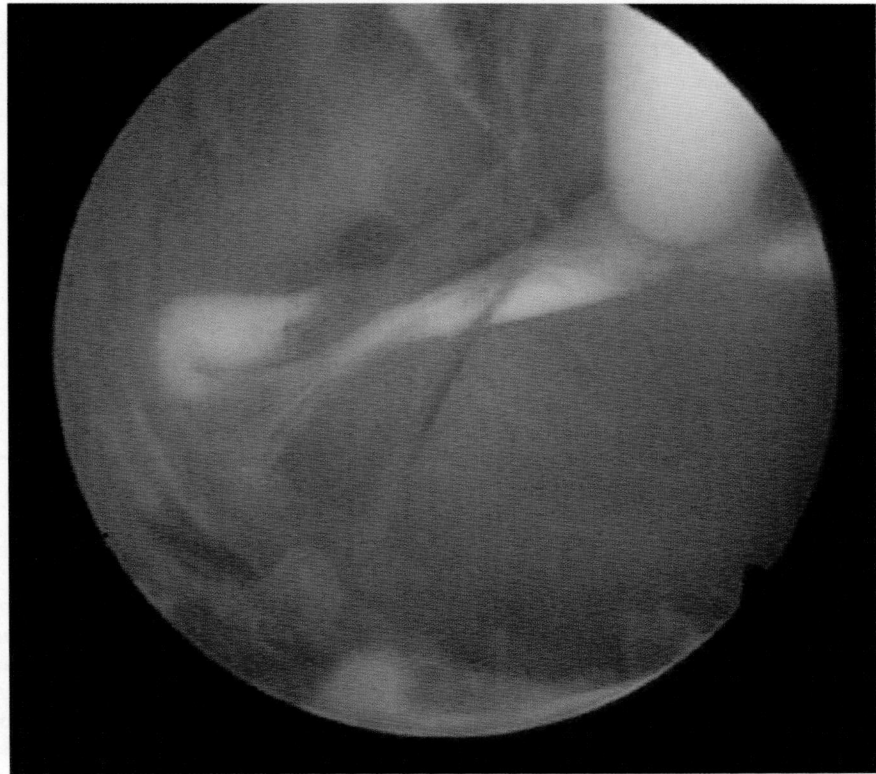

Tech Figure 17.12. Intrauterine Mirena IUD.

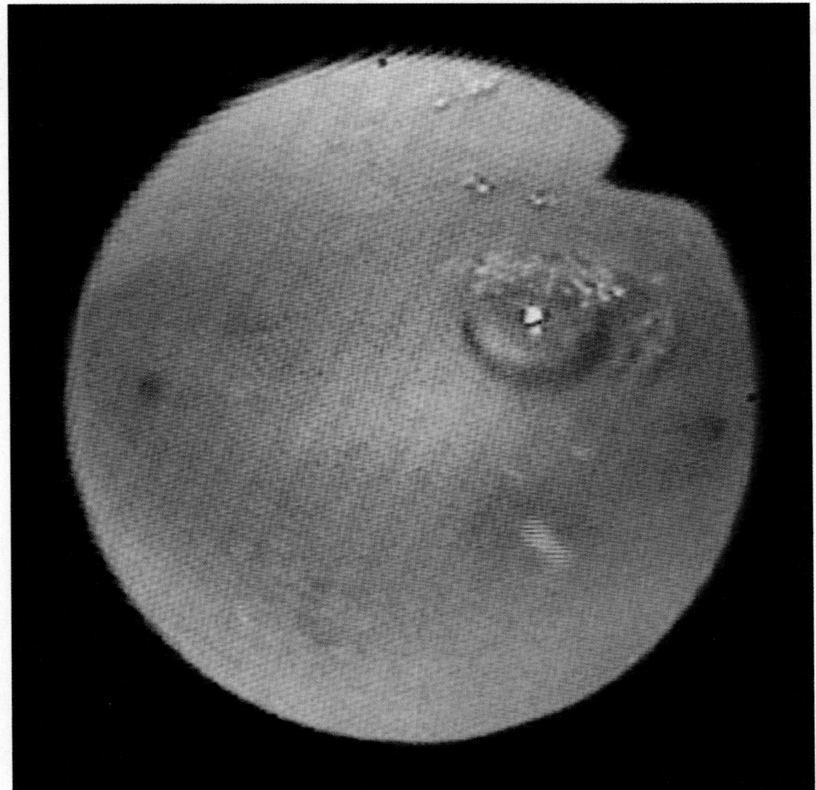

Tech Figure 17.13. Panoramic view of tubal ostia bilaterally.

PEARLS AND PITFALLS

- ○ Schedule in early proliferative phase for patients with ovulatory menses.
- ✕ Scheduling during the secretory phase is associated with more false positive findings and possible early pregnancy.
- ○ Consider hysteroscopy when abnormal bleeding persists despite a trial of medical therapy and negative endometrial biopsy.
- ✕ Missing an intracavitary lesion.
- ○ Evaluate the patient in the office if she presents with postprocedural pain, fever, or discharge.
- ✕ Phone triage may miss evidence of early pelvic infection.
- ○ Educate your office staff on the benefits of office hysteroscopy, safety, and outcomes.
- ✕ A misinformed office staff will convey unrealistic expectations and fear to the patient.
- ○ Have an emergency cart available and practice mock emergency drills.
- ✕ Pandemonium if nursing staff and physicians do not know basic steps for resuscitation.

POSTOPERATIVE CARE

- The patient may drive home if narcotics were not used.
- Most patients have mild cramping for a few hours after the procedure.
- Vaginal spotting or vaginal drainage may last several days.
- Nonsteroidal anti-inflammatory drugs or acetaminophen can be prescribed for the first 24 hours after the procedure.
- Patient may resume all activities except that she should avoid coitus for 48 to 72 hours.
- Patient may shower or take a tub bath.
- Instructed to contact office if persistent pain, increased bleeding, fever, or foul smelling discharge.
- Arrange for follow-up to discuss findings, endometrial biopsy, or response to medical therapy.
- If the patient calls with pain, fever, and persistent bleeding, she should be seen in the office for pelvic examination and further testing as clinically indicated.

OUTCOMES

- Diagnostic hysteroscopy is helpful in evaluation of the endocervix, endometrial cavity, and tubal ostia.
- Diagnostic hysteroscopy facilitates the triage of patients who need operative hysteroscopy.
  - The length of surgery, type of operative hysteroscopic equipment needed, operative hysteroscopic fluid selected, surgical risks and complications can be anticipated by preoperative evaluation with diagnostic hysteroscopy.
- Ideally, diagnostic hysteroscopy should be performed in the office setting as it decreases the costs by triaging patients who need an operative hysteroscopic procedure.
- Patients tolerate office hysteroscopy very well with small-caliber hysteroscopes currently available.

COMPLICATIONS

- A multicenter study of 13,600 procedures involving 82 hospitals noted a low complication rate of 0.13%
- Uterine perforation
- Pelvic infection
- Cervical laceration
- Hemorrhage
- Excessive fluid absorption
- Air or carbon dioxide embolism

Hysteroscopic Myomectomy and Polypectomy, and Removal of Retained Products of Conception

18

Linda D. Bradley

GENERAL PRINCIPLES

Definition

- **Uterine leiomyomas** also called uterine fibroids, myomas, or fibromyomas are benign proliferative, well-circumscribed, pseudoencapsulated benign growths composed of smooth muscle and fibrous connective tissue. They are the most common benign growth of the uterus. These benign growths may be located in the body of the uterus and cervix including endocervical, intracavitary, submucosal, intramural, transmural, subserosal exophytic may pedunculated positions, and may prolapse through the cervix. The size, number, and location of fibroids are unique to each patient and may be associated with a variety of clinical symptoms or menstrual aberrations. The pathogenesis of leiomyomas remains unknown.
- **Endometrial polyps** are benign growths of the endometrium. They are common throughout the lifespan of women. Most endometrial polyps are asymptomatic. Generally, they are single and may occur anywhere within the uterine cavity or near the tubal ostia. Polyps may occur also within the endocervix and ectocervix. They are usually single, sessile, but may be on a stalk, pedunculated, or prolapse through the ectocervix. In reproductive-aged women, the risk of coexisting endometrial hyperplasia (simple, complex without atypia, or complex hyperplasia with atypia) or malignancy within a polyp is approximately 1.7%. However, among women older than 60 years of age with symptomatic postmenopausal bleeding, there is an 8.3-fold increased risk of premalignant changes. Symptomatic polyps detected during the menopause may be associated with a 5% risk of malignancy. The pathogenesis of endometrial polyps remains elusive; however, increased risk is noted in women who use tamoxifen, are overweight/obese, hypertensive, diabetic, and associated with hormone replacement therapy.
- **Retained products of conception** can be seen following miscarriage, termination of pregnancy (first or second trimester), anembryonic first-trimester miscarriage, incomplete miscarriage, missed abortion, postpartum hemorrhage with "blind suction D&C," vaginal delivery, manual removal of placenta, C/section, or in pregnancies complicated by Müllerian anomalies.
  - Most often patients are counseled to undergo expectant management which is associated with 81% success.
  - However, one out of five women may have persistent bleeding, cramping, leukorrhea, fever, abdominal pain, incessant menstrual bleeding, or transvaginal sonographic findings suggestive of RPOC (homogeneous or heterogeneous echogenic foci or endometrial fluid collection with echogenic foci, coupled with high-velocity, low-resistance flow at color Doppler ultrasonography).
- Among women who become pregnant after vigorous curettage, there is an increased risk of abnormal placentation in future pregnancies predisposing patients to placenta accreta/increta/percreta.
  - For these women, historically, a "blind D&C" with vacuum aspiration has been performed. However, surrounding healthy, normal, viable endometrial tissue may be altered leading to Asherman's syndrome (mild, moderate, or severe) or resultant hypomenorrhea due to extensive alteration of the endometrial basalis layer.

Differential Diagnosis

- Endometrial polyps
- Adenomyomatous polyp
- Leiomyosarcoma
- Endometrial stromal tumor
- Stromal tumor of uncertain malignant potential
- Calcified retained products of conception
- Intracavitary endometrial blood clots
- Intracavitary leiomyoma
- Atypical leiomyoma
- Adenomyoma

Anatomic Considerations

- The FIGO classification system is useful in determining the position of the uterine fibroid within the endometrium and the depth of penetration into the myometrium.
- Hysteroscopic removal of uterine fibroids in general is limited to patients with FIGO classification type 0 and type 1 leiomyomas. Expert hysteroscopic surgical experience may permit removal of small type 2 leiomyomas (Fig. 18.1).
  - Type 0 leiomyomas are entirely within the uterine cavity with no myometrial extension. The base can be pedunculated, narrow, or wide (Fig. 18.2).
  - Type 1 leiomyomas involve <50% of the myometrium. When viewed hysteroscopically, there is >90-degree angle of the leiomyoma surface to the uterine wall (Fig. 18.3).
  - Type 2 leiomyomas involve >50% myometrial extension. When viewed hysteroscopically, there is a <90-degree angle of the leiomyoma surface to the uterine wall (Fig. 18.4).
    - While some type 2 leiomyomas may be performed hysteroscopically, expert surgical experience is needed. More commonly, they are removed by a laparoscopic/robotic or laparotomic approach.
    - It is important to determine the distance from the outer edge of the leiomyoma to the serosa with ultrasound or

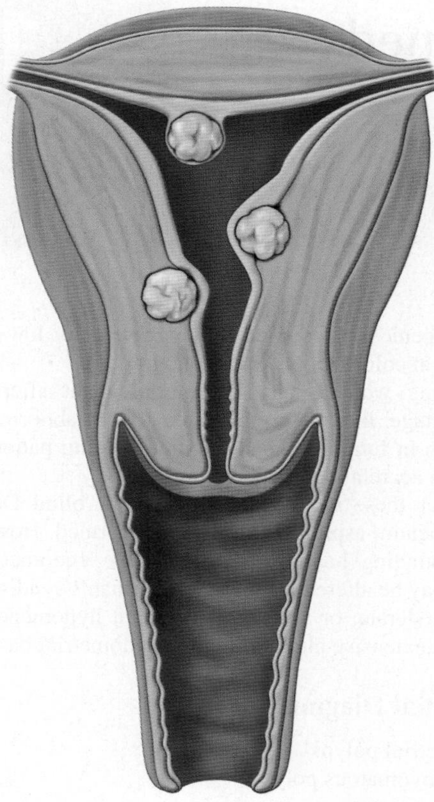

Figure 18.1. FIGO classification of types 0 and 1 fibroids.

pelvic MRI with and without contrast to determine if a hysteroscopic approach is feasible.

- The myometrium remodels during and after hysteroscopic myomectomy. It is advisable to exclude hysteroscopic resection of a leiomyoma that is within 1.0 cm from the serosal edge. Adherence to this guideline decreases the risk of uterine perforation.

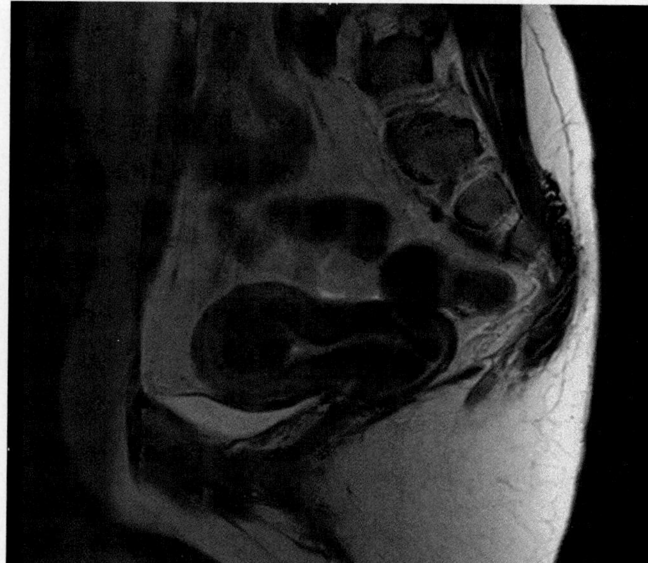

Figure 18.2. MRI with well-defined FIGO type 0 fibroid.

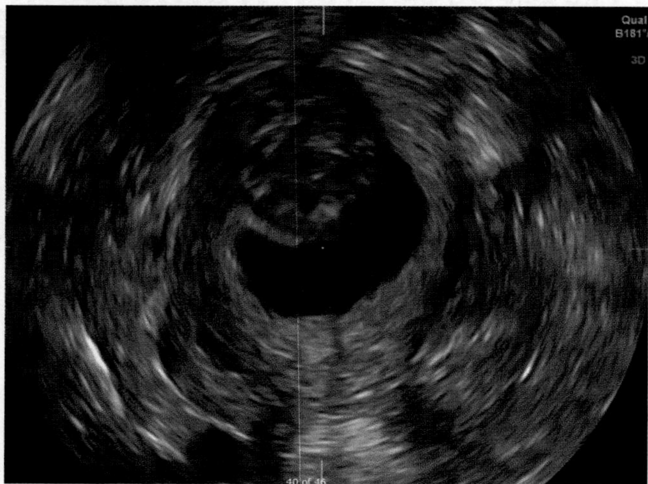

Figure 18.3. SIS demonstrates FIGO type 1 fibroid.

- Fluid absorption during hysteroscopic myomectomy is influenced by length of surgery, intrauterine pressure, fibroid size, number of fibroids treated, depth of myometrial involvement, breach of myometrial venous sinuses during surgery, and less significantly transtubal reflux.
    - The myometrium contains many venous sinuses. When these are opened by resection or morcellation technique, the fluid used during hysteroscopy is absorbed intravascularly. Thus, increased risk of fluid absorption occurs when type 1 and type 2 leiomyomas are treated.
    - Exceeding fluid absorption guidelines is associated with risks unique to the type of fluid used (isotonic or nonisotonic fluid).

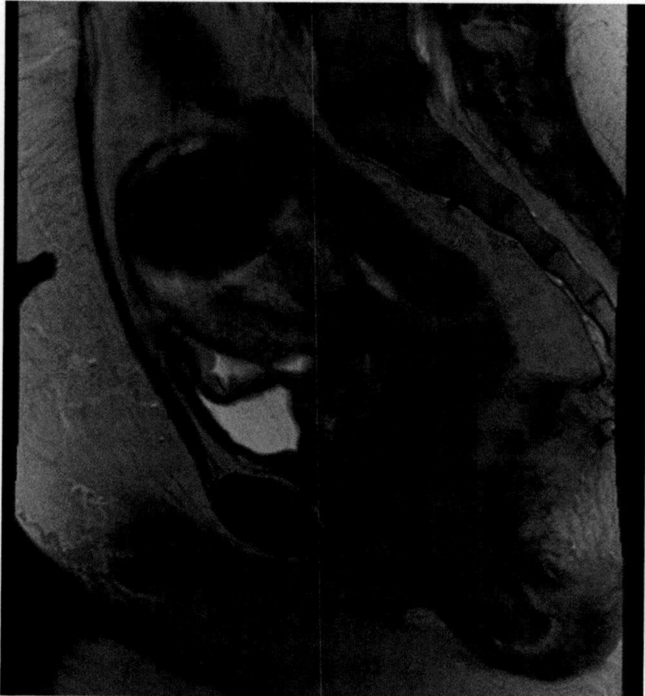

Figure 18.4. MRI depicts FIGO type 2 fibroid.

- Leiomyoma size, depth of myometrial involvement, number and location of intracavitary fibroids, and surgical expertise determines feasibility, safety, and ability to perform hysteroscopic removal as a single surgical procedure.
- Some hysteroscopic myomectomy procedures will require a two-stage procedure due to the inability to complete the initial surgery due to excessive fluid absorption.
  - With expert preoperative evaluation, the informed consent will reflect the discussion regarding the possibility of incomplete or two-staged hysteroscopic treatment.
- As the size of the leiomyoma increases, so does the volume of resected tissue. This affects the length of surgery, amount of fluid used, ability to complete the hysteroscopic resection, and risk of surgical complications.
  - The volumetric formula that describes the volume of hysteroscopic tissue removed is:
    - $4/dr^3$
      - 1 cm = 1/2 cm^3 tissue
      - 2 cm = 4 cm^3 tissue
      - 3 cm = 14 cm^3 tissue
      - 4 cm = 33 cm^3 tissue
- Anatomic and surgical considerations particular to hysteroscopic resection include:
  - Presence of blood, clots, and endometrial tissue debris
  - Endometrium (especially secretory or exaggerated proliferative endometrium)
  - Intracavitary bubbles
  - Tissue or "chip" management
  - Ability to anatomically recognize the pseudocapsule and myometrial fascicles
  - Navigation within the uterine cavity and determining the depth of fibroid resection
  - Uterine walls collapsing and increased juxtaposition of the uterine walls as hysteroscopic resection progresses
  - Fluid absorption
  - Uterine perforation
  - Uterine distensibility
  - C/section scar
  - Uterine size
  - Uterine position
    - Retroversion
    - Retroflexed
    - Axial
    - Deviated
    - Fixed position
  - Cervix
    - Cervical perforation
    - Cervical stenosis
      - With multiple insertions and removal of the hysteroscope in women with a stenotic cervix, risk of cervical lacerations, creation of false tracks, or uterine perforation may occur.
    - Tortuous cervical canal
    - Cervical laceration
    - Creation of cervical false tracks
    - The cervix may become more patulous with multiple insertions of the hysteroscope making it more difficult to maintain intrauterine pressure and intrauterine distention.
      - Placement of additional cervical tenaculum may be required to occlude a patulous cervix.

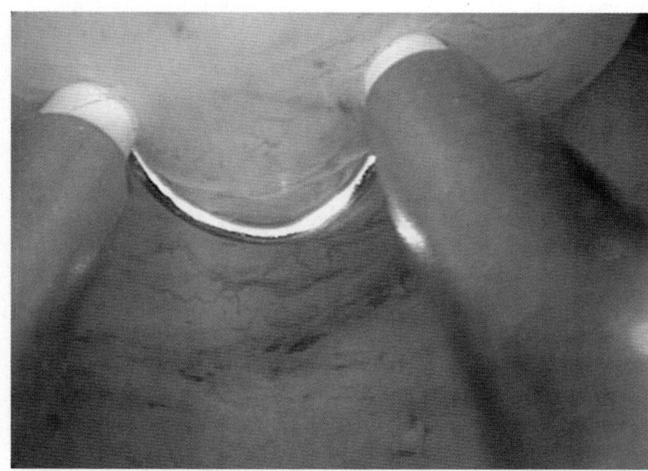

Figure 18.5. Monpolar resectoscope.

- Hysteroscopic removal of leiomyomas can be accomplished with a hysteroscopic resectoscope: monopolar or bipolar devices (Figs. 18.5 and 18.6).
- Increasingly, hysteroscopic morcellators are available and utilize saline as the distension medium and are more commonly employed for type 0 leiomyomas (Figs. 18.7 and 18.8).
  - Complete removal of type 0 and type 1 fundal leiomyomas and fundal endometrial polyps is more difficult with a hysteroscopic morcellator.
  - It is more difficult because the fibroid or polyp is flushed with the fundus and the morcellator operating device can not conform to reach the fundal location as well. Use of intermittent uterine decompression may facilitate complete removal.
- Increased surgical expertise and experience permits removal of deeper leiomyomas.
- Ideally, both hysteroscopic resection surgical expertise and hysteroscopic morcellation should be within a surgeon's armamentarium, as anatomic variations define choice of surgical equipment and fluid used.

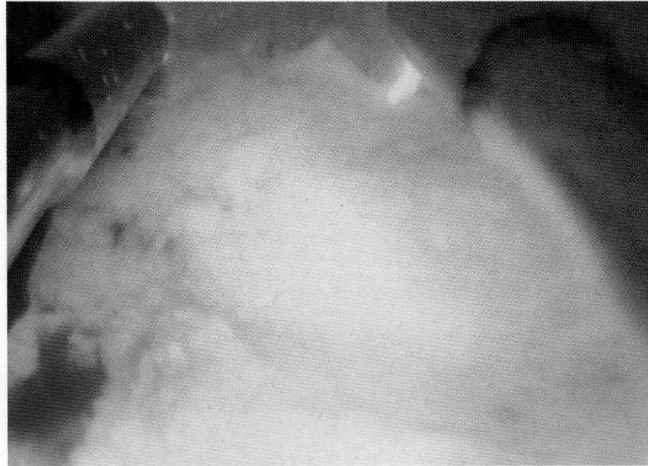

Figure 18.6. Bipolar resectoscope; note the golden orange halo produced by the energy source.

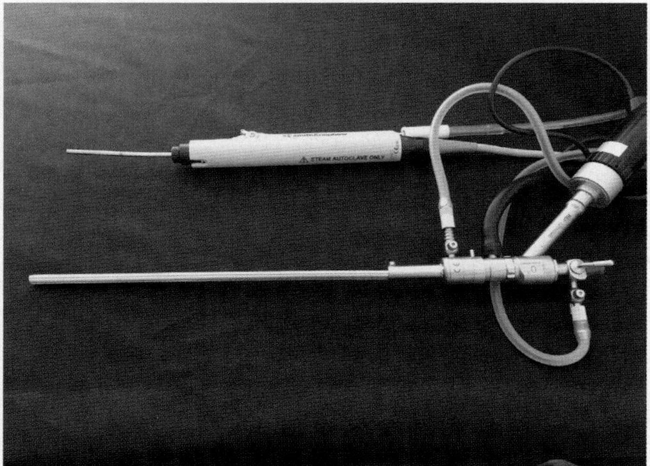

Figure 18.7. Smith & Nephew hysteroscopic morcellator equipment.

Nonoperative Management

- The prevalence of uterine fibroids varies between 20% and 80% in the female population. Risks of developing uterine fibroids are influenced by age, ethnicity, family history, and parity.
  - The majority of women with uterine fibroids are asymptomatic.
  - Surgery should not be offered to asymptomatic women, unless the location of the fibroid is clearly associated with infertility or impair fertility treatments such as *in vitro* fertilization (IVF).
- Among patients with recurrent pregnancy loss and preterm labor consultation with a maternal fetal medicine physician or reproductive infertility physician is advisable to determine if the surgical removal would improve pregnancy outcomes.
- Medical therapy for heavy menstrual bleeding can include a trial of tranexamic acid (for women with ovulatory heavy menstrual bleeding without thromboembolic risk factors), low-dose oral contraceptive pills, or nonsteroidal medications.
- Intrauterine contraceptive progesterone containing devices should not be placed in women with known intracavitary fibroids as it may be associated with increased risk of IUD expulsion, inaccurate placement, malposition, or uterine perforation.
- Patients may also have coexisting anovulatory cycles with intracavitary fibroids or endometrial polyps. Medical therapy for anovulatory may also need to be included.
- Expectant management
- Anatomic consideration for endometrial polyps differs from uterine fibroids because endometrial polyps are soft growths attached to the endometrium, endocervix, or ectocervix.
- More commonly, they are single; however, they can be multiple.
- May be associated with other intracavitary pathology including uterine fibroids, endometrial hyperplasia, or malignancy.
- If they are asymptomatic and found coincidentally, they usually do not need to be removed.
- Endometrial polyps associated with infertile patient should be removed hysteroscopically.
- Patients who develop endometrial polyps while using tamoxifen and have abnormal uterine bleeding or leukorrhea should have them removed.
- Removal of endometrial polyps should be performed with a hysteroscopic approach to increase the chance of complete removal.
  - Blind approaches for removal of endometrial polyps such as dilation and curettage are associated with incomplete resection and remnants.
  - Incomplete resection may be associated with recurrent or persistent symptoms.
- Endometrial polyps may be removed with hysteroscopic wire loop resection or a hysteroscopic morcellator. They should not be treated with desiccation technology because tissue sampling would not be possible.
- In general, hysteroscopic polypectomy procedures have the same risks as noted in hysteroscopic removal of uterine fibroids.
  - The same surgical principles and considerations should be followed as hysteroscopic myomectomy.
  - Endometrial polyps do not involve the myometrium; therefore, hysteroscopic resection or morcellation of polyps should be limited to the endometrium only.
- When asymptomatic endometrial polyps are coincidentally found with TVUS, they can be followed for a short length of time 6 to 12 months with repeat TVUS.
  - If there are no clinical symptoms including pelvic pain, leukorrhea, vaginal spotting, or heavy menstrual bleeding, then imaging can be discontinued.
  - If the endometrial echo increases, hysteroscopic surgical removal is recommended.
- Some endometrial polyps regress over time.

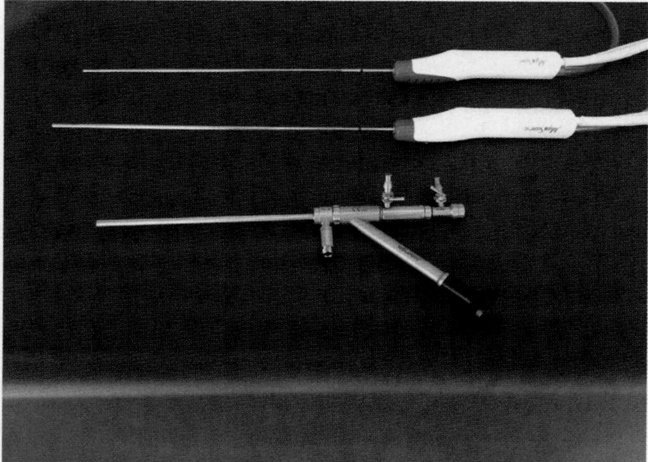

Figure 18.8. Hologic hysteroscopic morcellator equipment.

IMAGING AND OTHER DIAGNOSTICS

- Evaluation of the endometrial cavity in patients with suspected intracavitary fibroids, endometrial polyps, and retained products of conception may include:
  - office hysteroscopy;
  - diagnostic hysteroscopy in an office or ambulatory surgical center;
  - transvaginal ultrasound (TVUS);
  - saline infusion sonography (SIS) with 2D transvaginal ultrasound;

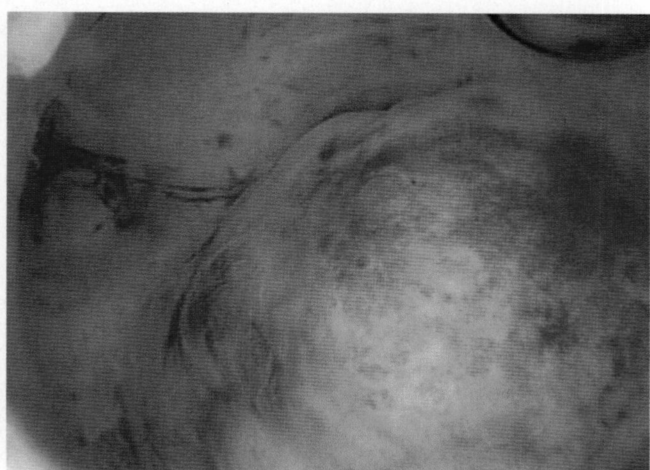

Figure 18.9. Diagnostic hysteroscopy reveals fundal myoma.

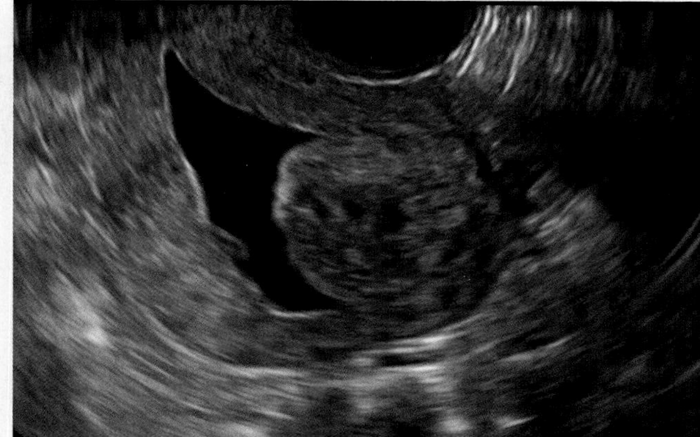

Figure 18.10. Two-dimensional saline-infused sonogram, sagittal view, demonstrates FIGO type 1 fibroid.

    - 3D saline infusion images with transvaginal ultrasound;
    - MRI of the pelvis with and without contrast (not indicated for primary evaluation of endometrial polyps and retained products of conception unless placental accreta/percreta/increta is suspected).
- Diagnostic hysteroscopy can determine the presence of type 0, type 1, and some type 2 leiomyomas (Fig. 18.9).
    - Type 1 and type 2 leiomyomas viewed hysteroscopically can be suspected by the angle of inclination of a fibroid that abuts the endometrial cavity.
    - However, if the size of the entire fibroid and the depth of myometrial penetration cannot be ascertained by hysteroscopy, additional imaging is needed.
        - If there is uncertainty about the depth of myometrial involvement, utilize SIS with 2D or 3D ultrasound.
        - The 3D SIS coronal view is extremely useful in determining the depth of leiomyoma penetration.
    - When 2D or 3D SIS is unsatisfactory or cannot be performed, then MRI of the pelvis with and without contrast helps delineate the boundaries of the leiomyoma.
    - Endometrial polyps are well visualized during diagnostic hysteroscopy, 2D SIS, and 3D SIS ultrasound.
- MRI with and without contrast may be considered when bimanual uterine fibroid size is greater than 12 to 14 gestational week size, limited uterine distention with SIS, or in patients who do not tolerate pelvic examinations.
    - Consider MRI when there are symptoms and signs of adenomyosis:
        - Boggy and tender uterus on clinical examination
        - Significant dysmenorrhea
        - Dysmenorrhea and irregular menstruation
    - MRI of the pelvis may be considered in virginal patients and those who do not tolerate pelvic examinations and transvaginal imaging.
    - MRI of the pelvis is useful in cases where uterine distention is limited including:
        - Patulous cervix
        - Large intracavitary lesions
        - Prior endometrial ablation
        - Adenomyosis
        - Uterine size greater than 12 to 14 weeks
    - Limited view of the endometrium due to copious bleeding which is associated with increased false positive results.
    - MRI is not indicated for the evaluation of endometrial polyps. While endometrial polyps may be visualized when MRI is performed for uterine fibroids, the expense of MRI and decreased sensitivity make it impractical for clinical use.
- While TVUS is helpful in determining the presence of uterine fibroids, the location and depth of myometrial penetration are more difficult. Therefore, we recommend 2D and 3D SIS for more accurate characterization of leiomyomas (Figs. 18.10 and 18.11).
    - SIS with both 2D and 3D images helps define the topography of the leiomyoma including: size, number, location, and depth of myometrial penetration of the leiomyoma.
    - SIS has greater sensitivity and specificity compared to TVUS in detecting endometrial pathology.
    - In patients who have an inconclusive TVUS SIS is advisable.
    - Endometrial polyps are well imaged with 2D SIS and 3D SIS.
- Accurate preop determination of the topography of intracavitary fibroids, endometrial polyps, and retained products of conception enhances surgical informed consent; predicts length of

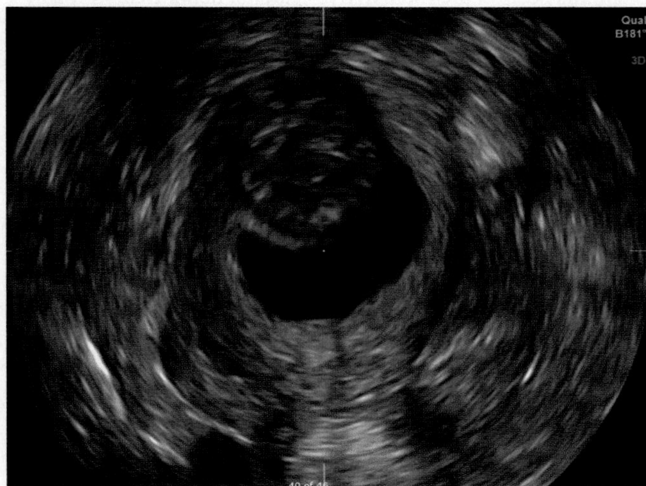

Figure 18.11. Three-dimensional, saline-infused sonogram with FIGO type 2 fibroid.

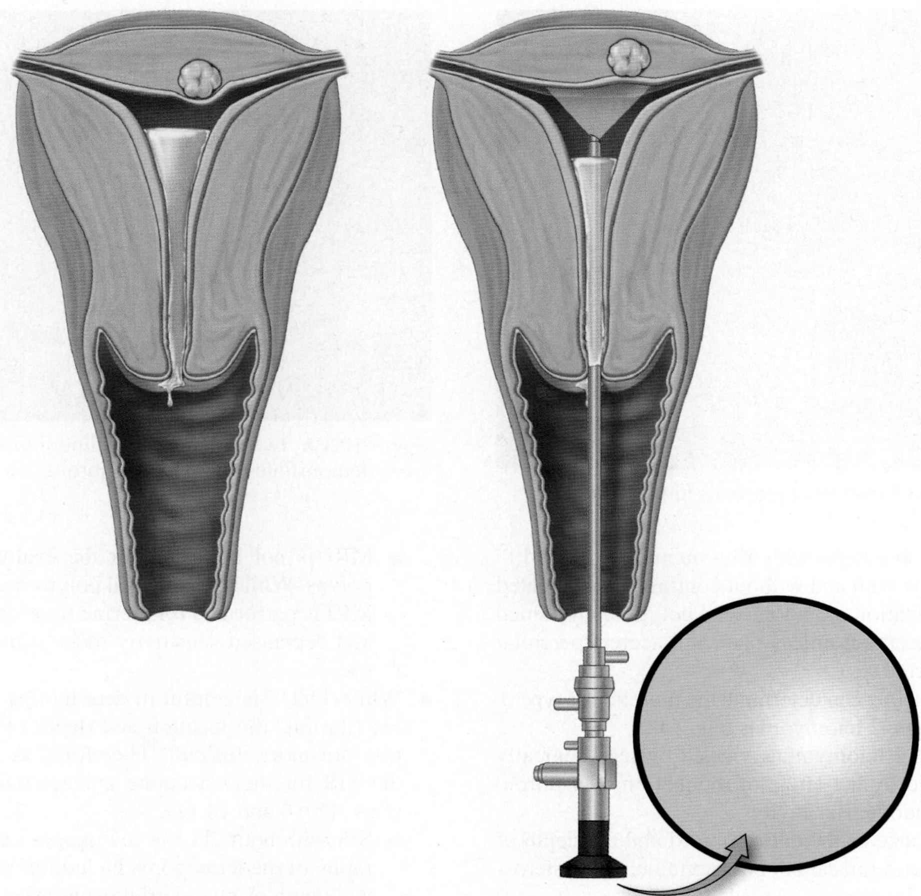

Figure 18.12. Intracavitary distention of fluid or CO_2 may flatten lesions and make them disappear, often referred to as "the disappearing act."

surgery, surgical expertise needed, likelihood of incomplete hysteroscopic resection/morcellation, complications, selection of hysteroscopic equipment and fluid needed (Fig. 18.12).

PREOPERATIVE PLANNING

- The preoperative planning caveats and principles discussed in this section are inclusive to patients being treated for hysteroscopic myomectomy, hysteroscopic polypectomy, and hysteroscopic treatment of retained products of conception.
- Operative hysteroscopy requires continuous infusion of fluid in order to distend the uterine cavity and provide clear visualization during surgery. The amount of fluid absorption and length of surgery will vary depending on the pathology encountered.
- Pulmonary, cardiac, and renal status should be assessed prior to surgery.
- While blood loss is minimal during most hysteroscopic surgical procedures it is important to replete iron stores prior to surgery. This can be accomplished with oral iron supplementation or IV iron infusion symptomatic patients.
- Hysteroscopy should not be performed if a patient has active pelvic inflammatory disease, acute endometritis, active herpes infection, or pyometra.
- Hysteroscopy should not be performed in febrile patients whose source of fever is attributable to a tubal–ovarian abscess, pelvic inflammatory disease, or acute endometritis.
- Patient should not have a viable intrauterine pregnancy.
- When possible, hysteroscopy should be scheduled during the proliferative phase of the menstrual cycle due to improved visualization.
- Operative hysteroscopic surgery should not be canceled in women that are actively bleeding.
  - The intraoperative use of a fluid management system irrigates blood, blood clots, and debris, and provides uterine distention.
  - The ability to vary the intrauterine pressure can facilitate visualization by tamponade of endometrial/myometrial arterioles in patients who are actively bleeding.
  - Intracervical injection of dilute vasopressin may decrease active bleeding.
- Consider misoprostol prior to hysteroscopic surgery because it:
  - facilitates cervical dilation;
  - decreases risk of cervical lacerations;
  - decreases risk of creating of false tracks;
  - decreases risks of uterine perforation;
  - enhances myometrial contractility.
    - Misoprostol-associated myometrial contractions may cause a type 1 leiomyoma become a type 0 or facilitate complete resection of deeper leiomyomas as they are pushed into the endometrial cavity.
    - Occasionally a type 0 leiomyoma may fully prolapse through the ectocervix and vaginal myomectomy can be performed.

- Mix 20 units of vasopressin in 200 mL normal saline and inject in 5 mL aliquots into the intracervical stromal (1 cm depth) at 11, 2, 4, and 8 o'clock position.
  - Prior to intracervical injection, confirm with the anesthesiologist that patient is hemodynamically stable.
  - Aspirate and inject the dilute vasopressin slowly into the cervical stroma. Do not inject when blood is aspirated.
  - Monitor vital signs closely during the injection as vasopressin may cause bradycardia, cardiac arrhythmias, hypertension, and death.
  - Inform the anesthesiologist of the total amount of vasopressin used.
- Perform a pelvic examination and visualize the cervix in the office prior to scheduling surgery. This allows the surgeon to anticipate potential difficulties intraoperatively with cervical dilation or visualization of the cervix.
  - In addition to prescribing misoprostol for cervical priming, the surgeon may also want to have a transabdominal ultrasound available to facilitate safe cervical dilation in potentially difficult cases.
- Cervical stenosis can be anticipated under the following circumstances:
  - Difficulty in performing a pap smear
  - Apical vaginal agglutination
  - The cervix is flushed against the vaginal vault
  - Prior LEEP or cone biopsy
  - Nulliparity
  - Menopausal status with atrophic vaginal changes
  - Prior Cesarean sections
- Consider a two day preoperative course of oral or vaginal misoprostol prior to operative hysteroscopy to facilitate cervical dilation.
  - Prescribe misoprostol 400 mcg by mouth or vaginally at bedtime 2 days before surgery and misoprostol 400 mcg by orally or vaginally at bedtime the night before surgery.
    - Side effects of misoprostol may include nausea, uterine cramping, pelvic pain vaginal bleeding, diarrhea, or pyrexia.
    - Patients may take an NSAID to mitigate these side effects.
- Historically laminara has been used as an osmotic cervical dilator; however, it has become less practical due to the need for an additional office visit for placement. Additionally, attempts at placement of an extra thin laminara may not be possible with marked cervical stenosis.
- A shallow or "mini" LEEP cone biopsy may be needed to excise the ectocervix in order to successfully dilate the endocervix.
  - Preoperative anticipation of a difficult dilation allows the surgeon to request ancillary equipment such as the LEEP machine and disposable LEEP wire loop.
  - Informed consent for a LEEP procedure should be obtained when cervical stenosis is anticipated.
- Consider intraoperative transabdominal ultrasound guidance when marked cervical stenosis is anticipated. This permits real-time transabdominal ultrasound guidance during cervical dilation and decreases the creation of false tracts and uterine perforation.
  - With a full bladder a transabdominal ultrasound probe utilizing the sagittal view permits continuous visualization as cervical dilators are serially inserted.
  - Transabdominal imaging is continued until serial dilation is completed.
- Intraoperative flexible hysteroscopy is often helpful when a circuitous endocervical canal or marked cervical stenosis is encountered.
  - Most flexible hysteroscopes are less than 3.5 mm and have less risk of uterine perforation than rigid hysteroscopy.
  - A small flexible hysteroscope has the advantage in that it can navigate a tortuous cervical canal more easily than a rigid hysteroscope.
  - Utilizing a flexible hysteroscope during difficult cervical dilation provides tactile discrimination of the pathway needed to dilate the cervix.
  - Once the endocervix is visualized with the flexible hysteroscope, the surgeon using tactile discrimination with Hegar dilators can progressively dilate the cervix.
- The cervix should only be dilated to the size needed for the operative hysteroscope used. Overdilation may lead to fluid leakage around the hysteroscope precluding adequate uterine distension.

SURGICAL MANAGEMENT

- Indications for surgical management of intracavitary leiomyoma may include:
  - Abnormal uterine bleeding
  - Postmenopausal bleeding
  - Abnormal bleeding on hormone replacement therapy, tamoxifen therapy, or with hormonal contraceptive therapy
  - Leukorrhea
  - Dysmenorrhea
  - Postcoital bleeding
  - Abnormal uterine bleeding following uterine fibroid embolization
  - Reproductive disorders
    - Infertility
    - Recurrent pregnancy loss
    - Premature labor
    - Uterine leiomyomas in women with Müllerian anomalies
- Indications for the surgical management of symptomatic endometrial polyps may include:
  - Abnormal uterine bleeding
  - Intermenstrual bleeding
  - Abnormal uterine bleeding on hormone replacement therapy, tamoxifen therapy, or with hormonal contraceptive therapy
  - Postcoital bleeding
  - Leukorrhea
  - May coexist with other endometrial pathology:
    - Intracavitary fibroids
    - Intramural fibroids
    - Endometrial hyperplasia
    - Endometrial cancer
  - IVF and infertility treatment
  - Postmenopausal bleeding
  - Endometrial polyps in women with a family history of Lynch syndrome or Cowden syndrome
  - Failure to respond to medical therapy for treatments of abnormal uterine bleeding who have coexisting endometrial polyps

- Complete enucleation of type 0 and/or type 1 leiomyoma is the goal of hysteroscopic myomectomy in women with menstrual dysfunction, infertility, desire fertility preservation, or who will undergo IVF treatment.
- An important caveat and clinical pearl for all hysteroscopic procedures is to incorporate intermittent uterine decompression during hysteroscopic surgery.
  - Intermittent uterine decompression increases the likelihood of complete leiomyoma enucleation and decreases the risk of incomplete hysteroscopic resection by identifying the pseudocapsule and enhancing myometrial contractions.
  - It is performed by intermittently lowering the intrauterine pressure on the hysteroscopic infusion pump below the mean arterial pressure (MAP) and increasing the intrauterine pressure to the maximum amount. This creates "yo-yo" effect of the myometrium and enhances myometrial contractility which effectively pushes the fibroid from its intramural location into the endometrium.
    - This technique is very helpful if the fibroid is shaved until it is flushed with the endometrium, yet the entire fibroid has not been removed. When intermittent uterine decompression is performed prior to complete enucleation, it will appear that the fibroid is larger and growing. This will permit continued resection/morcellation of the leiomyoma.
    - Another technique to employ with type 1 and type 2 leiomyoma is watchful waiting. Remove the hysteroscope entirely for 2 to 5 minutes and allow the uterus to decompress and remodel. Then replace the hysteroscope and redistend with the lowest intrauterine pressure for adequate visualization. Upon replacement of the hysteroscope, sometimes more of the leiomyoma can be seen within the endometrial cavity. Continue to resect or morcellate the tissue until the entire myoma is shelled out.
- The intraoperative surgical technique for uterine decompression is also helpful in patients with endometrial polyps.
  - Endometrial polyps conform to the endometrial cavity. With increased intrauterine pressure the polyps may disappear creating a "negative hysteroscopic view" because they become flushed with the endometrium.
  - Periodic lowering of the intrauterine pressure enhances the hysteroscopic view of endometrial polyps and permits increased removal of the entire endometrial polyp.
- Restoration of the normal endometrial cavity without postoperative adhesions is the goal of uterine-sparing procedures when pregnancy is desired. Avoid applying electrical energy to normal endometrium that is not associated with the uterine fibroid, endometrial polyp, or retained products of conception.
  - Women with "kissing lesions" or intracavitary lesions that abut each other and are removed, consider placement of a pediatric Foley catheter filled with 3 to 10 mL sterile water.
  - The Foley catheter keeps the walls from being opposed together and may decrease the risk of intrauterine adhesions.
    - Remove the intrauterine Foley to 10 days after surgery.
    - Consider prescribing conjugated estrogen for 30 days followed by withdrawal progesterone.
- Minimize hysteroscopic resection complications by avoiding hysteroscopic resection deeper than the pseudocapsule:
  - Identify the whorled appearance of the fibrous leiomyoma and limit resection only to the fibroid.
  - Identify the pink soft fleshy consistency of the myometrium that is below the leiomyoma. Do not breach this tissue plane.
  - Identify venous sinuses that are in the myometrium. Once breached anticipate increased and rapid fluid absorption. Work safely and quickly to complete the myomectomy before the fluid deficit limit is reached.
- With each bag of fluid that is used ask the nurse to audibly inform you of the type of fluid that is being hung. This will prevent iatrogenic complications of inadvertently infusing the incorrect fluid media.
  - Ideally keep only the type of 3-L fluid bags that will be used for the case in your operating room. The 3-L bags look very similar to one another and with dimmed ambient lights in the room the wrong fluid could be hung.
  - When there is a change in nursing staff it is important to have a sign off that informs the new nurse of the importance of fluid monitoring, how to handle hysteroscopic fluid on the floor, and the maximum fluid deficit allowable for the case.
    - Nurses should suction any hysteroscopic fluid on the floor with a "puddle vac" and return it to a canister that measures the outflow.
    - Nurses should never place blankets or towels on the floor to absorb fluid that leaks from the vagina because this will lead to inaccurate calculation of fluid deficit.
- Close and frequent assessment of hysteroscopic fluid deficit is essential to minimize intraoperative and postoperative complications.
- Communicate with the anesthesiologist the type of hysteroscopic fluid distention media that will be used during surgery:
  - Ionic
  - Nonionic
  - The amount of fluid deficit must be communicated frequently with the anesthesiologist.
  - Ideally minimal intravenous fluid should be given during the procedure if larger fluid absorption and deficit is anticipated.
- A continuous hysteroscopic fluid management system should be used during all operative hysteroscopic cases to constantly tabulate fluid deficit.
  - The ideal fluid management system employs audible alerts and halts the procedure when the preset fluid deficit is reached.
  - An ideal fluid management system provides the ability to vary the intrauterine pressure manually so that the surgeon can employ intermittent uterine decompression easily throughout the case.
- Abandon the hysteroscopic approach with or without electrosurgery when perforation is identified.
- If fundal perforation occurs without use of energy, then observation is adequate.
- If lateral, anterior, or posterior perforation occurs, then laparoscope is advised to assess the bladder and rectum.
- Throughout surgery, communication between all team members is essential to improve patient safety.
  - The anesthesiologist should pay particular attention to:
    - end-tidal CO_2
    - lung sounds
    - "wheel-mill" murmur
    - monitor for cardiac arrhythmias
    - oxygen desaturation
    - continuously evaluate for signs of fluid overload

- Easy access for venipuncture is necessary. The arms do not need to be tucked during operative hysteroscopy.
- Rapid access to venipuncture is needed during cases that might require stat labs, IV Lasix, or stat blood gases in the event of a surgical complication or fluid overload.
- Nurses play an integral component for patient safety during hysteroscopy in the following capacity:
  - Vigilantly monitor fluid deficit.
  - Determine if there is fluid on the floor—if so it should be collected with a puddle-vac and returned to the outflow canister.
  - They should not place blankets or towels on the floor to wipe up fluid spills because it prevents accurate calculation of the fluid deficit.

Positioning

- The patient should lie flat on the surgical table during hysteroscopy.
- The arms can be extended or safely padded at the patient's side during hysteroscopy. Rapid access to the arms must be available in the event of a hysteroscopic emergency (**Fig. 18.13**).
- Trendelenburg position is contraindicated during hysteroscopic surgery to decrease risk of air embolism.
- PAS stocking placed prior to induction of anesthesia.
- Allen stirrups utilized and foam padding placed by the knees to avoid neurologic injury.
- Buttock should be at the end of the surgical table.

Approach

- Hysteroscopic myomectomy and hysteroscopic polypectomy may be performed with a conventional operative hysteroscopic resectoscope.
  - Monopolar and bipolar devices are currently available.

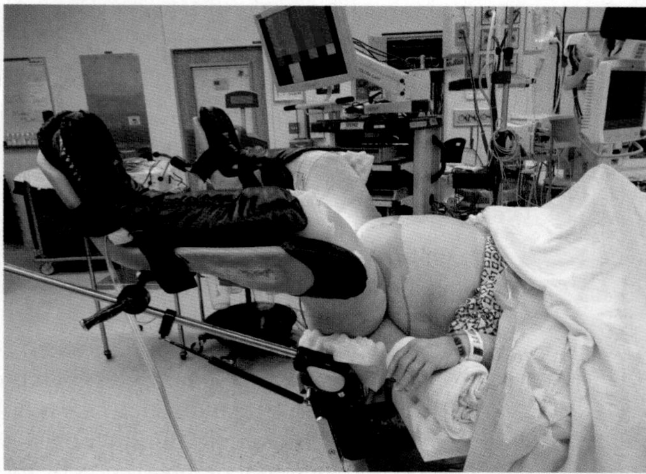

Figure 18.13. Patient positioning for hysteroscopy, note arms.

- Wire loop electrodes of varying angles can be selected depending on the location of the leiomyoma or endometrial polyp.
- Hysteroscopic straight loops are available and are helpful when intracavitary pedunculated leiomyomas are visualized. Large fibroids with a narrow pedunculated stalk can be transected and the fibroid grasped with Lehey clamps and removed via the cervix.
- Monopolar and bipolar barrel probes are available and helpful in desiccating or vaporizing large intracavitary fibroids.
  - Once the fibroid is smaller, a wire loop can be used to resect the remaining fibroid for histologic evaluation.
  - Vaporization probes should not be used for endometrial polyps because histologic analysis is needed to exclude coexisting hyperplasia or malignancy.

PROCEDURES AND TECHNIQUES

Procedures and Techniques (Video 18.1) 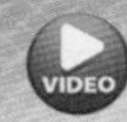

Team huddle

- A team huddle is necessary to confirm the patient and the planned procedure.
  - Specifically ensure that all hysteroscopic equipment and ancillary components are available and in working order.
  - Utilize a continuous hysteroscopic fluid pump during the entire duration of the procedure.
  - Confirm a negative pregnancy test in reproductive-aged women.
- Routine use of prophylactic antibiotics is not required.
- Involve the anesthesiologist during the team huddle:
  - Discuss the length of planned surgery, the type of hysteroscopic fluid that will be used, and the likely amount of fluid absorption during the case.
  - Keep the anesthesiologist aware of fluid deficit throughout the case.
  - Request notification if signs of fluid overload or decreased oxygenation.

Examination under anesthesia

- Once the patient is under adequate anesthesia, visualize the cervix, vagina, and perform a bimanual and rectal examination.
- It is important to note vaginal length (especially in overweight or obese women), uterine mobility, position, and size of the uterus. Extra-long vaginal weighted speculum or extra-long hysteroscope may be needed to access the uterine cavity.

Surgical prep

- A wide surgical prep should be performed including the mons pubis, vulva, vagina, cervix, mid-thigh, and buttock.

Sterile draping

- A sterile drape with a funnel pouch placed under the buttock to securely collect all fluids.
- Sterile drapes also used to cover thighs and abdomen (**Tech Fig. 18.1**).

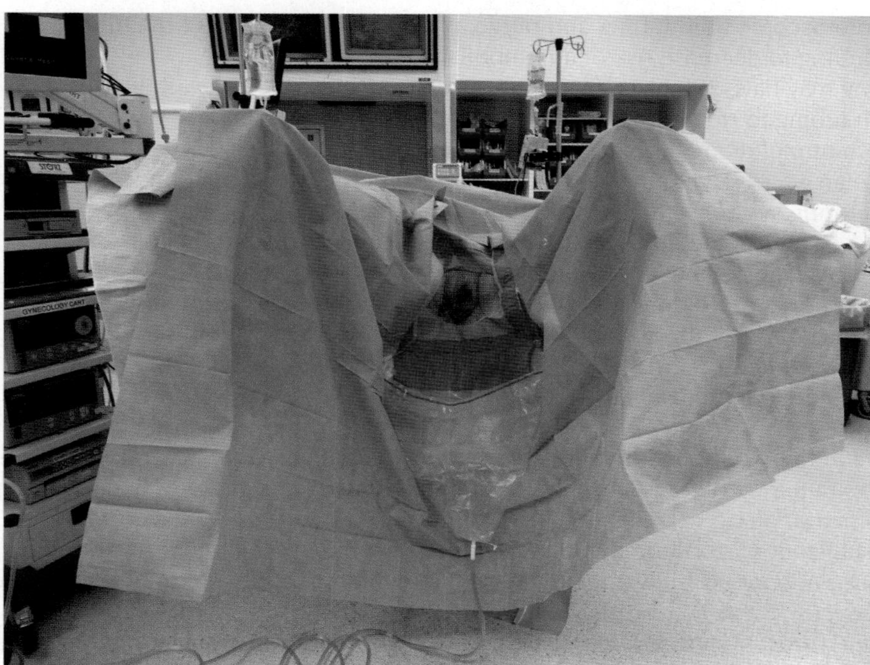

Tech Figure 18.1. Sterile draping for hysteroscopic procedure.

Gaining visual exposure to the cervix

- Heavy-weighted speculum or open-sided speculum utilized to visualize the cervix.
- Remove the heavy-weighted speculum or open-sided speculum when ready for hysteroscopic resection or hysteroscopic morcellation.

Cervical dilation

- Grasp the cervix with a single-toothed tenaculum, dilate with Hegar dilators to the appropriate diameter to accommodate the hysteroscope. Avoid overdilation to decrease risk of leakage of fluid from the cervix during the procedure.
- If overdilation occurs, then grasp the cervix with two single-toothed tenaculums placed at the 11 and 7 o'clock positions and 1 and 5 o'clock positions to occlude the cervix.
- If it is difficult to dilate the cervix, employ transabdominal ultrasound imaging to guide dilation.

Assemble hysteroscope, tubing, and attach fluid monitoring device

- Assemble all hysteroscopic equipment.
- Choose a 12- or 30-degree hysteroscope when a rigid hysteroscope is used:
  - Surgeon preference
  - A wider-angled scope may be helpful when lesions originate near the tubal cornua.
  - The lens for all hysteroscopic morcellators is 0 degrees.
- Light source and camera
  - Do not turn on the hysteroscopic light until the light cord is connected to the hysteroscope.
    - This minimizes the risk of igniting the surgical drape and causing a fire in the operating theatre.
    - Prevents skin burns to the patient risk.
    - Minimizes risk of physician or assistant burn.
    - Attach the camera and white balance.

- Attach hysteroscopic fluid tubing and purge all bubbles and air out of the tubing:
  - Prime tubing to decrease risk of air embolism.
    - Tubing may have 200 cc of dead space which can enter the intravascular space if not purged.
    - Flush tubing to rid it of bubbles which can impair visualization.
    - Attach funnel drape tubing to collection canister.
    - Place an accessory fluid absorption map or "puddle vac" that connects to the fluid monitoring system so that spills of fluid on the floor can be calculated.
      - Never collect the fluid on the floor with a blanket, towel, or drapes.
        - This leads to inaccurate fluid deficit calculations.
        - Sometimes fluid leaks will accumulate near the anesthesiologist. Remind them to inform you if they notice fluid in their workspace. They too should not place towels or blankets on the fluid; rather attach the puddle-vac to collect the fluid.
  - Attach tubing to hysteroscopic fluid monitoring device for accurate calculation of input and deficit.
  - Set intrauterine fluid pressure after determining the patient's MAP.
    - The intrauterine pressure must be greater than the MAP in order to tamponade the myometrial blood vessels.
    - If visualization is obscured and the surgeon is confident that uterine perforation is not a cause of poor visibility, then increase the intrauterine pressure until visualization is improved.
  - In general, most hysteroscopic infusion pumps provide a wide range of intrauterine pressure options ranging between 30 and 150 mm Hg (Tech Fig. 18.2). Many operative hysteroscopic cases can be performed with intrauterine pressures between 70 and 80 mm Hg.

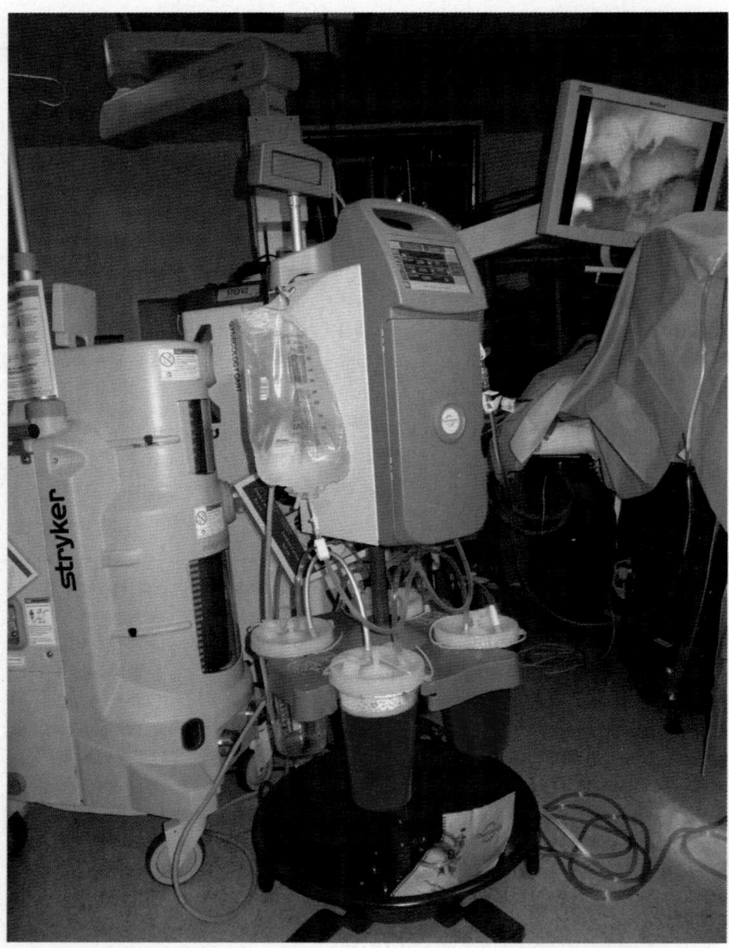

Tech Figure 18.2. Hysteroscopic fluid management system.

    - Increasing the intrauterine pressure should be encouraged when there is poor visibility.
        - Closing the outflow valve on the hysteroscope can also increase the intrauterine pressure.
        - Periodic opening and closing of the outflow valve is a great technique to improve visualization.
        - Removing the hysteroscope entirely and deflating the uterus of debris, clots, and tissue is helpful to clear bloody fluid from the uterus. Replace the hysteroscope and redistend the uterus with fluid.
        - The old surgical adage "the solution to pollution is dilution" is an important caveat in cases with excessive bleeding.
    - Higher intrauterine pressure may be required:
        - to clear debris, bubbles, and blood clots;
        - to clear tissue fragments;
        - if there is active bleeding or the patient is menstruating;
        - when the uterine walls collapse;
        - with increasing uterine size or size of intracavitary pathology.
    - Don't be reluctant to utilize higher intrauterine pressure in order to maintain visualization. Remain diligent in monitoring the fluid deficit throughout the procedure.
    - Realize that the intrauterine pressure may need to be varied during surgery to improve visualization and avoid the "negative hysteroscopic view" that hampers full enucleation of type 1 and type 2 leiomyomas and endometrial polyps.
    - Alternatively, patients with type 1 and type 2 myomas may increase successful enucleation by rapid and frequent uterine decompression by changing the intrauterine pressure from the preset value to the lowest intrauterine pressure.
        - Ostensibly, this creates a "yo-yo" effect within the myometrium and helps push the fibroid out of its pseudocapsule and into the endometrium thereby permitting resection or morcellation of the leiomyoma.
- Determine the preset allowable fluid deficit limit:
    - This is based on patient's risk factors, clinical history, and comorbidities.
    - Patients with cardiac, pulmonary, or renal disease may require a lower set point.
    - Choose fluid media based on the type of electrical energy used:
        - Ionic
            - Saline (bipolar or morcellation devices)
            - Lactated Ringer's (bipolar or morcellation devices)
        - Nonionic (monopolar devices)
            - 1.5% glycine
            - 3% sorbitol
            - Mannitol 5%
    - Do not exceed preset fluid limit.

Attach cords for electrical energy to the generator

- Select default settings for electrical energy (bipolar systems).
- Select cutting current for monopolar devices.
    - Usually 60 W cutting current is adequate; an increase in wattage may be needed depending on:
        - density of tissue;
        - CALCIFICATION of leiomyoma;
        - firmness of fibroid.

Insert the hysteroscope

- Always insert the hysteroscope under direct visualization into the endocervix:
  - Look for the "black hole" that safely ensures direct placement into the endocervix and uterine cavity.
  - If only white is seen, remove the hysteroscope and redirect. Seeing only white tissue indicates close proximity to the cervix, fundus, or endometrium.
    - Continuing to advance the hysteroscope when only "white" is seen increases the risk of uterine or cervical perforation.
  - Once within the endometrial cavity, recognize anatomic landmarks:
    - Identify the tubal ostia
    - Identify fundus
    - Identify lower uterine cavity
    - Identify suspected intrauterine pathology
  - Survey the entire endometrial cavity and endocervix to determine if there are any unanticipated findings.
  - If anatomic landmarks are not identified, it is likely that a false track has been created.
    - Do not advance the hysteroscope when anatomic landmarks are not seen because it will increase the risk of uterine perforation.
    - Slowly remove the hysteroscope and look for the black hole. Once seen, redirect the hysteroscope to the correct anatomic location.

Operative resectoscopy considerations

- Consider intracervical injection of a dilute solution of vasopressin when removing uterine fibroids, retained products of conception or if the patient has significant bleeding on the day of surgery.
- Generally, vasopressin is not needed in patients with single endometrial polyps as these cases are generally brief. However, reconsider vasopressin use case-by-case in women with polyps.
- Vasopressin formula:
  - Mix 20 units (1 ampule) of vasopressin in 200 mL saline.
  - Inject in 5 mL aliquots intracervically at the 11, 2, 4, and 7 o'clock positions and wait 5 to 10 minutes before starting the resection or morcellation. Insert the needle approximately 1.0 to 1.5 cm into the cervical stroma (**Tech Fig. 18.3**).
  - Alert the anesthesia team prior to injection and determine that the patient's vital signs are normal and that there a no pre-existing cardiac arrhythmias or abnormal vital signs.
  - Use cautiously or not at all in patients with uncontrolled hypertension, coronary artery disease, or pre-existing cardiac arrhythmias.
  - Intracervical vasopressin has several advantages during hysteroscopic myomectomy including:
    - Decreases absorption of hysteroscopic fluids
    - Decreases bleeding
    - Decreases operative time
    - Helps to soften the cervix in patients with cervical stenosis
    - Increases myometrial contractility

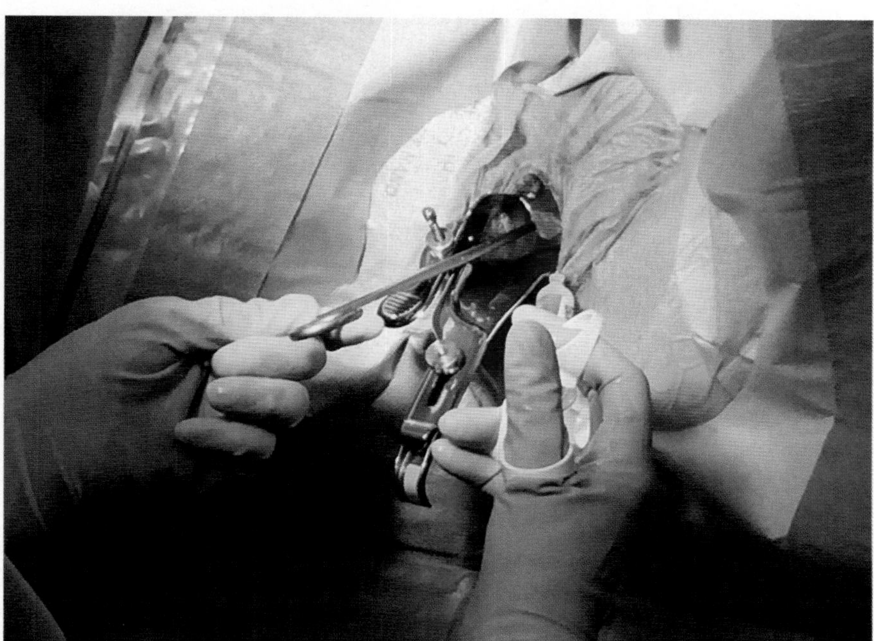

Tech Figure 18.3. Intracervical dilute vasopressin injection.

Operative hysteroscopic resectoscopy principles and caveats

- Always activate the electrode toward the surgeon.
- Place the wire loop behind the lesion and activate the electrode toward the surgeon (**Tech Figs. 18.4** and **18.5**).

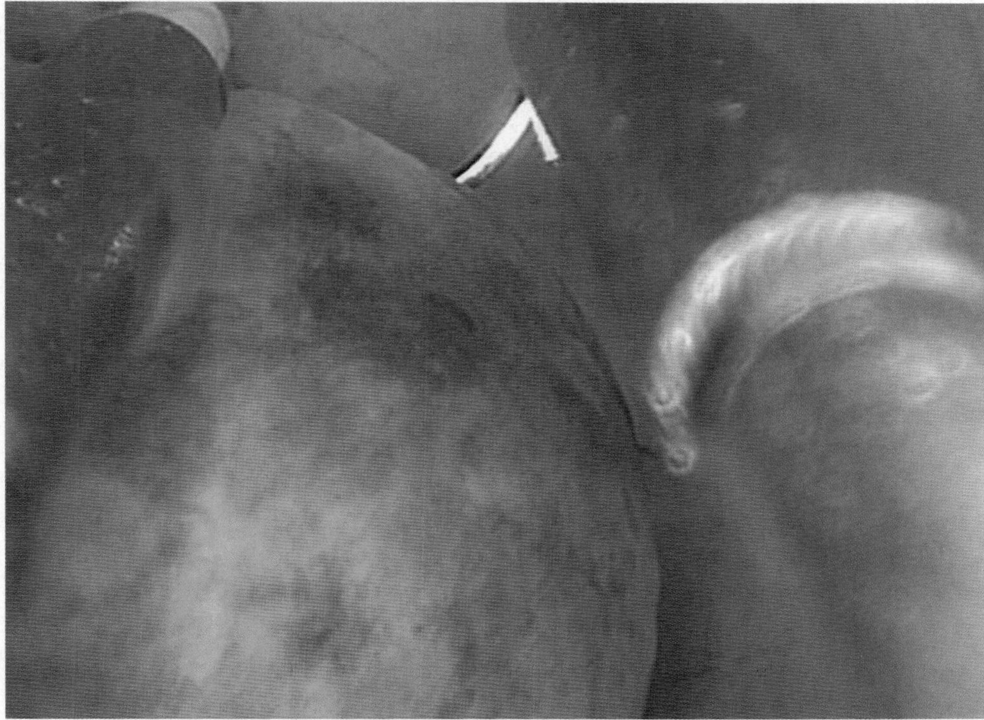

Tech Figure 18.4. Electrode activation with wire loop behind the lesion.

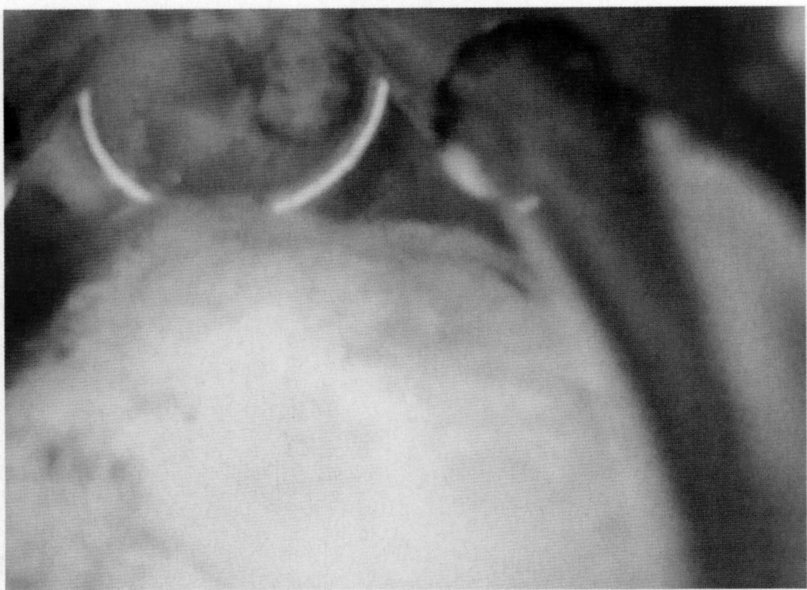

Tech Figure 18.5. Bipolar electroenergy activation, note loop is behind the lesion and activated as the loop is pulled toward the surgeon.

- Make long excursions with the wire loop in order to retrieve larger tissue fragments.
  - When using bipolar energy, the loop must be in contact with the lesion in order to activate the loop and cut tissue.
  - An "orange halo" is often seen when direct contact with the tissue is encountered with bipolar resection.
- Inspect uterine landmarks including the fundus and tubal ostia periodically throughout the case.
  - Once the fibroid is cut, it appears to have a white fibrous appearance or red fibrous appearance (indicates degeneration).
  - The myometrial fascicles appear pink and have longitudinal white grooves (**Tech Figs. 18.6** and **18.7**). Continue to resect until the pseudocapsule is reached. Monitor fluid absorption as it will quickly increase when the myometrium is breached.
- Continue to resect leiomyoma and endometrial polyps until visualization is hampered.

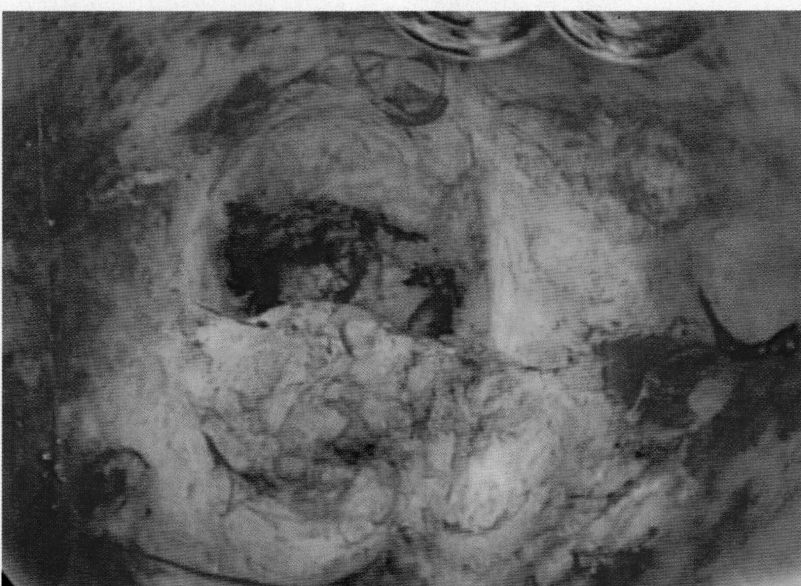

Tech Figure 18.6. Myometrial defect and fascicles.

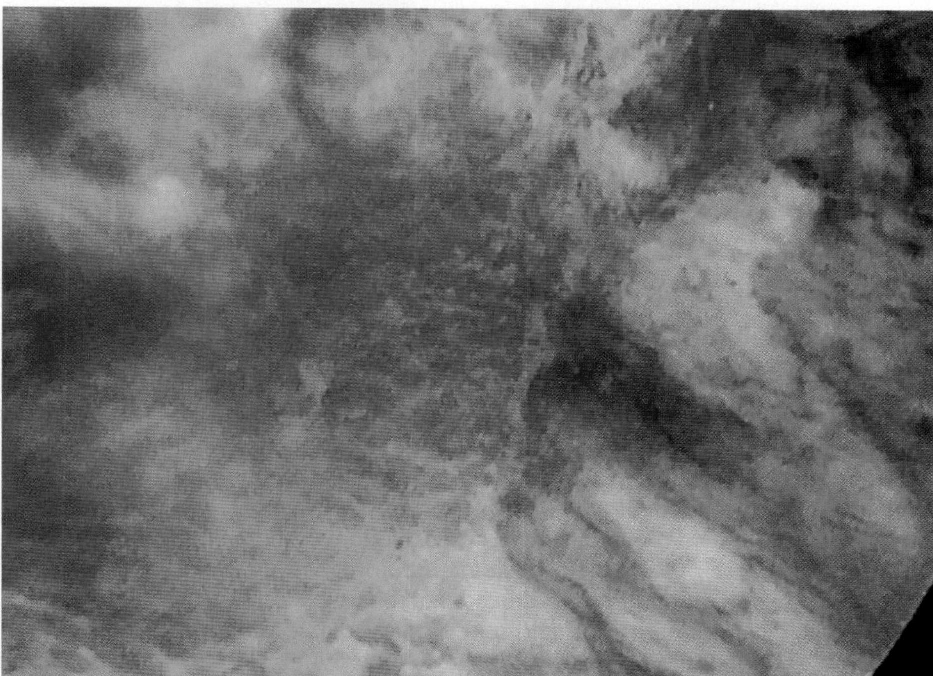

Tech Figure 18.7. Myometrium status postfibroid resection.

Resectoscopic tissue retrieval methods

- When visualization is not adequate, stop the resection and remove the tissue fragments.
  - It is safer to remove the fragments under direct hysteroscopic view than blindly with polyp forceps or myoma graspers.
  - With the hysteroscope in place advance the wire loop and grasp as many floating tissue fragments with the wire loop as possible.
    - Retract the wire loop toward the hysteroscope so that it hugs the distal aperture snuggly.
    - Keep the loop retracted (to keep the fragment from floating away) and remove the entire hysteroscope.
    - Remove the tissue fragments from the end of the wire loop.
  - Replace the hysteroscope and repeat this until technique until visualization is no longer obscured and additional resection can continue.
  - Continue to resect until all tissue fragments are removed.
  - Alternatively, remove tissue fragments with polyp forceps or Corson myoma graspers. This is done blindly and care must be taken to avoid uterine perforation.
  - Another method to retrieve tissue fragment is to remove the wire loop from the operating channel and allow tissue fragment to passively traverse the channel. The tissue fragments tumble out through the inner sheath of the hysteroscope.
  - The final method to retrieve tissue fragments involves slowly removing the entire hysteroscope and allowing the tissue fragments to tumble out through the dilated cervix.
  - Avoid use of curettage to remove tissue fragments as they increase endometrial bleeding and obscure visualization.
  - At the end of the surgical procedure, inspect the surgical drapes and funnel to collect any additional tissue fragments.
  - Endometrial polyps and retained products of conception originate from the endometrium and hysteroscopic resection should not involve the myometrium (especially in patients desirous of future fertility).
    - Shave the endometrial polyp until it is flushed with the endometrium.
    - Utilize intermittent uterine decompression to confirm complete retrieval of the fibroid.

- Removal of retained products employs the same technique as removal of endometrial polyps.
  - Retrieval of retained products can be performed without electrical energy.
  - Retained products are necrotic, friable, and decidualized tissue.
  - Use the wire loop as if performing a blind curettage, however, do not use electrical energy unless tissue is adherent.
- Do not leave tissue fragments in the uterine cavity as they will cause persistent leukorrhea, bleeding, potentially undergo metaplastic changes and ossification, and will not survive tissue processing and render a histologic diagnosis.

Hysteroscopic morcellation

- Hysteroscopic myomectomy, hysteroscopic polypectomy, and hysteroscopic retrieval of retained products of conception may be performed with a hysteroscopic morcellator device.
  - Currently, there are two mechanical morcellator devices available that mechanically remove leiomyomas without energy via suction-based mechanical technology.
  - These devices include:
    - Truclear™ hysteroscopic morcellator (Smith & Nephew, Andover, MA) approved in 2005.
    - Myosure™ Tissue Removal System (Hologic, Bedford, MA) in 2009.
    - Tissue removal is via suction-based mechanical energy.
    - Tissue is collected in a tissue trap and sent for histologic evaluation.
  - Currently, there is one radiofrequency (RF) morcellator Symphion™ (Boston Scientific) available (**Tech Fig. 18.8**).
    - Tissue removal is via a suction-based technology that can utilize RF energy during the procedure.
    - Directed RF energy can be used with Symphion cauterize tissue that bleeds.
  - Generally, hysteroscopic procedures are associated with minimal bleeding.
  - All three current devices utilize saline as the distension medium.
  - Strict attention to fluid deficit is required with all fluid media used.

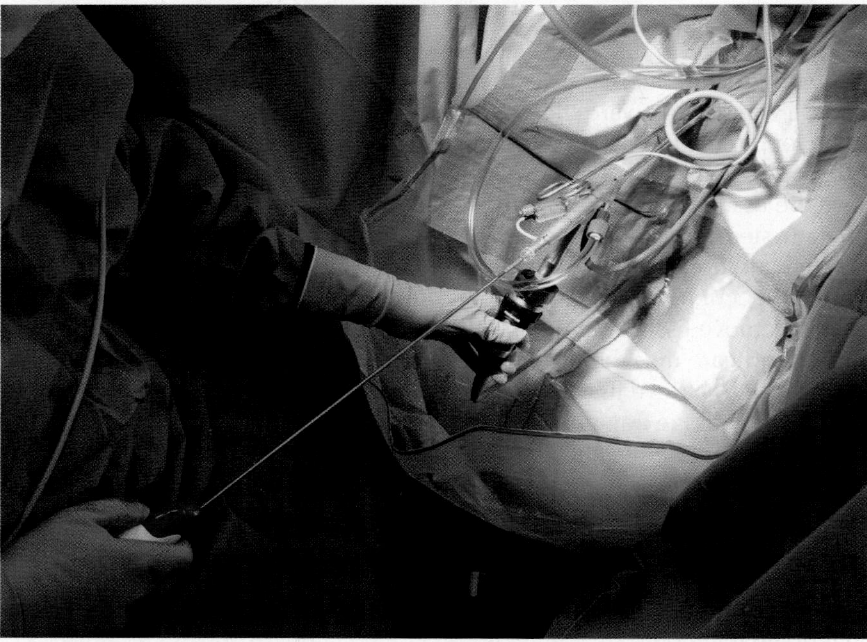

Tech Figure 18.8. Symphion hysteroscopic morcellator.

- Hysteroscopic morcellation devices can mechanically remove intracavitary lesions.
  - Ideally suited for type 0 and small (<3 cm) type 1 leiomyomas
  - Ideally suited for endometrial polyps
  - Ideally suited for retained products of conception
  - Ideally suited for visually directed dilation and curettage
  - All utilize a 0-degree hysteroscopic lens
  - Fundal lesions are more difficult to remove with a hysteroscopic morcellator because the morcellator cannot conform to the fundus.
    - To increase the success in removing fundal lesions with the morcellator, intermittent uterine decompression is needed.
    - Blind curettage of the fundus often misses lesions and is associated with uterine perforation, incomplete removal of lesions, and leaving remnants.
    - This author converts to wire loop resectoscopy to remove fundal lesions if incomplete removal occurs with the morcellator. More often, the initial instrumentation selected with fundal lesions would be hysteroscopy resection with a wire loop.
- Align the morcellator with the open aperture to the fibroid, endometrial polyp, or retained products of conception (**Tech Fig. 18.9**).
  - Maintain constant contact and pressure against the lesion for optimal mechanical tissue removal.
  - Rotate the reciprocating blade as the tissue is being morcellated (**Tech Figs. 18.10** and **18.11**).
- Utilize intermittent uterine decompression to facilitate complete excision of the tissue.

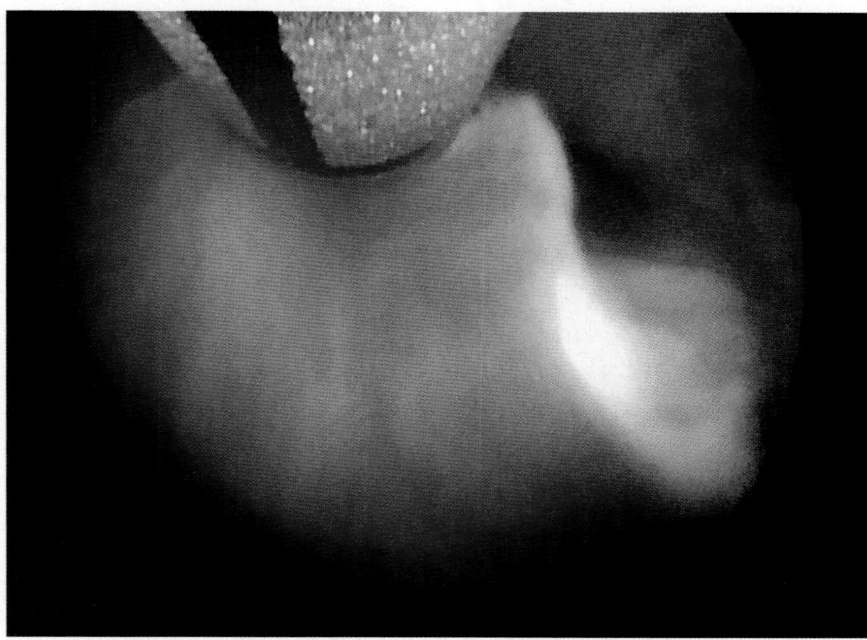

Tech Figure 18.9. Morcellation of posterior myoma. Align the morcellator with the open aperture to the fibroid.

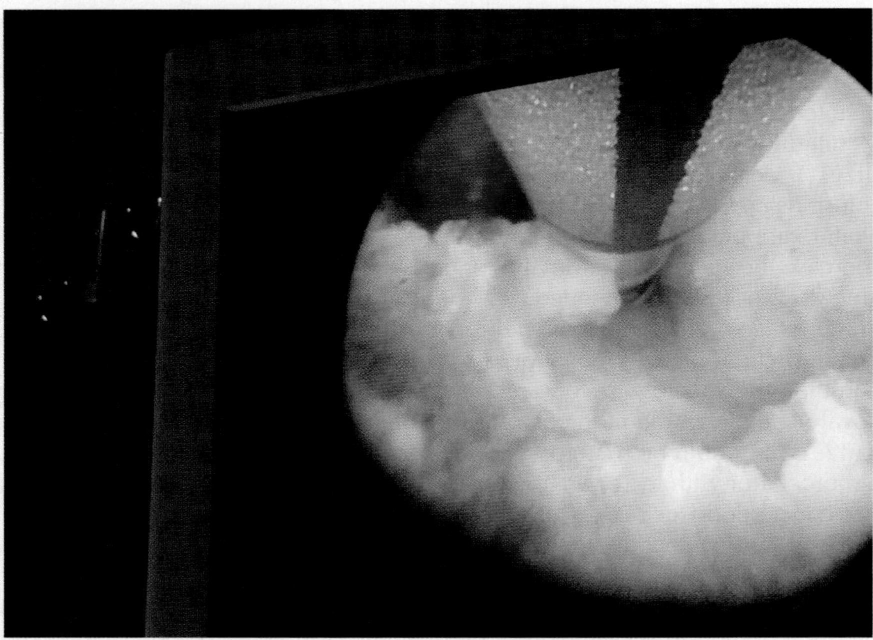

Tech Figure 18.10. Hysteroscopic morcellation, rotate the reciprocating blade.

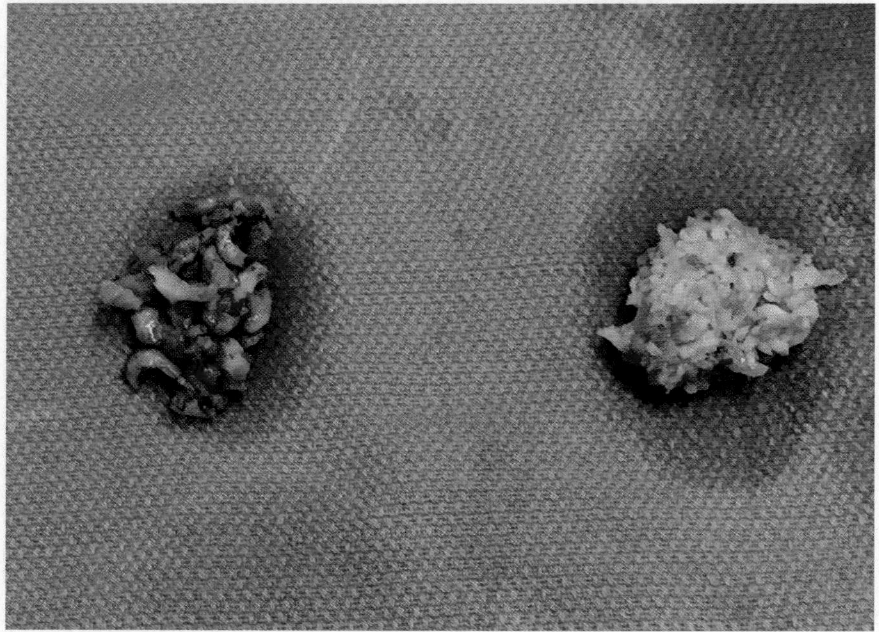

Tech Figure 18.11. Excised myoma tissue by resectoscope (*left*) and morcellator (*right*) techniques respectively.

Uterine decompression is essential

- Once hysteroscopic resection is complete, remove the operative hysteroscope and wait 3 to 5 minutes to facilitate uterine decompression. This technique is particularly helpful in patients with type 1 and type 2 leiomyomas.
  - Reinsert the hysteroscope and determine if any additional fibroid enucleates within the uterine cavity. If so, continue to resect (as long as the fluid limits have not been exceeded) until all the leiomyomas are removed.
  - If remnants of an endometrial polyp are seen, then continue with the hysteroscopic resection as described above.

Reaching fluid deficit: Considerations

- If incomplete resection occurs due to reaching preset fluid deficit, heavy bleeding, or anesthetic issues, document in the operative note, what percentage of the leiomyoma was removed and remains *in situ*.
- Request weight of the pathology specimen in addition to the histologic analysis. As surgical expertise improves, larger specimens will become increasingly able to be removed. Surgeons will be able to determine their upper limits of hysteroscopic surgical removal as their surgical acumen and case volume increases.

Postoperative surgical considerations

- Women desirous of fertility and treated who have opposing fibroids on opposite walls may be at risk for postop intrauterine adhesions.
  - Consider postoperative placement of a pediatric intrauterine Foley catheter to decrease the risk of intrauterine adhesion and synechiae.
  - At the conclusion of surgery, place a pediatric Foley and distend with 5 to 10 cc of water.
    - Remove 7 to 10 days after surgery in the office.
    - If possible, perform office hysteroscopy after the Foley catheter is removed to confirm complete removal of the leiomyoma and to exclude adhesions. If present, most adhesions are filmy and can be lysed with the distal tip of the hysteroscope.
    - On a case-by-case basis, a final hysteroscopy is performed 6 to 8 weeks after surgery to confirm normal uterine anatomy and resolution menstrual disturbances.
  - Consider oral conjugated estrogen 1.25 mg by mouth twice a day for 30 days. Followed by medroxyprogesterone 5 mg by mouth daily for 12 days to induce withdrawal menstrual bleeding in women who desire future fertility. This may decrease risk of intrauterine adhesions.

Completing hysteroscopic procedure

- Once surgery is completed, replace the heavy-weighted speculum or open-sided speculum. Remove the single-toothed tenaculum and observe for bleeding. Wait 3 to 5 minutes to determine if gushing of blood, passage of large blood clots, and inspect the cervix for lacerations.
- Immediate postoperative bleeding is rare following hysteroscopic myomectomy, polypectomy, or retrieval of retained products of conception. Increased bleeding may occur with deeper myometrial resection. If increased bleeding is noted in the following guidelines initiated:
  - Inform anesthesia of the amount of bleeding.
  - Inform the nursing staff that you need a 10 to 30 mL Foley catheter with a Foley-wire catheter guide. The rigid catheter guide placed into the Foley makes the Foley rigid and facilitates intrauterine placement, especially in women with uterine size greater than 10 to 12 gestational weeks' size.

- If heavy bleeding persists and the surgeon is confident that there is no uterine perforation, reinject intracervical vasopressin as described above.
- If bleeding persists, then place intrauterine Foley catheter and fill with sterile water until resistance is met.
  - Document the amount of fluid placed.
  - Attach Foley catheter to a Foley bag to measure blood loss.
  - Leave for 4 to 6 hours until the surgeon has re-evaluated the patient.
  - Once bleeding has stopped, the intrauterine Foley catheter can be deflated and removed.
  - Patient monitored and discharged if appropriate.

Procedures and Techniques: Polypectomy Techniques

Hysteroscopic polypectomy techniques

- Hysteroscopic polypectomy techniques performed with the resectoscope or hysteroscopic morcellator device is similar to performing a hysteroscopic myomectomy procedure. Follow the same guidelines outlined for hysteroscopic myomectomy.
  - The important caveat is that the entire polyp must be removed to restore the uterine cavity anatomy, treat infertility, resolve menstrual dysfunction, and to obtain complete pathology. Polyp remnants should be avoided.
    - Any tissue that floats within the endometrial cavity should be removed entirely with the wire loop or morcellator for histologic analysis.
  - If a surgeon prefers to look with the hysteroscope and then blindly place polyp forceps or perform blind curettage, it is important to replace the hysteroscope after a blind attempt and confirm complete retrieval of the polyp.
    - Intuitively, there is a greater risk of uterine perforation with blind attempts at retrieval of tissue.
    - The most ideal method of removing polyps is under direct visualization for the entire surgical procedure.
- Studies indicate that use of the hysteroscopic morcellator for the treatment of intrauterine lesions may be easier to master than conventional resectoscopy by physicians in training.
  - There is a minimal learning curve.
  - Fewer insertions are needed with the hysteroscopic morcellator.
    - Shorter operating time.

Procedures and Techniques: Removal of Retained Products of Conception

Utilize same positioning and surgical principles as hysteroscopic myomectomy and hysteroscopic polypectomy

- Techniques for selective removal of placental remnants are similar to performing hysteroscopic myomectomy and polypectomy.
- Cold loop hysteroscopic treatment of RPOC involves use of the operative hysteroscopic loop, without electrical current, to atraumatically curette the endometrium that only involves the placental fragments.
  - It is advisable to use a standard 22 to 26 F continuous-flow bipolar system equipped with an electrical loop.
  - A continuous-flow hysteroscopic fluid management system is utilized.
  - Selective direct "curettage" is performed using the loop electrode as a curette. No electrical energy is used unless very densely adherent placental fragments are noted.
  - Extra caution is needed in postpartum patients when involution of the uterus is not complete.
    - Postpartum removal of retained products of conception is practical when the uterine size has involuted between 12 and 14 week size.
    - Hysteroscopic retrieval of RPOC is not practical immediately postpartum because the cervix is too patulous, the uterus is too boggy and enlarged making it difficult to maintain intrauterine distention.
    - When compared to ultrasound-guided curettage with a metal curette, cold loop hysteroscopic resection and morcellation are associated with lower rates of intrauterine adhesion formation.
- Hysteroscopic morcellation has also been reported to removal residual retained products of conception.
  - In one detailed study that summarized the experience of its authors, the number of days of bleeding after the end of the pregnancy and performance of hysteroscopic morcellation was 1 to 46 weeks, with the median range of 10 weeks.
  - The diameter of the residual tissue ranged from 0.8 to 9.7 cm, with the median diameter of 2.0 cm.
  - Procedure time was 10 to 60 minutes, with the median being 10 minutes.
  - Complete removal at the first hysteroscopic morcellation approach was 94.3% and 85.7% were performed without any adverse side effects.
  - In 2% of cases, complete removal was not possible due to reaching the maximal fluid deficit.
  - Two percent had a perforation at the time of the procedure and 2% had retained products of conception noted at the time of follow-up and required a repeat procedure.
  - The benefits of hysteroscopic morcellation removal compared to cold loop resectoscopic removal are multifactorial including:
    - Fewer insertions of the operative hysteroscope; therefore, uterine perforation is less likely.
    - If there is a perforation, there is no thermal risk to peritoneal structures as the device is suction based. However, mechanical injury to intraperitoneal structures is still possible.
  - It is easy to remove associated intracavitary clots and direct removal of intrauterine placental RPOC with continuous visualization.
  - The use of saline decreases the risk of electrolyte disturbances; however, fluid monitoring is still needed to decrease risks of fluid overload.

- If the cervical os is patulous consider occluding the cervix with a Gimpelson double-toothed tenaculum or two single-toothed tenacula.
- Aspirated tissue sent for histologic analysis.
- Theoretically, the risk of Asherman's syndrome is decreased since only retained products of conception are treated.
- Routine postoperative office hysteroscopy is encouraged to evaluate the endometrium a few weeks after hysteroscopic morcellation to rule out intrauterine synechiae. If noted early, it is often very easy to lyse adhesions under direct visualization in the office.
- Theoretically, there may be an increased risk of intraoperative and postoperative bleeding during hysteroscopic tissue removal of RPOC.
- This author uses a dilute solution (as previously described) of intracervical vasopressin prior to performing hysteroscopic morcellation or resectoscopy of RPOC.

PEARLS AND PITFALLS

○ Expert preoperative evaluation using hysteroscopy, saline infusion sonography, or MRI to accurately determine the FIGO classification of uterine leiomyomas. This classification symptom coupled with the gynecologist's surgical acumen determines if hysteroscopic resection or hysteroscopic morcellation is feasible.

✖ Failure to know the size, number, and location of uterine fibroids can lead to the inappropriate selection of surgical technique/approach or hysteroscopic method selected. Not all intracavitary and type 1 or type 2 leiomyomas are amenable to a hysteroscopic approach.

○ Obtain an in-depth preoperative informed consent.

✖ Inadequate informed consent can be associated with patient dissatisfaction, distrust, and displeasure when a complication occurs or incomplete hysteroscopic resection occurs. Increased patient expense and additional recovery required if multiple procedures are required to complete a hysteroscopic procedure.

○ Perform a bimanual examination under anesthesia.

✖ Without knowledge of uterine position anatomic distortion may be due to prior cesarean section, severe endometriosis, extensive pelvic inflammatory disease, adnexal pathology, or enlarged uterus due to multiple fibroids. These factors may affect cervical dilation. If not anticipated, this may lead to an increased risk of uterine perforation during cervical dilation.

○ Insert hysteroscope only under direct visualization.

✖ Blind insertion of the hysteroscope can lead to increased risk of uterine perforation. Endocervical deviation may be associated with a circuitous route and requires vigilant insertion techniques in order to gain entrance to endometrial cavity.

○ Avoid overdilation of the cervix.

✖ Failure to know the diameter of the hysteroscope selected can be associated with over dilation and difficulty in maintaining uterine distension.

○ Strict attention to inflow and deficit.

✖ Failure to adhere to AAGL guidelines recommended for operative hysteroscopy can be associated with increased surgical morbidity and mortality. Pulmonary, cardiac, laryngeal, and cerebral edema can occur with fluid overload (ionic and nonionic). When nonionic fluid is used, severe electrolyte abnormalities, seizures, hyperammonemia, transient blindness, mental confusion, delirium, and death have been reported.

○ Operative field must always be clear.

✖ When visualization is hampered, quickly determine:
- if inflow and outflow bags are properly connected to inflow tubing;
- if the fluid bag is empty;
- obstruction (kinking) in the inflow tubing;
- outflow or inflow valves closed;
- fluid pump is turned on;
- if uterine perforation has occurred.

○ Tissues fragments obscure visualization.

✖ Remove tissue fragments when hysteroscopic visualization is hampered. Techniques to remove tissue fragments include:
- grasping directly with wire loop electrode;
- insertion of polyp or myoma graspers to blindly grasp tissue fragments;
- passive removal by slowly removing the hysteroscope and allowing fragments to exit via cervix.

Use hysteroscopic tissue morcellator as the initial surgical option to decrease accumulation of tissue fragments.

POSTOPERATIVE CARE

- Most hysteroscopic procedures are performed in an outpatient surgical center. Planned postoperative admission may be needed in patients with significant comorbidities including need for uninterrupted anticoagulation, significant pulmonary, renal or cardiac disease that require postoperative monitoring.
- Infectious morbidity is low following hysteroscopic excision of leiomyomas, endometrial polyps, and retained products of conception. Postoperative antibiotics are not routinely indicated.
- Since the majority of healthy women undergoing admission can be discharged within 2 to 4 hours of surgery, gynecologists must closely evaluate, monitor, and personally re-evaluate patients who do not meet discharge criteria to exclude complications:
  - Increasing pain
  - Increasing bleeding
  - Unstable vital signs

- Unplanned admissions may be needed when uterine perforation occurs, unanticipated large blood loss, fluid overload and electrolyte imbalances that cannot be promptly corrected, severe postoperative pain, unstable intra- and postoperative vital signs, or decompensated pulmonary, cardiac, or renal status.
- Inform the patient and family of any unanticipated intraoperative findings and how they will be evaluated.
- Write the brief operative note immediately after surgery and dictate operative note.
- Important aspects of the brief operative note and dictated note includes:
  - Operative time of the procedure
  - Was the planned surgery completed?
    - If not why?
    - What percentage of the planned procedure was completed?
  - Fluid deficit and type of fluid used during surgery
  - Urine output if measured

Table 18.1 Hysteroscopic Clinic Caveats

Device	Energy Source/ Mechanism of Action	Distension Medium	Max Deficit	Complication Tips
Resectoscope (rigid and varying sizes from 22–31 F)	Monopolar (causes resection or desiccation of tissue) Operates at 60–120 W with a monopolar resectoscope	Glycine 1.5% Sorbitol 3% Mannitol 5%	1,500 mL However, pause the procedure at 1,000 mL deficit and obtain stat electrolytes. If evidence of hyponatremia stops the case immediately. Maximum deficit in healthy patient without renal or cardiac problems is 1,500 mL	Notify Anesthesia Team, Strict Is/Os, STAT sodium, administer LASIX 20 mg IV. Place Foley catheter. Involve intensivist if profound hyponatremia. Monitor for pulmonary edema. Monitor for signs of confusion, upper motor neuron disorders, agitation, seizures. If present, also obtain stat ammonia level. Unrecognized hyponatremia may be associated with death and central pontine myelinolysis
Hysteroscopic morcellator (tissue extraction device) • Smith–Nephew • Hologic • Symphion	Utilizes a rotary blade for resection and suction tubing to remove tissue fragments. The Symphion system utilizes a bladeless resection technology, with RF energy and has a proprietary self-contained recirculating fluid management fluid and internal uterine pressure monitoring system.	Saline Lactated Ringer's	Maximum saline deficit 2,500 mL in patients without cardiac or renal comorbidities	Fluid overload including pulmonary edema, congestive heart failure, laryngeal edema, death. Administer Lasix 20 mg IV and place Foley catheter. Limit intravenous fluids.
Vaporization electrodes (e.g., Vaportrobe, Force FX, and Gyne-Pro Perforated roller barrel electrode) can be used with a monopolar or bipolar hysteroscope.	Operate at a higher power density (120–220 W versus 60–120 W with a monopolar resectoscope).	Monopolar vaporization electrodes utilize: glycine 1.5%, sorbitol 3%, or mannitol 5% Bipolar vaporization electrodes utilize: Saline or lactated Ringer's solution	See above	See above
Hysteroscope bipolar resectoscope	Bipolar energy and utilizes the default settings on controller	Saline Lactated Ringer's	Maximum saline deficit 2,500 mL in patients without cardiac or renal comorbidities	Fluid overload including pulmonary edema, congestive heart failure, laryngeal edema, death. Administer Lasix 20 mg IV and place Foley catheter. Limit intravenous fluids.

- Was Lasix used intra-operatively? If so, how much and why given?
- Estimated blood loss
- Amount of IV fluids given intraoperatively
- Complications
  - How was the complication recognized
  - What was the surgical response to the recognized to complication
  - Proposed follow up to any complication
- If the patient is admitted, it is critical that a staff to staff sign out of the case, and proposed postop management discussed in detail.

OUTCOMES

- Most women who undergo hysteroscopic myomectomy, polypectomy, and removal of retained products of conception may resume work and activities in 48 to 72 hours.
- All activities may be promptly resumed except for vaginal coitus which should be abstained for 1 week.
- With complete removal of intracavitary pathology, women with otherwise normal uterine anatomy will have restoration of normal menstruation, resolution of leukorrhea, and low risk of postoperative synchiae.
- Patient's desirous of pregnancy and who have type 0 and type 1 leiomyomas can deliver vaginally unless there is an obstetrical indication for cesarean section.
- Recurrence of leiomyomas following myomectomy is associated with:
  - Age,
  - Subsequent pregnancy,
  - Number of fibroids initially treated.
- Overall 5 to 10 year risk of leiomyoma recurrence is 20%, but highly correlated to patient age.
  - Menopausal women who undergo complete hysteroscopic excision have the lowest rate of recurrence, followed by perimenopausal women, followed by the reproductive-aged patient.
  - If fibroids do recur treatment, re-evaluation is necessary and treats only patients with recurrent symptoms.
- Hysteroscopic myoma excision should be offered to women with an enlarged uterus if there are no bulk symptoms and whose primary symptom is menstrual dysfunction. Resolution of bleeding is often the outcome.
- Recurrence of endometrial polyps is less than 5%.
- Resumption of normal menstruation and fertility preservation is possible with hysteroscopic myomectomy, polypectomy, and retained products of conception.

COMPLICATIONS

- A prospective multicenter trial involving 13,600 procedures noted a low complication rate of 0.95% during operative hysteroscopy.
- The most common complication is perforation due to blunt dilation or due to thermal energy.
- Other less common complications include incomplete removal of leiomyoma, cervical lacerations, and creation of false tracts, fluid overload, dilutional hyponatremia, hypoosmolality, infection, postoperative synechiae, neurologic positional injury, deep venous thrombosis, and death.
- Anesthesia
- Uterine access
  - Perforation
  - Inability to dilate the cervix
- Distention medium
  - Fluid overload
  - Electrolyte imbalance
- Electrosurgical burns
- Gas emboli
- Perforation
- Bleeding
- Infection

(Table 18.1)

KEY READINGS

Cooper NA, Smith P, Khan KS, Clark TJ. Does cervical preparation before outpatient hysteroscopy reduce women's pain experience? *BJOG.* 2011; 118(11):1292–1301.

Golan A, Dishi M, Shalev A, Keidar R, Ginath S, Sagiv R. Operative hysteroscopy to remove retained products of conception: novel treatment of an old problem. *J Minim Invasive Gynecol.* 2011;18:100–103.

Haber K, Hawkins E, Levie M, Chudnoff S. Hysteroscopic morcellation: review of the manufacturer and user facility device experience (MAUDE) database. *J Minim Invasive Gynecol.* 2015;22:110–114.

Hamerlynck TW, Blikkendaal MD, Schoot BC, Hansted MF, Jansen W. An alternative approach for removal of placental remnants: hysteroscopic morcellation. *J Minim Invasive Gynecol.* 2013;20(6):796–802.

Loffer FD, Bradley LD, Brill AI, Brooks PG, Cooper JM. Hysteroscopic fluid monitoring guidelines. *J Am Assoc Gynecol Laparosc.* 2000;7:438–442.

Munro MG. Complications of hysteroscopic and uterine resectoscopic surgery. *Obstet Gynecol Clin N Am.* 2010;37:399–425.

Pampalona JR, Bastos M, Moreno GM, et al. A Comparison of hysteroscopic mechanical tissue removal with bipolar electrical resection for the management of endometrial polyps in an ambulatory care setting: preliminary results. *J Minim Invasive Gynecol.* 2015;22:439–445.

Polena V, Mergui JL, Perrot N, Poncelet C, Barranger E, Uzan S. Long-term results of hysteroscopic myomectomy in 235 patients. *Eur J Obstet Gynecol Reprod Biol.* 2007;130:232–237.

Smith PP, Middleton LJ, Connor M, Clark TJ. Hysteroscopic morcellation compared with electrical resection of endometrial polyps: a randomized controlled trial. *Obstet Gynecol.* 2014;123:745–751.

van Dongen H, Emanuel MH, Wolterbeek R, Trimbos JB, Jansen W. Hysteroscopic morcellator for removal of intrauterine polyps and myomas: a randomized controlled pilot study among residents in training. *J Minim Invasive Gynecol.* 2008;115:466–471.

Widrich T, Bradley LD, Mitchinson AR, Collins, R. Comparison of saline infusion sonography with office hysteroscopy for the evaluation of the endometrium. *Am J Obstet Gynecol.* 1996;174:1327–1334.

Ablation Procedures

Linda D. Bradley, Jonathan D. Emery

19

GENERAL PRINCIPLES

Definition

- Endometrial ablation is a minimally invasive gynecologic surgical treatment that destroys the endometrium, endometrial basalis layer, spiral arterioles, and superficial myometrium. Energy applied to the endometrium leads to tissue necrosis, contracture, scarring and fibrosis of the uterine cavity and endometrium. Anatomic alterations in the endometrium result in menstrual changes that may include: amenorrhea, hypomenorrhea, or eumenorrhea. This procedure is limited to women who have completed childbearing and who have patient perceived heavy menstrual bleeding.
- Endometrial ablation technology has evolved over the past two decades. Manually performed and hysteroscopic-dependent resectoscopic endometrial ablation (REA), include: rollerball/roller-barrel ablation electrodes that desiccate the endometrium and wire loop electrodes that resect the endometrium and is called transcervical resection of the endometrium (TCRE). These first-generation technology ablation devices require fluid management awareness and expert hysteroscopic skills. Monopolar and bipolar hysteroscopic ablation technology are currently available. Automated endometrial ablation technology has evolved and requires less skill-intensive hysteroscopic ability and can be performed in the office under local anesthesia. These technical approaches are called nonresectoscopic endometrial ablation (NREA).
  - Current NREA ablative methods include; hydrothermal ablation (freely circulated hot fluid saline performed hysteroscopically), cryoablation (utilizing intra-uterine freezing probe with transabdominal ultrasound guidance), bipolar radiofrequency, microwave energy and Minerva (bipolar RF electrical current which ionizes argon gas within a sealed silicone membrane array).

Differential Diagnosis

Abnormal uterine bleeding may be attributed to a number of causes:

- Anatomic
  - Adenomyosis
  - Endometrial polyps
  - Endocervical and cervical polyps
  - Leiomyoma
  - Endometritis
  - Caesarean section niche
  - Endometrial hyperplasia
  - Endometrial cancer
  - Endometrial sarcomas
  - Leiomyosarcoma
  - Endometrial stromal sarcomas
  - Uterine vascular lesions (arteriovenous malformations)
- Hematologic
  - von Willebrand's disease
  - Platelet dysfunction
  - ITP
  - Rare blood dyscrasia's
- Endocrinologic disorders
  - Hypothalamic–pituitary disorders
  - Polycystic ovarian syndrome
  - Prolactin disorders
  - Obesity and overweight
  - Thyroid dysfunction
    - Hypothyroidism
    - Hyperthyroidism
  - Adrenal dysfunction
- Medication side effects
- Eating disorders including anorexia or bulimia
- Chronic diseases and systemic diseases
  - Liver disorder
  - Renal dysfunction
  - Cardiac
  - Pulmonary
  - Autoimmune diseases
- Foreign bodies
  - Intrauterine devices
  - Suture
  - Hysteroscopic sterilization inserts

Anatomic Considerations

- Endometrial ablation is an option for women with patient perceived heavy ovulatory menstrual bleeding with a normal uterine size, no Müllerian anomalies, normal uterine cavity (without intracavitary fibroids or endometrial polyps), negative endometrial biopsy without evidence of endometrial hyperplasia, and who have completed childbearing.
- It is essential to evaluate the uterine cavity with hysteroscopy or saline infusion sonography to exclude intracavitary lesions such as endometrial polyps, type 0 or type 1 leiomyomas, endometrial hyperplasia or malignancy, and adenomyosis (Fig. 19.1A–D).
- Ideally, women should be offered medical therapy initially for the treatment of heavy menstrual bleeding when there are no focal intracavitary lesions (Fig. 19.2). If medical therapy or the levonorgestrel intrauterine device is contraindicated, fails or patient refuses medical therapy, endometrial ablation or minimally invasive hysterectomy are therapeutic options.

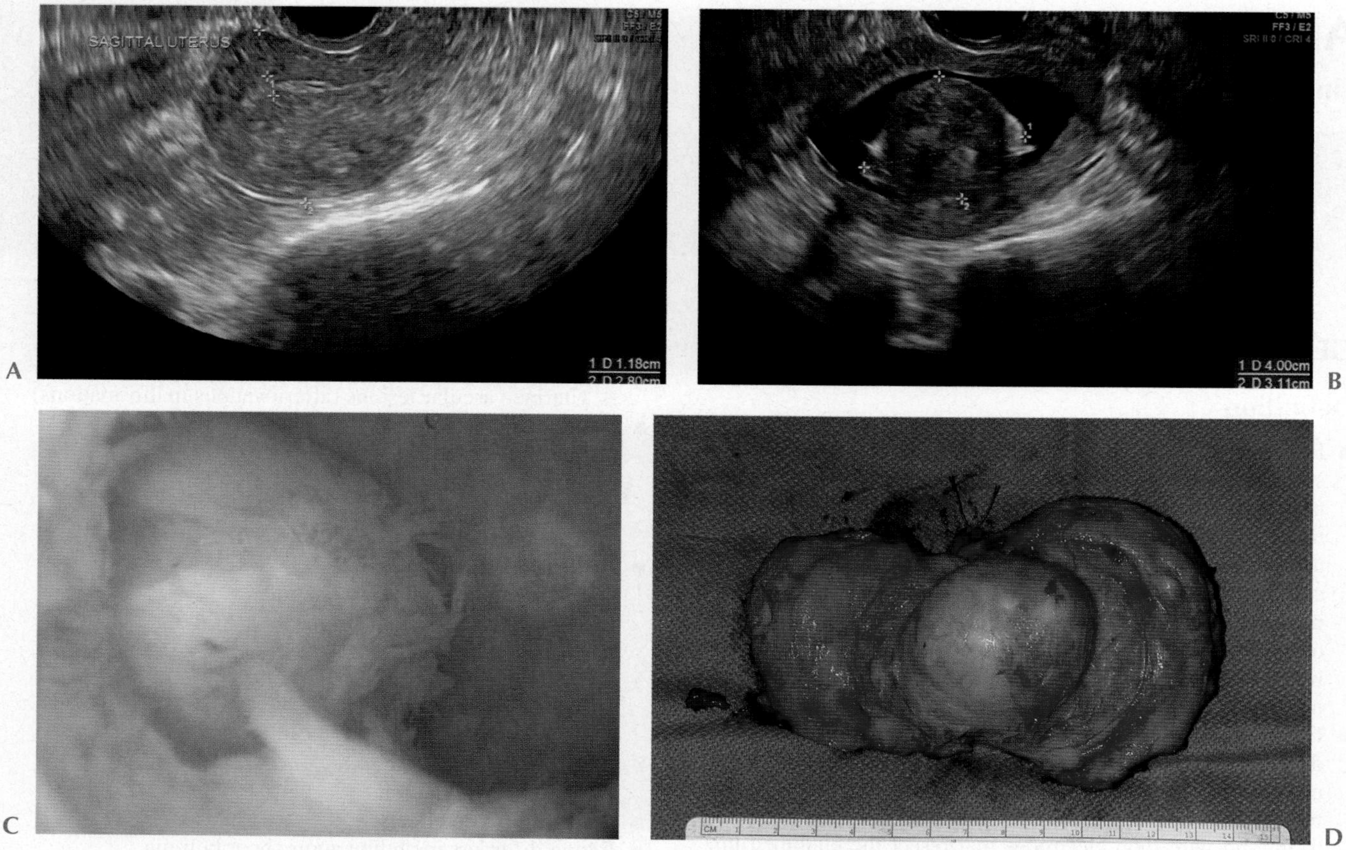

Figure 19.1. **A:** Transvaginal ultrasound adenomyosis a contraindication for endometrial ablation. **B:** Preoperative imaging excluded this patient from endometrial ablation. Coronal SIS view revealing a 4-cm intracavitary fibroid. **C:** Contraindication: intracavitary fibroid must be excised prior to endometrial ablation. **D:** Failed endometrial ablation due to large intracavitary fibroid.

- Failure and need for additional treatment following endometrial ablation is greater in women less than age 40 years, those who have had a tubal ligation, larger uterine cavities, and adenomyosis.
  - Hysterectomy risk increases with each decreasing stratum of age and exceeded 40% in women aged 40 years or younger.

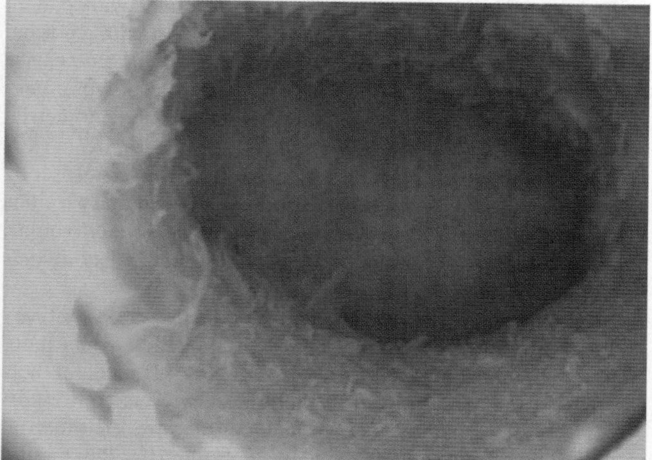

Figure 19.2. Ideal endometrial cavity for endometrial ablation. Note: There are no intracavitary lesions identified.

  - Women less than age 45 years were 2.1 times more likely to have a subsequent hysterectomy. The risk increases through the first 8 years of follow-up.
  - The type of endometrial ablation procedure (first-generation or NREA ablative methods), setting of procedure (inpatient or outpatient), and leiomyomas were not predictors of hysterectomy.

Nonoperative Management

- While the causes of abnormal uterine bleeding are diverse, treatment should be tailored specifically to the most likely etiology obtained with a patient-centric focused history and physical examination. The patient's clinical narrative, imaging results, desire for future childbearing, quality of life, and personal preferences will determine treatment options for heavy menstrual bleeding.
- Bleeding disorders must be considered and included in the differential diagnosis in order to offer appropriate therapeutic intervention and improved outcomes.
- Patients who are overweight or obese are at greater risk for polycystic ovarian syndrome, menstrual dysfunction, endometrial hyperplasia, endometrial cancer, diabetes, and hypertension. Additional laboratory testing in this high-risk patient population may include fasting glucose or hemoglobin A1C, lipid panel, and endometrial biopsy.
- A patient-focused history should be obtained in women with abnormal uterine bleeding.

- Quality-of-life determinants must be addressed including the impact of heavy menstrual bleeding on work, social embarrassment, sexuality, body image, and cost of hygiene products, pain, and impact on daily functioning.
- Tailored laboratory evaluation is selected based on the physical and pelvic examination, clinical history, quality-of-life indicators, family history, and duration of abnormal uterine bleeding.

- Laboratory testing should be individualized and may include:
  - CBC with platelets
  - TSH
  - Prolactin
  - Androgen testing
  - von Willebrand's assay
  - Complete metabolic profile
  - Pregnancy testing
- Patients with regular predictable heavy menstrual bleeding are likely ovulatory. Treatment options for women needing contraception, without risk factors include hormonal contraception or levonorgestrel intrauterine devices.
- Options for ovulatory bleeding in patient's without a history of pulmonary embolism, deep venous vein thrombosis, myocardial infarct or stroke may be offered and include:
  - Tranexamic acid
  - Mirena intrauterine device
  - Progesterone therapy beginning day 5 of menses for 21 days
  - Combined oral or vaginal contraception (estrogen and progesterone)
  - Mini-pill (progesterone only)
  - Injectable medroxyprogesterone acetate
  - Nonsteroidals during menses in women without known platelet disorders
- If the patient has anovulatory bleeding based upon a detailed history, then hormonal therapy is an option (excluding patients with known contraindications):
  - Oral contraceptive pills (consider continuous hormonal suppression for women who wish to avoid menses)
  - Levonorgestrel intrauterine device
  - Cyclic oral progesterone therapy (medroxyprogesterone, norethindrone acetate, megestrol)
  - Injectable medroxyprogesterone acetate
  - Nonsteroidal therapy in women without a known platelet disorder
  - Tranexamic acid has not been approved for anovulatory menstruation.
  - Short-term treatment (up to 6 months) with gonadotropin-releasing hormone (GNRH) agonist.

IMAGING AND OTHER DIAGNOSTICS

- Prior to performing hysteroscopic ablation or NREA. Appropriate radiologic studies are needed to evaluate the uterus, endometrial cavity, and endometrium.
- Available diagnostic procedures include:
  - Transvaginal ultrasound (TVUS)
    - While routine transvaginal imaging universally available—it is less sensitive in detecting intracavitary lesions in reproductive aged women compared to SIS.
    - In fact, in reproductive-aged patients one out of six patients with a "normal" endometrial echo may have an intracavitary lesion missed when only TVUS is performed.
  - Saline-infusion sonography (SIS)
  - 3D saline infusion sonography
    - SIS is recommended to evaluate menstrual aberrations, because the instillation of saline provides an acoustic window permitting increased detection of intracavitary lesions and evaluates the relationship of fibroids to the endometrial/myometrial/serosal interface.
    - The International Federation of Gynecology and Obstetrics (FIGO) universal terminology and diagnostic schema provides great surgical guidance for gynecologists who perform endometrial ablation or hysteroscopic myomectomy. Incorporating SIS in the evaluation of women with abnormal uterine bleeding is essential. Endometrial ablation should not be performed in women with endometrial polyps or intracavitary fibroids.
    - The FIGO classification system facilitates triage and selection of appropriate patients for hysteroscopic myomectomy, enhances patient communication during informed consent, and improves surgical outcomes.
    - The FIGO classification system helps to identify patients with anatomic contraindications to endometrial ablation.
  - Diagnostic hysteroscopy
    - It is more cost-effective to perform hysteroscopy in the office setting.
    - Small-caliber flexible or rigid hysteroscopes permit excellent visualization of the endocervix and endometrial cavity.
    - If other imaging modalities are equivocal, nondiagnostic, or indeterminate, then office hysteroscopy can be used for further evaluation.
- Endometrial biopsy is required to rule out endometrial hyperplasia and malignancy.

PREOPERATIVE PLANNING

- Endometrial ablation is an alternative to hysterectomy for women with ovulatory heavy menstrual periods who ideally have failed medical therapy. It is also offered to women who perceive their menstrual periods to be heavy and have a normal-sized uterine cavity. Childbearing must be complete in women who desire endometrial ablation.
- Patient should understand that the expected outcome of surgery is not permanent amenorrhea as less than 50% of women will develop amenorrhea. Managing patient expectation prior to surgery is essential. If a patient requests or expects amenorrhea she should be counseled for minimally invasive hysterectomy with removal of her cervix.
- Due to the difficulty in evaluating the endometrium after endometrial ablation, caution should be taken when offering the procedure to women at increased risk of endometrial hyperplasia including women who are: nulliparous, obese, history of chronic anovulation, diabetes mellitus, tamoxifen therapy, or have a family history of hereditary nonpolyposis colorectal cancer. The risk/benefit profile should be discussed in detail and included in the informed consent.
- Obtain a pregnancy test on the day of surgery.
- Ideally, schedule the procedure in the early proliferative phase when the endometrium is thin or medically prepared with hormonal contraception (except for Novasure or Minerva devices).

- Endometrial biopsy must be negative for endometrial hyperplasia (including simple or complex), endometrial hyperplasia with atypia, or endometrial cancer.
- CBC with platelet count, TSH, and if clinically indicated by history, von Willebrand's diagnostic panel.
- Negative Pap test.
- The endometrial cavity also evaluated by diagnostic hysteroscopy or saline infusion sonography to exclude intracavitary type 0 or type 1 leiomyomas, and endometrial polyps.
- Müllerian anomalies must be excluded.
- Hysteroscopic sterilization should not be performed concomitantly with endometrial ablation procedures due to the inability to obtain interpretable HSG at the required 3-month interval. If sterilization and ablation are requested, first perform hysteroscopic sterilization, then obtain the 3-month HSG. If tubal occlusion is demonstrated, endometrial ablation can then be scheduled.
- Endometrial ablation should not be offered to women with postmenopausal bleeding.
- Endometrial ablation should not be offered to women with postpartum bleeding.
- Exclude patients with current evidence of pelvic inflammatory disease, endometritis, hematometra and sexually transmitted disease, suspected abdominal or pelvic cancer.

SURGICAL MANAGEMENT

- Endometrial ablation may be accomplished using one of three operative techniques: rollerball/rollerbarrel endometrial ablation, transcervical resection of the endometrium (TCRE), and nonhysteroscopic endometrial ablation technology (Fig. 19.3).
- Historically, endometrial ablation was performed utilizing the operative hysteroscope with monopolar or bipolar technology. Later, nonhysteroscopic technology emerged including thermal balloon ablation (ThermaChoice® Uterine Balloon Therapy; Johnson & Johnson, New Brunswick, NJ, USA [FDA approval obtained in 1997]), cryoablation (Her Option™; Cooper Surgical, Trumbull, CT, USA [FDA approval obtained in 2001]), heated free fluid (Hydro ThermAblator [Hydro ThermAblator [HTA™] System; Boston Scientific, Natick, MA, USA [FDA approval obtained in 2001]), bipolar radiofrequency ablation (NovaSure® endometrial ablation; Hologic, Inc., Bedford, MA, USA [FDA approval obtained in 2001]), microwave ablation (MEA® System, previously produced by Microsulis Medical Limited, Denmead, UK [FDA approval obtained in 2003]), and radiofrequency bipolar electrical current utilizes ionized argon gas within a sealed silicone membrane array (Minerva®; Minerva Surgical, Inc., Redwood City, CA [FDA approval in 2015]). These techniques do not require hysteroscopic assistance during performance of the procedure with the exception of hydrothermal ablation.
- While the original hysteroscopically assisted techniques have been in use since the late 1980s, use of nonhysteroscopic devices for endometrial ablation have surpassed resectoscopic techniques due to ease of use, shorter learning curve, do not require a fluid management system, and typically involve a shorter procedural time than traditional hysteroscopic ablation technology.
- Nonhysteroscopic devices have been adopted for use in the office setting as well as ambulatory surgical centers.

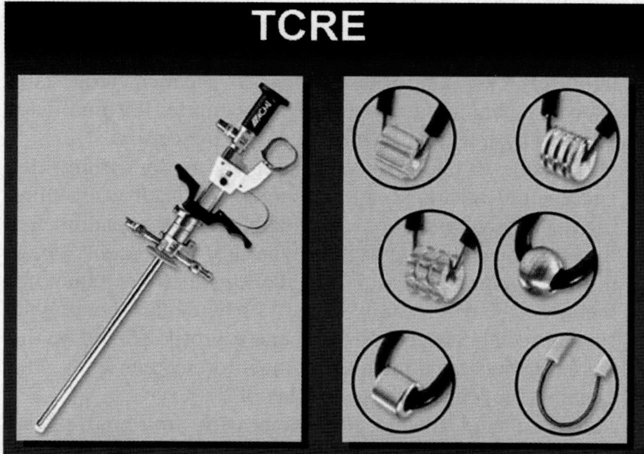

Figure 19.3. Instrumentation for transcervical resection of endometrium.

Positioning

- Endometrial ablation procedures may be done in the office or outpatient surgical center. The caveats of surgical positioning are applicable to both locations.
- Once the patient is under adequate anesthesia, proper patient positioning begins with placing the legs in Allen stirrups or appropriate leg rests in the dorsal lithotomy position. The buttocks should be at the edge of the operating table as this facilitates placement of vaginal retractors or an open-sided speculum.
- The operating table should be flat at all times during the procedure in order to decrease the risk of intraoperative air or fluid embolism
  - Air or fluid embolism can occur if the uterus is positioned higher than the heart (Trendelenburg position).
- If a prolonged procedure is anticipated anti-thromboembolic stockings or sequential compression devices is advised.
- Appropriate sterile draping should be utilized.
  - When first-generation endometrial ablation is performed that requires fluid media, utilize a funnel bag beneath the buttocks to capture excess fluid and measure.

Approach

- Endometrial ablation may be accomplished by a variety of techniques including:
  - Resectoscopic techniques
    - Rollerball or rollerbarrel endometrial ablation (Fig. 19.4).
    - Hysteroscopic transcervical resection of the endometrium (TCRE)
    - Nonhysteroscopic or global approaches
      - Novasure
      - Hydrothermal ablation
      - Cryoablation
      - Microwave
      - Minerva
- A description of the procedure of each nonhysteroscopic device is outside the scope of this chapter. Each device uses a specific form of energy to systematically ablate the endometrium in a uniform manner.
  - Gynecologists should thoroughly understand the indications for use (IFU) for each device.

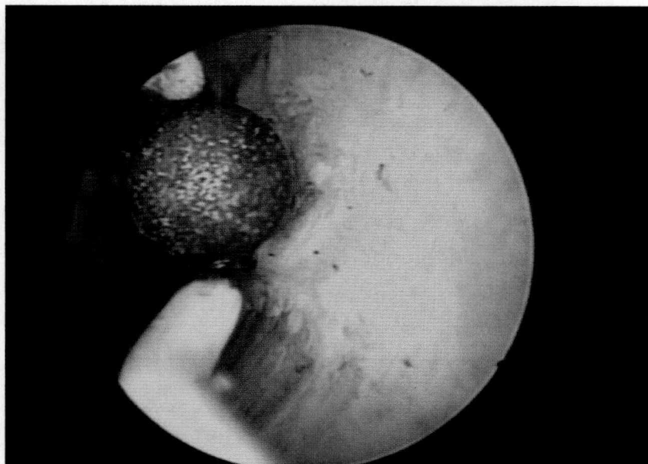

Figure 19.4. Rollerball endometrial ablation.

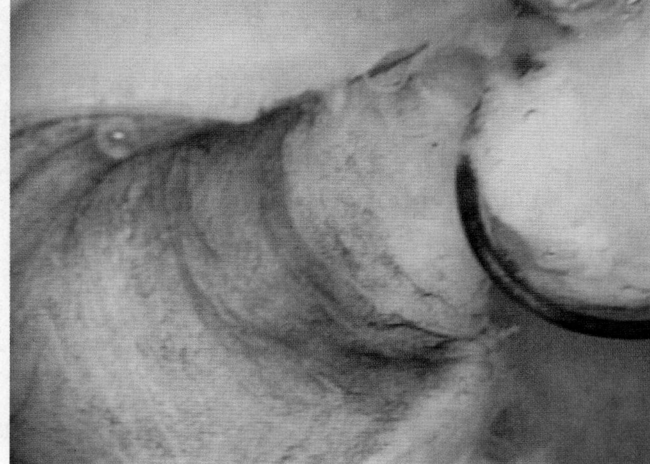

Figure 19.6. Endomyometrial resection.

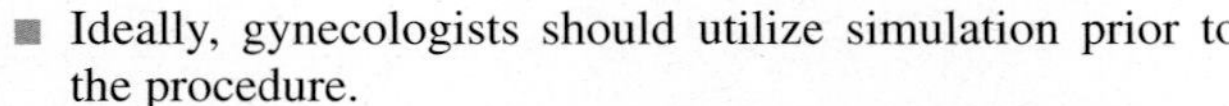

  - Ideally, gynecologists should utilize simulation prior to the procedure.
  - Consider working with a mentor or proctor for the first several cases.
- Hysteroscopically guided endometrial ablation allows the surgeon to treat a uterine cavity that has minor anatomic changes (arcuate uterus, concave tubal ostia, larger uterine cavity). Additionally, removal of intracavitary lesions that were not detected preoperatively is possible when the operative hysteroscope is utilized.
- Ancillary equipment to perform hysteroscopic endometrial ablation includes rollerball, rollerbarrel, or wire loop.
  - The rollerball and rollerbarrel are used to ablate the endometrium (Fig. 19.5).
  - The rollerball attachment does not produce these tissue fragments but rather desiccates endometrial tissue and the basalis layer.
  - Whereas, the wire loop can be used to perform endomyometrial resection, a procedure that resects the endometrium and superficial portion of the myometrium. Samples of this tissue can also aid in the diagnosis of adenomyosis and provide another opportunity to evaluate endometrial pathology (Figs. 19.6 and 19.7).
- Bipolar and monopolar technologies are widely available for endometrial ablation. When monopolar endometrial ablation or endomyometrial resection is performed, the energy should be set to between 60 and 80 W of cutting current. When monopolar current is used, hypo-osmolar distending media is utilized. Bipolar instrumentation utilizes of saline as the distending media.
- A hysteroscopic fluid management system is mandatory during operative hysteroscopic procedures that utilize fluid. Fluid management systems increase patient safety because they decrease the risk of fluid overload by providing instantaneous fluid deficit feedback, are automated to stop fluid inflow if perforation occurs (rapid fluid loss), and permit adjustment in the intrauterine pressure.

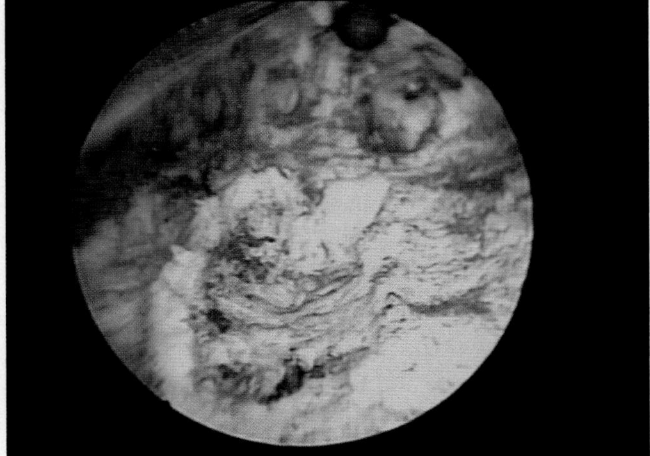

Figure 19.5. Rollerball endometrial ablation posterior wall completed.

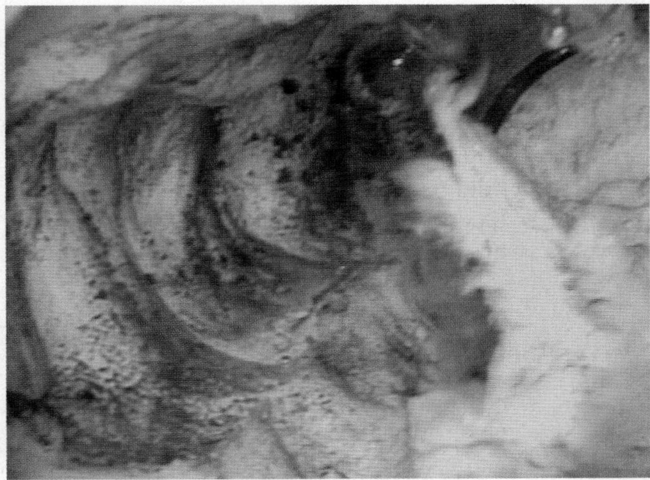

Figure 19.7. Endomyometrial posterior wall resection completed.

Procedures and Techniques (Video 19.1) 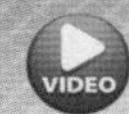

Placement of dispersive pads

- Once the patient is anesthetized and placed in proper position, placement of a dispersive grounding pad is required if using monopolar current.

Examination under anesthesia

- Bimanual examination is mandatory prior to surgery to confirm uterine position and uterine size.

Surgical pep

- Antiseptic preparation of the vagina and perineum.

Sterile draping

- A sterile drape with a funnel pouch in placed under the buttock to securely collect all hysteroscopic fluids.
- Confirm that funnel draping is secure to minimize fluid leaking onto the floor.

Fluid monitor setting

- At the outset determine the upper limits of fluid deficit that will be permitted based on the patients pulmonary, cardiac, and renal status.
- For patients with normal renal, pulmonary, and cardiac status, preset fluid monitors to stop the procedure if the fluid deficit exceeds 1,500 mL of a hypotonic solution (1.5% glycine or 3% sorbitol) or 2,500 mL of an isotonic solution (saline).
- Lower fluid deficit thresholds may be required in women with cardiac, pulmonary, or renal comorbidities.

Assemble the hysteroscope

- Assemble the hysteroscope with resectoscopic attachments, light source, distending media pump, and tubing. Connect outflow tubing to fluid management system canisters to calculate fluid deficit.
- Open the inflow channel and purge all air from the inflow tubing prior to insertion of the hysteroscope to decrease risk of air emboli.

Set power settings

- Set power generator to 60 to 80 W of electrosurgical cutting capacity and 60 to 80 W electrosurgical coagulation capacity when a monopolar device is used.
- Utilize the default setting for bipolar devices.

Begin procedure

- Place an appropriately sized open-sided speculum (or weighted vaginal retractor) into the vagina to allow for visualization of the uterine cervix.
- If a "vaginoscopic approach" is utilized, eliminate this step.
- Once the cervix is visualized, placement of a single-toothed at the anterior lip of the cervix. Consider, placement on the posterior lip if a markedly retroverted/retroflexed uterus is encountered.
- Using cervical dilators, sequential dilatation of the cervix to accommodate the diameter of the preferred operative hysteroscope. Do not "over dilate" the cervix as this will led to egress of fluid and prevent uterine distention resulting in poor intraoperative visualization.

Set intrauterine pressure

- Set the intrauterine pressure to reflect the patient's mean arterial pressure (MAP). The anesthesiologist can provide this information.
- This will usually range between 70 and 125 mg. The intrauterine pressure settings are not static. Adjustments in the intrauterine pressure are an inherent component of surgery and are encouraged.
- Variation in intrauterine pressure facilitates excellent visualization throughout surgery and is influenced by blood, uterine distensibility, and the presence of intracavitary lesions. Operate in a visible field. Do not be hesitant to increase the intrauterine fluid pressure.
- Remember that it's not how much fluid you need to complete the surgical procedure; it is the amount of fluid deficit that matters most.

Insert the hysteroscope

- Insert the hysteroscope into the cervix under direct visualization with the inflow valve open. Look for the "black hole" while advancing the hysteroscope. When the surgeon only sees white it means that the hysteroscope is too close to the cervix, fundus or endometrial tissue.
- Once in the endometrial cavity, identify all intrauterine landmarks including the tubal ostia, fundus, anterior and lateral walls, and endocervix. Do not proceed with endometrial ablation if landmarks are not clearly identified as a false track could have been created.
- During surgery, manipulate the inflow and outflow valves as well in order to maintain a clear view, dissipate bubbles, debris, and blood. On occasion if poor visualization occurs despite these maneuvers, remove the entire hysteroscope and re-insert.
- Endometrial ablation begins by marking the endometrium at the lower uterine segment circumferentially in order to delineate the limits of the ablation.
  - The endocervix should not be ablated. Marking the endpoint of the endometrial ablation simply means touching the lower uterine segment with the rollerball/rollerbarrel which creates a visual char and will define the endpoint of the ablation procedure (**Tech Fig. 19.1**).
  - Endometrial ablation begins by ablating each tubal ostium. Then rollerball across the fundus, or incorporate the technique of "pointillism," which means connecting tiny rollerball dots across the fundus and tubal ostia in order to completely ablate the fundus.
  - Place the rollerball on the posterior wall and slowly move the rollerball to the lower uterine segment where the previously defined limits of the endometrium were marked.
    - Then rollerball the lateral walls and finally the anterior wall. The endocervix is never ablated.
    - Always keep the rollerball in view at all times and activate the energy only when the loop is being returned to the hysteroscope. This decreases the risk of injury.
    - Sequential rollerball endometrial ablation creates a furrow of desiccated tissue with each pass of the rollerball.
    - Slightly overlap each rollerball pass with the prior pass, to minimize untreated endometrium. This technique will treat the endometrium in a uniform manner to a depth of 5 to 6 mm.

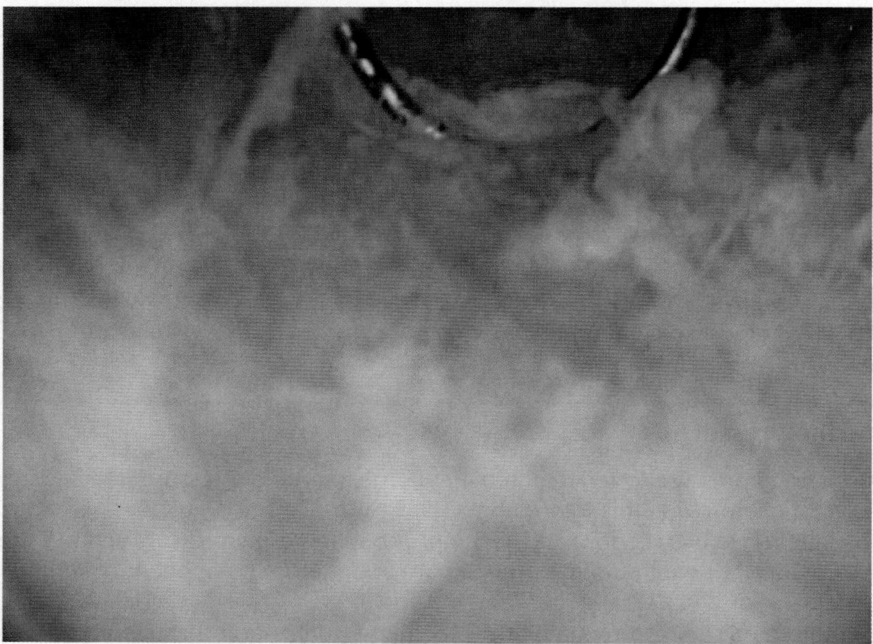

Tech Figure 19.1. Mark the lower uterine segment to prevent cauterization of the endocervical canal and hematometria.

- This same technique applies to use of the wire loop for performing endomyometrial ablation (EMR). This will create floating chips and will need to be removed with the hysteroscope periodically to maintain vision.
- At the completion of the procedure, record the total IV fluids used, type of hysteroscopic fluid used, total hysteroscopic fluid used, hysteroscopic fluid deficit, estimated blood loss, and complications. This should be recorded in the brief operative note and included in the final surgical report. If endomyometrial resection is performed, remove all tissue fragments for histopathology analysis.

Completing the procedure

- Remove all surgical instruments from the vagina after assessing for excessive blood loss. Once the tenaculum is removed from the cervical stroma, assess the tenaculum site and apply pressure if needed. Confirm correct surgical counts and labeling of the pathologic specimen. Perform a vaginal inspection "vaginal sweep" to confirm that no foreign bodies are left in the vagina. Remove the patient from lithotomy position.

Intraoperative surgical caveats

- Throughout the surgical procedure, be vigilant to monitor fluid deficits, vital signs, and blood loss.
- In the event of excessive bleeding at the completion of the procedure, reassess for uterine perforation, cervical laceration, or myometrial bleeding. Do not awaken the patient from anesthesia. Inform the anesthesiologist, circulating nurse, and scrub nurse of the concerns and potential next steps.
  - Consider injection of a dilute solution of vasopressin (20 units vasopressin mixed in 200 mL saline) and injection of 5 mL into the cervical stroma at 11, 2, 4, and 7 o'clock positions.

This will help decrease bleeding from the endomyometrial interface. If the bleeding does not significantly decrease within 5 minutes, then consider the following:

- Reinsert the hysteroscope and distend the uterine cavity to quickly survey the endometrial cavity. If visualization is poor with a rapid fluid deficit noted on infusion pump and bowel or omentum are seen then uterine perforation is likely.
- Determine if a laparoscopic/laparotomic approach is needed if significant hemodynamic changes or if there is a high concern for bowel injury.
- Inform the anesthesiologist and nursing team of your concerns and next steps. Determine if colorectal or general surgery intraoperative consultation is required. If blood transfusion is likely inform the blood bank.
- If there is concern about hemodynamic status or bowel injury, the patient should be prepped for laparoscopy. If uterine perforation is confirmed, then the entire bowel should be evaluated for burns, perforation, mesenteric bleeding, or other intra-abdominal injury. If the uterine perforation site is bleeding, then it should be sutured to ensure hemostasis.
- If no evidence of uterine perforation and brisk bleeding continues despite vasopressin, would advise placement of an intrauterine Foley catheter to tamponade the endomyometrial interface. Chose a Foley that distends to at least 10 to 30 mL and inflate until resistance is met. Document the amount of fluid used to distend the balloon. If the patient is very uncomfortable after she awakens from anesthesia, deflate a few milliliters at a time and keep *in situ* for 2 to 4 hours. Then deflate by half of the initial volume, leave 1 to 2 hours. If no additional bleeding, then remove completely. Maintain a pad count throughout the postoperative period. Follow hemodynamic status and serial CBCs.

PEARLS AND PITFALLS

- ○ Treatment should only include the endometrium.
- ✕ Avoid treating the cervix, to minimize the development of central hematometra. Treat only to the lower uterine segment.
- ○ Comprehensive preop imaging with saline infusion sonography, hysteroscopy, or MRI.
- ✕ Do not rely on endometrial biopsy alone without imaging. It is important to exclude intracavitary pathology such as endometrial polyps, intracavitary fibroids, endometrial hyperplasia. or malignancy.
- ○ Counsel patients regarding the need for lifelong contraception.
- ✕ Do not tell the patient that endometrial ablation is a method of contraception. Pregnancies have been reported up to one decade after endometrial ablation. Pregnancies following endometrial ablation can be complicated and associated with prematurity, postpartum hemorrhage, retained products of conception, ectopic pregnancy, and death.
- ○ Re-evaluate the patient who presents months or years later after ablation with pain—even in the absence of menstruation.
- ✕ Patients may develop central uterine hematometra, cervical stenosis, retrograde endometriosis, or cornual hematometra, and present with chronic or cyclical pain. Evaluate with pelvic imaging such as TVUS or MRI. Passage of a uterine sound may disrupt intrauterine adhesions and egress of blood from the hematometra.
- ○ Recurrence of heavy menses after endometrial ablation, should be offered conservative medical therapy or minimally invasive hysterectomy.
- ✕ Avoid offering a repeat endometrial ablation, as this is an off-label FDA indication. Serious complications have been reported in patients who have been treated with another endometrial ablation including: uterine perforation, hemorrhage, excessive fluid absorption, and genital tract burns.

POSTOPERATIVE CARE

- Patients should have pelvic rest including avoiding intercourse, tub bathing, and use of tampons for one week.
- Generally, patients may return to work 2 to 3 days following endometrial ablation.
- Clear or serosanguinous leukorrhea is common for several weeks after the procedure. If it persists more than 4 weeks after surgery, gently sound the uterus in the office, as filmy intrauterine adhesions may occur that prevent egress of blood or transudate.
- Most patients need nonsteroidal medication for 2 to 7 days after procedure.
- Generally minimal need for narcotics beyond 1 to 3 days following surgery.
- Patients should contact office for low grade fever, foul smelling discharge, or increasing pelvic pain.
- Continue contraception if needed until menopausal.
- If abnormal uterine bleeding or postmenopausal bleeding occurs, then reassessment is mandatory.

OUTCOMES

- Outcomes will vary by the age of the patient when the procedure was initially performed and length of time from when the procedure was performed.
- Randomized clinical trials demonstrate amenorrhea in less than 50% of most patients. MRI imaging has demonstrated persistent endometrial tissue after ablation.
- Many women have improvement in dysmenorrhea.
- Long-term failure of endometrial ablation may be up to 40% of women who undergo endometrial ablation under the age 40.
- Failures are higher in:
  - women younger than age 45;
  - parity of greater than five;
  - prior tubal sterilization;
  - history of dysmenorrhea;
  - preoperative ultrasound consistent with adenomyosis;
  - intramural fibroids greater than 3 cm.
- The most common indications for hysterectomy after ablation are due to bleeding, pain, and pain and bleeding. Surgical findings in postendometrial ablation hysterectomized patients include hematometra, intramural fibroids, adenomyosis, and endometriosis.

COMPLICATIONS

- Immediate complications intraoperatively:
  - Uterine perforation
  - Fluid overload
  - Bowel, bladder, or vessel injury due to perforation
- Pregnancy-related complications:
  - Pregnancy may occur following endometrial ablation. Endometrial ablation is not a form of contraception.
  - Asherman's syndrome
  - Miscarriage
  - Ectopic pregnancy
  - Placentation complications including:
    - Placenta accreta
    - Placenta increta
    - Placenta percreta
  - Intrauterine growth restriction
  - Amniotic band syndrome
  - Preterm rupture of membranes

- Increased rate of cesarean delivery
- Fetal death
- Postpartum hemorrhage and retained products of conception
- Uterine rupture
- Increased risk of postpartum hysterectomy due to hemorrhage and retained products of conception

- Long-term complications
  - Postablation tubal sterilization syndrome
    - Unilateral or bilateral pelvic pain or cramping with or without bleeding
    - Vaginal spotting
    - Swollen fallopian tubes with the etiology linked to retrograde menstruation of cornual hematometra.
  - Persistent endometrial tissue after endometrial ablation
  - Chronic pelvic pain
  - Cyclical pelvic pain
  - Adenomyosis
  - Hematometra at the cornual region
  - Hematosalpinx—unilateral or bilateral
  - Recurrent bleeding necessitating hysterectomy
  - Dysmenorrhea
  - Cervical stenosis
  - Inability to evaluate endometrium with hysteroscopy, endomerial biopsy, transvaginal ultrasound, saline infusion sonography, or MRI
    - The endometrium may be ill-defined, indeterminate, or not visualized completely.
    - Adenomyosis may be noted with imaging.
  - Inability to sample the endometrium due to iatrogenic synechiae following endometrial ablation.
  - Pregnancy

KEY READINGS

AlHilli MM, Wall DJ, Brown DL, Weaver AL, Hopkins MR, Famuyide AO. Uterine ultrasound findings after radiofrequency endometrial ablation correlation with symptoms. *Ultrasound Q.* 2012;28(4):261–268.

Copher R, Le Nestour E, Law A, Pocoski J, Zampaglione E. Retrospective analysis of variation in heavy menstrual bleeding treatments by age and underlying cause. *Curr Med Res Opin.* 2013;29(2):127–139.

Corona LE, Swenson CW, Sheetz KH, et al. Use of other treatments before hysterectomy for benign conditions in a statewide hospital collaborative. *Am J Obstet Gynecol.* 2015;212:304:e1–e7.

Daub CA, Sepmeyer JA, Hathuc V, et al. Endometrial ablation: normal imaging appearance and delayed complications. *AJR Am J Roentgenol.* 2015;205(4):451–460.

Gupta J, Kai J, Middleton L, Pattison H, Gray R, Daniels J; ECLIPSE Trial Collaborative Group. Levonorgestrel intrauterine system versus medical therapy for menorrhagia. *N Engl J Med.* 2013;368:128–137.

James AH, Kouides, PA, Abdul-Kadir R, et al. von Willebrand disease and other bleeding disorders in women: consensus on diagnosis and management from an international expert panel. *Am J Obstet Gynecol.* 2009;201:12:e1–e8.

Longinotti MK, Jacobson GF, Hung YY, Learman LA. Probability of hysterectomy after endometrial ablation. *Obstet Gynecol.* 2008;112:1214–1220.

Matteson KA, Clark MA. Questioning our questions: do frequently asked questions adequately cover the aspects of women's lives most affected by abnormal uterine bleeding? Opinions of women with abnormal uterine bleeding participating in focus group discussions. *Women Health.* 2010;50:195–211.

Munro MG, Critchley H, Broder MS, Fraser IS; FIGO Working Group on Menstrual Disorders. FIGO classification system (PALM-COEIN) for causes of abnormal uterine bleeding in nongravid women of reproductive age. *Int J Gynaecol Obstet.* 2011;113:3–13.

Sharp HT, Endometrial ablation: postoperative complications. *Am J Obstet Gynecol.* 2012;207:242–247.

Index

Note: Page numbers followed by *f* indicate figures, those followed by *p* indicate procedure material, and those followed by *t* indicate tables.